Immunology of Diabetes

Immunology of Diabetes

Editor: Quentin Furman

AMERICAN
MEDICAL PUBLISHERS
www.americanmedicalpublishers.com

AMERICAN
MEDICAL PUBLISHERS
www.americanmedicalpublishers.com

Cataloging-in-Publication Data

Immunology of diabetes / edited by Quentin Furman.
p. cm.
Includes bibliographical references and index.
ISBN 979-8-88740-205-5
1. Diabetes--Immunological aspects. 2. Autoimmunity. 3. Diabetes--Immunotherapy.
4. Diabetes. 5. Immunogenetics. I. Furman, Quentin.
RC660 .I43 2023
616.462--dc23

American Medical Publishers,
41 Flatbush Avenue,
1st Floor, New York,
NY 11217, USA

ISBN 979-8-88740-205-5 (Hardback)

Contents

Preface

Diabetes is a group of metabolic diseases caused by chronic high glucose levels in the blood. In this disease, beta cells (β cells) of the pancreas lose their ability to produce adequate insulin, or there is ineffective utilization of insulin by cells in the body. Type 1 diabetes (T1D) and type 2 diabetes (T2D) are the two prevalent types of diabetes. Type 1 diabetes is an autoimmune disorder in which the immune system attacks and damages the insulin producing beta cells. In type 2 diabetes the body becomes insulin resistant and there is an accumulation of sugar. Insulin resistance that is a result of insulin signaling inhibition leads to a series of immune responses that intensify the inflammatory state, leading to the condition of hyperglycemia. This book includes some of the vital pieces of work being conducted across the world, on various topics related to diabetes and it immunology. Its extensive content provides the readers with a thorough understanding of the subject. This book will prove to be immensely beneficial to students and researchers in this field.

After months of intensive research and writing, this book is the end result of all who devoted their time and efforts in the initiation and progress of this book. It will surely be a source of reference in enhancing the required knowledge of the new developments in the area. During the course of developing this book, certain measures such as accuracy, authenticity and research focused analytical studies were given preference in order to produce a comprehensive book in the area of study.

This book would not have been possible without the efforts of the authors and the publisher. I extend my sincere thanks to them. Secondly, I express my gratitude to my family and well-wishers. And most importantly, I thank my students for constantly expressing their willingness and curiosity in enhancing their knowledge in the field, which encourages me to take up further research projects for the advancement of the area.

Editor

1

Means, Motive and Opportunity: Do Non-Islet-Reactive Infiltrating T Cells Contribute to Autoimmunity in Type 1 Diabetes?

Teresa Rodriguez-Calvo , Gustaf Christoffersson[3,4], Christine Bender[5], Matthias G. von Herrath[5], Roberto Mallone[6,7], Sally C. Kent[8] and Eddie A. James[9]*

[1] Institute of Diabetes Research, Helmholtz Zentrum München, German Research Center for Environmental Health, Munich-Neuherberg, Germany, [2] German Center for Diabetes Research (DZD), Neuherberg, Germany, [3] Science for Life Laboratory, Uppsala University, Uppsala, Sweden, [4] Department of Medical Cell Biology, Uppsala University, Uppsala, Sweden, [5] Center for Autoimmunity and Inflammation, Type 1 Diabetes Center at La Jolla Institute for Immunology, La Jolla, CA, United States, [6] Université de Paris, Institut Cochin, CNRS, INSERM, Paris, France, [7] Assistance Publique Hôpitaux de Paris, Cochin Hospital, Service de Diabétologie et Immunologie Clinique, Paris, France, [8] Department of Medicine, Division of Diabetes, Diabetes Center of Excellence, University of Massachusetts Medical School, Worcester, MA, United States, [9] Translatonal Research Program, Benaroya Research Institute, Seattle WA, United States

Correspondence:
Sally C. Kent
sally.kent@umassmed.edu

In human type 1 diabetes and animal models of the disease, a diverse assortment of immune cells infiltrates the pancreatic islets. $CD8^+$ T cells are well represented within infiltrates and HLA multimer staining of pancreas sections provides clear evidence that islet epitope reactive T cells are present within autoimmune lesions. These *bona fide* effectors have been a key research focus because these cells represent an intellectually attractive culprit for β cell destruction. However, T cell receptors are highly diverse in human insulitis. This suggests correspondingly broad antigen specificity, which includes a majority of T cells for which there is no evidence of islet-specific reactivity. The presence of "non-cognate" T cells in insulitis raises suspicion that their role could be beyond that of an innocent bystander. In this perspective, we consider the potential pathogenic contribution of non-islet-reactive T cells. Our intellectual framework will be that of a criminal investigation. Having arraigned islet-specific $CD8^+$ T cells for the murder of pancreatic β cells, we then turn our attention to the non-target immune cells present in human insulitis and consider the possible regulatory, benign, or effector roles that they may play in disease. Considering available evidence, we overview the case that can be made that non-islet-reactive infiltrating T cells should be suspected as co-conspirators or accessories to the crime and suggest some possible routes forward for reaching a better understanding of their role in disease.

Keywords: type 1 diabetes, insulitis, autoreactive T cells, non-islet reactive T cells, β cell destruction

INTRODUCTION

In criminal investigations, establishing means, motive, and opportunity are necessary elements to prove a suspect's guilt. In this construct, means refers to available tools or methods to commit the crime; motive refers to a plausible reason for committing the crime, and opportunity is the occasion that presents itself to allow the crime to occur (1). In this perspective, we explore the role and function of non-islet-reactive immune cells in human insulitis. Type 1 diabetes (T1D) involves the criminal activity of murder of the insulin-producing pancreatic islet β cells. In this context, "means" is established by showing that a suspect possesses an adequately potent murder weapon (effector function); "motive" is established by showing that the suspect was driven by some plausible impulse to commit the crime (typically, an islet-reactive antigen receptor); and "opportunity" is demonstrated by placing the suspect at the scene of the crime and eliminating any "alibi". There is increasing evidence suggesting that β-cell metabolic dysfunction may directly contribute to β-cell stress and demise (2), and, potentially, to the autoimmune attack ("assisted suicide") (3, 4). Furthermore, some evidence suggests that neonatal remodeling events (waves of apoptosis) may lead to "incompetent repairmen", leaving vulnerabilities that set the stage for the crime (revealed when the perpetrators "case the joint") (5). However, the focus of this mini-review is to investigate the role of T cells at the scene of the crime. We will present ample evidence of opportunity: cells with no discernable evidence of islet antigen reactivity that may be non-self-reactive, are present in human insulitic lesions. Establishing means and motive is a more nuanced venture, as their possible roles could be either pathogenic or protective, passive, or co-conspirators to the crime. Nevertheless, we will conclude that credible evidence exists for a role of non-islet-reactive T cells in disease.

INVESTIGATING THE SCENE OF THE CRIME: EVIDENCE OF CRIMINAL ACTION WITHIN ISLETS IN T1D

The Victims: Pancreatic Islet β Cells

In T1D, a scenario in which the scene of the crime is the pancreatic islet and the victim is the β cell can be contemplated. Arriving on this scene, our investigator is confronted by a chilling scene: a small crowd of infiltrating cells has gathered (first termed insulitis in 1902 by Schmidt (6), observing the pancreas of a 10-year-old child with diabetes). These infiltrates are diverse in location and composition. Insulitis is present in a small percentage of islets (even at diagnosis), making it easy to miss when examining small numbers of islets. The nature of β-cell destruction seems sporadic, almost random. Analysis of pancreas biopsies from adult living individuals taken only weeks from diagnosis (7) showed that insulitis [defined as ≥15 $CD45^+$ cells/islet (8)] affected only 11% of the islets at diagnosis. At onset, insulitis is present in 25.8% of the insulin containing islets (ICIs) versus 2.9% of the insulin deficient islets (IDIs) (8). Thus, these snapshots of evidence of insulitis are concentrated in islets with insulin expression, indicating focused aggression against functional β cells.

Factors in the islet microenvironment that could serve to provoke immune attack remain under study. As mentioned above, remodeling events (waves of apoptosis that prime the immune system: "remodeling gone wrong") that occur early in life could set the stage for subsequent unlawful entry (5). Once the stage has been set, islet α and β cells in T1D could express the CXCL10 chemokine. CXCR3 expression in T cells has been identified in inflamed pancreata and pancreatic draining lymph nodes from donors with T1D (9, 10) along with islet β-cell expression of monocyte chemoattractant protein-1 [MCP-1 (11)]. Further potential contributors to a chemoattractive/pro-inflammatory environment are the expression of IFN-α (12), and later in disease progression, IL-1β (13), the latter potentially secreted by virally infected β cells or by α cells (14). In addition, the scene in the islets appears altered with increased HLA Class I (HLA-I) expression in both α and β cells (15) and changes in the extracellular matrix (16) (among others) that can be interpreted as signs of a confrontation.

Gathering Evidence at the Scene of the Crime

A survey of human insulitis reveals a diverse array of suspects, composed of $CD8^+$ and $CD4^+$ T cells, B cells, macrophages, and other immune cells (17–22) [along with data sets from consortia such as the Network of Pancreatic Organ Donors with Diabetes (nPOD; https://www.jdrfnpod.org/), the Exeter Archival Diabetes Biobank (EADB; https://foulis.vub.ac.be/) and the Human Islet Research Network (HIRN; https://hirnetwork.org/)]. Islet-reactive T cells emerge as prime suspects of β cell killing. These have been unambiguously identified in the pancreas using HLA-I multimers (MMrs) (23–27), and implicated through *in vitro* assays using HLA class II restricted peptides with many specificities defined in peripheral blood which have been confirmed among islet infiltrating T cells (28–30). Insulitic $CD8^+$ T cells are present in higher numbers than other immune cell types. They increase in number as insulin decreases and decline once insulin positive cells can no longer be detected (21). This suggests a major role, but did these prime suspects act alone or with assistance from co-conspirators? This surge in T cell numbers represents an 'opportunity' for non-islet reactive T cells to also enter the islets (in response to the chemoattractive and pro-inflammatory factors), interact with antigen presenting cells (APCs) and reinforce islet-reactive T cell responses.

Other immune cell populations follow a similar trend, albeit in lower numbers. These include $CD4^+$ T cells with only a few detected in human islets. Their numbers are slightly increased in the pancreas at the autoantibody positive stage, along with an increase in $CD11c^+$ cells (31). This could indicate that $CD4^+$

cells and APCs play a role in disease initiation, which would be consistent with Non Obese Diabetic (NOD) mouse studies (32) and a recent single cell analysis that demonstrated a progressive increase of intra-islet leukocyte infiltration and significant heterogeneity in cell type and function (33). $CD20^+$ B cells, macrophages and other immune cells are also present in insulitis or in peri-insulitis. Their presence and numbers are associated with length of disease and age at disease diagnosis (18–20, 34–37). Only a few studies have attempted to identify $CD4^+$ regulatory T cells (Tregs) in the human pancreas with some success (38), but other studies did not confirm the presence of conventional $CD4^+$ Tregs in human insulitis (18, 20). It remains to be demonstrated (with better tools) whether regulatory cells are overwhelmed by the developing effector response, incapable of providing adequate T cell regulation, or if they are absent altogether. Such dereliction of duty by immune regulation/Tregs would be a notable contributing factor to the crime that took place.

Arraigning the Key Perpetrators/Prime Suspects: Islet Reactive T Cells in Human T1D

Although the number of antigens reported to be recognized by insulitic $CD4^+$ and $CD8^+$ T cells from donors with T1D is limited, $CD8^+$ epitopes from native and neoepitopes from islet-derived proteins have been identified (25, 26, 39) along with broad $CD4^+$ T cell reactivity (28–30); see (40) for a review of islet proteins with native and neoantigen epitope targets. Two reports documented higher numbers of pancreas-infiltrating cells reactive to zinc transporter 8 and epitopes derived from previously unidentified targets in donors with T1D than healthy controls (25, 26). Bender et al. demonstrated that preproinsulin reactive $CD8^+$ T cells were enriched in the islets of donors with T1D. These cells preferably infiltrated ICI, with a mean frequency of 40% (of total $CD8^+$ T) cells compared to 22% in IDIs. Preproinsulin-reactive $CD8^+$ T cells were also present in the exocrine pancreas of non-diabetic donors, and their numbers increased in donors with islet autoantibodies and T1D (23). What is the role of T cells found in the pancreatic exocrine tissue in T1D? To date, this is unknow, but the identification of the reactivity and extended phenotype of these T cells, their possible reactivity to islet targets, or exocrine or duct components, will require investigation to understand their role in T1D. Rodriguez-Calvo et al. showed that 10% of $CD8^+$ T cells react against preproinsulin in the pancreas of living individuals with T1D whose specimens were obtained only weeks from diagnosis (27). Although some of these $CD8^+$ T cells express the memory marker CD45RO in human pancreas specimens (23, 26), the question of whether this memory phenotype is a universal feature and its precise nature remains unsettled. Islet-reactive $CD8^+$ T cells have been shown to produce inflammatory and cytotoxic mediators (25, 26), indicating sufficient means to commit the crime. Thus, islet-reactive T cells have the means, motive, and opportunity to commit the crime of β cell damage.

INVESTIGATING ALLEGED CO-CONSPIRATORS: EVIDENCE OF CRIMINAL ACTION BY NON-ISLET-REACTIVE T CELLS IN T1D

Islet reactive T cells were arraigned as our prime suspects but did these suspects act alone or with assistance from accomplices? Here, we consider potential roles for non-islet-reactive T cells, including active involvement, indirect contributions that either promoted or potentiated the crime, and modestly heroic attempts to regulate the aggressiveness of the islet-reactive T cell attack on β cells. To build our case, we will draw on T cell data from animal models and from human T1D.

Non-Islet-Reactive T Cells in Animal Models

Although animal models of T1D do not completely reflect the human disease, they are a crucial tool to perform real-time exploration of mechanisms of immune regulation in the pancreas and associated lymphoid organs. In the lymphocytic choriomeningitis virus-rat insulin promotor-glycoprotein (LCMV-RIP-GP) mouse model of T1D, as little as 1% of the islet T cell infiltrate consists of $CD8^+$ T cells specific for the driver antigen in this monospecific model (41). In this transgenic (i.e. β cells transgenically expressing experimental driver antigens), non-islet-reactive $CD8^+$ T cells with known specificity towards irrelevant antigens were transferred and activated *in vivo* during disease onset (42). Titration of the numbers of non-islet-reactive $CD8^+$ T cells revealed that these cells halted T1D onset in a dose-dependent manner. High numbers of non-islet-reactive infiltrating $CD8^+$ T cells left β cells largely unharmed despite islet-specific $CD8^+$ T cells being also present at the site. Another study showed that inflammation induced by diabetogenic CD4+ T cells alone was not sufficient to mediate non-islet reactive CD4+ T cell islet entry and/or retention (43). In addition, islet antigen expression was a key factor in determining the ability of a given T cell population to accumulate in the islets (43). Some evidence suggests that non-islet-reactive T cells may have different entry requirements than islet-reactive T cells. For example, in one study, the entrance of non-islet-reactive T cells required a chemokine response and VCAM-1 expression by the islets (44).

In multiple sclerosis (MS) and the experimental autoimmune encephalomyelitis (EAE) mouse model of the disease, the Davis lab reported an opposing immune response against the autoimmune $CD4^+$ T cells driving the disease (45). Clonal expansion of endogenous $CD8^+$ T cells not reactive to the myelin driver antigen was found, and the target peptides were identified for two clones. Co-immunization of mice with the disease-driving antigen myelin oligodendrocyte glycoprotein and the newly discovered peptides protected mice from EAE through expansion of regulatory CD8+ T cells expressing CD122 and Ly49. These markers have been found to be expressed on regulatory $CD8^+$ T cells in other studies (46).

It is evident from these model studies and others on islet-infiltrating T cells (and from those infiltrating most other inflammatory sites) that T-cell recruitment to islets (or other sites of inflammation) is antigen independent (e.g., viral reactive cells at autoimmune sites), with an antigen-dependent component (43), with the likelihood that both mechanisms rely on diverse interstitial chemokines and upregulation of integrins on the vascular endothelium (47, 48).

Non-Islet-Reactive T Cells in Insulitis in Humans

Establishing an opportunity that would allow the crime to occur boils down to showing that the suspect was present at the scene of the crime. Non-islet-reactive T cells would be drawn to a pro-inflammatory and chemoattractive environment in islets: this establishes 'opportunity' for non-islet-reactive T cells to be present *in situ*. Although informative, the strategies [MMr staining (23–27), growth from islets (28, 30), sorted T cells for T cell receptor (TCR) transductant generation (29)] to identify the targets of autoreactive T cells in human insulitis have not yet defined the relative representation of islet specificities among the total number of islet-infiltrating $CD4^+$ and/or $CD8^+$ T cells. Moreover, these strategies are inherently biased by their focus on epitopes known to be targeted by circulating T cells, which could be different in the pancreas (26). The antigen specificities for a large fraction (96%) of TCR transductants generated from single T cells seen in (29) or T cell lines and clones derived from insulitis remain unassigned (23, 25–28). This raises two possibilities: 1) a significant proportion of islet infiltrating T cells recognize self-antigens that are not yet appreciated as being disease relevant or 2) a significant proportion of T cells found in the islets are not islet-reactive. Collectively, the relative representation of islet-infiltrating T cells recognizing islet *vs.* non-islet antigens and the hierarchy of the islet antigens recognized remain open questions.

Interacting With the Crime in Progress: Indirect Roles for Non-Islet-Reactive T Cells in T1D

Non-islet-reactive T cells are present at the scene of the crime in animal models of T1D, in human T1D, and in other human autoimmune diseases, but what are their possible roles in the disease process? We consider three: 1) active regulatory cell function or secretion of regulatory cytokines/factors, 2) potentiation of the pro-inflammatory environment, and 3) bystander consumption of cytokines/growth factors/nutrients *in situ* (potentially dampening autoreactive T cell function) (**Figure 1**).

Regulation of the Microenvironment

As well-meaning citizens, active Tregs or T cells with regulatory cytokine secretory, or 'exhausted' properties may suppress autoreactive T cells *in situ*. In NOD mice, the suppressive mechanism of infiltrating Tregs seems to be of a less specific nature. Islet-reactive $CD8^+$ T cells in the pancreas of protected mice showed greatly reduced proliferation rates and lower amounts of islet-reactive cells present, with some signs of exhaustion (42). In EAE, on the other hand, a perforin-dependent mechanism of suppression was found (45). Tregs strongly impact T1D pathogenesis in mouse models, with a gradual decrease in the Treg:T conventional (Tconv) cell ratio in inflamed islets (49). Tang et al. suggested that the decline in pancreatic Tregs reflected apoptosis; a reduced influx of Treg *vs.* Tconv cells may also be possible. In human insulitis, the data point to an absence of classical $CD4^+FOXP3^+$ Tregs. Current data from animal models supports multiple regulatory mechanisms, but the common thread is that Treg activity is inadequate to prevent the crime.

Another mode of microenvironment regulation in diverse mouse model systems is the local secretion of IL-4. Expression of IL-4 in β cells under the control of the human insulin promoter abrogated development of T1D (50, 51), but conversely, increased antigen presentation within islets (52). The use of an IL-4-Ig fusion protein suppressed proinflammatory cytokine production, but augmented islet infiltration (53). Interestingly, expression of CD1d, the ligand for NKT cells, under the control of the insulin promoter in β cells in NOD mice was associated with an IL-4-secreting phenotype of NKT cells and abrogation of T1D development (54). Collectively, these data in murine models suggest that skewing of the microenvironment with regulatory cytokines can have a beneficial effect for the development of T1D, but requires its own regulation.

Potentiation of the Proinflammatory Microenvironment

Non-islet-reactive T cells may be propagators of violence ("egging on the perpetrators") by secretion of pro-inflammatory cytokines (e.g. IFN-γ) or IL-2, which can potentiate and support the replication and function of $CD8^+$ autoreactive T cells. IL-6 has an unclear role in the development of T1D as the expression of IL-6 from both α and β cells was found to be reduced in islets of donors with T1D as compared to those of control donors (55). In mouse models, overexpression of IL-6 has been found to be insufficient to induce T1D, but rather increased islet infiltration by predominantly B cells, but also $CD4^+$ T cells and macrophages (56) whereas IL-6 inhibition has been found to reduce incidence (57). Proinflammatory cytokines, possibly secreted by bystander T cells, are known to contribute to β cell stress (58–60) and to directly damage β cells (61–63).

A potential source of bystander T cell activation in the pancreas is viral infection. Bystander activated $CD8^+$ T cells have been investigated in NOD mice infected with Coxsackievirus B3 and diabetes acceleration was observed. However, this required a pre-existing level of insulitis at the time of infection (62, 63). Of note, viral infections have also been found to be protective in T1D models (64), suggesting that the specific influence from non-islet reactive T cells may be largely dependent on situation and timing. In different models, bystander activated $CD8^+$ T cells have been implicated as either benefiting or harming the microenvironment (65), but the strongest evidence seems to suggest a harmful role.

Depletion of Nutrients and Growth Factors

Non-islet-reactive T cells could contribute to the crime scene by "taking up space". The tumor microenvironment is highly metabolically active to support tumor growth. This leads to a rapid depletion of nutrients in tumors with high glycolytic rates,

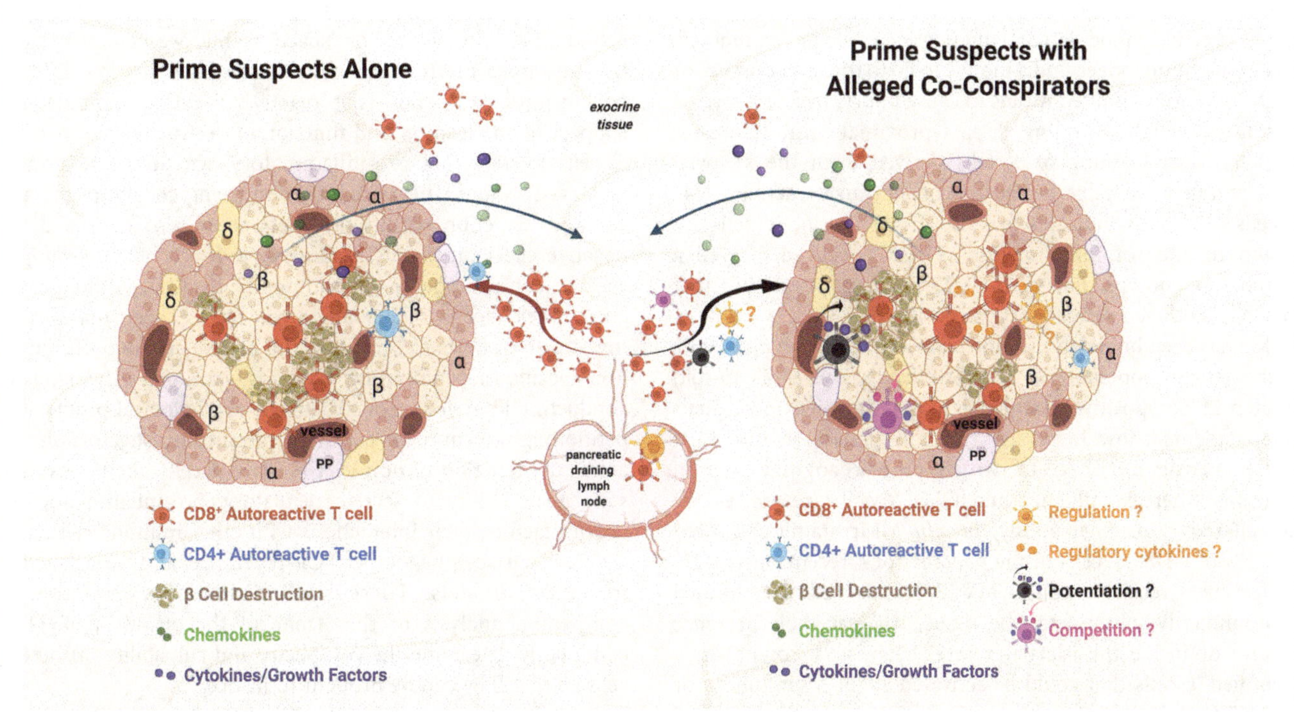

FIGURE 1 | Prime suspects and alleged co-conspirators at the scene of the crime: function of islet-reactive T cells and potential function(s) of non-islet-reactive T cells in insulitis. Proposed schema for islet and non-islet cell reactive T cell functions in insulitis. Representative alpha (α), beta, (β) and delta (δ); cells, and blood vessels are labeled and shown in the represented islet on the left and on the right. The islets are depicted as sources of chemoattractants/cytokines gradients (depicted in green and purple symbols, respectively) through venules with the resultant egress of lymphocytes from the pancreatic draining lymph nodes (pLN) and migration to the islets. Autoreactive CD4⁺ T cells are depicted in blue. On the left, the prime suspects, β–cell cytolytic function of islet-reactive CD8⁺ T cells (depicted in brick red) with β cell destruction depicted in brown. For both representative islets, auto-reactive CD8⁺ T cells are shown in the exocrine tissue. On the right, three potential functions of the alleged co-conspirators, non-islet-reactive T cells, on β–cell destruction by the prime suspects, are depicted. A pro-inflammation 'potentiating' T cell (depicted in black) with cytokine/growth factor secretion (depicted in green and purple) and increased β–cell destruction are depicted in brown. The potential suppressive function of a Treg on β–cell destruction and the potential regulatory effects of cytokines are depicted in orange. The competitive function(s) of a resource/nutrient/growth factor consuming T cells are depicted. The three proposed functions of non-islet-reactive T cells in insulitis are not necessarily mutually exclusive.

and the microenvironment becomes metabolically restrictive for infiltrating T cells leading to resistance to T cell cytotoxicity (64). Could similar mechanisms be at play in an islet infiltrate consisting of a large amount of non-islet-reactive cells? Competition over nutrients can occur between immune cells. One example is the interaction between T cells and APCs, where APCs can become nutrient-starved by clusters of neighboring activating CD8⁺ T cells (65). Similar clustering was observed in mouse models of suppression (42). Depletion of arginine and tryptophan in the microenvironment may also shift the inflammatory response. Arginine is utilized for nitric oxide (NO) production in inflammatory macrophages, and is important for T cell responses (66). Tryptophan is depleted by the enzyme indoleamine 2,3-dioxygenase (IDO), and the expression of IDO, for example, in tolerogenic APCs leads to inhibition of T cells through both lack of tryptophan and the presence of the resulting metabolite kynurenine (67). T cells increase their metabolic demand upon stimulation and activation. Consequently, depletion of nutrients is a potential regulatory factor worthy of further exploration in the context of insulitis. Competition for nutrients and growth factors by non-islet reactive T cells in insulitis could contribute to the indolent nature of T1D development in humans.

EVIDENCE OF CRIMINAL ACTION BY NON-TARGET REACTIVE T CELLS IN OTHER AUTOIMMUNE DISEASES AND IN VIRAL INFECTIONS: IS THERE A COMMON MODE OF ACTION?

In rheumatoid arthritis (RA), epidemiologic and clinical observations suggest that Th1 responses are primary drivers of disease (68). This is illustrated by the amelioration of RA in pregnant women, who present improved symptoms and diminished inflammation driven by a shift from Th1 to Th2 T cell responses (69). However, given that relapses occur six months after delivery in most cases, the beneficial Th2 response is not maintained long term. These observations have implications for disease pathogenesis, as they indicate that T cell responses (antigen-specific and bystander) have plasticity and can be effectively modulated. If modulation could be maintained, T cells might no longer find a motive to go to the target tissues or might have more limited means to cause injury. In RA, a disease setting in which sampling disease-proximal joint tissues is feasible, MMr staining of T cells derived from the synovial fluid revealed a notable population of influenza-reactive $CD4^+$ T cells (70). This indicates that non-tissue specific T cells are drawn to sites of inflammation. These T cells displayed a memory phenotype, but were CD25-negative, suggesting that they had not been recently activated.

MS has been linked to EBV infection and, although up to 95% of the general population is seropositive, disease risk is 15-fold greater in seropositive compared to seronegative individuals (71). Patients show increased T cell responses against EBV nuclear antigen (EBNA1), which cross-recognize myelin antigens, whereas influenza and CMV-specific responses are not altered (72). Analogously, *in situ* MMr staining showed that 5% of $CD8^+$ T cells in the pancreas of 4 recent onset T1D subjects were reactive against CMV (27). These cells were located predominantly in the exocrine tissue, whereas their presence around or inside the islets was rare. Likewise, a recent study identified T cells that could be activated either by influenza or GAD65 (73), but these cross-reactive cells were from peripheral blood and not documented within the islets.

The role of virus-reactive T cells in the pathogenesis of human autoimmune diseases remains unclear. Given the potential cyclical activation of T cells due to new infections or viral reactivation, virus-reactive T cells might be important contributors to tissue inflammation. T1D has been historically associated with enterovirus infections (74). Investigating the location and phenotype of enterovirus-reactive cells has potentially important implications for disease pathogenesis and prevention. Although molecular mimicry between microbial and β-cell epitopes has been described, the arrival of virus-reactive T cells could be driven by viral antigens and/or chemokines/cytokines, with the aim of eliminating infected β cells. Their ongoing activity could contribute to islet inflammation by activating anti-viral responses (interferon-mediated), favoring antigen presentation (increasing HLA-I expression), and inducing β cell destruction. With ~96% of the reactivities of islet infiltrating T cells undefined, the question remains open as to the identity and *in situ* function of this large portion of T cells.

CONCLUSIONS AND FUTURE PERSPECTIVES

Collectively, there is some consensus that in T1D (and other autoimmune diseases), T cells that lack any documented self-reactivity are present within inflamed tissues. Some of these might recognize unknown self-antigens, but others have been shown to recognize epitopes from common viruses. It cannot be completely ruled out that non-islet reactive infiltrating T cells could actively suppress autoreactive T cells or restrain their activity by depleting nutrients and growth factors/regulatory cytokines or competing for 'space'. While we cannot exclude that multiple mechanisms may be at play, the most likely conclusion is that non-islet reactive T cells potentiate and support the replication and function of destructive autoreactive T cells by secreting pro-inflammatory cytokines and growth factors. It should be noted that nutrient consumption and cytokine secretion within the islets could also have a direct negative effect on β cells, leading to a direct, but non-antigen specific contribution to autoimmunity in T1D. Although the current evidence is inadequate to convict, we assert that further investigative efforts to scrutinize the motive and opportunity of non-specific islet infiltrating T cells is warranted. Analogous to conducting interviews, constructing a psychological profile, and petitioning the court for a search warrant, investigators should assess the function of non-islet-reactive T cells, their activation state, their ability to secrete regulatory, pro-inflammatory or growth factors, their interactions with other immune cell types, their cell surface phenotype, TCR repertoire, and their function in animal models. These studies should be paired with companion analysis of the 'scene of the crime' in T1D to confidently determine the complicity and culpability of these T cells so that they can be brought to justice.

AUTHOR CONTRIBUTIONS

All authors actively contributed to writing and revising the article and approved the submitted version. All authors are accountable for the content of the work.

FUNDING

GC is supported by grants from the Swedish Research Council, the Swedish Society for Medical Research, the Göran Gustafsson Foundation, and the Science for Life Laboratory. EJ is supported by the National Institute of Diabetes and Digestive and Kidney Diseases (Human Islet Research Network U24 DK104162). SK is supported by the National Institute of Diabetes and Digestive and Kidney Diseases (UC4 DK116284), and SK is the George F. and Sybil H. Fuller Term Chair in Diabetes. RM is funded by grants from The Leona M. and Harry B. Helmsley Charitable Trust (Helmsley no. 1901-03689), the Fondation pour la Recherche Médicale (EQU20193007831) and the Agence Nationale de la Recherche (ANR-19-CE15-0014-01). RM and TR-C are funded by the Innovative Medicines Initiative 2 Joint Undertaking under grant agreements 115797 and 945268 (INNODIA and INNODIA HARVEST). These Joint Undertakings receive support from the Union's Horizon 2020 research and innovation programme, European Federation of Pharmaceutical Industries Associations, JDRF and The Leona M. and Harry B. Helmsley Charitable Trust. MH is supported by NIH R01 AI134971 and NIH R01 AI092453.

Research in the laboratories of authors (SK, RM, TR-C, MH) is performed with the support of the Network for Pancreatic Organ donors with Diabetes (nPOD; RRID : SCR_014641), a collaborative type 1 diabetes research project supported by JDRF (nPOD: 5-SRA-2018-557-Q-R) and The Leona M. & Harry B. Helmsley Charitable Trust (Grant#2018PG-T1D053). Organ Procurement Organizations (OPO) partnering with nPOD to provide research resources are listed at http://www.jdrfnpod.org/for-partners/npod-partners/.

ACKNOWLEDGMENTS

Figure 1 was created with BioRender.com.

REFERENCES

1. Herbert R, Aird C, Reilly JM. *The Oxford Companion to Crime and Mystery Writing*. New York: Oxford University Press (1999).
2. Sims EK, Mirmira RG, Evans-Molina C. The Role of Beta-Cell Dysfunction in Early Type 1 Diabetes. *Curr Opin Endocrinol Diabetes Obes* (2020) 27:215–24. doi: 10.1097/MED.0000000000000548
3. Atkinson MA, Bluestone JA, Eisenbarth GS, F HM, Herold KC, Accili D, et al. How Does Type 1 Diabetes Develop?: The Notion of Homicide or β-Cell Suicide Revisited. *Diabetes* (2011) 60:1370–9. doi: 10.2337/db10-1797
4. Bottazzo GF. Lawrence Lecture. Death of a Beta Cell: Homicide or Suicide? *Diabetes Med* (1986) 3:119–30. doi: 10.1111/j.1464-5491.1986.tb00722.x
5. Trudeau JD, Dutz JP, Arany E, Hill DJ, Fieldus WE, Finegood DT. Neonatal Beta-Cell Apoptosis: A Trigger for Autoimmune Diabetes? *Diabetes* (2000) 49:1–7. doi: 10.2337/diabetes.49.1.1
6. Schmidt MB. Ueber Die Beziehung Der Langenhans'schen Inseln Des Pankreas Zum Diabetes Mellitus. *München Med Wochenschr (Ger)* (1902) 49:51–4.
7. Krogvold L, Wiberg A, Edwin B, Buanes T, Jahnsen FL, Hanssen KF, et al. Insulitis and Characterisation of Infiltrating T Cells in Surgical Pancreatic Tail Resections From Patients At Onset of Type 1 Diabetes. *Diabetologia* (2016) 59:492–501. doi: 10.1007/s00125-015-3820-4
8. Campbell-Thompson ML, Atkinson MA, Butler AE, Chapman NM, Frisk G, Gianani R, et al. The Diagnosis of Insulitis in Human Type 1 Diabetes. *Diabetologia* (2013) 56:2541–3. doi: 10.1007/s00125-013-3043-5
9. Nigi L, Brusco N, Grieco GE, Licata G, Krogvold L, Marselli L, et al. Pancreatic Alpha-Cells Contribute Together With Beta-Cells to CXCL10 Expression in Type 1 Diabetes. *Front Endocrinol* (2020) 11:630. doi: 10.3389/fendo.2020.00630
10. Roep BO, Kleijwegt FS, Van Halteren AGS, Bonato V, Boggi U, Vendrame F, et al. Islet Inflammation and CXCL10 in Recent-Onset Type 1 Diabetes. *Clin Exp Immunol* (2010) 159:338–43. doi: 10.1111/j.1365-2249.2009.04087.x
11. Kutlu B, Darville MI, Cardozo AK, Eizirik DL. Molecular Regulation of Monocyte Chemoattractant Protein-1 Expression in Pancreatic Beta-Cells. *Diabetes* (2003) 52:348–55. doi: 10.2337/diabetes.52.2.348
12. Foulis AK, Farquharson MA, Meager A. Immunoreactive Alpha-Interferon in Insulin-Secreting Beta Cells in Type 1 Diabetes Mellitus. *Lancet* (1987) 2:1423–7. doi: 10.1016/s0140-6736(87)91128-7
13. Anquetil F, Sabouri S, Thivolet C, Rodriguez-Calvo T, Zapardiel-Gonzalo J, Amirian N, et al. Alpha Cells, the Main Source of IL-1β in Human Pancreas. *J Autoimmun* (2017) 81:68–73. doi: 10.1016/j.jaut.2017.03.006
14. Colli ML, Szymczak F, Eizirik DL. Molecular Footprints of the Immune Assault on Pancreatic Beta Cells in Type 1 Diabetes. *Front Endocrinol* (2020) 11:568446. doi: 10.3389/fendo.2020.568446
15. Richardson SJ, Rodriguez-Calvo T, Gerling IC, Mathews CE, Kaddis JS, Russell MA, et al. Islet Cell Hyperexpression of HLA Class I Antigens: A Defining Feature in Type 1 Diabetes. *Diabetologia* (2016) 59:2448–58. doi: 10.1007/s00125-016-4067-4
16. Bogdani M, Korpos E, Simeonovic CJ, Parish CR, Sorokin L, Wight TN. Extracellular Matrix Components in the Pathogenesis of Type 1 Diabetes. *Curr Diabetes Rep* (2014) 14:552. doi: 10.1007/s11892-014-0552-7
17. Campbell-Thompson M, Fu A, Kaddis JS, Wasserfall C, Schatz DA, Pugliese A, et al. Insulitis and β-Cell Mass in the Natural History of Type 1 Diabetes. *Diabetes* (2016) 65:719–31. doi: 10.2337/db15-0779
18. Damond N, Engler S, Zanotelli VRT, Schapiro D, Wasserfall CH, Kusmartseva I, et al. A Map of Human Type 1 Diabetes Progression by Imaging Mass Cytometry. *Cell Metab* (2019) 29:755–768.e5. doi: 10.1016/j.cmet.2018.11.014
19. Foulis AK, Mcgill M, Farquharson MA. Insulitis in Type 1 (Insulin-Dependent) Diabetes Mellitus in Man–Macrophages, Lymphocytes, and Interferon-Gamma Containing Cells. *J Pathol* (1991) 165:97–103. doi: 10.1002/path.1711650203
20. Wang YJ, Traum D, Schug J, Gao L, Liu C, Atkinson MA, et al. Multiplexed In Situ Imaging Mass Cytometry Analysis of the Human Endocrine Pancreas and Immune System in Type 1 Diabetes. *Cell Metab* (2019) 29:769–783.e4. doi: 10.1016/j.cmet.2019.01.003
21. Willcox A, Richardson SJ, Bone AJ, Foulis AK, Morgan NG. Analysis of Islet Inflammation in Human Type 1 Diabetes. *Clin Exp Immunol* (2009) 155:173–81. doi: 10.1111/j.1365-2249.2008.03860.x
22. In't Veld P. Insulitis in Human Type 1 Diabetes: The Quest for an Elusive Lesion. *Islets* (2011) 3:131–8. doi: 10.4161/isl.3.4.15728
23. Bender C, Rodriguez-Calvo T, Amirian N, Coppieters KT, Von Herrath MG. The Healthy Exocrine Pancreas Contains Preproinsulin-Specific CD8 T Cells That Attack Islets in Type 1 Diabetes. *Sci Adv* (2020) 6:eabc5586. doi: 10.1126/sciadv.abc5586
24. Coppieters KT, Dotta F, Amirian N, Campbell PD, Kay TWH, Atkinson MA, et al. Demonstration of Islet-Autoreactive CD8 T Cells in Insulitic Lesions From Recent Onset and Long-Term Type 1 Diabetes Patients. *J Exp Med* (2012) 209:51–60. doi: 10.1084/jem.20111187
25. Culina S, Lalanne AI, Afonso G, Cerosaletti K, Pinto S, Sebastiani G, et al. Islet-Reactive CD8(+) T Cell Frequencies in the Pancreas, But Not in Blood, Distinguish Type 1 Diabetic Patients From Healthy Donors. *Sci Immunol* (2018) 3:eaao4013. doi: 10.1126/sciimmunol.aao4013
26. Gonzalez-Duque S, Azoury ME, Colli ML, Afonso G, Turatsinze JV, Nigi L, et al. Conventional and Neo-Antigenic Peptides Presented by β Cells Are Targeted by Circulating Naïve Cd8+ T Cells in Type 1 Diabetic and Healthy Donors. *Cell Metab* (2018) 28:946–960.e6. doi: 10.1016/j.cmet.2018.07.007
27. Rodriguez-Calvo T, Krogvold L, Amirian N, Dahl-Jørgensen K, Von Herrath M. One in Ten Cd8+ Cells in the Pancreas of Living Individuals With Recent Onset Type 1 Diabetes Recognizes the Preproinsulin Epitope Ppi(15-24). *Diabetes* (2021) 70:752–8. doi: 10.2337/db20-0908
28. Babon JAB, Denicola ME, Blodgett DM, Crèvecoeur I, Buttrick TS, Maehr R, et al. Analysis of Self-Antigen Specificity of Islet-Infiltrating T Cells From Human Donors With Type 1 Diabetes. *Nat Med* (2016) 22:1482–7. doi: 10.1038/nm.4203
29. Michels AW, Landry LG, Mcdaniel KA, Yu L, Campbell-Thompson M, Kwok WW, et al. Islet-Derived Cd4 T Cells Targeting Proinsulin in Human Autoimmune Diabetes. *Diabetes* (2017) 66:722–34. doi: 10.2337/db16-1025
30. Pathiraja V, Kuehlich JP, Campbell PD, Krishnamurthy B, Loudovaris T, Coates PT, et al. Proinsulin-Specific, HLA-DQ8, and HLA-DQ8-Transdimer-Restricted Cd4+ T Cells Infiltrate Islets in Type 1 Diabetes. *Diabetes* (2015) 64:172–82. doi: 10.2337/db14-0858
31. Rodriguez-Calvo T, Ekwall O, Amirian N, Zapardiel-Gonzalo J, Von Herrath MG. Increased Immune Cell Infiltration of the Exocrine Pancreas: A Possible Contribution to the Pathogenesis of Type 1 Diabetes. *Diabetes* (2014) 63:3880–90. doi: 10.2337/db14-0549
32. Unanue ER, Ferris ST, Carrero JA. The Role of Islet Antigen Presenting Cells and the Presentation of Insulin in the Initiation of Autoimmune Diabetes in the NOD Mouse. *Immunol Rev* (2016) 272:183–201. doi: 10.1111/imr.12430
33. Zakharov PN, Hu H, Wan X, Unanue ER. Single-Cell RNA Sequencing of Murine Islets Shows High Cellular Complexity at All Stages of Autoimmune Diabetes. *J Exp Med* (2020) 217:e20192362. doi: 10.1084/jem.20192362

34. Carré A, Richardson SJ, Larger E, Mallone R. Presumption of Guilt for T Cells in Type 1 Diabetes: Lead Culprits or Partners in Crime Depending on Age of Onset? *Diabetologia* (2021) 64:15–25. doi: 10.1007/s00125-020-05298-y
35. Leete P, Oram RA, Mcdonald TJ, Shields BM, Ziller C, Hattersley AT, et al. Studies of Insulin and Proinsulin in Pancreas and Serum Support the Existence of Aetiopathological Endotypes of Type 1 Diabetes Associated With Age At Diagnosis. *Diabetologia* (2020) 63:1258–67. doi: 10.1007/s00125-020-05115-6
36. Leete P, Willcox A, Krogvold L, Dahl-Jørgensen K, Foulis AK, Richardson SJ, et al. Differential Insulitic Profiles Determine the Extent of β-Cell Destruction and the Age At Onset of Type 1 Diabetes. *Diabetes* (2016) 65:1362–9. doi: 10.2337/db15-1615
37. Lu J, Zhang C, Li L, Xue W, Zhang C, Zhang X. Unique Features of Pancreatic-Resident Regulatory T Cells in Autoimmune Type 1 Diabetes. *Front Immunol* (2017) 8:1235. doi: 10.3389/fimmu.2017.01235
38. Seay HR, Yusko E, Rothweiler SJ, Zhang L, Posgai AL, Campbell-Thompson M, et al. Tissue Distribution and Clonal Diversity of the T and B Cell Repertoire in Type 1 Diabetes. *JCI Insight* (2016) 1:e88242. doi: 10.1172/jci.insight.88242
39. Azoury ME, Tarayrah M, Afonso G, Pais A, Colli ML, Maillard C, et al. Peptides Derived From Insulin Granule Proteins Are Targeted by CD8(+) T Cells Across Mhc Class I Restrictions in Humans and NOD Mice. *Diabetes* (2020) 69:2678–90. doi: 10.2337/db20-0013
40. James EA, Mallone R, Kent SC, Dilorenzo TP. T-Cell Epitopes and Neo-Epitopes in Type 1 Diabetes: A Comprehensive Update and Reappraisal. *Diabetes* (2020) 69:1311–35. doi: 10.2337/dbi19-0022
41. Oldstone MBA, Edelmann KH, Mcgavern DB, Cruite JT, Welch MJ. Molecular Anatomy and Number of Antigen Specific CD8 T Cells Required to Cause Type 1 Diabetes. *PloS Pathog* (2012) 8:e1003044. doi: 10.1371/journal.ppat.1003044
42. Christoffersson G, Chodaczek G, Ratliff SS, Coppieters K, Von Herrath MG. Suppression of Diabetes by Accumulation of Non-Islet-Specific CD8(+) Effector T Cells in Pancreatic Islets. *Sci Immunol* (2018) 3:eaam6533. doi: 10.1126/sciimmunol.aam6533
43. Lennon GP, Bettini M, Burton AR, Vincent E, Arnold PY, Santamaria P, et al. T Cell Islet Accumulation in Type 1 Diabetes Is a Tightly Regulated, Cell-Autonomous Event. *Immunity* (2009) 31:643–53. doi: 10.1016/j.immuni.2009.07.008
44. Calderon B, Carrero JA, Miller MJ, Unanue ER. Entry of Diabetogenic T Cells Into Islets Induces Changes That Lead to Amplification of the Cellular Response. *Proc Natl Acad Sci USA* (2011) 108:1567–72. doi: 10.1073/pnas.1018975108
45. Saligrama N, Zhao F, Sikora MJ, Serratelli WS, Fernandes RA, Louis DM, et al. Opposing T Cell Responses in Experimental Autoimmune Encephalomyelitis. *Nature* (2019) 572:481–7. doi: 10.1038/s41586-019-1467-x
46. Kim H-J, Wang X, Radfar S, Sproule TJ, Roopenian DC, Cantor H. Cd8+ T Regulatory Cells Express the Ly49 Class I MHC Receptor and Are Defective in Autoimmune Prone B6-Yaa Mice. *Proc Natl Acad Sci USA* (2011) 108:2010–5. doi: 10.1073/pnas.1018974108
47. Lindsay RS, Corbin K, Mahne A, Levitt BE, Gebert MJ, Wigton EJ, et al. Antigen Recognition in the Islets Changes With Progression of Autoimmune Islet Infiltration. *J Immunol* (2015) 194:522–30. doi: 10.4049/jimmunol.1400626
48. Sandor AM, Lindsay RS, Dyjack N, Whitesell JC, Rios C, Bradley BJ, et al. Cd11c(+) Cells Are Gatekeepers for Lymphocyte Trafficking to Infiltrated Islets During Type 1 Diabetes. *Front Immunol* (2019) 10:99. doi: 10.3389/fimmu.2019.00099
49. Tang Q, Adams JY, Penaranda C, Melli K, Piaggio E, Sgouroudis E, et al. Central Role of Defective Interleukin-2 Production in the Triggering of Islet Autoimmune Destruction. *Immunity* (2008) 28:687–97. doi: 10.1016/j.immuni.2008.03.016
50. Gallichan WS, Balasa B, Davies JD, Sarvetnick N. Pancreatic IL-4 Expression Results in Islet-Reactive Th2 Cells That Inhibit Diabetogenic Lymphocytes in the Nonobese Diabetic Mouse. *J Immunol* (1999) 163:1696–703.
51. Mueller R, Krahl T, Sarvetnick N. Pancreatic Expression of Interleukin-4 Abrogates Insulitis and Autoimmune Diabetes in Nonobese Diabetic (NOD) Mice. *J Exp Med* (1996) 184:1093–9. doi: 10.1084/jem.184.3.1093
52. Falcone M, Yeung B, Tucker L, Rodriguez E, Krahl T, Sarvetnick N. IL-4 Triggers Autoimmune Diabetes by Increasing Self-Antigen Presentation Within the Pancreatic Islets. *Clin Immunol* (2001) 98:190–9. doi: 10.1006/clim.2000.4979
53. Walz M, Overbergh L, Mathieu C, Kolb H, Martin S. A Murine Interleukin-4-Ig Fusion Protein Regulates the Expression of Th1- and Th2-Specific Cytokines in the Pancreas of NOD Mice. *Horm Metab Res* (2002) 34:561–9. doi: 10.1055/s-2002-35417
54. Falcone M, Facciotti F, Ghidoli N, Monti P, Olivieri S, Zaccagnino L, et al. Up-Regulation of CD1d Expression Restores the Immunoregulatory Function of NKT Cells and Prevents Autoimmune Diabetes in Nonobese Diabetic Mice. *J Immunol* (2004) 172:5908–16. doi: 10.4049/jimmunol.172.10.5908
55. Rajendran S, Anquetil F, Quesada-Masachs E, Graef M, Gonzalez N, Mcardle S, et al. IL-6 Is Present in Beta and Alpha Cells in Human Pancreatic Islets: Expression Is Reduced in Subjects With Type 1 Diabetes. *Clin Immunol* (2020) 211:108320. doi: 10.1016/j.clim.2019.108320
56. Campbell IL, Hobbs MV, Dockter J, Oldstone MB, Allison J. Islet Inflammation and Hyperplasia Induced by the Pancreatic Islet-Specific Overexpression of Interleukin-6 in Transgenic Mice. *Am J Pathol* (1994) 145:157–66.
57. Campbell IL, Kay TW, Oxbrow L, Harrison LC. Essential Role for Interferon-Gamma and Interleukin-6 in Autoimmune Insulin-Dependent Diabetes in NOD/Wehi Mice. *J Clin Invest* (1991) 87:739–42. doi: 10.1172/JCI115055
58. Brozzi F, Nardelli TR, Lopes M, Millard I, Barthson J, Igoillo-Esteve M, et al. Cytokines Induce Endoplasmic Reticulum Stress in Human, Rat and Mouse Beta Cells Via Different Mechanisms. *Diabetologia* (2015) 58:2307–16. doi: 10.1007/s00125-015-3669-6
59. Colli MI, Ramos-Rodríguez M, Nakayasu ES, Alvelos MI, Lopes M, Hill JLE, et al. An Integrated Multi-Omics Approach Identifies the Landscape of Interferon-α-Mediated Responses of Human Pancreatic Beta Cells. *Nat Commun* (2020) 11:2584. doi: 10.1038/s41467-020-16327-0
60. Demine S, Schiavo AA, Marín-Cañas S, Marchetti P, Cnop M, Eizirik DL. Pro-Inflammatory Cytokines Induce Cell Death, Inflammatory Responses, and Endoplasmic Reticulum Stress in Human iPSC-Derived Beta Cells. *Stem Cell Res Ther* (2020) 11:7. doi: 10.1186/s13287-019-1523-3
61. Feduska JM, Tse HM. The Proinflammatory Effects of Macrophage-Derived NADPH Oxidase Function in Autoimmune Diabetes. *Free Radic Biol Med* (2018) 125:81–9. doi: 10.1016/j.freeradbiomed.2018.04.581
62. Horwitz E, Krogvold L, Zhitomirsky S, Swisa A, Fischman M, Lax T, et al. β-Cell DNA Damage Response Promotes Islet Inflammation in Type 1 Diabetes. *Diabetes* (2018) 67:2305–18. doi: 10.2337/db17-1006
63. Rabinovitch A, Suarez-Pinzon W, Strynadka K, Ju Q, Edelstein D, Brownlee M, et al. Transfection of Human Pancreatic Islets With an Anti-Apoptotic Gene (bcl-2) Protects Beta-Cells From Cytokine-Induced Destruction. *Diabetes* (1999) 48:1223–9. doi: 10.2337/diabetes.48.6.1223
64. Cascone T, Mckenzie JA, Mbofung RM, Punt S, Wang Z, Xu C, et al. Increased Tumor Glycolysis Characterizes Immune Resistance to Adoptive T Cell Therapy. *Cell Metab* (2018) 27:977–87. doi: 10.1016/j.cmet.2018.02.024
65. Lawless SJ, Kedia-Mehta N, Walls JF, Mcgarrigle R, Convery O, Sinclair LV, et al. Glucose Represses Dendritic Cell-Induced T Cell Responses. *Nat Commun* (2017) 8:15620. doi: 10.1038/ncomms15620
66. Geiger R, Rieckmann JC, Wolf T, Basso C, Feng Y, Fuhrer T, et al. L-Arginine Modulates T Cell Metabolism and Enhances Survival and Anti-tumor Activity. *Cell Metab* (2016) 167:829–42. doi: 10.1016/j.cell.2016.09.031
67. Prendergast GC, Smith C, Thomas S, Mandik-Nayak L, Laury-Kleintop L, Metz R, et al. Indoleamine 2,3-Dioxygenase Pathways of Pathogenic Inflammation and Immune Escape in Cancer. *Cancer Immunol Immunother* (2014) 63:721–35. doi: 10.1007/s00262-014-1549-4
68. Skapenko A, Leipe J, Lipsky PE, Schulze-Koops H. The Role of the T Cell in Autoimmune Inflammation. *Arthritis Res Ther* (2005) 7:S4–14. doi: 10.1186/ar1703
69. Da Silva JA, Spector TD. The Role of Pregnancy in the Course and Aetiology of Rheumatoid Arthritis. *Clin Rheumatol* (1992) 11:189–94. doi: 10.1007/BF02207955
70. Pieper J, Dubnovitsky A, Gerstner C, James EA, Rieck M, Kozhukh G, et al. Memory T Cells Specific to Citrullinated α-Enolase Are Enriched in the Rheumatic Joint. *J Autoimmun* (2018) 92:47–56. doi: 10.1016/j.jaut.2018.04.004
71. Ascherio A, Munger KL. Environmental Risk Factors for Multiple Sclerosis. Part I: The Role of Infection. *Ann Neurol* (2007) 61:288–99. doi: 10.1002/ana.21117

72. Lünemann JD, Jelcić I, Roberts S, Lutterotti A, Tackenberg B, Martin R, et al. EBNA1-Specific T Cells From Patients With Multiple Sclerosis Cross React With Myelin Antigens and Co-Produce IFN-Gamma and IL-2. *J Exp Med* (2008) 205:1763–73. doi: 10.1084/jem.20072397
73. Yang J, Jing L, James EA, Gebe JA, Koelle DM, Kwok WW. A Novel Approach of Identifying Immunodominant Self and Viral Antigen Cross-Reactive T Cells and Defining the Epitopes They Recognize. *Front Immunol* (2018) 9:2811. doi: 10.3389/fimmu.2018.02811
74. Rodriguez-Calvo T. Enterovirus Infection and Type 1 Diabetes: Unraveling the Crime Scene. *Clin Exp Immunol* (2019) 195:15–24. doi: 10.1111/cei.13223

2

Type I Interferon is a Catastrophic Feature of the Diabetic Islet Microenvironment

*Brittney N. Newby and Clayton E. Mathews**

Department of Pathology, Immunology and Laboratory Medicine, University of Florida, Gainesville, FL, United States

***Correspondence:**
Clayton E. Mathews
clayton.mathews@pathology.ufl.edu

A detailed understanding of the molecular pathways and cellular interactions that result in islet beta cell (β cell) destruction is essential for the development and implementation of effective therapies for prevention or reversal of type 1 diabetes (T1D). However, events that define the pathogenesis of human T1D have remained elusive. This gap in our knowledge results from the complex interaction between genetics, the immune system, and environmental factors that precipitate T1D in humans. A link between genetics, the immune system, and environmental factors are type 1 interferons (T1-IFNs). These cytokines are well known for inducing antiviral factors that limit infection by regulating innate and adaptive immune responses. Further, several T1D genetic risk loci are within genes that link innate and adaptive immune cell responses to T1-IFN. An additional clue that links T1-IFN to T1D is that these cytokines are a known constituent of the autoinflammatory milieu within the pancreas of patients with T1D. The presence of IFNα/β is correlated with characteristic MHC class I (MHC-I) hyperexpression found in the islets of patients with T1D, suggesting that T1-IFNs modulate the cross-talk between autoreactive cytotoxic CD8$^+$ T lymphocytes and insulin-producing pancreatic β cells. Here, we review the evidence supporting the diabetogenic potential of T1-IFN in the islet microenvironment.

Keywords: type 1 diabetes, type 1 interferons, humans, CD8$^+$ T cell, beta cells

INTRODUCTION

Type 1 diabetes (T1D) results from an autoimmune-mediated attack that specifically targets insulin (INS)-secreting pancreatic beta (β) cells. Through the interactions of β cell antigen-specific T cell receptors (TCR) with MHC-peptide complexes, β cells are destroyed leading to aberrant glucose homeostasis and persistent hyperglycemia. Critical to T1D pathogenesis is the targeted destruction of pancreatic β cells mass by autoreactive cytotoxic CD8$^+$ T lymphocytes (CTLs) (1–6). Although responses in T1D are directed toward autoantigens, the activation of the β cell specific CTLs is expected to be similar to activation of CD8$^+$ T cells observed during a typical response to infectious agents. Following activation, autoreactive CTLs clonally expand, home into the pancreatic islets, and survey the surface of β cells for antigen presented in the context of MHC class I (MHC-I). Recognition of the specific cognate peptide- human leukocyte antigen (HLA) class I complex results in the induction of TCR signaling, formation of the immunological synapse, and targeted destruction of β cells. While the immune system plays a significant role in perpetuating disease pathology, a large body of literature supports the notion that development of T1D is dependent upon a complex network of determinants including those of genetic and environmental etiologies (7–15). Tissue microenvironments influence immune responses in models of tumor biology and infectious disease. However, this notion remains largely been unexplored in the target tissues of autoimmune diabetes.

Type 1 interferons (T1-IFNs), classically known for interfering with viral infection, have been implicated in the early stages of T1D autoimmunity (16–21). Transcriptome analysis reveals a T1-IFN signature in the peripheral blood of patients prior to the development of autoantibodies (16, 17). Additionally, these cytokines have been identified as being expressed in the pancreata of deceased tissue/organ donors with T1D versus non-diabetic donors (18, 19, 21). GWAS studies reveal several T1D-associated genes that are involved in the production, signaling, and regulation of the T1-IFN pathway (12, 22). Moreover, induction of T1D has been reported in patients receiving T1-IFN therapy for various conditions including hepatitis C, multiple sclerosis, and hairy cell leukemia (23–30) supporting the idea that these cytokines may actively exacerbate T1D progression. Despite the growing evidence for the role of T1-IFNs in T1D, little is known about how these cytokines contribute to the inflammatory environment of the human autoimmune diabetic islet (16, 17, 31–36). This review will consider the current paradigms in the natural history of T1D as well as T1-IFN action while summarizing the published literature regarding a role for T1-IFNs in T1D pathogenesis. Additionally, we highlight the exciting new avenues of research suggesting that T1-IFNs may be a catastrophic feature within the diabetic microenvironment.

SETTING THE STAGE FOR AUTOIMMUNITY: ROLE OF GENETIC SUSCEPTIBILITY

Genetic predisposition constitutes a primary risk factor for the initiation of β cell autoimmunity and can be attributed to the complex interplay of more than 50 genetic loci that may impact immune function, INS expression, and β cell function (11, 37, 38). Identified as the first genetic locus associated with T1D in the 1970s, the HLA region on chromosome 6p21 confers approximately 50% of the genetic risk for disease development (39). This region, also referred to as (it) IDDM1 (it), is highly polymorphic, containing over 200 identified genes that can be categorized as class I, II, or III genes that play an important role in antigen presentation as well as regulation of this process. Particularly, class I and II genes encode the classical HLA cell surface proteins that are involved in presenting antigen to CD8+ and CD4+ lymphocytes, respectively. In fact, the strongest association is found in patients harboring the specific HLA class II haplotypes, DR3-DQ2 (DRB*301-DQB*201) and DR4-DQ8 (DRB*401-DQA*301-DQB*302) with the highest risk seen in DR3/DR4 compound heterozygotes (40, 41). Conversely, strong protection from T1D is observed in individuals with the DQB*602 allele, which is reported in less than 1% of patients with T1D (42, 43). Comparison of high- and low-risk DQ alleles in humans and mouse models reveal key differences in peptide binding, as predisposing alleles contain a substitution of non-charged amino acids (alanine, valine, or serine) for aspartate at position 57, which destabilizes binding of antigenic epitopes (44–46). While most studies assessing HLA risk haplotypes have been carried out in Caucasian individuals, recent efforts have begun to characterize HLA susceptibility in other ethnic groups. For example, HLA genotyping in African American patients found that the African-specific DR9 (DRB1*09:01-DQA1*03:01-DQB1*02:01g) haplotype in combination with DR4 mimics risk for T1D seen in patients with DR3/DR4 heterozygosity in European populations. Alternatively, the African-specific "DR3" haplotype (DRB1*03:02-DQA1*04:01-DQB1*04:02) confers significant protection (47). Future studies in this area should be geared toward understanding HLA risk haplotypes in individuals of diverse ethnic backgrounds. Although not as widely studied, HLA class I alleles, HLA A*24 and HLA B*39, appear to be associated with increased susceptibility for T1D, decreased age of onset, and fulminant β cell destruction (48–50).

Numerous additional loci outside of the HLA region summate the remaining genetic risk for diabetes development, although the individual odds ratios conferred by these regions are modest (11, 12). Several of these genes are thought to influence tolerance mechanisms facilitating the escape of autoreactive T cells into the periphery. For instance, variants within the INS gene are known to modulate thymic INS expression, which comprises about 10% of the genetic risk for T1D and carry an odds ratio of 2.2 (51–53). Extensive mapping of this region associates variable number of tandem repeats in the 5′ promoter of INS with diabetes risk (53–55). Shorter class I alleles [23–63 repeats] predispose for diabetes, while longer class III alleles [140–210 repeats] are protective (55). The number of tandem repetitions determines INS transcription in the thymus through interactions with the autoimmune regulator, AIRE, which is essential for appropriate T cell education and provides strong evidence that central tolerance to INS, the primary autoantigen in T1D, is impaired in patients who harbor this risk variant (56).

Protein tyrosine phosphatase non-receptor type 22 (PTPN22) is another well-known example, as this locus confers the third highest genetic association for T1D and is also known to be a regulator of signaling in a variety of immune cell types including lymphocytes, monocytes, dendritic cells (DCs), and neutrophils (57). Case-control and association studies show that this coding variant causes a non-synonymous substitution from an arginine to a tryptophan (R620W) located within the protein-binding domain of PTPN22. Biochemical studies in lymphocytes demonstrate the PTPN22*W620 allele behaves as a gain-of-function mutant with dampened TCR signaling (58). In contrast, the same variant in myeloid derived cell types is highly controversial with some models demonstrating hyper-responsive DC phenotypes with increased T cell activation while others exhibit reduced function and selective impairment of T1-IFN responses following TLR stimulation (59, 60). How might seemingly paradoxical functions be contributing to onset of T1D? On one hand, diminished TCR signaling by the risk variant could impair central and peripheral T cell tolerance, while reduced T1-IFN production by TLRs may hinder effective clearance of β-cell tropic viruses triggering self-reactivity (61). Studies remain ongoing to determine the full gamut of functional consequences induced by this variant.

Like PTPN22, many T1D-associated genes play multiple roles in immune sensing and signaling especially in response to environmental ques, which supports the hypothesis that genetic risk coupled to permissive environmental determinants collectively contribute to diabetes progression. Diabetogenic viruses signify a highly postulated candidate for initiation and potentiation of islet autoimmunity. Critical for the innate immune response to viral infection are T1-IFNs. Several identified genetic loci for T1D also have prominent roles in the induction and signaling of this pathway, including IFIH1 (rs1990760), TYK2 (rs2304256), and STAT4 (rs7574865) (62–64). TYK2 is a tyrosine kinase involved in proximal TI-IFN signal transduction as well as regulation of IFNAR1 surface expression (65–67). Similarly, STAT4 is a key mediator of T1-IFN signaling essential for the generation of Th1 responses, which contribute to the T cell-mediated pathology observed in diabetes (68, 69). Also associated with several other autoimmune disorders, protective variants for each of these genes is associated with reduced T1-IFN signaling (67, 70). IFIH1 encodes the protein MDA5, a cytoplasmic sensor of viral double-stranded RNA. The non-synonymous SNP found in IFIH1 results in alanine to threonine amino acid substitution at position 946 (A946T) and may diminish ATPase activity of MDA5 activity leading to deranged constitutive provocation of T1-IFN as well as blunted viral sensing (62, 71, 72). Compelling evidence in primary human islets reveals that presence of the homozygous risk allele decreases the autonomous innate response to Coxsackievirus B3 (73). Collectively, these data suggest that the A946T risk variant in IFIH1 may act as a double-edged sword, predisposing β cells to persistent enteroviral infection while concurrently promoting deleterious T1-IFN production in and around the islet microenvironment.

EVOLUTION OF ISLET DESTRUCTION IN HUMAN DIABETES

Human β cells act as quintessential metabolic sensors working to integrate environmental cues for rapid and efficient glycemic control (74). Reports of decreased C-peptide responses and reduced glucose tolerance in autoantibody positive individuals suggest that ongoing inflammation precipitates the deterioration of β cell function prior to diabetes onset (75–77). Additionally, β cells are also widely believed to be active participants in promoting a diabetogenic islet microenvironment. For example, MHC-I is known to be hyperexpressed within the islets of T1D patients, suggesting that β cells may be more visible to infiltrating CTL (1, 20, 21, 78). Increasing data insinuates that signals arising from the islet microenvironment, such as T1-IFNs, could trigger such disease promoting adaptations. Additionally, active inflammatory signals within the islet microenvironment prompt substantial variation in the β cell transcriptome and proteome as well as augmenting the capacity for cytokine and chemokine production by islet or β cells (79).

The conceptual model proposed by George Eisenbarth for the natural history of T1D has shaped theories regarding the evolution of T1D pathogenesis (80, 81). Many facets of this paradigm have been tested and updated over the past 3 decades. The amalgamation of genetic pre-disposition and initiating environmental triggers create the framework for models that describe the insurgence of β cell autoimmunity. Though the nature of the instigating insult is not completely understood, once initiated, active immune-onslaught can be indicated by the presence of autoantibodies and histological detection of the pathognomonic lesion termed insulitis (82). Found in or around the islets, insulitis is a heterogeneous inflammatory infiltrate comprised of T lymphocytes, B lymphocytes, macrophages, and DCs, however CD8$^+$ T cells form the primary constituent [(1, 2, 83) and **Figure 1A**]. First noted by German pathologist Martin Schmidt in the early 1900s, this lesion was not considered a prominent feature of T1D until the landmark paper by Willy Gepts in 1965 where the presence of insulitic lesions were observed in 15/22 recent onset T1D cases (82, 84, 85). Further evaluation of these samples using immunohistochemical techniques and additional data from subsequent studies revealed that inflammation was primarily observed in islets with INS immunoreactivity. Further, in cases with long-standing disease, many islets appear to be devoid of INS containing β cells without active insulitis, alluding to the role of these cells as the inciting antigen in T1D (1, 2, 20, 82, 86–88).

Until recently, efforts aimed at characterizing the nature, composition, and frequency of insulitis have been challenging. This is due to the anatomical inaccessibility of the pancreas for direct study in living subjects as well as a dearth of well-preserved human cadaveric tissues for analysis (84, 89). The inception of the Network for Pancreatic Organ Donors with Diabetes (nPOD) has dramatically advanced our understanding of β cell/Islet autoimmunity (89–92). Moreover, studies of human pancreata have allowed for the emergence of new paradigms in T1D, including the current consensus definition of insulitis, defined as the presence of more than 15 peri- or intrainsulitic CD45$^+$ cells within a minimum of three islets (93). The most comprehensive screening and characterization of insulitis to date was recently described using the nPOD collection where a total of 159 pancreata were screened (61 controls, 18 autoantibody positive cases without a diagnosis of T1D, and 80 T1D cases) (88). Investigators presented confirmatory findings that insulitis is present most frequently in recent-onset patients within INS-containing islets and inversely correlates with disease duration. The presence of adaptive-immune infiltration into the islets of individuals with autoantibodies is a rare event, observed only in individuals with multiple antibodies (94). Additionally, patients with T1D display tremendous heterogeneity in terms nature, distribution, and severity of insulitis in addition to the amount of residual β mass present following diagnosis (88, 95).

A critical cell-to-cell interaction during the development of T1D occurs when β cells and islet-antigen specific CTLs come into contact. Strong evidence has supported a crucial role for CD8$^+$ T cells in T1D. First reported by Bottazzo in 1985, histological characterization of pancreas sections from T1D cases demonstrated that CTL are the most abundant immune cell type found in human insulitis [(20) and **Figure 1A**]. Additional studies have confirmed that CD8$^+$ T cells have a prominent role in T1D as well as recurrent T1D that occurs after transplantation of islets, pancreas (pancreas alone, or SPK recipients) into patients with T1D.

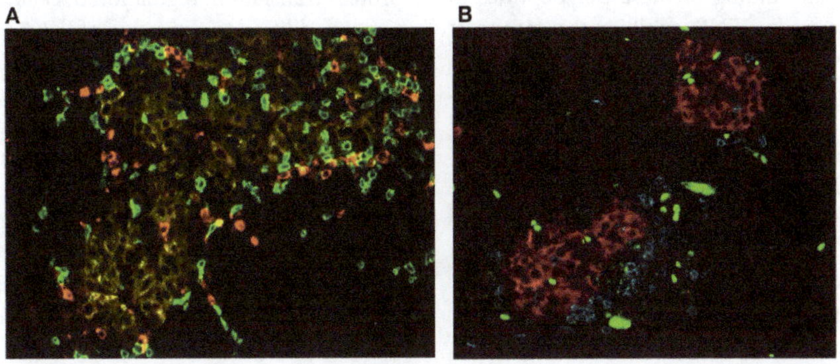

FIGURE 1 | CD8 T cells are the major leukocyte component of the insulitis lesion in type 1 diabetes (T1D) as well as recurrent disease. Pancreatic sections [courtesy of Network for Pancreatic Organ Donors with Diabetes (nPOD)] were examine histologically for the presence of islet invading immune cells. **(A)** Section taken from a pancreas organ donor with T1D (nPOD case 6052). The tissue section was immunofluorescently stained for glucagon (yellow) to identify the islet, CD4 T lymphocytes (red), and CD8 T lymphocytes (green). Within this islet cytotoxic CD8+ T lymphocytes (CTLs) are the predominant T cell type observed. Image courtesy of Martha Campbell-Thompson, DVM/PhD (University of Florida). **(B)** Section taken from a pancreas transplant biopsy, from an simultaneous pancreas and kidney (SPK) recipient who had developed recurrence of T1D. Tissues were stained for insulin (red), CD4 T lymphocytes (blue), and CD8 T lymphocytes (teal). Within the insulitic lesions, CTLs represented the dominant T cell found. Figure shows islets with both CD8 than CD4 T cells, but most islets were primarily infiltrated by CD8 T cells. Green/yellow bright stains represent non-specific fluorescence from red blood cells. Image courtesy of Alberto Pugliese, MD, Francesco Vendrame, MD, and George Burke, III, MD, University of Miami.

Biopsy and histological examination of the transplanted pancreas demonstrate the accumulation of high numbers of CD8+ T cells into INS positive islets in patients who are undergoing active islet autoimmunity (**Figure 1B**).

Regarded as the final executioner in T1D, CTLs mediate direct β cell destruction through the recognition of epitopes from proteins that are selectively expressed in β cells and are presented by these INS-producing cells the context of MHC-I. Following recognition of cognate antigen, CTLs create a close contact with the target β cell by forming an immunological synapse, where several cytotoxic mechanisms are employed to induce death of β cells. These include the induction of molecules involved in the granule exocytosis pathway such as perforin, granzyme, or granulysin as well as increased surface expression of death ligands such as Fas Ligand and TNF-related apoptosis inducing ligand (96–98). The presence of CTLs specific for well-known autoantigens such as IGRP, preproinsulin, and IA-2, have been documented in islets with augmented MHC-I expression (1, 2, 88). CD8+ T cells bearing TCR that are specific for β cell antigens have been detected in circulation of patients. These TCRs imbue CTL with the ability to destroy human β cells *in vitro* (99–102). In patients undergoing recurrent autoimmunity following islet transplantation, autoreactive CD8+ T cells are associated with β cell destruction resulting in graft failure (103). This evidence for an essential role of CTL in T1D in humans is further bolstered by studies in mice. Spontaneous diabetes fails to develop in non-obese diabetic (NOD) mice lacking MHC-I or β2 microglobulin (4, 6), while diabetes onset can be accelerated by adoptive transfer of diabetogenic CTL (104, 105).

Mounting evidence suggests that stimuli from the diabetic islet microenvironment likely contribute to autoreactive CTL-mediated β cell cytotoxicity. For example, using NOD adoptive transfer systems with IGRP-specific NY8.3 CD8+ T cells, it has been demonstrated that CD8+ T cells acquire greater cytolytic capacity and an effector-memory phenotype upon migration into the NOD islet (106–108). As T1-IFNs are linked to increased HLA expression in the pancreatic islets of patients with T1D, suggesting that these cytokines contribute to autoimmune surveillance and promote insulitis. While the effect of T1-IFNs on human islets have only recently begun to emerge, evidence suggests that T1-IFNs are involved in the cross talk between the adaptive immune effectors and the microenvironment of the diabetic islet (16, 17, 31–36, 109, 110).

TYPE 1 INTERFERONS

Type 1 interferons belong to a large family of cytokines that were originally described by Alick Issacs and Jean Lindenmann in 1957 as soluble factors responsible for mediating viral interference following a primary virus exposure (111–113). Since then, this large family of cytokines has been further categorized into three distinct classes that play essential roles in cellular-mediated defense against viral and microbial infections as well as in autoimmunity (113–116). Differing in structural homology and signaling receptor complexes, these categories include the T1-IFNs as well as the type 2 interferon [interferon gamma (IFNγ)] and the recently identified type III IFNs including IFNλ1 (IL-29), IFNλ2 (IL-28A), IFNλ3 (IL-28B), and IFNλ4 (114, 117–121). T1-IFNs signal through the heterodimeric IFNAR1-IFNAR2 receptor [IFNAR] and comprises the largest class of IFN including thirteen IFNα subtypes in addition to IFNβ, IFNε, IFNκ, and IFNω. Though multiple T1-IFN subtypes may appear redundant, these distinct entities display unique binding affinities to the IFNAR that result in diverse functional outcomes with respect to antiviral, immunomodulatory, and growth inhibitory activity (122–128). While all T1-IFN subtypes contain several conserved "anchoring" residues that are important for receptor binding, the contribution of residues flanking these anchor points determine the overall binding of these polypeptides to IFNAR1/2 (126–130). As such, IFNβ exhibits the strongest interaction with the receptor out of all T1-IFN subtypes (130).

Type 1 interferons represent an early line of defense against viral infection and can be produced by virtually every cell in the body (131–134). Induction of T1-IFNs are initiated by stimulation of pattern recognition receptors (PRRs) that recognize conserved motifs found on viruses, including toll-like receptors (TLR3, TLR4, TLR7, and TLR9), cytosolic RNA helicases (RIG-I and MDA-5), and cytosolic DNA sensors (131, 133, 134). Following activation of these distinct pathways, the adaptor molecules MAVS (cytosolic RNA sensors), STING (cytosolic DNA sensors), TRIF (TLR3/4), and MyD88 (TLR7/8/9) transduce signals that converge on the activation of TBK-1, which phosphorylates IRF-3 leading to transcription of T1-IFN and IRF-7 that engage in a positive feedback loop for amplification of this response (134–136).

Following production, T1-IFNs signal in an autocrine or paracrine fashion through IFNAR. Engagement of the receptor leads to trans-phosphorylation as well as activation of the tyrosine kinases TYK2 and JAK1 that are constitutively associated with the IFNAR subunits, IFNAR1 and IFNAR2, respectively. Signaling downstream of IFNAR can lead to the activation of several pathways that contribute to the widespread range of effects by T1-IFNs depending upon the cell type and the context in which the TI-IFN signal was received (117, 133, 137, 138). Classically, T1-IFN signaling invokes the activation of STAT1-STAT2 heterodimers that rapidly translocate to the nucleus and complex with IRF9 to form the interferon-stimulated gene factor 3 (ISGF3) complex. Formation of ISGF3 leads to binding of the interferon response element (consensus sequence: TTTCNNTTTC) for the transcription of interferon-stimulated genes (ISGs) that mediate a diverse range of functions (117, 133, 139). Alternatively, T1-IFNs are capable of activating all seven members of the STAT family that can manifest as homodimers or heterodimers to induce downstream signaling and transcription. For instance, T1-IFN induced STAT1 homodimers are known to bind IFNγ activated sequences (GAS; consensus sequence: TTCNNNGAA) to initiate proinflammatory programs similar to IFNγ, whereas T1-IFN induced STAT3 homodimers have been reported to interact with the corepressor complex SIN3A to indirectly counteract inflammatory responses (133, 140–142). Utilization of these alternative T1-IFN signaling pathways is partially determined by the expression of individual STAT family members (143). This concept is clearly evident in lymphocytes. The balance between STAT1 and STAT4 dictates T cell responses following T1-IFN exposure (144). This is highly dependent upon STAT4 expression within the T cell, which is initially induced through activation of TCR signaling. This induces a switch from the "classical" anti-proliferative and proapoptotic actions of STAT1 signaling to STAT4 that promotes T cell proliferation, differentiation, and survival (143–145).

In addition to JAK-STAT signaling, several other noncanonical pathways are known to be induced by T1-IFNs. For example, activation of JAK1 and TYK2 after T1-IFN engagement has been shown to induce the PI3K-AKT pathway that leads to activation of mTOR, which leads to downstream control of protein translation, regulation of cellular division, and proliferation, in addition to activation of IKKβ resulting in NF-κB activity (117, 137). In lymphocytes, the MAPK pathway mediates cross-talk between T1-IFN signaling and the TCR complex resulting in growth inhibition (117). While studies are still ongoing to unmask the complex signaling networks induced by T1-IFNs, the ability of these cytokines to induce a wide array of signaling pathways explains their pleiotropic and sometimes paradoxical biological activities.

Type 1 interferons signaling culminates in the induction of a robust antiviral program. Several key components required for T1-IFN signaling, including STAT1 and IRF9, are also well-known ISGs that act to reinforce and amplify the IFN response. T1-IFNs also act to enhance host defense and pathogen detection by increasing the expression of several PRRs involved in viral sensing, expression of 2,5 oligoadenylate synthetase (OAS) that facilitates eradication viral RNA, as well as upregulation of proteins that interfere at various steps of the viral life cycle, including viral entry, replication, and viral egress from infected cells (146).

Type 1 interferons dynamically regulate the actions of innate and adaptive immune cells, including the ability to enhance NK cell cytotoxicity as well as the production of IL-1β and IL-18 by macrophages (147). These cytokines are also well known for directly and indirectly influencing T cell responses that assist in the eradication of invading pathogens or malignant cells (132, 138, 147, 148). IFNα/β promote the differentiation and maturation of DCs by enhancing the expression of MHC-I and II along with costimulatory molecules (CD40, CD80, CD83, CD86, 4-1BBL) required for efficient $CD4^+$ and $CD8^+$ T cell priming (138, 149–151). These cytokines promote trafficking of DCs to lymphoid organs, stimulate expression of adhesion molecules, and induce the secretion of chemoattractant molecules that promote communication between DCs and T lymphocytes (138, 152–154). In line with their effects on DCs, T1-IFNs promote the activity of antigen-exposed $CD8^+$ T cells, by inciting proliferation, enhancing survival, and increasing effector function. Conversely, in antigen-inexperienced $CD8^+$ T cells the T1-IFNs prevent growth and differentiation in an effort to direct a specific T cell response toward the inciting pathogen (138). While T1-IFNs act to implement numerous mechanisms aimed at thwarting the spread of infection, aberrant activation of this pathway, as seen in autoimmunity, can lead to overactivation of immune cells and perpetuation of tissue damage.

T1-IFNs AND PATHOGENESIS OF T1D

Evidence in Humans

The characterization of insulitis in seminal studies by Gepts and Foulis altered the landscape regarding the pathogenesis of T1D to one of an immune etiology. Soon after, it was reported that there was a striking genetic association between the HLA DR locus and T1D onset (155). These findings, along with the notion that class II antigens could be expressed abnormally in other organ-specific autoimmune diseases prompted investigators to hypothesize that altered antigen presentation by pancreatic β cells in T1D might explain activation and infiltration of autoimmune T cells found within insulitic lesions (156–158). In 1985, Bottazzo et al. reported that residual β cells found in a 12-year-old recent onset donor were selectively positive for HLA-DR. In addition to noting enhanced expression of HLA-DR, this was also the first report to note enhanced HLA class I expression in insulitic islets the same donor (20). Since the aberrant expression of MHC-II molecules could be induced by IFNγ on thyroid follicular cells in autoimmune thyroiditis, it was postulated that IFNγ could be acting in a similar manner to induce this uncharacteristic expression in pancreatic β cells. While subsequent studies showed that interferons were incapable of directly inducing ectopic expression of MHC-II on pancreatic β cells, they were found to be potent inducers of MHC-I expression (21). Subsequent analyses confirmed that MHC-I expression was a prominent phenotype found in patients undergoing islet autoimmunity, especially in normal appearing or inflamed islets containing residual β cells (1, 78, 159–162). Based on the heterogeneity of insulitis in T1D, it was hypothesized that β cells could be actively generating soluble mediators that are capable of acting in a paracrine manner to exert affects within the diabetic microenvironment. IFNα represented a prime candidate, as it was known to induce MHC-I in islet tissue and was known to be produced by a wide range of cells (21). The first report to correlate the presence of IFNα in the islets of patients with recent-onset T1D diabetes was published in 1987. Investigators examined 37 pancreata from cadaveric donors with T1D and found that 34 of 37 samples displayed MHC-I hyperexpression. Further, 97% of patients displaying this feature concurrently exhibited positivity for IFNα by immunocytochemistry (18). Transcript expression of various cytokines, including IFNα, IFNβ, IFNγ, IL-1β, TNFα, were compared in diabetic and control pancreata. Among the panel of cytokines tested, only IFNα displayed a clear and consistent pattern of augmented expression in patients (19).

Additional lines of evidence implicate a pathogenic role for T1-IFNs in human autoimmune diabetes. The presence of β cell-specific autoantibodies signifies the preclinical phase of T1D and serves as an essential biomarker for identifying at-risk individuals (163). Long-term follow up of at risk children enrolled in the BABYDIET and DIPP longitudinal studies reveal T1-IFN inducible signatures in the peripheral blood, which was positively correlated with episodes of upper respiratory infections. The signature was strongest immediately prior to seroconversion and began to decline after the detection of autoantibodies. This time course suggests that activation and production of T1-IFNs may be involved in the early stages of islet autoimmunity (16, 17). In accordance with these findings, IFNα in the plasma of patients with T1D was shown to be elevated when compared to controls (10.1 U/mL; 69.6% positivity vs. 0.4 U/mL, 0% positivity, respectively) and plasmacytoid dendritic cells (pDCs), well known for producing T1-IFNs, were observed in the peripheral blood of new-onset patients during diagnosis (164, 165). Furthermore, enterovirus RNA, particularly Coxsackievirus B, was identified in 50% of patients who displayed positivity for IFNα (165).

The half-life of cytokines within the T1-IFN family is relatively short (IFNα: 4–16 h; IFNβ 1–2 h) and serum levels of IFN begin to decline very rapidly once secreted (166, 167). Due to rapid clearance, detection of IFNs in circulation can prove challenging. To circumvent this, investigators have attempted to use T1-IFN induction pathways, such as Poly(I:C), or the measurement of ISGs in PBMC as surrogate markers for T1-IFN activation when comparing patients and controls (168, 169). For example, patients display a higher basal expression of the ISG OAS, as well as increased sensitivity to IFNα exhibited by maximal induction at lower IFNα concentrations when compared to control subjects (168). T1-IFN production was higher from PBMC isolated from patients with T1D compared to controls, whereas IFNγ production by isolated PBMC in response to concanavalin A was not different between control and T1D patient samples (169). With respect to the IFNα response, there was no correlation to blood glucose levels, HbA1c, age of onset, disease duration, or ICA positivity, which may point to the importance of genes associated with T1D that are involved in signaling of this pathway (169).

Initiation of islet autoimmunity has been noted in individuals following T1-IFN therapy for chronic hepatitis, multiple sclerosis, as well as hematologic malignancies (23, 24). First reported in 1992, T1-IFN-induced autoimmune diabetes was described in a patient with Hepatitis C, who was seropositive before treatment for autoantibodies against both GAD and INS (30). While this complication occurs in a minor subset of patients, half of all cases reporting T1D following IFN therapy were positive for autoantibodies. This suggests that T1-IFNs may precipitate loss of tolerance and self-reactivity in at-risk patients (170). Studies investigating β cell function in these patients suggest that T1-IFNs can reduce INS secretion, impair carbohydrate metabolism during an oral glucose challenge, and induce INS dependency over the course of treatment (171, 172). Patients who incur T1-IFN-induced autoimmune diabetes to not exhibit normoglycemia when T1-IFN therapy is arrested suggesting that in these patients β cell mass is lost to an extent that metabolic control cannot be reestablished.

Evidence In Animal Models of T1D

Animal models have been indispensable for ascertaining knowledge regarding the cellular and molecular events involved in T1D pathogenesis. Likewise, these models have also been instrumental in elucidating how T1-IFNs contribute to diabetes pathogenesis. One example includes the diabetes prone biobreeding rat (BB-DP rat). These animals emulate some pathologic features observed in human diabetes including polygenic inheritance [including the MHC], peripubescent onset, and β cell destruction characterized by mononuclear infiltration (173, 174). Initial studies conducted in this model demonstrate a dose dependent stimulation of IFNα production by Poly(I:C) that correlates with accelerated diabetes incidence and severity (175, 176). Conversely, elevation of serum IFNα in non-diabetes prone Wistar rats did not instigate diabetes, suggesting that T1-IFNs are not pathogenic without an inherent risk for diabetes (175, 176). Additionally, investigation into the natural history of diabetes in BBDP rats revealed spontaneous expression of IFNα in the islets of Langerhans prior to insulitis proposing that induction of T1-IFNs in the islet microenvironment may disrupt self-tolerance in this preclinical model (177).

The NOD mouse model has served as the principal animal model for the investigation of causative mechanisms leading to autoimmune diabetes (178). Several lines of evidence in the NOD support an association for T1-IFNs in T1D. One of the most striking is the presence of a T1-IFN signature in NOD islets prior to diabetes onset, reminiscent of the signature observed in humans and BBDP rats (31). In 4- to 6-week-old NOD females, T1-IFNs serve as one of the first distinctive signs of pathology in these animals followed by lymphocytic infiltration and synchronized elevation of activation markers in the islet tissue (31). Elevated levels of IFNα and pDC in the pancreatic draining lymph nodes are also reported in 2- to 3-week-old NOD mice (36). This argues that aberrant activation of pDCs, a DC subset that specializes in T1-IFN production, may contribute to the development of this signature, perhaps through ineffective clearance of islet cell debris (36, 179, 180). Moreover, innate sensing by TLRs represents an essential pathway for the stimulation of T1-IFNs. Accordingly, ablation of MDA-5 (encoded by *Ifih1*) in NOD mice results in protection from spontaneous T1D development, while NOD mice carrying a single allele of MDA-5 experience slowed progression and reduced incidence (181). MDA-$5^{+/-}$ animals also displayed protection from Coxsackie B4 virus-induced T1D when compared to MDA-$5^{+/+}$ littermates that developed disease despite being able to efficiently clear the virus (181). Further investigations have revealed that CB4 infection of MDA-$5^{+/-}$ mice resulted in a transient increase in IFNβ that returned to baseline by 7 days postinfection, while IFNβ levels in MDA-$5^{+/+}$ mice remain consistently elevated after infection (181). These data suggest that protective allotypes of MDA-5 may act in a similar manner to tightly regulate IFN production while keeping antiviral defense mechanisms intact (181). Accordingly, stimulation of TLR7, which recognizes ssRNA to promote T1-IFN production, results in accelerated T1D onset in NOD animals, whereas abrogation of TLR9 signaling, important for the response to unmethylated DNA, retards progressive islet destruction (182, 183). Inhibition of T1-IFN signaling through the heterodimeric IFNAR has presented conflicted results. Incidence in NOD and NOD.IFNAR$1^{-/-}$ was indistinguishable, however short-course administration of an IFNAR1 blocking antibody to NOD animals 15–25 postpartum significantly delayed the onset of diabetes (36, 184, 185). Recently, CRISPR-Cas9 deletion of the IFNAR1 subunit in LEW.1WR1 rats, a newly described animal model for T1D, caused delayed onset and frequency of Poly(I:C) induced diabetes (186, 187). Taken together, these data support the idea that coordinated activation of T1-IFN is an early event in autoimmune diabetes but its role in disease progression is likely heavily influenced by the immune response to environmental cues and inheritance of risk/resistance alleles in genes that impact T1-IFN production or signaling.

Utilization of transgenic model systems during the late 20th century provided strong evidence that T1-IFNs may act to accelerate diabetes pathogenesis. Overexpression of IFNα or IFNκ in pancreatic β cells of mice not normally prone to T1D leads to onset of diabetes with severe insulitis, hypoinsulinemia, and diabetes (35, 188). Transgenic mice expressing of IFNβ under the control of the rat INS promoter display various phenotypes depending on genetic background. For example, C57BL6/SJL mice with the RIP-IFNβ transgene do not develop overt diabetes, but display mild hyperglycemia with decreased glucose-stimulated INS secretion and impaired glucose tolerance characteristic of a prediabetic state (34). However, overexpression of IFNβ in the islets of other mouse strains that are not prone to developing T1D, including the non-obese diabetes resistant, induced spontaneous diabetes development (34, 189). Moreover, NOD RIP-IFNβ mice had accelerated and fulminant onset of T1D (189). Taken together, these data demonstrate that T1-IFNs can act as a spark leading to autoimmunity but only in individuals that possess an inherent risk for development of T1D. Further, these data demonstrate that T1-IFNs in the islet microenvironment result in deleterious effects on β cell function and viability by promoting islet inflammation.

T1-IFNs ARE MAJOR PLAYERS IN T1D

Although T1-IFNs have been associated with the induction of T1D and have been identified as a consistent component of the islet autoinflammatory milieu, the direct impact of these cytokines on the pancreatic β cell, cytotoxic T-lymphocytes, and other cellular constituents within the islet that facilitate ongoing islet autoimmunity have only recently been studied using human systems (18, 19, 160, 190). The defining feature observed in T1D is the hyper expression of MHC-I in the islets of patients with T1D, suggesting enhanced β cell immunogenicity and increased susceptibility for targeting by CTLs (1, 2, 18, 19, 190). T1-IFN represent a likely candidate within the local microenvironment capable of mediating this effect, as IFNα/β have been shown to directly induce MHC expression on primary human islet cells [**Figure 2** and (21, 109)]. Recent findings by Marroqui et al. demonstrate that IFNα induced HLA is dependent upon canonical T1-IFN signaling, with TYK2, STAT2, and IRF9 being critically required for induction of HLA class I (109). Another notable finding within the islets of new onset T1D patients is elevated levels of the chemoattractant, CXCL10 (191, 192). Touted as a well-known ISG, CXCL10 is induced by IFNα in primary human islets (109). Our laboratory has corroborated these data, showing that exposure of primary islets to T1-IFN results in significant increases in cell surface Class I HLA by flow cytometry as well as increased mRNA expression of MHC-I and CXCL10 by transcriptome analysis (193). Furthermore, we also find upregulation of transcripts critically required for the MHC-I antigen processing and presentation. Enhanced expression of immunoproteasome subunits PSMB8 and PSMB9 (**Figure 2**) along with proteasome activator subunits PSME1 and PSME2 by T1-IFN suggests an increased efficiency of peptide generation under conditions of inflammatory stress and ATP depletion (194–196). Analysis of constituents of the peptide loading complex following T1-IFN exposure reveal a significant increase in TAP1, TAP2, TAPBP, chaperones, and the editing enzyme ERAP1 suggesting increased transport, stable processing, and loading of peptides onto MHC-I within the endoplasmic reticulum (ER) [(196) and **Figure 2**]. Additionally, there is a global augmentation of antigen processing and enhanced surface MHC-I with functional reductions in β cell mass, as priming of β cells with T1-IFN results in enhanced CTL-induced lysis by chromium release assay [(193) and **Figure 2**].

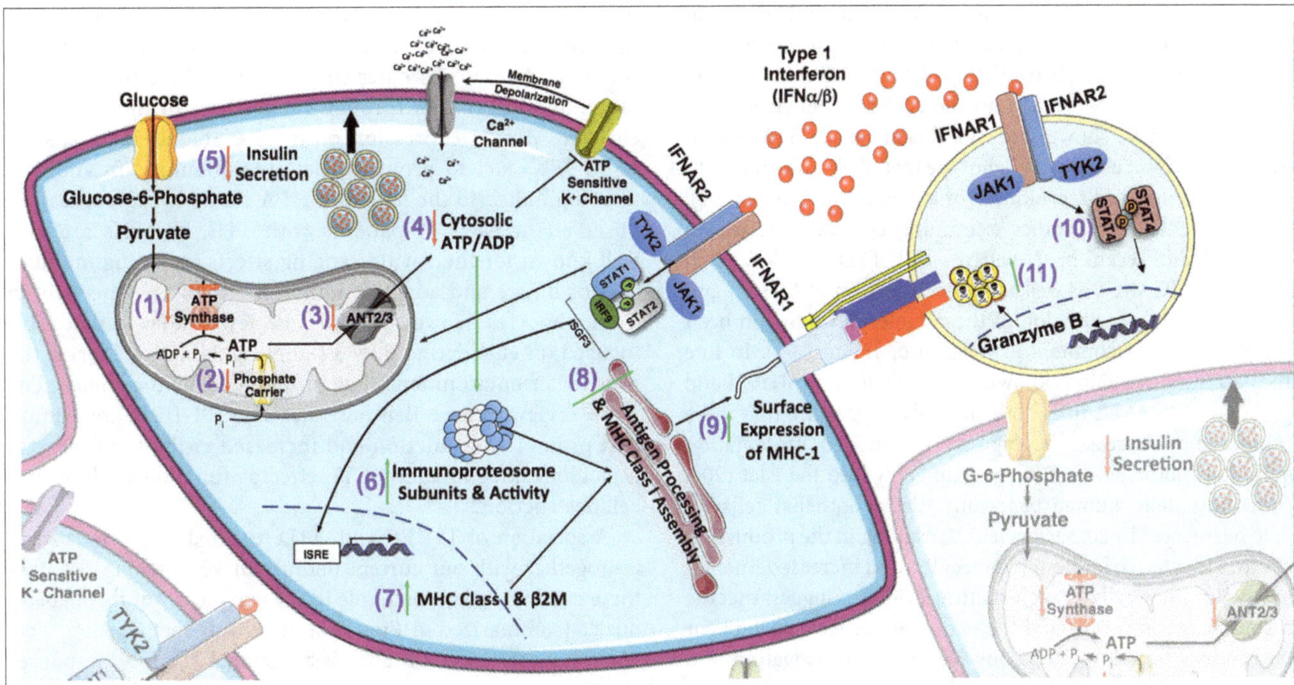

FIGURE 2 | Type 1 interferons (T1-IFNs) are a catastrophic feature of the islet microenvironment in type 1 diabetes (T1D). Based on previous literature and current findings, T1-IFNs are consistently found in the islet autoinflammatory milieu and represent a viable signal that may precipitate diabetogenicity in T1D. With respect to β cells, these cytokines can impair insulin secretory function, possibly through the induction of endoplasmic reticulum (ER) stress as well as by impairing mitochondrial bioenergetics. Whole transcriptome analysis reveals decreased expression of genes involved in the regulation of ATP production and transport, including ATP5A (1), SLC25A3 (2), and SLC25A5/6 (3). Reduction in these transcripts likely lead to decreases in the cytosolic ATP/ADP ratio (4) that is required for glucose-stimulated insulin secretion by β cells (5). T1-IFNs also enhance the autoimmune surveillance of pancreatic β cells through induction of the immunoproteasome (6), *de novo* synthesis of MHC class I and genes responsible for the peptide loading complex (7 and 8), as well as enhanced surface expression of MHC class I (9). This increased capacity for antigen presentation results in a functional ability of cytotoxic CD8+ T lymphocyte (CTL)-mediated β cell destruction, which is further augmented by the ability of T1-IFN to amplify infiltrating CTL cytotoxic capacity through STAT4-induced granzyme B production (10 and 11).

Two recent studies have noted the impact of IFNα on β cells. Using IFNα both groups determined that this cytokine induced the unfolded protein response (UPR) leading to ER stress. However, neither publication reported negative impacts on β cell viability, suggesting that ER stress induced by IFNα did not impact cell death, and there was no reported functional changes (109, 110). While these two studies demonstrate increased expression of markers that signal ER stress, the induction of this response differed in timing and severity, which likely points to differences in experimental design and methodology (109, 110). Indeed, these reports utilized different culture conditions including different media formulations as well as very different time courses of study. For instance, Marroqui et al. revealed an elevated expression of ATF3 and CHOP in primary human islets following 24 h of IFNα (2,000 U/mL) exposure (109). The study conducted by Lombardi and Tomer more widespread induction of the UPR and also assessed INS secretory function in primary human islets and EndoC-βH1 cells after 2 days of exposure to 1,000 U/mL of IFNα. They detected no alterations in glucose stimulated INS secretion, but did correlate the induction of ER stress with reductions in INS content, increased proinsulin to INS ratio, in addition to reduced expression of prohormone convertases, PC1, and PC2 (110). Although ER stress has been a frequently hypothesized explanation for β cell dysfunction in T1D, the idea that IFNα elicits expression of genes involved in the UPR presents a conundrum (197, 198). Previous reports demonstrate that ER stress actually impairs MHC-I expression. These differences in findings of these two recent publications with the discordance of coexisting ER stress and enhanced ER antigen processing highlight the need for a greater understanding of how the numerous signals provoked by T1-IFN alter the β cell in T1D (199–201). Further inspection of metabolic pathways responsible for coordinating INS secretion in β cells by transcriptome analysis revealed a decreased expression ATP5A1, a subunit required for ATP production by ATP synthase; decreased expression of adenine nucleotide translocases 2 and 3 (SLC25A5 and SLC25A6), responsible for regulating mitochondrial ATP export, and decreased expression of the mitochondrial phosphate carrier, SLC25A3 [(193) and **Figure 2**]. A reduction in these genes will likely have major implications on regulation of glucose-stimulated secretion as they directly alter ATP/ADP ratios that are required to trigger islet cell depolarization that leads to release of INS secretory granules.

Another very important component of the islet microenvironment is vascular endothelial cells that facilitate delivery of oxygen and enable the rapid exchange of nutrients and hormones between the blood and the endocrine pancreas. These cells also act as a barrier to intricately regulate trafficking and extravasation of autoreactive immune cells into the islet microenvironment. Several studies have shown that endothelial cells in and around the islets display an activated phenotype that likely contributes to increased homing and recruitment of autoreactive T cells (202). Immunohistochemical studies examining endothelium within the pancreata of recent onset patients with T1D reveal elevated expression of ICAM-1 as well as hyperexpression of MHC-I and -II (83, 190, 203). Expression of these molecules has also been associated with concomitant expression of IFNα (190). In line with these studies, IFNα is known to directly induce MHC-I and expression of ICAM-1 in endothelial cells, suggesting that these cytokines may increase the capacity for antigen presentation required for autoreactive CTLs to gain entry into the islet (204, 205). Additionally, human pancreatic islet endothelial cells are able to be infected by coxsackievirus B resulting in the production of IFNα, induction of adhesion molecules, and increased interaction with immune cells (206). Mounting evidence suggest that the crosstalk between β cells and the endothelium is important for INS secretory function (207). However, more investigation into the role of T1-IFNs in modulating this interaction is warranted.

It is well known that tissue microenvironments are key determinants in driving local immune responses models of cancer and infectious disease. While armed with the ability to modulate the innate and adaptive arms of the immune system, the impact of T1-IFN within the islet microenvironment has not been fully elucidated. Known to contribute to T cell priming and activation through their effects on DCs, T1-IFNs have been directly shown to mediate DC maturation and migration even in the absence of PPR engagement (208, 209). Specifically, they facilitate the metabolic switch from oxidative phosphorylation to glycolysis through regulation of the transcription factor HIF-1α, inducing the upregulation of MHC-I in these cells as well as costimulatory molecules (208, 209). In the case of the autoimmune diabetogenic microenvironment, the presence of T1-IFNs may act to promote DC immunogenicity skewing toward proinflammatory immune activation in addition to augmenting the function of islet infiltrating immune cells, such as $CD8^+$ T cells. Studies completed in our laboratory suggest that T1-IFN drastically augment cytotoxicity elicited by human islet-reactive CTLs. Extensive characterization of T1-IFN signaling mechanisms within these cells show that these cytokines can induce a remarkably rapid acquisition of effector function through induction and direct binding of pSTAT4 to the promoter of Granzyme B (**Figure 2**). In accordance with studies exhibiting full acquisition of autoreactive CTL effector function within the pancreatic microenvironment, these novel studies implicate T1-IFN as a putative innate signal capable of driving CTL differentiation in the islet (106).

CONCLUSION AND MODEL DETAILING HOW IFNα CAN WREAK HAVOC IN THE DIABETIC MICROENVIRONMENT

Several determinants predict an individual's susceptibility to T1D. It is well appreciated that the immune system plays a critical role in diminishing β cell mass, precipitating the onset of persistent hyperglycemia. Critical to this destruction is the presence of $CD8^+$ T cells within the diabetic microenvironment. These cells enter the pancreas where they directly target and kill β cells through interactions of the TCR with elevated MHC-I expression on β cells. Soluble factors, such as T1-IFNs, act to promote islet autoimmunity. In addition to being linked to the hallmark HLA class I hyper-expression observed in islets of patients with T1D, T1-IFNs are also well known for their wide-ranging effects including modulation of innate and adaptive immune responses, especially in T lymphocytes. However, until now, few studies to date have focused on elucidating how T1-IFN signaling transforms the islet to an environment that promotes diabetogenicity. The work reviewed here demonstrates that T1-IFNs are stimuli that promote dysfunction and increased visibility of target β cells alongside enhanced CTL effector function leading to β cell destruction.

Association of T1-IFN with T1D reported in previous studies together with our current findings makes a strong case that these cytokines play some role in the complexity of the diabetes puzzle (summarized in **Figure 2**). It is likely that a genetic predisposition skewed toward dysfunctional T1-IFN responses create an islet environment permissive to enhanced autoantigen presentation, augmented human β cell-specific cytotoxicity by autoreactive CTLs and resulting β cell dysfunction. While the pleiotropic actions of T1-IFNs are designed to strengthen the immune response to viral pathogens, this response proves detrimental in the case of autoimmunity where the immune response is misdirected toward self and in this way can promote β cell death in T1D.

AUTHOR CONTRIBUTIONS

This manuscript was conceived by BN and CM. Interpretation of data/results and discussion were completed by BN and CM. Manuscript was written and revised by BN and CM.

ACKNOWLEDGMENTS

The authors would like to graciously thank Dr. Martha Campbell-Thompson (University of Florida, Gainesville, FL, USA) and Dr. Alberto Pugliese (University of Miami, Miami, FL, USA) for providing us with the images of the pancreatic sections containing insulitis. In addition, the authors thank nPOD staff members for donor recovery, data collection, and helpful discussions. This work was supported by grants from the National Institutes of Health National Institute of Diabetes, Digestive, and Kidney Diseases (NIH-NIDDK): UC4-DK104194 (CEM), UC4-DK104155 (CEM), and F30-DK105788 (BNN) as well as the NIH National Institute of Allergy and Infectious Diseases (NIH-NIAID): P01-A1042288 (CEM). Human organ donor tissue samples were collected by nPOD according to UF IRB approved protocols following the provision of written informed consent by the donor's family as described at https://www.jdrfnpod.org/for-investigators/standard-operating-procedures/.

REFERENCES

1. Coppieters KT, Dotta F, Amirian N, Campbell PD, Kay TW, Atkinson MA, et al. Demonstration of islet-autoreactive CD8 T cells in insulitic lesions from recent onset and long-term type 1 diabetes patients. *J Exp Med* (2012) 209:51–60. doi:10.1084/jem.20111187
2. Willcox A, Richardson SJ, Bone AJ, Foulis AK, Morgan NG. Analysis of islet inflammation in human type 1 diabetes. *Clin Exp Immunol* (2009) 155:173–81. doi:10.1111/j.1365-2249.2008.03860.x
3. Katz J, Benoist C, Mathis D. Major histocompatibility complex class I molecules are required for the development of insulitis in non-obese diabetic mice. *Eur J Immunol* (1993) 23:3358–60. doi:10.1002/eji.1830231244
4. Serreze DV, Leiter EH, Christianson GJ, Greiner D, Roopenian DC. Major histocompatibility complex class I-deficient NOD-B2mnull mice are diabetes and insulitis resistant. *Diabetes* (1994) 43:505–9. doi:10.2337/diabetes.43.3.505
5. Sumida T, Furukawa M, Sakamoto A, Namekawa T, Maeda T, Zijlstra M, et al. Prevention of insulitis and diabetes in beta 2-microglobulin-deficient non-obese diabetic mice. *Int Immunol* (1994) 6:1445–9. doi:10.1093/intimm/6.9.1445
6. Wicker LS, Leiter EH, Todd JA, Renjilian RJ, Peterson E, Fischer PA, et al. Beta 2-microglobulin-deficient NOD mice do not develop insulitis or diabetes. *Diabetes* (1994) 43:500–4. doi:10.2337/diab.43.3.500
7. Dabelea D, Mayer-Davis EJ, Saydah S, Imperatore G, Linder B, Divers J, et al. Prevalence of type 1 and type 2 diabetes among children and adolescents from 2001 to 2009. *JAMA* (2014) 311:1778–86. doi:10.1001/jama.2014.3201
8. Patterson CC, Dahlquist GG, Gyurus E, Green A, Soltesz G, EURODIAB Study Group. Incidence trends for childhood type 1 diabetes in Europe during 1989–2003 and predicted new cases 2005–20: a multicentre prospective registration study. *Lancet* (2009) 373:2027–33. doi:10.1016/S0140-6736(09)60568-7
9. Patterson CC, Gyurus E, Rosenbauer J, Cinek O, Neu A, Schober E, et al. Trends in childhood type 1 diabetes incidence in Europe during 1989–2008: evidence of non-uniformity over time in rates of increase. *Diabetologia* (2012) 55:2142–7. doi:10.1007/s00125-012-2571-8
10. Harjutsalo V, Sjoberg L, Tuomilehto J. Time trends in the incidence of type 1 diabetes in Finnish children: a cohort study. *Lancet* (2008) 371:1777–82. doi:10.1016/S0140-6736(08)60765-5
11. Barrett JC, Clayton DG, Concannon P, Akolkar B, Cooper JD, Erlich HA, et al. Genome-wide association study and meta-analysis find that over 40 loci affect risk of type 1 diabetes. *Nat Genet* (2009) 41:703–7. doi:10.1038/ng.381
12. Concannon P, Rich SS, Nepom GT. Genetics of type 1A diabetes. *N Engl J Med* (2009) 360:1646–54. doi:10.1056/NEJMra0808284
13. Eringsmark Regnéll S, Lernmark A. The environment and the origins of islet autoimmunity and type 1 diabetes. *Diabet Med* (2013) 30:155–60. doi:10.1111/dme.12099
14. Craig ME, Nair S, Stein H, Rawlinson WD. Viruses and type 1 diabetes: a new look at an old story. *Pediatr Diabetes* (2013) 14:149–58. doi:10.1111/pedi.12033
15. Stene LC, Gale EA. The prenatal environment and type 1 diabetes. *Diabetologia* (2013) 56:1888–97. doi:10.1007/s00125-013-2929-6
16. Ferreira RC, Guo H, Coulson RM, Smyth DJ, Pekalski ML, Burren OS, et al. A type I interferon transcriptional signature precedes autoimmunity in children genetically at-risk of type 1 diabetes. *Diabetes* (2014) 63(7):2538–50. doi:10.2337/db13-1777
17. Kallionpaa H, Elo LL, Laajala E, Mykkanen J, Ricano-Ponce I, Vaarma M, et al. Innate immune activity is detected prior to seroconversion in children with HLA-conferred type 1 diabetes susceptibility. *Diabetes* (2014) 63(7):2402–14. doi:10.2337/db13-1775
18. Foulis AK, Farquharson MA, Meager A. Immunoreactive alpha-interferon in insulin-secreting beta cells in type 1 diabetes mellitus. *Lancet* (1987) 2:1423–7. doi:10.1016/S0140-6736(87)91128-7
19. Huang X, Yuang J, Goddard A, Foulis A, James RF, Lernmark A, et al. Interferon expression in the pancreases of patients with type I diabetes. *Diabetes* (1995) 44:658–64. doi:10.2337/diabetes.44.6.658
20. Bottazzo GF, Dean BM, McNally JM, MacKay EH, Swift PG, Gamble DR. In situ characterization of autoimmune phenomena and expression of HLA molecules in the pancreas in diabetic insulitis. *N Engl J Med* (1985) 313:353–60. doi:10.1056/NEJM198508083130604
21. Pujol-Borrell R, Todd I, Doshi M, Gray D, Feldmann M, Bottazzo GF. Differential expression and regulation of MHC products in the endocrine and exocrine cells of the human pancreas. *Clin Exp Immunol* (1986) 65:128–39.
22. Todd JA. Etiology of type 1 diabetes. *Immunity* (2010) 32:457–67. doi:10.1016/j.immuni.2010.04.001
23. Uonaga T, Yoshida K, Harada T, Shimodahira M, Nakamura Y. Case of type 1 diabetes mellitus following interferon beta-1a treatment for multiple sclerosis. *Intern Med* (2012) 51:1875–7. doi:10.2169/internalmedicine.51.7609
24. Nakamura K, Kawasaki E, Imagawa A, Awata T, Ikegami H, Uchigata Y, et al. Type 1 diabetes and interferon therapy: a nationwide survey in Japan. *Diabetes Care* (2011) 34:2084–9. doi:10.2337/dc10-2274
25. Oka R, Hiroi N, Shigemitsu R, Sue M, Oshima Y, Yoshida-Hiroi M. Type 1 diabetes mellitus associated with pegylated interferon-alpha plus Ribavirin treatment for chronic hepatitis C: case report and literature review. *Clin Med Insights Endocrinol Diabetes* (2011) 4:39–45. doi:10.4137/CMED.S7815
26. Kado S, Miyamoto J, Komatsu N, Iwaki Y, Ozaki H, Taguchi H, et al. Type 1 diabetes mellitus caused by treatment with interferon-beta. *Intern Med* (2000) 39:146–9. doi:10.2169/internalmedicine.39.146
27. Fabris P, Betterle C, Greggio NA, Zanchetta R, Bosi E, Biasin MR, et al. Insulin-dependent diabetes mellitus during alpha-interferon therapy for chronic viral hepatitis. *J Hepatol* (1998) 28:514–7. doi:10.1016/S0168-8278(98)80328-0
28. Shiba T, Morino Y, Tagawa K, Fujino H, Unuma T. Onset of diabetes with high titer anti-GAD antibody after IFN therapy for chronic hepatitis. *Diabetes Res Clin Pract* (1995) 30:237–41. doi:10.1016/0168-8227(95)01188-9
29. Guerci AP, Guerci B, Levy-Marchal C, Ongagna J, Ziegler O,Candiloros H, et al. Onset of insulin-dependent diabetes mellitus after interferon-alfa therapy for hairy cell leukaemia. *Lancet* (1994) 343:1167–8. doi:10.1016/S0140-6736(94)90276-3
30. Fabris P, Betterle C, Floreani A, Greggio NA, de Lazzari F, Naccarato R, et al. Development of type 1 diabetes mellitus during interferon alfa therapy for chronic HCV hepatitis. *Lancet* (1992) 340:548. doi:10.1016/0140-6736(92)91744-S
31. Carrero JA, Calderon B, Towfic F, Artyomov MN, Unanue ER. Defining the transcriptional and cellular landscape of type 1 diabetes in the NOD mouse. *PLoS One* (2013) 8:e59701. doi:10.1371/journal.pone.0059701
32. Santin I, Moore F, Grieco FA, Marchetti P, Brancolini C, Eizirik DL. USP18 is a key regulator of the interferon-driven gene network modulating pancreatic beta cell inflammation and apoptosis. *Cell Death Dis* (2012) 3:e419. doi:10.1038/cddis.2012.158
33. Nakanishi K, Saitoh S. Clinical and genetic characteristics of patients with type 1 diabetes associated with interferon therapy. *Diabetes Care* (2011) 34:471–3. doi:10.2337/dc10-1237
34. Pelegrin M, Devedjian JC, Costa C, Visa J, Solanes G, Pujol A, et al. Evidence from transgenic mice that interferon-beta may be involved in the onset of diabetes mellitus. *J Biol Chem* (1998) 273:12332–40. doi:10.1074/jbc.273.20.12332
35. Stewart TA, Hultgren B, Huang X, Pitts-Meek S, Hully J, MacLachlan NJ. Induction of type I diabetes by interferon-alpha in transgenic mice. *Science* (1993) 260:1942–6. doi:10.1126/science.8100367
36. Li Q, Xu B, Michie SA, Rubins KH, Schreriber RD, McDevitt HO. Interferon-alpha initiates type 1 diabetes in nonobese diabetic mice. *Proc Natl Acad Sci U S A* (2008) 105:12439–44. doi:10.1073/pnas.0806439105
37. Bradfield JP, Qu HQ, Wang K, Zhang H, Sleiman PM, Kim CE, et al. A genome-wide meta-analysis of six type 1 diabetes cohorts identifies multiple associated loci. *PLoS Genet* (2011) 7:e1002293. doi:10.1371/journal.pgen.1002293
38. Pociot F. Lernmark Å: genetic risk factors for type 1 diabetes. *Lancet* (2016) 387:2331–9. doi:10.1016/S0140-6736(16)30582-7
39. Clayton DG. Prediction and interaction in complex disease genetics: experience in type 1 diabetes. *PLoS Genet* (2009) 5:e1000540. doi:10.1371/journal.pgen.1000540
40. Erlich H, Valdes AM, Noble J, Carlson JA, Varney M, Concannon P, et al. HLA DR-DQ haplotypes and genotypes and type 1 diabetes risk: analysis of the type 1 diabetes genetics consortium families. *Diabetes* (2008) 57:1084–92. doi:10.2337/db07-1331

41. Sheehy MJ, Scharf SJ, Rowe JR, Neme de Gimenez MH, Meske LM, Erlich HA, et al. A diabetes-susceptible HLA haplotype is best defined by a combination of HLA-DR and -DQ alleles. *J Clin Invest* (1989) 83:830–5. doi:10.1172/JCI113965
42. Ettinger RA, Kwok WW. A peptide binding motif for HLA-DQA1*0102/DQB1*0602, the class II MHC molecule associated with dominant protection in insulin-dependent diabetes mellitus. *J Immunol* (1998) 160:2365–73.
43. Ettinger RA, Papadopoulos GK, Moustakas AK, Nepom GT, Kwok WW. Allelic variation in key peptide-binding pockets discriminates between closely related diabetes-protective and diabetes-susceptible HLA-DQB1*06 alleles. *J Immunol* (2006) 176:1988–98. doi:10.4049/jimmunol.176.3.1988
44. Todd JA, Bell JI, McDevitt HO. HLA-DQ beta gene contributes to susceptibility and resistance to insulin-dependent diabetes mellitus. *Nature* (1987) 329:599–604. doi:10.1038/329599a0
45. Horn GT, Bugawan TL, Long CM, Erlich HA. Allelic sequence variation of the HLA-DQ loci: relationship to serology and to insulin-dependent diabetes susceptibility. *Proc Natl Acad Sci U S A* (1988) 85:6012–6. doi:10.1073/pnas.85.16.6012
46. Corper AL, Stratmann T, Apostolopoulos V, Scott CA, Garcia KC, Kang AS, et al. A structural framework for deciphering the link between I-Ag7 and autoimmune diabetes. *Science* (2000) 288:505–11. doi:10.1126/science.288.5465.505
47. Noble JA, Johnson J, Lane JA, Valdes AM. HLA class II genotyping of African American type 1 diabetic patients reveals associations unique to African haplotypes. *Diabetes* (2013) 62:3292–9. doi:10.2337/db13-0094
48. Noble JA, Valdes AM, Bugawan TL, Apple RJ, Thomson G, Erlich HA. The HLA class I A locus affects susceptibility to type 1 diabetes. *Hum Immunol* (2002) 63:657–64. doi:10.1016/S0198-8859(02)00421-4
49. Nakanishi K, Kobayashi T, Murase T, Nakatsuji T, Inoko H, Tsuji K, et al. Association of HLA-A24 with complete beta-cell destruction in IDDM. *Diabetes* (1993) 42:1086–93. doi:10.2337/diab.42.7.1086
50. Valdes AM, Erlich HA, Noble JA. Human leukocyte antigen class I B and C loci contribute to type 1 diabetes (T1D) susceptibility and age at T1D onset. *Hum Immunol* (2005) 66:301–13. doi:10.1016/j.humimm.2004.12.001
51. Concannon P, Chen WM, Julier C, Morahan G, Akolkar B, Erlich HA, et al. Genome-wide scan for linkage to type 1 diabetes in 2,496 multiplex families from the type 1 diabetes genetics consortium. *Diabetes* (2009) 58:1018–22. doi:10.2337/db08-1551
52. Bell GI, Horita S, Karam JH. A polymorphic locus near the human insulin gene is associated with insulin-dependent diabetes mellitus. *Diabetes* (1984) 33:176–83. doi:10.2337/diabetes.33.2.176
53. Bennett ST, Lucassen AM, Gough SC, Powell EE, Undlien DE, Pritchard LE, et al. Susceptibility to human type 1 diabetes at IDDM2 is determined by tandem repeat variation at the insulin gene minisatellite locus. *Nat Genet* (1995) 9:284–92. doi:10.1038/ng0395-284
54. Kennedy GC, German MS, Rutter WJ. The minisatellite in the diabetes susceptibility locus IDDM2 regulates insulin transcription. *Nat Genet* (1995) 9:293–8. doi:10.1038/ng0395-293
55. Pugliese A, Zeller M, Fernandez A, Zalcberg LJ, Bartlett RJ, Ricordi C, et al. The insulin gene is transcribed in the human thymus and transcription levels correlated with allelic variation at the INS VNTR-IDDM2 susceptibility locus for type 1 diabetes. *Nat Genet* (1997) 15:293–7. doi:10.1038/ng0397-293
56. Cai CQ, Zhang T, Breslin MB, Giraud M, Lan MS. Both polymorphic variable number of tandem repeats and autoimmune regulator modulate differential expression of insulin in human thymic epithelial cells. *Diabetes* (2011) 60:336–44. doi:10.2337/db10-0255
57. Bottini N, Musumeci L, Alonso A, Rahmouni S, Nika K, Rostamkhani M, et al. A functional variant of lymphoid tyrosine phosphatase is associated with type I diabetes. *Nat Genet* (2004) 36:337–8. doi:10.1038/ng1323
58. Vang T, Congia M, Macis MD, Musumeci L, Orrú V, Zavattari P, et al. Autoimmune-associated lymphoid tyrosine phosphatase is a gain-of-function variant. *Nat Genet* (2005) 37:1317–9. doi:10.1038/ng1673
59. Zhang J, Zahir N, Jiang Q, Miliotis H, Heyraud S, Meng X, et al. The autoimmune disease-associated PTPN22 variant promotes calpain-mediated Lyp/Pep degradation associated with lymphocyte and dendritic cell hyperresponsiveness. *Nat Genet* (2011) 43:902–7. doi:10.1038/ng.904
60. Wang Y, Shaked I, Stanford SM, Zhou W, Curtsinger JM, Mikulski Z, et al. The autoimmunity-associated gene PTPN22 potentiates toll-like receptor-driven, type 1 interferon-dependent immunity. *Immunity* (2013) 39:111–22. doi:10.1016/j.immuni.2013.06.013
61. Bottini N, Peterson EJ. Tyrosine phosphatase PTPN22: multifunctional regulator of immune signaling, development, and disease. *Annu Rev Immunol* (2014) 32:83–119. doi:10.1146/annurev-immunol-032713-120249
62. Smyth DJ, Cooper JD, Bailey R, Field S, Burren O, Smink LJ, et al. A genome-wide association study of nonsynonymous SNPs identifies a type 1 diabetes locus in the interferon-induced helicase (IFIH1) region. *Nat Genet* (2006) 38:617–9. doi:10.1038/ng1800
63. Wallace C, Smyth DJ, Maisuria-Armer M, Walker NM, Todd JA,Clayton DG. The imprinted DLK1-MEG3 gene region on chromosome 14q32.2 alters susceptibility to type 1 diabetes. *Nat Genet* (2010) 42:68–71. doi:10.1038/ng.493
64. Martínez A, Varadé J, Márquez A, Cénit MC, Espino L, Perdigones N, et al. Association of the STAT4 gene with increased susceptibility for some immune-mediated diseases. *Arthritis Rheum* (2008) 58:2598–602. doi:10.1002/art.23792
65. Richter MF, Duménil G, Uzé G, Fellous M, Pellegrini S. Specific contribution of Tyk2 JH regions to the binding and the expression of the interferon alpha/beta receptor component IFNAR1. *J Biol Chem* (1998) 273:24723–9. doi:10.1074/jbc.273.38.24723
66. Ragimbeau J, Dondi E, Alcover A, Eid P, Uzé G, Pellegrini S. The tyrosine kinase Tyk2 controls IFNAR1 cell surface expression. *EMBO J* (2003) 22:537–47. doi:10.1093/emboj/cdg038
67. Marroqui L, Dos Santos RS, Fløyel T, Grieco FA, Santin I, Op de Beeck A, et al. TYK2, a candidate gene for type 1 diabetes, modulates apoptosis and the innate immune response in human pancreatic β-cells. *Diabetes* (2015) 64:3808–17. doi:10.2337/db15-0362
68. Holz A, Bot A, Coon B, Wolfe T, Grusby MJ, von Herrath MG. Disruption of the STAT4 signaling pathway protects from autoimmune diabetes while retaining antiviral immune competence. *J Immunol* (1999) 163:5374–82.
69. Yang Z, Chen M, Ellett JD, Fialkow LB, Carter JD, McDuffie M, et al. Autoimmune diabetes is blocked in Stat4-deficient mice. *J Autoimmun* (2004) 22:191–200. doi:10.1016/j.jaut.2003.08.006
70. Kariuki SN, Kirou KA, MacDermott EJ, Barillas-Arias L, Crow MK, Niewold TB. Cutting edge: autoimmune disease risk variant of STAT4 confers increased sensitivity to IFN-alpha in lupus patients in vivo. *J Immunol* (2009) 182:34–8. doi:10.4049/jimmunol.182.1.34
71. Funabiki M, Kato H, Miyachi Y, Toki H, Motegi H, Inoue M, et al. Autoimmune disorders associated with gain of function of the intracellular sensor MDA5. *Immunity* (2014) 40:199–212. doi:10.1016/j.immuni.2013.12.014
72. Looney BM, Xia CQ, Concannon P, Ostrov DA, Clare-Salzler MJ. Effects of type 1 diabetes-associated IFIH1 polymorphisms on MDA5 function and expression. *Curr Diab Rep* (2015) 15:96. doi:10.1007/s11892-015-0656-8
73. Domsgen E, Lind K, Kong L, Hühn MH, Rasool O, van Kuppeveld F, et al. Flodström-Tullberg M: An IFIH1 gene polymorphism associated with risk for autoimmunity regulates canonical antiviral defence pathways in Coxsackievirus infected human pancreatic islets. *Sci Rep* (2016) 6:39378. doi:10.1038/srep39378
74. Nicholls DG. The pancreatic β-cell: a bioenergetic perspective. *Physiol Rev* (2016) 96:1385–447. doi:10.1152/physrev.00009.2016
75. Sosenko JM, Palmer JP, Greenbaum CJ, Mahon J, Cowie C, Krischer JP, et al. Increasing the accuracy of oral glucose tolerance testing and extending its application to individuals with normal glucose tolerance for the prediction of type 1 diabetes: the diabetes prevention trial-type 1. *Diabetes Care* (2007) 30:38–42. doi:10.2337/dc06-1615
76. Sosenko JM, Palmer JP, Rafkin-Mervis L, Krischer JP, Cuthbertson D, Matheson D, et al. Glucose and C-peptide changes in the perionset period of type 1 diabetes in the diabetes prevention trial-type 1. *Diabetes Care* (2008) 31:2188–92. doi:10.2337/dc08-0935
77. Xu P, Wu Y, Zhu Y, Dagne G, Johnson G, Cuthbertson D, et al. Prognostic performance of metabolic indexes in predicting onset of type 1 diabetes. *Diabetes Care* (2010) 33:2508–13. doi:10.2337/dc10-0802
78. Richardson SJ, Rodriguez-Calvo T, Gerling IC, Mathews CE, Kaddis JS, Russell MA, et al. Islet cell hyperexpression of HLA class I antigens: a defining feature in type 1 diabetes. *Diabetologia* (2016) 59:2448–58. doi:10.1007/s00125-016-4067-4
79. Eizirik DL, Sammeth M, Bouckenooghe T, Bottu G, Sisino G, Igoillo-Esteve M, et al. The human pancreatic islet transcriptome: expression of

candidate genes for type 1 diabetes and the impact of pro-inflammatory cytokines. *PLoS Genet* (2012) 8:e1002552. doi:10.1371/journal.pgen.1002552
80. Eisenbarth G. Autoimmune beta cell insufficiency: diabetes mellitus type 1. *Triangle* (1984) 23:111–23.
81. Eisenbarth GS. Type I diabetes mellitus. A chronic autoimmune disease. *N Engl J Med* (1986) 314:1360–8. doi:10.1056/NEJM198605223142106
82. Gepts W. Pathologic anatomy of the pancreas in juvenile diabetes mellitus. *Diabetes* (1965) 14:619–33. doi:10.2337/diab.14.10.619
83. Hänninen A, Jalkanen S, Salmi M, Toikkanen S, Nikolakaros G, Simell O. Macrophages, T cell receptor usage, and endothelial cell activation in the pancreas at the onset of insulin-dependent diabetes mellitus. *J Clin Invest* (1992) 90:1901–10. doi:10.1172/JCI116067
84. In't Veld P. Insulitis in human type 1 diabetes: the quest for an elusive lesion. *Islets* (2011) 3:131–8. doi:10.4161/isl.3.4.15728
85. Gale EA. The discovery of type 1 diabetes. *Diabetes* (2001) 50:217–26. doi:10.2337/diabetes.50.2.217
86. Gepts W, De Mey J. Islet cell survival determined by morphology. An immunocytochemical study of the islets of Langerhans in juvenile diabetes mellitus. *Diabetes* (1978) 27(Suppl 1):251–61. doi:10.2337/diab.27.1.S251
87. Foulis AK, Liddle CN, Farquharson MA, Richmond JA, Weir RS. The histopathology of the pancreas in type 1 (insulin-dependent) diabetes mellitus: a 25-year review of deaths in patients under 20 years of age in the United Kingdom. *Diabetologia* (1986) 29:267–74. doi:10.1007/BF00452061
88. Campbell-Thompson M, Fu A, Kaddis JS, Wasserfall C, Schatz DA, Pugliese A, et al. Insulitis and β-cell mass in the natural history of type 1 diabetes. *Diabetes* (2016) 65:719–31. doi:10.2337/db15-0779
89. Campbell-Thompson M. Organ donor specimens: what can they tell us about type 1 diabetes? *Pediatr Diabetes* (2015) 16:320–30. doi:10.1111/pedi.12286
90. Campbell-Thompson M, Wasserfall C, Kaddis J, Albanese-O'Neill A, Staeva T, Nierras C, et al. Network for Pancreatic Organ Donors with Diabetes (nPOD): developing a tissue biobank for type 1 diabetes. *Diabetes Metab Res Rev* (2012) 28:608–17. doi:10.1002/dmrr.2316
91. Pugliese A, Yang M, Kusmarteva I, Heiple T, Vendrame F, Wasserfall C, et al. The juvenile diabetes research foundation Network for Pancreatic Organ Donors with Diabetes (nPOD) program: goals, operational model and emerging findings. *Pediatr Diabetes* (2014) 15:1–9. doi:10.1111/pedi.12097
92. Kaddis JS, Pugliese A, Atkinson MA. A run on the biobank: what have we learned about type 1 diabetes from the nPOD tissue repository? *Curr Opin Endocrinol Diabetes Obes* (2015) 22:290–5. doi:10.1097/MED.0000000000000171
93. Campbell-Thompson ML, Atkinson MA, Butler AE, Chapman NM, Frisk G, Gianani R, et al. The diagnosis of insulitis in human type 1 diabetes. *Diabetologia* (2013) 56:2541–3. doi:10.1007/s00125-013-3043-5
94. In't Veld P, Lievens D, De Grijse J, Ling Z, Van der Auwera B, Pipeleers-Marichal M, et al. Screening for insulitis in adult autoantibody-positive organ donors. *Diabetes* (2007) 56:2400–4. doi:10.2337/db07-0416
95. Zheng S, Mathews CE. Metabolic abnormalities in the pathogenesis of type 1 diabetes. *Curr Diab Rep* (2014) 14:519. doi:10.1007/s11892-014-0519-8
96. Graham KL, Sutherland RM, Mannering SI, Zhao Y, Chee J, Krishnamurthy B, et al. Pathogenic mechanisms in type 1 diabetes: the islet is both target and driver of disease. *Rev Diabet Stud* (2012) 9:148–68. doi:10.1900/RDS.2012.9.148
97. Barry M, Bleackley RC. Cytotoxic T lymphocytes: all roads lead to death. *Nat Rev Immunol* (2002) 2:401–9. doi:10.1038/nri819
98. Fooksman DR, Vardhana S, Vasiliver-Shamis G, Liese J, Blair DA, Waite J, et al. Functional anatomy of T cell activation and synapse formation. *Annu Rev Immunol* (2010) 28:79–105. doi:10.1146/annurev-immunol-030409-101308
99. Campbell PD, Estella E, Dudek NL, Jhala G, Thomas HE, Kay TW, et al. Cytotoxic T-lymphocyte-mediated killing of human pancreatic islet cells in vitro. *Hum Immunol* (2008) 69:543–51. doi:10.1016/j.humimm.2008.06.008
100. Schloot NC, Willemen S, Duinkerken G, de Vries RR, Roep BO. Cloned T cells from a recent onset IDDM patient reactive with insulin B-chain. *J Autoimmun* (1998) 11:169–75. doi:10.1006/jaut.1997.0183
101. Abreu JR, Martina S, Verrijn Stuart AA, Fillié YE, Franken KL, Drijfhout JW, et al. CD8 T cell autoreactivity to preproinsulin epitopes with very low human leucocyte antigen class I binding affinity. *Clin Exp Immunol* (2012) 170:57–65. doi:10.1111/j.1365-2249.2012.04635.x
102. Unger WW, Velthuis J, Abreu JR, Laban S, Quinten E, Kester MG, et al. Discovery of low-affinity preproinsulin epitopes and detection of autoreactive CD8 T-cells using combinatorial MHC multimers. *J Autoimmun* (2011) 37:151–9. doi:10.1016/j.jaut.2011.05.012
103. Pinkse GG, Tysma OH, Bergen CA, Kester MG, Ossendorp F, van Veelen PA, et al. Autoreactive CD8 T cells associated with beta cell destruction in type 1 diabetes. *Proc Natl Acad Sci U S A* (2005) 102:18425–30. doi:10.1073/pnas.0508621102
104. Wong FS, Visintin I, Wen L, Flavell RA, Janeway CA. CD8 T cell clones from young nonobese diabetic (NOD) islets can transfer rapid onset of diabetes in NOD mice in the absence of CD4 cells. *J Exp Med* (1996) 183:67–76. doi:10.1084/jem.183.1.67
105. DiLorenzo TP, Graser RT, Ono T, Christianson GJ, Chapman HD, Roopenian DC, et al. Major histocompatibility complex class I-restricted T cells are required for all but the end stages of diabetes development in nonobese diabetic mice and use a prevalent T cell receptor alpha chain gene rearrangement. *Proc Natl Acad Sci U S A* (1998) 95:12538–43. doi:10.1073/pnas.95.21.12538
106. Graham KL, Krishnamurthy B, Fynch S, Mollah ZU, Slattery R, Santamaria P, et al. Autoreactive cytotoxic T lymphocytes acquire higher expression of cytotoxic effector markers in the islets of NOD mice after priming in pancreatic lymph nodes. *Am J Pathol* (2011) 178:2716–25. doi:10.1016/j.ajpath.2011.02.015
107. Chee J, Ko HJ, Skowera A, Jhala G, Catterall T, Graham KL, et al. Effector-memory T cells develop in islets and report islet pathology in type 1 diabetes. *J Immunol* (2014) 192:572–80. doi:10.4049/jimmunol.1302100
108. Graham KL, Krishnamurthy B, Fynch S, Ayala-Perez R, Slattery RM, Santamaria P, et al. Intra-islet proliferation of cytotoxic T lymphocytes contributes to insulitis progression. *Eur J Immunol* (2012) 42:1717–22. doi:10.1002/eji.201242435
109. Marroqui L, Dos Santos RS, Op de Beeck A, Coomans de Brachène A, Marselli L, Marchetti P, et al. Interferon-α mediates human beta cell HLA class I overexpression, endoplasmic reticulum stress and apoptosis, three hallmarks of early human type 1 diabetes. *Diabetologia* (2017) 60:656–67. doi:10.1007/s00125-016-4201-3
110. Lombardi A, Tomer Y. Interferon alpha impairs insulin production in human beta cells via endoplasmic reticulum stress. *J Autoimmun* (2017) 80:48–55. doi:10.1016/j.jaut.2017.02.002
111. Isaacs A, Lindenmann J. Pillars article: virus interference. I. The interferon. Proc R Soc Lond B Biol Sci. 1957. 147: 258–267. *J Immunol* (2015) 195:1911–20.
112. Isaacs A, Lindenmann J, Valentine RC. Pillars article: virus interference. II. Some properties of interferon. Proc R Soc Lond B Biol Sci. 1957. 147: 268–273. *J Immunol* (2015) 195:1921–8.
113. Pestka S. The interferons: 50 years after their discovery, there is much more to learn. *J Biol Chem* (2007) 282:20047–51. doi:10.1074/jbc.R700004200
114. Pestka S, Krause CD, Walter MR. Interferons, interferon-like cytokines, and their receptors. *Immunol Rev* (2004) 202:8–32. doi:10.1111/j.0105-2896.2004.00204.x
115. Di Domizio J, Cao W. Fueling autoimmunity: type I interferon in autoimmune diseases. *Expert Rev Clin Immunol* (2013) 9:201–10. doi:10.1586/eci.12.106
116. Niewold TB. Type I interferon in human autoimmunity. *Front Immunol* (2014) 5:306. doi:10.3389/fimmu.2014.00306
117. Platanias LC. Mechanisms of type-I- and type-II-interferon-mediated signalling. *Nat Rev Immunol* (2005) 5:375–86. doi:10.1038/nri1604
118. Kotenko SV, Gallagher G, Baurin VV, Lewis-Antes A, Shen M, Shah NK, et al. IFN-lambdas mediate antiviral protection through a distinct class II cytokine receptor complex. *Nat Immunol* (2003) 4:69–77. doi:10.1038/ni875
119. Sheppard P, Kindsvogel W, Xu W, Henderson K, Schlutsmeyer S, Whitmore TE, et al. IL-28, IL-29 and their class II cytokine receptor IL-28R. *Nat Immunol* (2003) 4:63–8. doi:10.1038/ni873
120. Egli A, Santer DM, O'Shea D, Tyrrell DL, Houghton M. The impact of the interferon-lambda family on the innate and adaptive immune response to viral infections. *Emerg Microbes Infect* (2014) 3:e51. doi:10.1038/emi.2014.51
121. O'Brien TR, Prokunina-Olsson L, Donnelly RP. IFN-λ4: the paradoxical new member of the interferon lambda family. *J Interferon Cytokine Res* (2014) 34:829–38. doi:10.1089/jir.2013.0136
122. Jaitin DA, Roisman LC, Jaks E, Gavutis M, Piehler J, Van der Heyden J, et al. Inquiring into the differential action of interferons (IFNs): an IFN-alpha2 mutant with enhanced affinity to IFNAR1 is functionally similar to IFN-beta. *Mol Cell Biol* (2006) 26:1888–97. doi:10.1128/MCB.26.5.1888-1897.2006

123. Kalie E, Jaitin DA, Podoplelova Y, Piehler J, Schreiber G. The stability of the ternary interferon-receptor complex rather than the affinity to the individual subunits dictates differential biological activities. *J Biol Chem* (2008) 283:32925–36. doi:10.1074/jbc.M806019200
124. Moraga I, Harari D, Schreiber G, Uzé G, Pellegrini S. Receptor density is key to the alpha2/beta interferon differential activities. *Mol Cell Biol* (2009) 29:4778–87. doi:10.1128/MCB.01808-08
125. Thomas C, Moraga I, Levin D, Krutzik PO, Podoplelova Y, Trejo A, et al. Structural linkage between ligand discrimination and receptor activation by type I interferons. *Cell* (2011) 146:621–32. doi:10.1016/j.cell.2011.06.048
126. de Weerd NA, Samarajiwa SA, Hertzog PJ. Type I interferon receptors: biochemistry and biological functions. *J Biol Chem* (2007) 282:20053–7. doi:10.1074/jbc.R700006200
127. de Weerd NA, Nguyen T. The interferons and their receptors – distribution and regulation. *Immunol Cell Biol* (2012) 90:483–91. doi:10.1038/icb.2012.9
128. de Weerd NA, Vivian JP, Nguyen TK, Mangan NE, Gould JA, Braniff SJ, et al. Structural basis of a unique interferon-beta signaling axis mediated via the receptor IFNAR1. *Nat Immunol* (2013) 14:901–7. doi:10.1038/ni.2667
129. Piehler J, Thomas C, Garcia KC, Schreiber G. Structural and dynamic determinants of type I interferon receptor assembly and their functional interpretation. *Immunol Rev* (2012) 250:317–34. doi:10.1111/imr.12001
130. Ng CT, Mendoza JL, Garcia KC, Oldstone MB. Alpha and beta type 1 interferon signaling: passage for diverse biologic outcomes. *Cell* (2016) 164:349–52. doi:10.1016/j.cell.2015.12.027
131. Gonzalez-Navajas JM, Lee J, David M, Raz E. Immunomodulatory functions of type I interferons. *Nat Rev Immunol* (2012) 12:125–35. doi:10.1038/nri3133
132. Welsh RM, Bahl K, Marshall HD, Urban SL. Type 1 interferons and antiviral CD8 T-cell responses. *PLoS Pathog* (2012) 8:e1002352. doi:10.1371/journal.ppat.1002352
133. Ivashkiv LB, Donlin LT. Regulation of type I interferon responses. *Nat Rev Immunol* (2014) 14:36–49. doi:10.1038/nri3581
134. McNab F, Mayer-Barber K, Sher A, Wack A, O'Garra A. Type I interferons in infectious disease. *Nat Rev Immunol* (2015) 15:87–103. doi:10.1038/nri3787
135. Honda K, Taniguchi T. IRFs: master regulators of signalling by toll-like receptors and cytosolic pattern-recognition receptors. *Nat Rev Immunol* (2006) 6:644–58. doi:10.1038/nri1900
136. Tamura T, Yanai H, Savitsky D, Taniguchi T. The IRF family transcription factors in immunity and oncogenesis. *Annu Rev Immunol* (2008) 26:535–84. doi:10.1146/annurev.immunol.26.021607.090400
137. Theofilopoulos AN, Baccala R, Beutler B, Kono DH. Type I interferons (alpha/beta) in immunity and autoimmunity. *Annu Rev Immunol* (2005) 23:307–36. doi:10.1146/annurev.immunol.23.021704.115843
138. Crouse J, Kalinke U, Oxenius A. Regulation of antiviral T cell responses by type I interferons. *Nat Rev Immunol* (2015) 15:231–42. doi:10.1038/nri3806
139. Stark GR, Darnell JE. The JAK-STAT pathway at twenty. *Immunity* (2012) 36:503–14. doi:10.1016/j.immuni.2012.03.013
140. Wang WB, Levy DE, Lee CK. STAT3 negatively regulates type I IFN-mediated antiviral response. *J Immunol* (2011) 187:2578–85. doi:10.4049/jimmunol.1004128
141. Murray PJ. The JAK-STAT signaling pathway: input and output integration. *J Immunol* (2007) 178:2623–9. doi:10.4049/jimmunol.178.5.2623
142. Ho HH, Ivashkiv LB. Role of STAT3 in type I interferon responses. Negative regulation of STAT1-dependent inflammatory gene activation. *J Biol Chem* (2006) 281:14111–8. doi:10.1074/jbc.M511797200
143. Kallal LE, Biron CA. Changing partners at the dance: variations in STAT concentrations for shaping cytokine function and immune responses to viral infections. *JAKSTAT* (2013) 2:e23504. doi:10.4161/jkst.23504
144. Gil MP, Ploquin MJY, Watford WT, Lee SH, Kim K, Wang X, et al. Regulating type 1 IFN effects in CD8 T cells during viral infections: changing STAT4 and STAT1 expression for function. *Blood* (2012) 120:3718–28. doi:10.1182/blood-2012-05-428672
145. Nguyen KB, Watford WT, Salomon R, Hofmann SR, Pien GC, Morinobu A, et al. Critical role for STAT4 activation by type 1 interferons in the interferon-gamma response to viral infection. *Science* (2002) 297:2063–6. doi:10.1126/science.1074900
146. Schneider WM, Chevillotte MD, Rice CM. Interferon-stimulated genes: a complex web of host defenses. *Annu Rev Immunol* (2014) 32:513–45. doi:10.1146/annurev-immunol-032713-120231
147. Zitvogel L, Galluzzi L, Kepp O, Smyth MJ, Kroemer G. Type I interferons in anticancer immunity. *Nat Rev Immunol* (2015) 15:405–14. doi:10.1038/nri3845
148. Tough DF. Modulation of T-cell function by type I interferon. *Immunol Cell Biol* (2012) 90:492–7. doi:10.1038/icb.2012.7
149. Santini SM, Lapenta C, Logozzi M, Parlato S, Spada M, Di Pucchio T, et al. Type I interferon as a powerful adjuvant for monocyte-derived dendritic cell development and activity in vitro and in Hu-PBL-SCID mice. *J Exp Med* (2000) 191:1777–88. doi:10.1084/jem.191.10.1777
150. Paquette RL, Hsu NC, Kiertscher SM, Park AN, Tran L, Roth MD, et al. Interferon-alpha and granulocyte-macrophage colony-stimulating factor differentiate peripheral blood monocytes into potent antigen-presenting cells. *J Leukoc Biol* (1998) 64:358–67.
151. Lee PK, Chang CJ, Lin CM. Lipopolysaccharide preferentially induces 4-1BB ligand expression on human monocyte-derived dendritic cells. *Immunol Lett* (2003) 90:215–21. doi:10.1016/j.imlet.2003.08.002
152. Rouzaut A, Garasa S, Teijeira A, González I, Martinez-Forero I, Suarez N, et al. Dendritic cells adhere to and transmigrate across lymphatic endothelium in response to IFN-α. *Eur J Immunol* (2010) 40:3054–63. doi:10.1002/eji.201040523
153. Padovan E, Spagnoli GC, Ferrantini M, Heberer M. IFN-alpha2a induces IP-10/CXCL10 and MIG/CXCL9 production in monocyte-derived dendritic cells and enhances their capacity to attract and stimulate CD8+ effector T cells. *J Leukoc Biol* (2002) 71:669–76.
154. Parlato S, Santini SM, Lapenta C, Di Pucchio T, Logozzi M, Spada M, et al. Expression of CCR-7, MIP-3beta, and Th-1 chemokines in type I IFN-induced monocyte-derived dendritic cells: importance for the rapid acquisition of potent migratory and functional activities. *Blood* (2001) 98:3022–9. doi:10.1182/blood.V98.10.3022
155. Wolf E, Spencer KM, Cudworth AG. The genetic susceptibility to type 1 (insulin-dependent) diabetes: analysis of the HLA-DR association. *Diabetologia* (1983) 24:224–30. doi:10.1007/BF00282704
156. Hanafusa T, Pujol-Borrell R, Chiovato L, Russell RC, Doniach D, Bottazzo GF. Aberrant expression of HLA-DR antigen on thyrocytes in Graves' disease: relevance for autoimmunity. *Lancet* (1983) 2:1111–5. doi:10.1016/S0140-6736(83)90628-1
157. Pujol-Borrell R, Hanafusa T, Chiovato L, Bottazzo GF. Lectin-induced expression of DR antigen on human cultured follicular thyroid cells. *Nature* (1983) 304:71–3. doi:10.1038/304071a0
158. Unanue ER. Antigen-presenting function of the macrophage. *Annu Rev Immunol* (1984) 2:395–428. doi:10.1146/annurev.iy.02.040184.002143
159. Foulis AK, Farquharson MA, Hardman R. Aberrant expression of class II major histocompatibility complex molecules by B cells and hyperexpression of class I major histocompatibility complex molecules by insulin containing islets in type 1 (insulin-dependent) diabetes mellitus. *Diabetologia* (1987) 30:333–43. doi:10.1007/BF00299027
160. Richardson SJ, Willcox A, Bone AJ, Morgan NG, Foulis AK. Immunopathology of the human pancreas in type-I diabetes. *Semin Immunopathol* (2011) 33:9–21. doi:10.1007/s00281-010-0205-0
161. Foulis AK. The pathology of the endocrine pancreas in type 1 (insulin-dependent) diabetes mellitus. *APMIS* (1996) 104:161–7. doi:10.1111/j.1699-0463.1996.tb00702.x
162. Rodriguez-Calvo T, Suwandi JS, Amirian N, Zapardiel-Gonzalo J, Anquetil F, Sabouri S, et al. Heterogeneity and lobularity of pancreatic pathology in type 1 diabetes during the prediabetic phase. *J Histochem Cytochem* (2015) 63:626–36. doi:10.1369/0022155415576543
163. Ziegler AG, Rewers M, Simell O, Simell T, Lempainen J, Steck A, et al. Seroconversion to multiple islet autoantibodies and risk of progression to diabetes in children. *JAMA* (2013) 309:2473–9. doi:10.1001/jama.2013.6285
164. Chehadeh W, Weill J, Vantyghem MC, Alm G, Lefèbvre J, Wattré P, et al. Increased level of interferon-alpha in blood of patients with insulin-dependent diabetes mellitus: relationship with coxsackievirus B infection. *J Infect Dis* (2000) 181:1929–39. doi:10.1086/315516
165. Xia CQ, Peng R, Chernatynskaya AV, Yuan L, Carter C, Valentine J, et al. Increased IFN-alpha-producing plasmacytoid dendritic cells (pDCs) in human Th1-mediated type 1 diabetes: pDCs augment Th1 responses

through IFN-alpha production. *J Immunol* (2014) 193:1024–34. doi:10.4049/jimmunol.1303230

166. Taylor JL, Grossberg SE. Recent progress in interferon research: molecular mechanisms of regulation, action, and virus circumvention. *Virus Res* (1990) 15:1–25. doi:10.1016/0168-1702(90)90010-9
167. Wills RJ. Clinical pharmacokinetics of interferons. *Clin Pharmacokinet* (1990) 19:390–9. doi:10.2165/00003088-199019050-00003
168. Bonnevie-Nielsen V, Larsen ML, Frifelt JJ, Michelsen B, Lernmark A. Association of IDDM and attenuated response of 2',5'-oligoadenylate synthetase to yellow fever vaccine. *Diabetes* (1989) 38:1636–42. doi:10.2337/diabetes.38.12.1636
169. Toms GC, Baker P, Boucher BJ. The production of immunoreactive alpha- and gamma-interferon by circulating mononuclear cells in type 1 diabetes. *Diabet Med* (1991) 8:547–50. doi:10.1111/j.1464-5491.1991.tb01649.x
170. Fabris P, Floreani A, Tositti G, Vergani D, De Lalla F, Betterle C. Type 1 diabetes mellitus in patients with chronic hepatitis C before and after interferon therapy. *Aliment Pharmacol Ther* (2003) 18:549–58. doi:10.1046/j.1365-2036.2003.01681.x
171. Tai TY, Lu JY, Chen CL, Lai MY, Chen PJ, Kao JH, et al. Interferon-alpha reduces insulin resistance and beta-cell secretion in responders among patients with chronic hepatitis B and C. *J Endocrinol* (2003) 178:457–65. doi:10.1677/joe.0.1780457
172. Nemesanszky E, Pusztay M, Csepregi A. Effects of interferon treatment on the glucose metabolism of patients with chronic hepatitis C. *Eur J Intern Med* (2000) 11:151–5. doi:10.1016/S0953-6205(00)00080-7
173. Nakhooda AF, Like AA, Chappel CI, Murray FT, Marliss EB. The spontaneously diabetic Wistar rat. Metabolic and morphologic studies. *Diabetes* (1977) 26:100–12. doi:10.2337/diabetes.26.2.100
174. Colle E, Guttmann RD, Seemayer T. Spontaneous diabetes mellitus syndrome in the rat. I. Association with the major histocompatibility complex. *J Exp Med* (1981) 154:1237–42. doi:10.1084/jem.154.4.1237
175. Ewel CH, Sobel DO, Zeligs BJ, Bellanti JA. Poly I:C accelerates development of diabetes mellitus in diabetes-prone BB rat. *Diabetes* (1992) 41:1016–21. doi:10.2337/diabetes.41.8.1016
176. Sobel DO, Ewel CH, Zeligs B, Abbassi V, Rossio J, Bellanti JA. Poly I:C induction of alpha-interferon in the diabetes-prone BB and normal Wistar rats. Dose-response relationships. *Diabetes* (1994) 43:518–22. doi:10.2337/diab.43.4.518
177. Huang X, Hultgren B, Dybdal N, Stewart TA. Islet expression of interferon-alpha precedes diabetes in both the BB rat and streptozotocin-treated mice. *Immunity* (1994) 1:469–78. doi:10.1016/1074-7613(94)90089-2
178. Makino S, Kunimoto K, Muraoka Y, Mizushima Y, Katagiri K, Tochino Y. Breeding of a non-obese, diabetic strain of mice. *Jikken Dobutsu* (1980) 29:1–13.
179. O'Brien BA, Geng X, Orteu CH, Huang Y, Ghoreishi M, Zhang Y, et al. A deficiency in the in vivo clearance of apoptotic cells is a feature of the NOD mouse. *J Autoimmun* (2006) 26:104–15. doi:10.1016/j.jaut.2005.11.006
180. Swiecki M, Colonna M. The multifaceted biology of plasmacytoid dendritic cells. *Nat Rev Immunol* (2015) 15:471–85. doi:10.1038/nri3865
181. Lincez PJ, Shanina I, Horwitz MS. Reduced expression of the MDA5 Gene IFIH1 prevents autoimmune diabetes. *Diabetes* (2015) 64:2184–93. doi:10.2337/db14-1223
182. Lee AS, Ghoreishi M, Cheng WK, Chang TY, Zhang YQ, Dutz JP. Toll-like receptor 7 stimulation promotes autoimmune diabetes in the NOD mouse. *Diabetologia* (2011) 54:1407–16. doi:10.1007/s00125-011-2083-y
183. Zhang Y, Lee AS, Shameli A, Geng X, Finegood D, Santamaria P, et al. TLR9 blockade inhibits activation of diabetogenic CD8+ T cells and delays autoimmune diabetes. *J Immunol* (2010) 184:5645–53. doi:10.4049/jimmunol.0901814
184. Li Q, McDevitt HO. The role of interferon alpha in initiation of type I diabetes in the NOD mouse. *Clin Immunol* (2011) 140:3–7. doi:10.1016/j.clim.2011.04.010
185. Quah HS, Miranda-Hernandez S, Khoo A, Harding A, Fynch S, Elkerbout L, et al. Deficiency in type I interferon signaling prevents the early interferon-induced gene signature in pancreatic islets but not type 1 diabetes in NOD mice. *Diabetes* (2014) 63:1032–40. doi:10.2337/db13-1210
186. Mordes JP, Guberski DL, Leif JH, Woda BA, Flanagan JF, Greiner DL, et al. LEW.1WR1 rats develop autoimmune diabetes spontaneously and in response to environmental perturbation. *Diabetes* (2005) 54:2727–33. doi:10.2337/diabetes.54.9.2727
187. Qaisar N, Lin S, Ryan G, Yang C, Oikemus SR, Brodsky MH, et al. A critical role for the type I interferon receptor in virus-induced autoimmune diabetes in rats. *Diabetes* (2017) 66:145–57. doi:10.2337/db16-0462
188. Vassileva G, Chen SC, Zeng M, Abbondanzo S, Jensen K, Gorman D, et al. Expression of a novel murine type I IFN in the pancreatic islets induces diabetes in mice. *J Immunol* (2003) 170:5748–55. doi:10.4049/jimmunol.170.11.5748
189. Alba A, Puertas MC, Carrillo J, Planas R, Ampudia R, Pastor X, et al. IFN beta accelerates autoimmune type 1 diabetes in nonobese diabetic mice and breaks the tolerance to beta cells in nondiabetes-prone mice. *J Immunol* (2004) 173:6667–75. doi:10.4049/jimmunol.173.11.6667
190. Somoza N, Vargas F, Roura-Mir C, Vives-Pi M, Fernandez-Figueras MT, Ariza A, et al. Pancreas in recent onset insulin-dependent diabetes mellitus. Changes in HLA, adhesion molecules and autoantigens, restricted T cell receptor V beta usage, and cytokine profile. *J Immunol* (1994) 153:1360–77.
191. Roep BO, Kleijwegt FS, van Halteren AG, Bonato V, Boggi U, Vendrame F, et al. Islet inflammation and CXCL10 in recent-onset type 1 diabetes. *Clin Exp Immunol* (2010) 159:338–43. doi:10.1111/j.1365-2249.2009.04087.x
192. Uno S, Imagawa A, Saisho K, Okita K, Iwahashi H, Hanafusa T, et al. Expression of chemokines, CXC chemokine ligand 10 (CXCL10) and CXCR3 in the inflamed islets of patients with recent-onset autoimmune type 1 diabetes. *Endocr J* (2010) 57:991–6. doi:10.1507/endocrj.K10E-076
193. Newby B, Annamali M, Brusko T, Gerling I, Mathews C. *Type 1 Interferons Create a Virulent Islet Microenvironment*. San Diego, CA: American Diabetes Association (ADA) 77th Scientific Sessions (2017).
194. Freudenburg W, Gautam M, Chakraborty P, James J, Richards J, Salvatori AS, et al. Reduction in ATP levels triggers immunoproteasome activation by the 11S (PA28) regulator during early antiviral response mediated by IFNbeta in mouse pancreatic beta-cells. *PLoS One* (2013) 8:e52408. doi:10.1371/journal.pone.0052408
195. Seifert U, Bialy LP, Ebstein F, Bech-Otschir D, Voigt A, Schröter F, et al. Immunoproteasomes preserve protein homeostasis upon interferon-induced oxidative stress. *Cell* (2010) 142:613–24. doi:10.1016/j.cell.2010.07.036
196. Neefjes J, Jongsma ML, Paul P, Bakke O. Towards a systems understanding of MHC class I and MHC class II antigen presentation. *Nat Rev Immunol* (2011) 11:823–36. doi:10.1038/nri3084
197. Eizirik DL, Cardozo AK, Cnop M. The role for endoplasmic reticulum stress in diabetes mellitus. *Endocr Rev* (2008) 29:42–61. doi:10.1210/er.2007-0015
198. Eizirik DL, Miani M, Cardozo AK. Signalling danger: endoplasmic reticulum stress and the unfolded protein response in pancreatic islet inflammation. *Diabetologia* (2013) 56:234–41. doi:10.1007/s00125-012-2762-3
199. Granados DP, Tanguay PL, Hardy MP, Caron E, de Verteuil D, Meloche S, et al. ER stress affects processing of MHC class I-associated peptides. *BMC Immunol* (2009) 10:10. doi:10.1186/1471-2172-10-10
200. Ulianich L, Terrazzano G, Annunziatella M, Ruggiero G, Beguinot F, Di Jeso B. ER stress impairs MHC class I surface expression and increases susceptibility of thyroid cells to NK-mediated cytotoxicity. *Biochim Biophys Acta* (2011) 1812:431–8. doi:10.1016/j.bbadis.2010.12.013
201. de Almeida SF, Fleming JV, Azevedo JE, Carmo-Fonseca M, de Sousa M. Stimulation of an unfolded protein response impairs MHC class I expression. *J Immunol* (2007) 178:3612–9. doi:10.4049/jimmunol.178.6.3612
202. Zanone MM, Favaro E, Camussi G. From endothelial to beta cells: insights into pancreatic islet microendothelium. *Curr Diabetes Rev* (2008) 4:1–9. doi:10.2174/157339908783502415
203. Itoh N, Hanafusa T, Miyazaki A, Miyagawa J, Yamagata K, Yamamoto K, et al. Mononuclear cell infiltration and its relation to the expression of major histocompatibility complex antigens and adhesion molecules in pancreas biopsy specimens from newly diagnosed insulin-dependent diabetes mellitus patients. *J Clin Invest* (1993) 92:2313–22. doi:10.1172/JCI116835
204. Chakrabarti D, Huang X, Beck J, Henrich J, McFarland N, James RF, et al. Control of islet intercellular adhesion molecule-1 expression by interferon-alpha and hypoxia. *Diabetes* (1996) 45:1336–43. doi:10.2337/diab.45.10.1336
205. Savinov AY, Wong FS, Stonebraker AC, Chervonsky AV. Presentation of antigen by endothelial cells and chemoattraction are required for homing of insulin-specific CD8+ T cells. *J Exp Med* (2003) 197:643–56. doi:10.1084/jem.20021378

206. Zanone MM, Favaro E, Ferioli E, Huang GC, Klein NJ, Perin PC, et al. Human pancreatic islet endothelial cells express coxsackievirus and adenovirus receptor and are activated by coxsackie B virus infection. *FASEB J* (2007) 21:3308–17. doi:10.1096/fj.06-7905com
207. Hogan MF, Hull RL. The islet endothelial cell: a novel contributor to beta cell secretory dysfunction in diabetes. *Diabetologia* (2017) 60:952–9. doi:10.1007/s00125-017-4272-9
208. Longhi MP, Trumpfheller C, Idoyaga J, Caskey M, Matos I, Kluger C, et al. Dendritic cells require a systemic type I interferon response to mature and induce CD4+ Th1 immunity with poly IC as adjuvant. *J Exp Med* (2009) 206:1589–602. doi:10.1084/jem.20090247
209. Pantel A, Teixeira A, Haddad E, Wood EG, Steinman RM, Longhi MP. Direct type I IFN but not MDA5/TLR3 activation of dendritic cells is required for maturation and metabolic shift to glycolysis after poly IC stimulation. *PLoS Biol* (2014) 12:e1001759. doi:10.1371/journal.pbio.1001759

3

Characterization of Human CD4 T Cells Specific for a C-Peptide/C-Peptide Hybrid Insulin Peptide

*Timothy A. Wiles[1], Anita Hohenstein[1,2], Laurie G. Landry[3], Mylinh Dang[1], Roger Powell[1], Perrin Guyer[4], Eddie A. James[4], Maki Nakayama[2,3], Kathryn Haskins[2], Thomas Delong[1] and Rocky L. Baker[2]**

[1] Department of Pharmaceutical Sciences, University of Colorado Skaggs School of Pharmacy and Pharmaceutical Sciences, Aurora, CO, United States, [2] Department of Immunology and Microbiology, University of Colorado School of Medicine, Aurora, CO, United States, [3] Barbara Davis Center for Childhood Diabetes, University of Colorado School of Medicine, Aurora, CO, United States, [4] Department of Translational Research, Benaroya Research Institute at Virginia Mason, Seattle, WA, United States

***Correspondence:**
Rocky L. Baker
Rocky.Baker@cuanschutz.edu*

Hybrid Insulin Peptides (HIPs), which consist of insulin fragments fused to other peptides from β-cell secretory granule proteins, are CD4 T cell autoantigens in type 1 diabetes (T1D). We have studied HIPs and HIP-reactive CD4 T cells extensively in the context of the non-obese diabetic (NOD) mouse model of autoimmune diabetes and have shown that CD4 T cells specific for HIPs are major contributors to disease pathogenesis. Additionally, in the human context, HIP-reactive CD4 T cells can be found in the islets and peripheral blood of T1D patients. Here, we performed an in-depth characterization of the CD4 T cell response to a C-peptide/C-peptide HIP (HIP11) in human T1D. We identified the TCR expressed by the previously-reported HIP11-reactive CD4 T cell clone E2, which was isolated from the peripheral blood of a T1D patient, and determined that it recognizes HIP11 in the context of HLA-DQ2. We also identified a HIP11-specific TCR directly in the islets of a T1D donor and demonstrated that this TCR recognizes a different minimal epitope of HIP11 presented by HLA-DQ8. We generated and tested an HLA-DQ2 tetramer loaded with HIP11 that will enable direct *ex vivo* interrogation of CD4 T cell responses to HIP11 in human patients and control subjects. Using mass spectrometric analysis, we confirmed that HIP11 is present in human islets. This work represents an important step in characterizing the role of CD4 T cell responses to HIPs in human T1D.

Keywords: CD4, hybrid insulin peptides, autoimmunity, mass spectrometry, type 1 diabetes, neoepitope, tetramer

INTRODUCTION

Type 1 diabetes (T1D) is an autoimmune disease driven by T cells specific for pancreatic β-cell autoantigens. Identifying β-cell antigens targeted by autoreactive T cells is an important step in understanding the etiopathogenesis of T1D. Post-translational modification of proteins can generate neo-epitopes in the periphery that are not represented in the thymus, providing a mechanism by which autoreactive T cells can evade central tolerance mechanisms and mediate β-cell destruction in the pancreatic islets. Hybrid Insulin Peptide (HIP) formation is a recently discovered modification that may play a key role in the generation of primary targets of autoimmunity in T1D (1). HIPs are formed by covalent fusion of the N-terminus of β-cell secretory granule peptides (a right peptide) to the C-terminus of truncated insulin peptides (a left peptide) through a peptide bond. The resulting HIPs contain amino acid sequences not encoded by the genome, making them plausible targets for autoreactive T cells in T1D. We have identified HIPs in murine and human islets by mass spectrometry (1, 2), and a separate group recently demonstrated that HIPs can be found in the major histocompatibility complex (MHC) class II peptidome of mice (3).

In contrast to conventional post-translational modifications, such as phosphorylation or deamidation, which alter the side chain of a single amino acid residue, HIP formation leads to the replacement of an entire sequence of amino acids within insulin. This could have marked consequences for how a HIP, when compared to the unmodified precursor, binds to a given human leukocyte antigen (HLA) molecule and interacts with a specific T cell receptor (TCR). This, in turn, could result in recognition of a HIP in the periphery by T cells that did not recognize the corresponding unmodified peptides in the thymus during negative selection.

The role of HIPs as autoantigens in the non-obese diabetic (NOD) mouse model of T1D is clearly established. We have demonstrated that HIPs are the peptide ligands of diabetogenic CD4 T cell clones isolated from NOD mice (1). HIP-specific CD4 T cells display an inflammatory phenotype and can be detected in the pancreatic lymph nodes (pLN), islets, and spleen of prediabetic and diabetic NOD mice using MHC class II tetramers (4). The frequency of HIP-specific CD4 T cells in the blood of NOD mice increases with age, as do the percentages of HIP-specific CD4 T cells that display an activated phenotype, suggesting that these cells may serve as biomarkers of disease progression (4).

Evidence supporting an important role for HIPs as autoantigens in human T1D is also mounting. Multiple CD4 T cell clones/lines specific for different HIPs have been isolated from the residual islets of human organ donors with T1D (1, 5–7). As recently reported, we screened peripheral blood mononuclear cells (PBMCs) from T1D patients or controls for reactivity to a panel of HIPs by IFN-γ enzyme-linked immunosorbent spot (ELISpot) analysis (6). We observed statistically significant responses from patient PBMC to four of the HIPs tested. One of those HIPs (HIP11) is a hybrid peptide formed by the fusion of a C-peptide fragment with the N-terminus of C-peptide. Robust responses to HIP11 were detected in samples from more than 20% of the 35 patients tested (6). Here, using the CD4 T cell clone E2 isolated from the PBMCs of a new onset T1D patient (6), we describe the further characterization of the CD4 T cell response to HIP11, advancing our understanding of HIPs as autoantigens in T1D and providing a foundation for future efforts to investigate responses to HIPs during the development of T1D.

MATERIALS AND METHODS

Peptides

The list of peptides used in this study were obtained commercially at >95% chromatographic purity and are listed in **Supplementary Table 1**.

HIP Nomenclature

To avoid ambiguity and confusion, we developed a systematic nomenclature to describe the large diversity of potential HIP sequences. HIPs are identified using standard abbreviations for the proteins from which the left and right peptides originated (*e.g.*, Ins, IAPP, CgA), separated by a dash. Next to each abbreviation, a subscript is used to describe the residues from the parent protein that span the sequence. For easy reference, insulin peptides are designated as "insA", "insB", or "insC", indicating that the peptide originated from the A-chain, B-chain, or C-peptide region of insulin, respectively, and numbering is based on the position of the residues within the specific peptide. For peptides from all other proteins, residues are numbered based on their position in the pre-proprotein, with position 1 being the N-terminal residue of the signal peptide. For example, the HIP sequences DLQVGQVELGGGPGA GSLQPLAL-EAE and SLQPLAL–EAEDLQV (hyphen indicates the HIP junction) referenced in this study are designated $insC_{4-26}$ – $insC_{1-3}$ and $insC_{20-26}$ – $insC_{1-7}$, respectively.

The defining feature of any individual HIP is its junction region. Trimming of a HIP – as may occur within an antigen-presenting cell, the proteasome, or with a protease used during sample preparation prior to LC-MS/MS analysis – could lead to the generation of peptides of different lengths that all represent the same HIP (*i.e.*, they contain the same junction). Common names can be used to refer to a specific HIP junction. For example, the HIP generated when an insulin C-peptide fragment ending with residue 26 is fused to the N-terminus of C-peptide ($insC_{x-26}$ – $insC_{1-x}$) has been designated HIP11 (1). Both $insC_{4-26}$ – $insC_{1-3}$ and $insC_{20-26}$ – $insC_{1-7}$ are considered HIP11 peptides.

Sequencing and Generation of E2a and E2b Transductants

TCRα and TCRβ chain genes were amplified by 5'RACE-PCR, followed by sequencing on an MiSEQ sequencer (Illumina) as previously described (6). V- and J-gene usages as well as CDR3 sequences were then analyzed by IMGT/V-QUEST (http://www.imgt.org). The determined TCRα and TCRβ chain genes were expressed on a 5KC hybridoma cell line transduced with the NFAT-ZsGreen-1 reporter construct using a retroviral expression system as previously described (8). Briefly, a murine stem cell virus-based retroviral vector encoding TCRα and TCRβ chain genes connected by a porcine-2A peptide was generated, and the reporter 5KC cell line was spinfected with a virus supernatant, followed by MACS-based enrichment of transduced cells using magnetic beads conjugated with anti-CD3 antibody. The E2a and E2b transductants (2 x 10^4 cells/well) were cultured with or without peptides along with K562 cells expressing DQ2 (DQA1*05:01-DQB1*02:01) or DR3 (DRA1*01:01-DRB1*03:01) at 5 x 10^4 cells/well in a round-bottom 96 well plate overnight, followed by evaluating ZsGreen-1 expression by the TCR transductants on a Cytoflex flow-cytometer (Beckman Coulter).

GSE.8E3 Transductant Activation Assay

GSE.8E3 transductant cells (2 x 10^4 cells/well), produced by the same method used to generate the E2a and E2b transductants, were cultured with various concentrations of peptides in the presence of K562 cells expressing DQ8 (DQA1*03:01-DQB1*03:02) or DQ8*trans* (DQA1*05:01-DQB1*03:02) at 5 x 10^4 cells/well in a round-bottom 96 well plate overnight. ZsGreen-1 expression by the TCR transductants was analyzed on a Cytoflex flow-cytometer (Beckman Coulter).

T Cell Clone Assays

Early-passage CD4 T cell clones (E2, a HIP11-reactive clone and B11b, a HIP4-reactive clone) were thawed and restimulated with HIP11 or HIP4, respectively, in the presence of irradiated autologous EBV-transformed B-cell line as antigen-presenting cells (APC). Twenty-four hours later, IL-2 and IL-4 were added to the T cell cultures for T cell expansion. T cells were maintained in culture for 14-28 days before functional assays were performed. For T cell assays, CD4 T cell clones (0.5 – 5 x 10^5) were incubated either with the irradiated autologous EBV-transformed B-cell line (0.5 – 5 x 10^5 cells) or with irradiated PBMC from a partially HLA matched donor, in the presence or absence of antigen at indicated concentrations. For IFN-γ and TNF-α ELISA, supernatants were collected 24-48 hours after culture and analyzed using a kit from eBiosciences according to manufacturer's protocol. To determine the DR- or DQ-HLA restriction of HIP responses, the antigen assay was performed in the presence and absence of anti-DR (L243) or anti-DQ (SPV-L3) antibodies. The EBV-transformed cell lines were first pulsed with peptide (50 μg/ml) and washed twice with AIM V medium. Antibodies were added at a final concentration of 1 μg/ml.

Flow Cytometry

For the CD25 upregulation assay, 1 x 10^5 CD4 T cells were cultured with an autologous EBV-transformed B cell line (1 x 10^5 cells) in the presence or absence of peptide. After 24 hours, cells were harvested, washed, and stained for CD4, CD25 and viability (efluor780, Invitrogen) before analysis. Antibodies used for staining of T cells were anti-CD4 BV711 (SK3; BD Biosciences) and anti-CD25 BV421 (M-A251; BD Biosciences). Gating strategies are indicated in each figure; the lymphocyte gate was based on FSC/SSC properties and the singlets gate was based on the FSC-A/FSC-H. Samples were run on a BD Fortessa X-20 flow cytometer (5 lasers), a Cytek Aurora (5 lasers) or a CytoFlex (Beckton Dickinson) flow cytometer (3 lasers), and 5,000 – 50,000 cells were acquired for analysis. Data were analyzed using FlowJo v10 software (Tree Star, USA).

Preparation of Islet Proteins

Islets from a non-diabetic human donor (64 year-old male) were obtained from the University of Alberta Diabetes Institute Islet Core (Edmonton, Alberta, Canada). Upon arrival, islets were washed with phosphate-buffered saline (PBS) and then pelleted. The supernatant was removed and tubes were placed in liquid nitrogen to rapidly freeze the islet pellets. Islets were stored at -80°C until use. Islets were processed as described previously (2). Briefly, islets were thawed and lysed in 50% trifluoroethanol with heat and sonication, and cellular debris was pelleted by high-speed centrifugation. The supernatant, which contained extracted islet proteins, was fractionated by size exclusion chromatography (SEC). SEC fractions were then digested overnight at 37°C with the endoproteinase AspN (cleaves at the N-terminal side of aspartic acid residues) in buffer supplemented with zinc sulfate. Digested samples were dried in a vacuum concentrator and then reconstituted in loading buffer (2.7% acetonitrile/0.1% formic acid/water), sonicated, and spun at 17,000 x g for 2 minutes to remove any insoluble material. The supernatant was then analyzed by liquid chromatography tandem-mass spectrometry (LC-MS/MS).

LC-MS/MS Analysis of Human Islet Proteins

Samples were analyzed by LC-MS/MS using an Agilent 1200 series UHPLC system with a nanoflow adapter and an Agilent 6550 Q-TOF equipped with a nano-ESI source. Samples were separated online by reversed-phase liquid chromatography using a trap forward-elute configuration (trap column: Thermo Acclaim Pepmap 100, 75 μm x 2 cm, 3 μm particles, 100Å pores; analytical column: Thermo Acclaim Pepmap RSLC C18 analytical column, 75 μm inner diameter, 2 μm particles, 100Å pores). A water/acetonitrile gradient was used (buffer A: 0.1% formic acid in water; buffer B: 0.1% formic acid and 90% acetonitrile in water). Mass spectrometric data was collected in positive ion mode with an MS scan range of 290-1700 m/z, an MS acquisition rate of 5 spectra/sec, an MS/MS scan range of 50-1700 m/z, and a minimum MS/MS scan rate of 3 spectra/sec. Abundance dependent accumulation was enabled with a target of 80,000 counts/spectrum. Using auto-MS/MS mode, the ten most abundant precursors per cycle were selected for fragmentation (absolute threshold: 3000 counts; relative threshold: 0.01%). Singly-charged precursors were excluded.

Analysis of Mass Spectrometric Data

Data were searched using the Spectrum Mill MS Proteomics Workbench (Agilent, Rev B.06.00.201) and the SwissProt human proteome database. For data extraction, spectrum merging was enabled based on precursor selection purity, spectral similarity, retention time (2-minute window), and m/z. Search settings were as follows: instrument = Agilent ESI Q-TOF; precursor mass tolerance = +/- 10 ppm; product ion mass tolerance = +/- 20 ppm; digest = no enzyme. Matches were considered valid if the following thresholds were satisfied: score > 10, percentage scored peak intensity (SPI) > 70%, and rank 1 minus rank 2 (R1-R2) score > 2.5. Spectra that could not be confidently matched to unmodified peptides in the SwissProt database were subjected to a second round of searches using the settings listed above, except oxidized methionine and deamidated asparagine/glutamine were considered as variable modifications and digest was set to AspN (maximum of two missed cleavages). Spectra that remained unmatched according to the validation filters listed above were searched against a custom database containing hypothetical human HIPs (2) using the same settings as in the first search.

Validation of HIP11 Identification Using Synthetic Peptide and the P-VIS Approach

The HIP11 peptide-spectrum match (PSM) was first evaluated by applying our previously-published criteria (2). A synthetic version of the HIP11 peptide (GenScript, >95% pure) was then used to validate the match by applying the novel PSM Validation with Internal Standards (P-VIS) approach recently developed by our group (9). In bottom-up proteomics, proteins from a biological spectrum are digested using a protease such as trypsin. The resultant peptides are analyzed by LC-MS/MS to generate fragmentation spectra. These spectra are then used to search a protein database, generating a large number of PSMs. Traditionally, to confirm that the correct sequence interpretation has been assigned to a particular fragmentation spectrum, the fragmentation spectrum of a synthetic version of the candidate sequence is compared to the fragmentation spectrum of the biological peptide in question using a metric such as the Pearson correlation coefficient. Since two spectra for the same peptide will not be entirely identical, the investigator decides subjectively if the similarity is high enough to indicate that the synthetic peptide and the biological peptide are the same. In the P-VIS approach (9), a set of internal standard peptides is spiked into both the biological sample and the synthetic peptide sample prior to LC-MS/MS analysis. For each internal standard peptide, the fragmentation spectra from the two samples are compared and the Pearson correlation coefficient is calculated. This information is used to determine a prediction interval for the Pearson correlation coefficient of a correct match. A similar process is used to determine if the chromatographic retention time of the biological peptide and synthetic peptide are close enough to indicate that the peptides are the same. PROCAL peptides (JPT Peptide Technologies) were used as internal standard peptides (10). LC-MS/MS analysis was performed as described above, except precursor selection was limited to those masses predicted for the peptides of interest. PSM_validator v1.4 (https://github.com/Delong-Lab/PSM_validator/releases) was used for data analysis with the following settings applied: pre_mz_tol = 20, pro_mz_tol = 20, abund_thresh = 500, PCC_abund_thresh = 10, min_score = 30, min_weighted_score = 25, min_pairs_PCC = 8, min _PCC = 0.7, RTtol = 0.6, min_RT = 10, max_RT = 90, manual_RTdev_thresh = 0, min_intstd = 10, percentile_thresh = 5, ion_type = "b/y".

RESULTS

Response to HIP11 by the E2 CD4 T Cell Clone Is DQ2-Restricted

The HIP11-reactive CD4 T cell clone E2 was isolated from the peripheral blood of a patient with T1D (patient 3196) and in a previous study, we determined that the E2 response to HIP11 was restricted to HLA-DQ (6). We further confirmed these findings using thymidine incorporation as a read-out for T cell proliferation (**Figure 1A**). Since patient 3196 carries one copy of the DQ2 haplotype (DQA1*05:01-DQB1*02:01) and one copy of the DQA1*03:02-DQB1*03:03 haplotype, our goal was to determine the presenting HLA element. Using donor PBMCs partially matched for each haplotype as APCs, we tested the ability of the two haplotypes to stimulate the E2 CD4 T cell clone to HIP11. The E2 T cell clone proliferated when stimulated with the HIP11 peptide $insC_{20-26}$ – $insC_{1-7}$ (SLQPLAL–EAEDLQV) presented by PBMCs homozygous for DQ2, but not when presented by PBMCs homozygous for DQA1*03:02-DQB1*03:03 (**Figure 1B**). As an additional control, we determined that mis-matched PBMCs homozygous for DQ8 (DQA2*0301-DQB2*0302) did not stimulate the E2 T cell clone either at the 1 μM or the 10 μM concentration. To provide additional evidence of the presenting element, we used an artificial antigen-presenting line (K562) devoid of any HLA molecules and transduced with DQ2 or HLA-DRB1*03:01 (DR3) as a negative control (8). Each K562 line (expressing either DQ2 or DR3) was pulsed with the HIP11 peptide and cultured with the E2 T cell clone (**Figure 1C**). After 18h, upregulation of CD25 was assessed by flow cytometry as a measure of T cell activation. The E2 CD4 T cell clone upregulated CD25 in response to HIP11 only when the K562 line was transduced with DQ2, but not DR3, confirming our previous observation that the E2 T cell clone is stimulated by HIP11 in the context of DQ2.

Identification of TCR Responsible for Recognition of HIP11 by the E2 Clone

TCR sequencing of the E2 CD4 T cell clone revealed that two different TCRα chains – along with a single TCRβ chain – were expressed at the RNA level (6). It has been shown that dual TCRα-expressing T cells can contribute to autoimmunity through different processes, including escape of central tolerance (11) and failure to generate thymically-derived Tregs reactive to self-antigens (12). To determine which TCRα was responsible for the recognition of HIP11, each TCRα chain was expressed individually in combination with the cognate TCRβ chain in a TCR-deficient hybridoma (5KC) engineered with a ZsGreen-1 fluorescent protein gene, under the NFAT promotor (8). Under these conditions, the TCR transductants express ZsGreen-1 when the TCR is engaged with the peptide-MHC complex, enabling monitoring of T cell activation by flow cytometry. The resulting transductants, E2a and E2b (expressing either TRAV6 or TRAV8-2/8-4 respectively), were then challenged with HIP11-pusled artificial APCs (K562 line expressing DQ2). The E2b – but not the E2a – transductant recognized HIP11 in the context of DQ2 (**Figure 1D**), demonstrating that the combination of the TRAV8-2/8-4 TCRα chain with the TRBV5-4 TCRβ chain is responsible for recognizing HIP11.

Characterization of a HIP11-Specific TCR From the Islets of a T1D Donor

We previously isolated T cell clones and lines from the residual islets of human T1D donors recognizing four different HIPs containing a sequence from the C-peptide linked to insulin A-chain, Islet Amyloid Polypeptide, or Neuropeptide Y (1, 5). Although the E2 clone, which was isolated from the peripheral blood of a T1D patient, is specific for HIP11, isolating a HIP11-reactive T cell clone from the islets – the actual site of autoimmune destruction – would further establish the relevance of HIP11 as an autoantigen in human T1D. Michels et al. previously generated transductants expressing TCRs identified by direct TCR sequencing of islet-infiltrating T cells

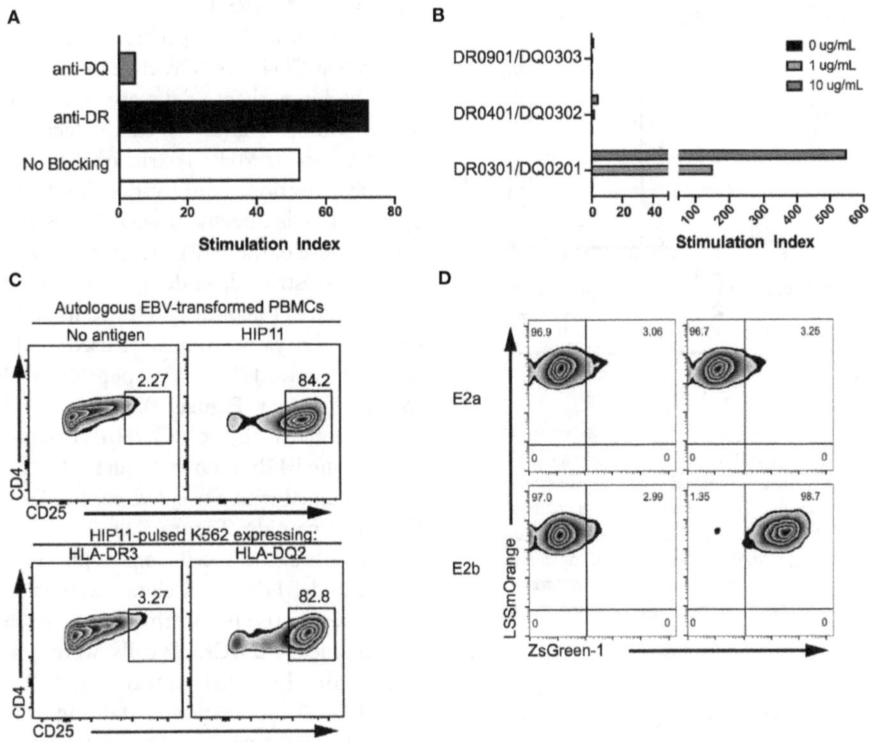

FIGURE 1 | The E2 TCR consisting of the TRAV8-2/8-4 TCRα chain and the TRBV5-4 TCRβ chain recognizes HIP11 in the context of DQ2. **(A)** Peptide-specific proliferation of the E2 T cell clone was assessed using cells from an autologous EBV transformed B cell line as antigen presenting cells and pulsing with 10 µg/mL of the cognate HIP11 peptide in the presence or absence of anti-DR (black bar) or anti-DQ (grey bar) blocking antibody. **(B)** HLA restriction was further defined using cells from partially HLA-matched third-party donors as antigen presenting cells. Irradiated PBMC from each third party donor were pulsed with the cognate HIP11 peptide at concentrations of 0, 1, and 10 µg/mL. Substantial proliferation was observed only in response to the DQA1*05:01-DQB1*02:01 (HLA-DQ2) positive antigen presenting cells, indicating a DQA1*05:01-DQB1*02:01-restricted response. All data are represented as stimulation index (SI) values, calculated by normalizing the proliferation of the T cell clone based on [3H] thymidine incorporation of un-stimulated wells. **(C)** To confirm DQ2 restriction, the E2 T cell clone was cultured in the presence of either an autologous B cell line or K562 lines expressing DR3 or DQ2. After 18h, cells were harvested and stained for CD4 and CD25, and CD25 expression was monitored by flow cytometry. Data is representative of 3 independent experiments. **(D)** Two TCR alpha sequences and one beta sequence were identified from the E2 clone. Each TCR alpha/beta combination, E2a and E2b, was expressed in 5KC T-hybridoma cells with an NFAT-reporter. ZsGreen-1 is expressed upon T cell activation. The E2a and E2b TCR transductants were cultured with the HIP-11 peptide in the presence of K562 cells expressing DQ2 followed by evaluation of ZsGreen-1 expression by flow cytometry.

in organ donors with T1D (13). Several of the CD4 T cell transductants were shown to be reactive to proinsulin peptides. The CD4 T cell transductant GSE.8E3 responded to the peptide insC$_{17-33}$ (GAGSLQPLALEGSLQKR), a region of the C-peptide prone to HIP formation (2). We previously tested reactivity of human PBMCs to eight HIPs containing that region of the C-peptide (6) and found that reactivity to two of them (HIP11 and HIP16) was increased (compared to no antigen) in T1D patients but not in control subjects (6). We hypothesized that post-translational modification of the C-peptide fragment through hybrid peptide formation would generate a more potent antigen for GSE.8E3. Eight HIPs containing the insulin C-peptide fragment insC$_{20-26}$ as the left peptide were tested for antigenicity. The GSE.8E3 transductant strongly reacted to the HIP11 peptide insC$_{20-26}$ – insC$_{1-7}$ (SLQPLAL–EAEDLQV) in the context of both DQ8 and DQ8*trans* (**Figure 2**). When DQ8 was the presenting element, GSE.8E3 did not respond to the native insulin peptide insC$_{16-31}$ (PGAGSLQPLALEGSLQ) (**Figure 3A**) except at very high concentrations (**Figure 2**). GSE.8E3 did respond to insC$_{16-31}$ when presented by DQ8-trans (**Figure 3B**). The E2 clone did not respond to native C-peptide when presented by DQ2 (**Figure 3C**).

E2 and GSE.8E3 Recognize Different Minimal Epitopes of HIP11

Although the E2 and GSE.8E3 TCRs both recognized HIP11, it was possible that they were specific for different HIP11 epitopes, particularly since recognition by these TCRs was restricted to different HLA molecules. Identifying the precise epitope recognized by each TCR could facilitate future efforts to characterize the immune response to HIP11. For example, it could enable the generation of HLA class II tetramers that allow for detection of different subsets of HIP11-reactive T cells in human subjects. To determine the minimal epitope recognized by the E2 T cell clone and the islet-derived GSE.8E3 transductant, we tested reactivity to HIP11 peptides truncated

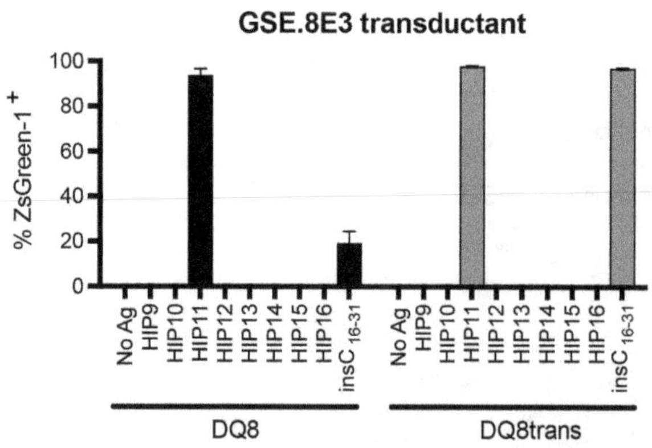

FIGURE 2 | The GSE.8E3 transductant recognizes HIP11 in the context of DQ8 and DQ8-trans. The GSE.8E3 TCR clonotype identified from a CD4 T cell in the islets of a T1D organ donor was expressed in 5KC T-hybridoma cells with an NFAT-reporter. The GSE.8E3 TCR transductant was cultured with or without various HIPs (10 μM) or a native proinsulin peptide (100 μM) in the presence of K562 cells expressing DQ8 (black bars) or DQ8-trans (gray bars). ZsGreen-1 expression was evaluated by flow cytometry. Each result is the mean for three independent experiments. Error bars indicate the standard error of the mean.

either on the N- or the C-terminus. Our data show that the response by the E2 T cell clone was completely abrogated when the glutamine on the N-terminus was missing (**Figure 4A**) and when the aspartic acid (D) on the C-terminal region was truncated (**Figure 4B**), indicating that the minimal HIP11 epitope seen by the E2 T cell clone is QPLALEAED. For the GSE.8E3 transductant, our data show that the minimal epitope presented by DQ8 is LQPLALEAE (**Figures 4A, B**). Results were similar when testing the GSE.8E3 response using DQ8*trans* as the presenting element (**Supplementary Figure 1**). Residues flanking these minimal epitopes also seem to contribute to overall activity, possibly as TCR contact residues outside of the peptide binding groove. Based on these data and published data regarding preferred binding residues for DQ2 and DQ8 (14, 15), we propose that HIP11 is presented in two different binding registers depending on whether DQ2 or DQ8 is the presenting element, as shown in **Figure 4C**.

Design and Validation of an HLA-DQ2/HIP11 Tetramer

The study of antigen-specific T cells is a high priority in T1D research as CD4 T cells reactive to islet antigens could potentially serve as biomarkers of disease progression in at-risk subjects. While ELISpot analysis can detect cytokine-secreting cells independent of MHC restriction, HLA class II tetramers allow for the detection, enumeration, and phenotyping of antigen-specific T cells directly *ex vivo* (16). Based on the discovery that the response of the HIP11-reactive CD4 T cell clone E2 to HIP11 was DQ2-restricted, we designed an HLA class II tetramer loaded with the HIP11 peptide and tested its ability to stain the E2 T cell clone. As a negative control we used the T cell clone B11b, which is reactive to HIP4, a C-peptide/A-chain hybrid peptide (**Supplementary Figure 2**). While the HIP11-reactive T cell clone stained with the DQ2/HIP11 tetramer, the HIP4-reactive T cell clone B11b did not (**Figure 5A**). Neither of the CD4 T cell clones stained with a negative control DQ2 tetramer loaded with the CLIP peptide (**Figure 5A**). To determine whether antigen stimulation of the T cell clone could improve tetramer binding, the E2 and B11b T cell clones were stimulated with HIP11 or HIP4 respectively in the presence of autologous EBV-transformed PBMCs. T cells were stained with either the HIP11 or the CLIP tetramers 8, 12 and 23 days after stimulation and tetramer staining was monitored by flow cytometry (**Figure 5A**). Our data indicate that the strongest staining is obtained within a week after stimulation. Finally, PBMCs from two DQ2+ T1D patients (with T1D onset less that 2 years) were cultured with medium only or in the presence of HIP4 or HIP11. After 10 days of culture, cells were harvested and stained with the HIP11 tetramer. A substantial population of CD4 T cells present in one of the patients stained with the HIP11/DQ2 tetramer when PBMCs were stimulated with HIP11, but not when stimulated with an irrelevant HIP (**Figure 5B**).

HIP11 Is Present in Human Islets

A critical step in confirming that HIP11 is a natural antigen in human T1D was to identify HIP11 in human islets by mass spectrometry (LC-MS/MS). Proteins were isolated from non-diabetic human donor islets and digested with the protease AspN to generate peptides suitable for mass spectrometric analysis. Resultant

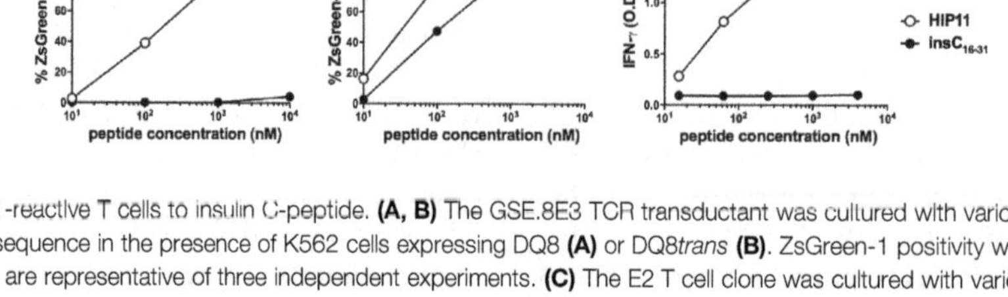

FIGURE 3 | Response of HIP11-reactive T cells to insulin C-peptide. **(A, B)** The GSE.8E3 TCR transductant was cultured with various concentrations of a HIP11 peptide or an insulin C-peptide sequence in the presence of K562 cells expressing DQ8 **(A)** or DQ8*trans* **(B)**. ZsGreen-1 positivity was assessed by flow cytometry as a measure of activation. Data are representative of three independent experiments. **(C)** The E2 T cell clone was cultured with various concentrations of a HIP11 peptide or an insulin C-peptide sequence in the presence of an autologous EBV-transformed B cell line. After 48 hours, supernatants from T cell cultures were harvested and IFN-γ concentrations were measured by ELISA. Results are representative of two independent experiments.

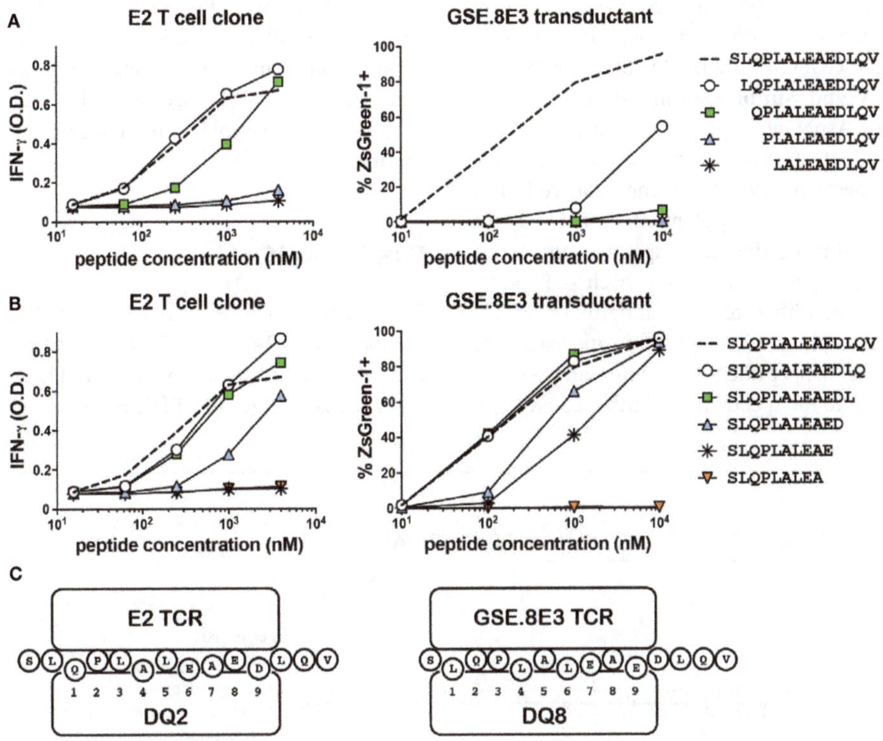

FIGURE 4 | The E2 CD4 T cell clone and the GSE.8E3 TCR transductant recognize different minimal epitopes. N-terminally **(A)** and C-terminally **(B)** truncated HIP11 peptides were tested with E2 and GSE.8E3 for antigenicity. Results are representative of three independent experiments. **(C)** Proposed binding registers for HIP11 in the context of DQ2 or DQ8 when recognized by E2 or GSE.8E3, respectively.

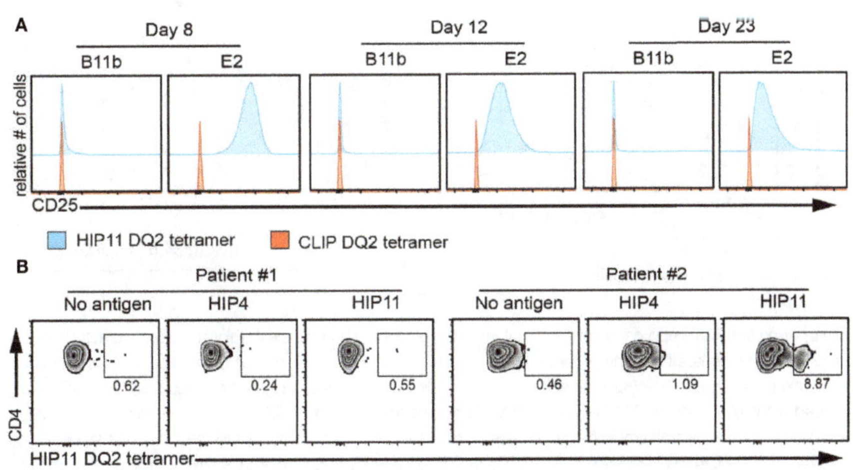

FIGURE 5 | HIP11/DQ2 tetramer stains the E2 T cell clone and PBMCs from a T1D patient. **(A)** The E2 or B11b T cell clones were stimulated with HIP11 or HIP4 respectively and an irradiated autologous EBV-transformed B cell line. T cells were then maintained in culture and harvested at 8, 12 and 23 days post-stimulation and stained with the DQ2/HIP11 tetramer (blue histograms) or DQ2/CLIP tetramer (red histograms), CD4, and a fixable viability dye. Tetramer staining was assessed by flow cytometry by gating on live, $CD4^+$ cells. Data are representative of two independent experiments. **(B)** PBMCs from two DQ2+ patients were isolated, stained with CFSE and cultured with medium only, HIP4, or HIP11. After 10 days, cells were harvested and stained with the DQ2/HIP11 tetramer, anti-CD4 and anti-CD25 antibodies, and a fixable viability dye before flow cytometry analysis. Gates were set on live, $CD4^+$ $CD25^+$ $CFSE^{low}$ events and the percentage of tetramer positive events is reported.

peptides were then analyzed by LC-MS/MS, and data were searched against a custom database to find peptides describing the HIP11 hybrid junction. Our analysis identified the peptide $insC_{4\text{-}26}$ – $insC_{1\text{-}3}$ (DLQVGQVELGGGPGAGSLQPLAL-EAE) with high confidence (**Figure 6A** and **Supplementary Table 2**). This peptide is the predicted AspN cleavage product of HIP11. We previously established a set of rigorous criteria to confidently identify HIPs by mass spectrometry (2), and the putative HIP11 match satisfied all of these criteria (**Supplementary Table 3**). To further confirm the validity of the mass spectrometry-based HIP11 identification, we applied a novel approach – Peptide-spectrum match Validation with Internal Standards (P-VIS) – recently developed by our group (9). Using this approach, the fragmentation spectrum of the peptide found in human islets was found to be highly similar to the spectrum of synthetic $insC_{4\text{-}26}$ – $insC_{1\text{-}3}$ peptide (**Figure 6A**), with a Pearson correlation coefficient of 0.953 (**Figure 6B**). Based on the data for internal standard peptides, this degree of correlation indicated that the peptide found in human islets was indeed the HIP11 peptide $insC_{4\text{-}26}$ – $insC_{1\text{-}3}$ (**Figure 6C**). This finding was confirmed by P-VIS chromatographic retention time analysis (**Supplementary Figure 3**).

DISCUSSION

The discovery of HIPs in human islets (2) and the detection and isolation of HIP-reactive CD4 T cells from the peripheral blood and islets of individuals with T1D (1, 5–7) indicate a role for HIPs as autoantigens in T1D. Here, we used LC-MS/MS analysis

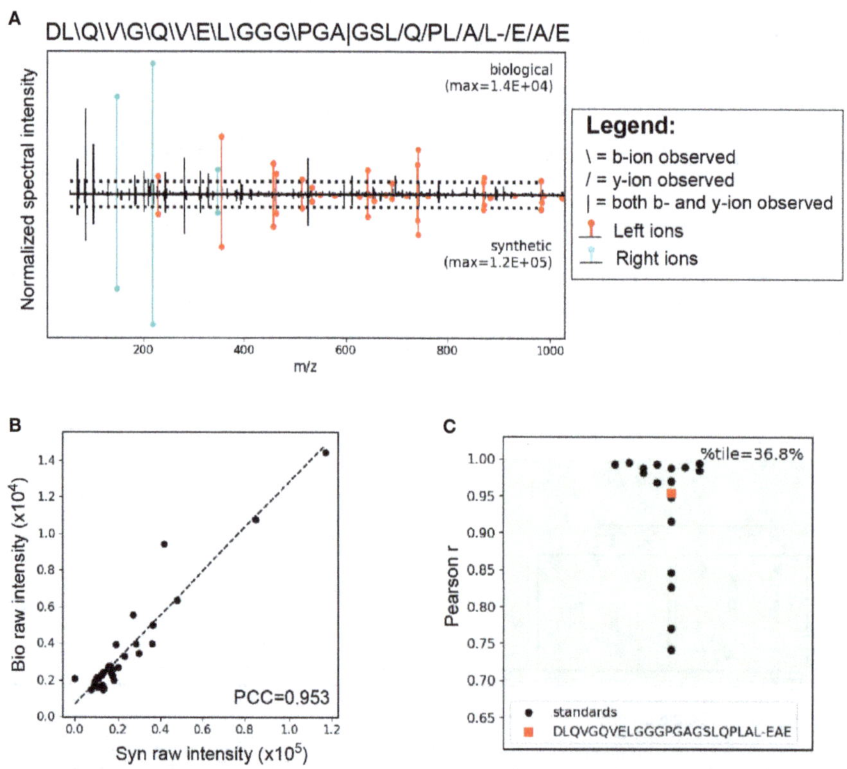

FIGURE 6 | LC-MS/MS analysis using the P-VIS approach confirms that HIP11 is present in human islets. Proteins were extracted from human islets, fractionated by size exclusion chromatography (SEC), and digested with the protease AspN, which cleaves at the N-terminus of aspartic acid (D) residues. Samples were analyzed by LC-MS/MS and data were searched using Agilent Spectrum Mill software. The predicted HIP11 AspN cleavage product DLQVGQVELGGGPGAGSLQPLAL-EAE was identified with high confidence and validated using the P-VIS approach. **(A)** Mirror plot generated by PSM_validator displaying the spectrum from the biological sample (positive y-axis) and the spectrum from the validation sample (negative y-axis). Peak intensities are normalized to the most intense peak in each spectrum. The intensity of the tallest peak in each spectrum is indicated. In the sequence map, "", "/", and "|" indicate that the spectrum from the biological sample contained a b-ion, y-ion, or both, respectively, corresponding to fragmentation at a given bond. Horizontal dotted lines indicate the user-defined threshold for consideration of peaks in the Pearson correlation coefficient (PCC) calculation. Ions corresponding to fragmentation of a bond to the left (L ions) or right (R ions) of the hybrid junction are labeled in red and cyan, respectively. **(B)** Peaks that were present above the intensity threshold in at least one of the spectra were used to calculate the Pearson correlation coefficient (PCC) between the two spectra. For each peak, the intensity in the biological peptide spectrum (bio raw intensity) and the intensity in the spectrum for the synthetic peptide (syn raw intensity) were paired, and the pairs for all peaks were plotted. Calculation of the PCC for these values indicated that the spectra were highly correlated (PCC = 0.953). **(C)** Comparison of the PCC for the HIP11 match to the distribution of PCCs for internal standard peptides (ISPs). Data for the ISPs passed the D'Agostino-Pearson omnibus normality test ($p = 0.229$; $p > 0.05$ indicates that the null hypothesis cannot be rejected and the data can be treated as normal). Green shading indicates the 95% prediction interval based on one-tailed analysis of Fisher's z-transformed PCC values. The PCC comparing the biological spectrum and the validation spectrum is shown (red square), and the percentile (%tile) is reported.

to report for the first time that HIP11, a C-peptide/C-peptide HIP, is present in human islets. We determined the TCR Vα and Vβ usage and the HLA class II restriction of the HIP11-reactive E2 clone previously isolated from the peripheral blood of a T1D donor. We also demonstrated that HIP11 is a potent epitope for a proinsulin-specific T cell receptor (GSE.8E3) identified by analysis of islet-infiltrating T cells from a T1D organ donor (13). Notably, we found that GSE.8E3 and the E2 clone each recognize a different minimal epitope of HIP11 and recognition by these clones was restricted to HLA-DQ8/HLA-DQ8*trans* or HLA-DQ2, respectively. HLA-DQ8 and HLA-DQ8*trans* consist of the same β chain paired with different α chains. A previous study (17) demonstrated that CD4 T cell clones (isolated from T1D donors and specific for immunodominant islet epitopes) could recognize their cognate peptide epitopes presented by either DQ8 or DQ8*trans*, with presentation by DQ8*trans* eliciting a stronger response. The DQ8*trans* α chain lacks the Arg52 residue present in the DQ8 α chain. The authors demonstrated that the absence of Arg52α led to differences in the orientation of TCR contact residues in the bound peptide, resulting in a higher affinity between the TCR and the peptide-DQ8*trans* complex (17). The GSE.8E3 transfectoma was more sensitive to N-terminal and C-terminal truncations of the HIP11 peptide SLQPLAL-EAEDLQV when DQ8 was the presenting element, also suggesting possible differences in the orientation of crucial TCR contacts when either DQ8 or *DQ8trans* was the presenting element. However, structural characterization, such as by X-ray crystallography, would be needed for definitive characterization of the interactions between the TCR, the peptide, and the different HLA molecules.

As more than 73% of all patients with T1D carry either HLA-DQ8 (DQA2*0301-DQB2*0302), HLA-DQ2 (DQA1*0501-DQB1*0201), or both (18), presentation by two different HLA molecules strongly associated with disease susceptibility further supports the case for HIP11 as a relevant autoantigen in T1D. Of note, individuals that carry both DQ2 and DQ8 alleles have a higher risk of developing T1D (19) and investigation of the relevance of HIP11 in this population is currently underway in our lab. Like I-A^{g7} in the NOD mouse model of autoimmune diabetes, position 57 of the β-chain of HLA-DQ8 and HLA-DQ2 has a non-aspartic acid (D) amino acid polymorphism that favors the presentation of an acidic amino acid in p9 of the binding groove (20). While there are clear amino acid preferences for binding to either molecule in pockets 1, 4, 6, 7 and 9 (14, 15, 21), the possibility of forming HLA trans dimers offers additional possibilities for peptide binding while maintaining the β57 non-D amino acid (22).

Formation of HIPs in pancreatic β-cells is likely the result of the cellular environment where unique peptides, such as the insulin C-peptide, are present at high local concentrations inside secretory granules. This could lead to the formation of specific HIPs that do not form in the thymus. Thus, central tolerance to these HIPs may not be established, allowing for the development of autoreactivity to HIPs in the periphery. Cross-reactivity of HIP-reactive T cells to unmodified peptides such as C-peptide may then lead to a break in tolerance to these unmodified insulin peptides, potentially resulting in a more robust autoimmune response. We observed, for example, that the GSE.8E3 transductant, which responded to HIP11 in the context of either HLA-DQ8 or HLA-DQ8*trans*, also responded to native C-peptide but only when presented by DQ8*trans* and not by DQ8. One could speculate that the ability of HLA-DQ8*trans* to present both a HIP and an unmodified insulin peptide to an autoreactive T cell clone in a stimulatory fashion suggests a possible mechanism in which carrying both the HLA-DQ2 and HLA-DQ8 alleles increases the risk of developing T1D by facilitating T cell cross reactivity to HIPs and unmodified peptides. It should be noted that HIP11 could be found in the islets of a non-T1D organ donor, suggesting that HIP formation is not limited to humans with autoimmunity. Similarly, insulin has long been recognized as an autoantigen in T1D, even though it is expressed in all individuals. Elucidating how various factors such as HIP formation and HLA genotype act in concert to promote disease development could be key to future progress in T1D research.

The former gold standard for validating mass spectrometry-based peptide identifications was to compare the fragmentation spectrum and chromatographic retention time for a synthetic version of a putative peptide sequence to those observed for the biological peptide. Our P-VIS approach (9) adds rigor and objectivity to this process by using comparisons for internal standard peptides to evaluate if the observed degree of similarity between the biological and synthetic peptides is high enough to indicate a correct match. Although we confidently identified HIP11 in human islets, the observed fragment provides limited information about the origin and mechanism of formation of the biological peptide since human islet proteins were digested with the AspN protease prior to LC-MS/MS analysis. Could HIP11 be the product of intramolecular transpeptidation and therefore the generation of a cis-hybrid? In this scenario, a protease would remove the five C-terminal residues from a C-peptide molecule and fuse the N-terminus of the same molecule to the newly-formed C-terminus, thereby generating a cyclic peptide. Cleavage of this cyclic peptide by a protease or the proteasome complex could then generate a linear HIP11 peptide suitable for presentation by MHC molecules. Alternatively, HIP11 could be formed by intermolecular transpeptidation (formation of a trans-hybrid), in which one C-peptide molecule is cleaved, generating the $insC_{1-26}$ fragment, and the N-terminus of a separate C-peptide molecule is fused to the C-terminus of the $insC_{1-26}$ fragment. Various other details of how HIP11 is formed are also unknown including for example, the specific enzyme responsible for formation of HIP11 in human islets.

In combination with our previous work, our results provide a thorough analysis of a disease-relevant HIP in human T1D, including identification of the HIP in islets, investigation of CD4 T cell responses, and molecular characterization of epitope recognition. The validation of an HLA-DQ2/HIP11 tetramer opens the path for further characterization of the role of HIP11-reactive T cells in T1D. To our knowledge, this is one of the first DQ2 tetramers loaded with a T1D disease-relevant antigen. This work provides a precedent for in-depth characterization of responses to HIPs as important components of the autoimmune response in T1D.

AUTHOR CONTRIBUTIONS

RB, TW, MN, and EJ designed experimental work. AH, RB, TW, MD, LL, RP, and MN performed experimental work. RB, TW, KH, and TD wrote and edited the manuscript. All authors contributed to the article and approved the submitted version.

ACKNOWLEDGMENTS

We would like to thank the NIH tetramer core for providing the tetramers used in this study, Dr. Peter Gottlieb for providing patients samples and James Dilisio for assistance with flow cytometry experiments.

REFERENCES

1. Delong T, Wiles TA, Baker RL, Bradley B, Barbour G, Reisdorph R, et al. Pathogenic CD4 T Cells in Type 1 Diabetes Recognize Epitopes Formed by Peptide Fusion. *Science (80-)* (2016) 351:711–4. doi: 10.1126/science.aad2791
2. Wiles TA, Powell R, Michel CR, Scott Beard K, Hohenstein A, Bradley B, et al. Identification of Hybrid Insulin Peptides (HIPs) in Mouse and Human Islets by Mass Spectrometry. *J Proteome Res* (2019) 18:814–25. doi: 10.1021/acs.jproteome.8b00875
3. Wan X, Vomund AN, Peterson OJ, Chervonsky AV, Lichti CF, Unanue ER. The MHC-II Peptidome of Pancreatic Islets Identifies Key Features of Autoimmune Peptides. *Nat Immunol* (2020) 21:455–63. doi: 10.1038/s41590-020-0623-7
4. Baker RL, Jamison BL, Wiles TA, Lindsay RS, Barbour G, Bradley B, et al. CD4 T Cells Reactive to Hybrid Insulin Peptides Are Indicators of Disease Activity in the NOD Mouse. *Diabetes* (2018) 67:1836–46. doi: 10.2337/db18-0200
5. Babon JAB, DeNicola ME, Blodgett DM, Crèvecoeur I, Buttrick TS, Maehr R, et al. Analysis of Self-Antigen Specificity of Islet-Infiltrating T Cells From Human Donors With Type 1 Diabetes. *Nat Med* (2016) 22:1482–7. doi: 10.1038/nm.4203
6. Baker RL, Rihanek M, Hohenstein AC, Nakayama M, Michels A, Gottlieb PA, et al. Hybrid Insulin Peptides Are Autoantigens in Type 1 Diabetes. *Diabetes* (2019) 68:1830–40. doi: 10.2337/db19-0128
7. Arribas-Layton D, Guyer P, Delong T, Dang M, Chow IT, Speake C, et al. Hybrid Insulin Peptides Are Recognized by Human T Cells in the Context of Drb1*04:01. *Diabetes* (2020) 69:1492–502. doi: 10.2337/db19-0620
8. Mann SE, Zhou Z, Landry LG, Anderson AM, Alkanani AK, Fischer J, et al. Multiplex T Cell Stimulation Assay Utilizing a T Cell Activation Reporter-Based Detection System. *Front Immunol* (2020) 11. doi: 10.3389/fimmu.2020.00633
9. Wiles TA, Saba LM, Delong T. Peptide-Spectrum Match Validation With Internal Standards (P–VIS): Internally-Controlled Validation of Mass Spectrometry-Based Peptide Identifications. *J Proteome Res* (2020) 20 (1):236–49. doi: 10.1021/acs.jproteome.0c00355
10. Zolg DP, Wilhelm M, Yu P, Knaute T, Zerweck J, Wenschuh H, et al. PROCAL: A Set of 40 Peptide Standards for Retention Time Indexing, Column Performance Monitoring, and Collision Energy Calibration. *Proteomics* (2017) 17. doi: 10.1002/pmic.201700263
11. Ji Q, Perchellet A, Goverman JM. Viral Infection Triggers Central Nervous System Autoimmunity Via Activation of CD8 + T Cells Expressing Dual TCRs. *Nat Immunol* (2010) 11:628–34. doi: 10.1038/ni.1888
12. Schuldt NJ, Auger JL, Spanier JA, Martinov T, Breed ER, Fife BT, et al. Cutting Edge: Dual TCRα Expression Poses an Autoimmune Hazard by Limiting Regulatory T Cell Generation. *J Immunol* (2017) 199:33–8. doi: 10.4049/jimmunol.1700406
13. Michels AW, Landry LG, McDaniel KA, Yu L, Campbell-Thompson M, Kwok WW, et al. Islet-Derived CD4 T Cells Targeting Proinsulin in Human Autoimmune Diabetes. *Diabetes* (2017) 66:722–34. doi: 10.2337/db16-1025
14. Vartdal F, Johansen BH, Friede T, Thorpe CJ, Stevanović S, Eriksen JE, et al. The Peptide Binding Motif of the Disease Associated HLA-DQ (α 1(*) 0501, β 1(*) 0201) Molecule. *Eur J Immunol* (1996) 26:2764–72. doi: 10.1002/eji.1830261132
15. Chang KY, Unanue ER. Prediction of HLA-DQ8 Cell Peptidome Using a Computational Program and Its Relationship to Autoreactive T Cells. *Int Immunol* (2009) 21:705–13. doi: 10.1093/intimm/dxp039
16. Nepom GT. MHC Class II Tetramers. *J Immunol* (2012) 188:2477–82. doi: 10.4049/jimmunol.1102398
17. Chow IT, Gates TJ, Papadopoulos GK, Moustakas AK, Kolawole EM, Notturno RJ, et al. Discriminative T Cell Recognition of Cross-Reactive Islet-Antigens Is Associated With HLA-DQ8 Transdimer–Mediated Autoimmune Diabetes. *Sci Adv* (2019) 5:eaaw9336. doi: 10.1126/sciadv.aaw9336
18. Erlich H, Valdes AM, Noble J, Carlson JA, Varney M, Concannon P, et al. HLA DR-DQ Haplotypes and Genotypes and Type 1 Diabetes Risk Analysis of the Type 1 Diabetes Genetics Consortium Families. *Diabetes* (2008) 57:1084–92. doi: 10.2337/db07-1331
19. Pociot F, McDermott MF. Genetics of Type 1 Diabetes Mellitus. *Genes Immun* (2002) 3:235–49. doi: 10.1038/sj.gene.6363875
20. Jones EY, Fugger L, Strominger JL, Siebold C. MHC Class II Proteins and Disease: A Structural Perspective. *Nat Rev Immunol* (2006) 6:271–82. doi: 10.1038/nri1805
21. Van De Wal Y, Kooy YMC, Drijfhout JW, Amons R, Koning F. Peptide Binding Characteristics of the Coeliac Disease Associated DQ(α1(*)0501, β1(*) 0201) Molecule. *Immunogenetics* (1996) 44:246–53. doi: 10.1007/BF02602553
22. Van Lummel M, Van Veelen PA, De Ru AH, Pool J, Nikolic T, Laban S, et al. Discovery of a Selective Islet Peptidome Presented by the Highest-Risk HLA-DQ8trans Molecule. *Diabetes* (2016) 65:732–41. doi: 10.2337/db15-1031

4

The Four-Way Stop Sign: Viruses, 12-Lipoxygenase, Islets and Natural Killer Cells in Type 1 Diabetes Progression

*Michele L. Semeraro, Lindsey M. Glenn and Margaret A. Morris**

Department of Internal Medicine, Strelitz Diabetes Center, Eastern Virginia Medical School, Norfolk, VA, United States

***Correspondence:**
Margaret A. Morris
morrisma@evms.edu

Natural killer (NK) cells represent an important effector arm against viral infection, and mounting evidence suggests that viral infection plays a role in the development of type 1 diabetes (T1D) in at least a portion of patients. NK cells recognize their target cells through a delicate balance of inhibitory and stimulatory receptors on their surface. If unbalanced, NK cells have great potential to wreak havoc in the pancreas due to the beta cell expression of the as-yet-defined NKp46 ligand through interactions with the activating NKp46 receptor found on the surface of most NK cells. Blocking interactions between NKp46 and its ligand protects mice from STZ-induced diabetes, but differential expression non-diabetic and diabetic donor samples have not been tested. Additional studies have shown that peripheral blood NK cells from human T1D patients have altered phenotypes that reduce the lytic and functional ability of the NK cells. Investigations of humanT1D pancreas tissues have indicated that the presence of NK cells may be beneficial despite their infrequent detection. In non-obese diabetic (NOD) mice, we have noted that NK cells express high levels of the proinflammatory mediator 12/15-lipoxygenase (12/15-LO), and decreased levels of stimulatory receptors. Conversely, NK cells of 12/15-LO deficient NOD mice, which are protected from diabetes development, express significantly higher levels of stimulatory receptors. Furthermore, the human NK92 cell line expresses the ALOX12 protein [human 12-lipoxygenase (12-LO), related to mouse 12/15-LO] *via* Western blotting. Human 12-LO is upregulated in the pancreas of both T1D and T2D human donors with insulin-containing islets, showing a link between 12-LO expression and diabetes progression. Therefore, our hypothesis is that NK cells in those susceptible to developing T1D are unable to function properly during viral infections of pancreatic beta cells due to increased 12-LO expression and activation, which contributes to increased interferon-gamma production and an imbalance in activating and inhibitory NK cell receptors, and may contribute to downstream autoimmune T cell responses. The work presented here outlines evidence from our lab, as well as published literature, supporting our hypothesis, including novel data.

Keywords: coxsackievirus infections, islets, natural killer cells, 12-lipoxygenase, type 1 diabetes

INTRODUCTION

Autoimmune destruction of the pancreatic beta cells leads to the development of Type 1 diabetes (T1D). The number of T1D cases is on the rise, with the relative risk for developing the disease ranging from 0.1% [no family history, protective human leukocyte antigen (HLA)] to up to 70% (monozygotic twin with susceptible HLA), and is dependent largely upon genetic susceptibility

(1). Importantly, the strongest genetic link to the development of T1D is the expression of certain HLA haplotypes. Class II HLA genes, especially DR3, DR4, and DQ8, are the strongest links; however, HLA Class I molecules also play a role in diabetes development (2, 3). Expression of both Class I and Class II molecules is the largest contributing factor in determining the immune response to a given pathogen, as peptides are processed and presented to T and natural killer (NK) cells *via* the proteins of the major histocompatibility complex (MHC) locus (4). Therefore, these molecules play a key role in directing immune responses, be they beneficial or detrimental. However, the genetic contributions to T1D development are unable to fully account for the increased rates, supporting the idea that environmental factors play a role in the development of T1D. Furthermore, susceptible siblings of T1D patients who are closely monitored frequently show signs of autoimmunity in the form of autoantibodies prior to metabolic dysfunction. Many believe, based on this evidence, that development of full-blown diabetes requires multiple insults to the system in order to manifest itself.

Patients with T1D currently depend upon treatment options that are limited to methods that replace the deficit in insulin production, either *via* injection or transplantation [reviewed in Ref. (5), in press]. While technological advances have helped improve these methods, they still do not provide a cure for the disease. Therefore, determining the mechanisms leading to immune damage of pancreatic beta (β) cells, and treatments to maintain β cell mass, are of the utmost importance.

Recently, perceptions of T1D development have evolved, with a greater attention being paid to islet inflammation as an important event propagating autoimmunity and further loss of β cell mass (6–8). Debates persist as to whether islets are independently inflamed prior to the autoimmune response or the autoimmune response brings about the islet inflammation. One of these recent studies described the incorrect processing of the insulin protein that led to the generation of abnormal peptides recognized by circulating $CD8^+$ T cells in T1D patients (8). This line of evidence certainly points to β cell defects contributing to diabetes pathogenesis; however, this study does not address what might cause β cells to produce this incorrectly processed protein. One study in non-obese diabetic (NOD) mice has suggested that incorrect protein processing in these mice causes an increase in endoplasmic reticulum (ER) stress, and results in the development of autoimmunity (9). Given the lack of complete concordance among monozygotic twins, many believe external environmental factors, such as viruses, strongly influence the development of islet inflammation leading to T1D. Trying to understand all of these data in concert brings researchers in the field to ponder the chicken and egg scenario. Are either islets or immune cells in susceptible individuals causing the initial insults that spark diabetes development, or does an environmental factor trigger the disease? Do we see signs of virus infections in patients with T1D because the infection is what precipitates diabetes development, or are patients with diabetes more susceptible to developing virus infections because of defects in their bodies' defense systems? With the data that are currently available, the order of events in the precipitation of T1D is unclear.

A NEW HYPOTHESIS

As we gather more evidence, it is becoming clear that we must look at the integrated physiology to fully understand the mechanism(s) of T1D development. Here, we outline an idea that incorporates early antiviral immune effectors, NK cells, with proinflammatory processes involving 12-lipoxygenase (12-LO) occurring in the pancreatic beta cells. We hypothesize that the activation of NK cell 12/15-LO (*Alox15,* in mice) or 12-LO (*ALOX12,* in humans) through environmental triggers, such as Coxsackievirus infection, contributes to T1D initiation by affecting the normal innate immune interplay between NK cells and islets, which primes downstream autoimmune responses leading to islet destruction. This may occur, in part, due to the effects of inflammation (including 12-LO) on the balance of NK cell receptor expression (10). Below, we will describe the evidence supporting this hypothesis, beginning with one of the suspected environmental triggers, enteroviruses.

DIRECT EVIDENCE FOR VIRUS INFECTIONS IN T1D

Over the past fifty years, there has been accumulating evidence linking viruses, and the patients' responses to these viruses, to the initiation of T1D. This idea that viruses contribute to the initiation and development of T1D was first introduced in the 1960s (11, 12). This is, of course, difficult to fully pinpoint, as the infection may occur long before disease onset, and scientists with access to human pancreas tissues are granted only a snapshot of the patient's final day as their window into the disease process. Additionally, as mentioned previously, it is unclear whether or not patients susceptible to developing T1D are also more susceptible to developing virus-mediated infections in the pancreatic islets, which might increase the viral signature in the islets of patients with T1D. Therefore, this might not be a causal relationship, but merely coincidental. Since we cannot directly test whether viruses initiate T1D in humans, researchers have used animal models to test this theory. NOD mouse models have been used to show that Coxsackievirus B1 and B4 (CVB1, CVB4) infection speeds diabetes pathogenesis (13), and is dependent upon host sensors of virus (14–16). Others have shown that these effects are highly age dependent, as infection at before 10 weeks of age can prevent diabetes development (17, 18). Additionally, studies of immunodeficient mice engrafted with human islets have shown that human islets can become infected with CVB4, which causes direct damage to the β cells, and results in diabetes. Gene expression profiles of these infected islets indicated significant increases in genes related to the Type 1 interferon (T1-IFN) pathway, as well as genes related to ER stress (19). While these data support the idea of viruses contributing to diabetes development, they do not answer the question about which occurs first: islet dysfunction or immune activation.

To address the role of virus infections in human T1D, groups such as Persistent Virus Infection in Diabetes Network and the Network for Pancreatic Organ Donors with Diabetes—Viral Working Group (nPOD-V) have approached the question with great coordination across multiple platforms (20) assessing the same donor samples (PCR, immunohistochemistry, proteomics, and ISH). These team science efforts have yielded results estimating that Coxsackievirus infections might contribute to diabetes development in over 50% of cases (21, 22). While certainly not causal, pancreas tissues, and specifically β cells, from T1D donors have been found to express viral VP1 proteins more frequently than non-diabetic (ND) donors (23, 24). These studies continue to progress, generating a wealth of information from human donor samples.

Mechanistically, enteroviruses can infect *via* a fecal/oral route, thereby implicating intestinal involvement during the infection process. Mounting evidence has shown a role for the gut microbiome as a contributing factor in autoimmune diabetes development. Viruses and microbiota are known to interact with one another, and shape the response of both parties, which may influence the development of T1D (25). Recent human studies of closely matched control and T1D experimental groups demonstrate both increased inflammation in the duodenum of T1D patients (26), and direct detection of enteroviruses (27). In the first study, donors were tested for markers of inflammation using histological techniques and PCR array, indicating significant inflammatory processes in T1D donors, including increased macrophage numbers in the duodenum of T1D (26). In the second study, T1D donors were much more likely to have markers of enterovirus infection than control donors independent of HLA haplotypes, as tested by *in situ* hybridization and histological techniques (27). This work could not conclude whether T1D patients were more susceptible to the virus infections, or the infections are persistent. Coxsackievirus infection of β cells with strains B1 (28) and B4 (13) may occur *via* β cell expression of the Coxsackie Adenovirus Receptor (29, 30) following viral migration from the duodenum to the pancreas through the common bile duct or affiliated vessels (27). Pursuant to the role of islet inflammation following environmental insult, *in vitro* studies indicate that infection could lead to ER stress in β cells, contributing to islet dysfunction that activates the autoimmune response (9, 31). Alternatively, the infection could also directly activate immune responses that become uncontrolled due to inherent immune defects. Until imaging of live T1D patients affords the ability to detect virus infection in real-time, other experimental avenues must be explored, including the use of cultured islets and mouse models.

INDIRECT EVIDENCE FOR VIRUS INFECTIONS IN T1D

While viruses themselves may be difficult to detect in our snapshot views of human T1D, there is ample "circumstantial" evidence that exists in the form of immune cells and mediators. Both mouse models and organ donors with T1D have provided clear evidence that islet inflammation is a key hallmark of this disease. Immune cells infiltrate the islets, albeit at different intensities, in both species. Many patients show signs of adaptive immunity against the pancreatic islets in the form of autoantibodies and islet-specific T cell clones.

Beyond cellular responses, cytokines and chemokines also contribute to islet demise and can stem from both innate and adaptive responses. T1-IFNs have recently gained more respect as effectors in the development of T1D (see the review by Newby and Mathews in this issue). Indeed, virus infections are strong stimulators of T1-IFN production, which leads to a subsequent upregulation of MHC Class I expression, another hallmark of T1D (32).

Downstream of this response, numerous proinflammatory cytokines and chemokines have been detected in patients with diabetes (33, 34). One of these, IFN-gamma (IFN-γ), has been shown to play an important, albeit controversial, role in T1D pathogenesis (7, 35). While absence of the cytokine itself leads to delayed disease development (36), absence of the receptor protects against the development of insulitis (37). IFN-γ has many points at which it can act in the development of T1D, from altering MHC/HLA expression on involved cells to altering endothelial cell function and signaling to immune cells to activate cytotoxic effectors (37). Diminished IFN-γ responses can prevent the recruitment of insulitic T cells, as well as their ability to respond to antigens, which might prevent diabetes progression. However, increased IFN-γ production by $CD4^+$ T cells can actually contribute to the resolution of $CD8^+$ T cell responses (35). While it is appreciated that $CD4^+$ T cells contribute to the IFN-γ production during T1D pathogenesis, this does not exclude the idea that NK cells may be the first producers of IFN-γ present in the islets. Interestingly, IFN-γ is also frequently detected following virus infections, and is used by the immune system to combat viral replication. Given these data, it is unclear whether IFN-γ is serving in a proinflammatory capacity or an unsuccessful attempt at tolerance induction during the development of T1D (35).

NK CELLS AND THEIR ROLE IN T1D

Natural killer cells are large granular lymphocytes that are considered part of the innate immune system. While they do not react as quickly as neutrophils and macrophages against invading pathogens, they mount a response more quickly than do T cells from the adaptive arm of the immune system. NK cells are known as key players in fighting off both tumor cells and virus-infected cells. Despite their small number (only 5–10% of leukocytes in the spleen and 1–6% in peripheral blood) (38), NK cells are powerful cytolytic effectors. Upon stimulation by a variety of cytokines, including T1-IFNs and IL-12 (39), NK cells utilize several different mechanisms to lyse their targets: the combination of perforin and granzymes, signaling through death receptors (i.e., Fas/FasL), and antibody-dependent cellular cytotoxicity leading to either apoptosis or necrosis (40). NK cells can also produce potent cytokines, such as IFN-γ and TNF-α (41). IFN-γ production by NK cells might also serve an antigen presenting capacity (42–44), which, along with their potent cytokine production abilities, would give them the power to stimulate immune responses downstream of their own activation.

In order to recognize their targets, NK cells have developed an intricate system of check and balances. As NK cells are expected to determine aberrant "self" cells (tumors and virus-infected cells), they must be able to distinguish which cells are healthy, and which are not. NK cells respond to virus infections in both mouse and man (4) through signaling mechanisms involving a delicate balance of inhibitory and stimulatory receptors expressed by NK cells. Normal expression of MHC Class I molecules (HLA in humans) send "self" signals to NK cells, inhibiting lytic responses (45). Virus infection can lead to the downregulation of MHC Class I molecules on the surface of infected cells. While this prevents CD8$^+$ T cells from responding to viral peptides, it also diminishes the inhibitory signal transmitted to NK cells [reviewed in Ref. (46)]. Subsequently, stimulatory signals to the NK cell are able to override inhibitory signals, leading to lysis of affected cells. In some instances, including during infection of pancreatic islets, viruses push the cellular machinery into overdrive and promote Type 1 IFN production (47), causing hyperexpression of the MHC Class I molecules (32). To circumvent this tactic, NK cells utilize receptors that recognize the upregulation of ligands for the natural cytotoxicity receptors, like NKp46, on the surface of infected cells (48, 49). Thus, NK cells can become "licensed to kill" through several mechanisms that allow them to detect alterations in MHC Class I molecules, as well as increased expression of stimulatory ligands, making them versatile effectors during virus infections (50).

Typically, T1D is thought to be dominated by autoimmune T cell responses; however, growing evidence suggests that NK cells are also involved (51). NK cells take up residence throughout the body (52), providing immune surveillance and protection against viruses wherever they enter the body. NK cells are plentiful in the intestines as compared to other organs (53), comprising 20–40% of Intestinal Epithelial Lymphocytes in healthy children (54), as compared to about 10% of the blood and spleen. This provides NK cells ample opportunity to respond to Coxsackievirus infections, as well as others (*Salmonella, Toxoplasma gondii,* other parasites, viruses, and bacteria) (55), transmitted *via* the fecal/oral route. Paired with the evidence of increased inflammation in duodenum of T1D patients, these data support our hypothesis. Furthermore, NK cells have been detected in the pancreas of both diabetic mice and humans. In mice, the cells appear shortly after macrophages (56). In human pancreatic samples, although NK cells are not frequently detected (57), they have been found in insulitic lesions, and show indications of having a protective effect (58). When one considers the frequency of NK cells in lymphocyte-rich organs (5–10% of leukocytes in the spleen), and also accounts for the number of cells required to define insulitis in humans [six or more CD3$^+$ cells in at least three islets (59)], then perhaps it is not surprising that NK cells are rarely detected in donor samples. Alternatively, it is possible that NK cells may prime the pancreatic environment for the entry of diabetogenic T cells, and subsequently depart. As we only have access to one time point for each human donor, we cannot currently distinguish these hypotheses. However, the use of mouse models made aid in this differentiation.

Natural killer cells themselves have recently been directly implicated in the development of T1D through additional expression quantitative trait loci analysis following genome-wide association studies, which further suggests that NK cells play a key role in T1D pathogenesis (60). Interestingly, this study indicates that NK cells may impact T1D development more than CD8$^+$ T cells. The carefully designed and executed study is limited to only 105 Japanese subjects, which might not apply to other ethnic backgrounds. However, it is comprehensive, and provides a solid approach for other ethnic backgrounds to be tested. Another data set investigating NK cell phenotypes from patients with T1D showed that NK cells from these patients express significantly reduced levels of activating receptors on their surface as compared to healthy controls (10).

It is unlikely that NK cells act independently in T1D development. Macrophages recognize environmental signals, and have been shown to enter pancreatic islets at 3–4 weeks of age in NOD mice (61, 62). Macrophage production of IL-12 and IL-18 can strongly activate NK cells, which are found in the pancreas of diabetes-prone NOD mice as early as 4 weeks of age (56, 63), to produce high levels of IFN-γ (64). Indeed, serum levels of both IL-12 and IL-18 are higher patients with T1D (65, 66), and IL-18 has been shown to participate in T1D pathogenesis of NOD mice (67). Despite a defect in IL-15 signaling in NOD mice (68), which affects NK cell development and function, others have shown in IL-15-deficient mice that increased IL-12 signaling may allow NK cells to overcome this deficit when faced with pathogenic stimuli (69, 70). The early appearance of NK cells in the pancreas may enable them to activate diabetogenic T cell responses.

Perhaps most importantly, NK cells can directly interact with pancreatic islets through expression of ligands for the NK activating receptors NKG2D and NKp46. Both of these receptors have been implicated in NK-mediated self-aggression in human NK cells that can be triggered by signaling through NKG2D and NKp46 (71). The NKG2D ligand, RAE-1 (72), is one of these ligands. Some speculate that NKG2D ligands cause down-modulation of the receptors, thereby making the NK cells less active (73); however, others have failed to validate this hypothesis (74). They instead showed that differential expression of NKG2D ligands did not hinder NK cytotoxicity through methodical assessment of receptor and ligand levels using genetic tools to dictate the alteration of expression.

Pancreatic islets also broadly express ligands for the NKp46 natural cytotoxicity receptor. NKp46 is a Type I transmembrane protein with two extracellular Ig-like domains followed by a short stalk region, a transmembrane domain containing a positively charged amino acid residue, and a short cytoplasmic tail (75, 76). However, the cellular ligands for NKp46 have not been identified or characterized. The only NKp46 ligands identified so far are the hemagglutinin of influenza virus and the hemagglutinin-neuraminidase of parainfluenza virus (48), suggesting a role for sugars in NKp46 ligand recognition. Studies of NKp46 ligands have utilized the NKp46 Fc chimeric protein in flow cytometry and histological techniques to examine expression over time in the islets of mice and humans (63). Functional studies from the same group showed that blockade of NKp46 receptor/ligand interactions protects against streptozotocin-induced diabetes (63). Although these studies have assessed expression over time, differential expression of the NKp46 ligands in human ND controls versus T1D donor samples has not been tested.

We recently studied ND, autoantibody positive (AAb+), and T1D donor samples from nPOD in order to determine whether there were expression differences in NKp46 ligands using the NKp46 Fc chimeric protein. **Figure 1A** highlights representative images from donors with different health statuses. Islet images from two ND, three AAb+, and three T1D donors were analyzed by NIH Image J to quantify the density of NKp46 Fc staining (red) within the islet area as determined by glucagon staining (**Figure 1B**). Islets from T1D donors frequently retain alpha cell mass longer than insulin-positive beta cell mass (77, 78). Therefore, we used glucagon staining to more accurately determine the islet area for each donor in order to calculate the intensity of NKp46 Fc staining in islets. Interestingly, NKp46 Fc levels were significantly higher in the AAb+ donors as compared to ND donors. Although the difference was not statistically significant when comparing T1D and AAb+ donors, there was a trend toward higher expression in the AAb+ donors. These data suggest that NKp46 ligands are upregulated during the development of T1D, and diminish as the islet health and mass decrease over the course of the disease. While this may be the result of ongoing immune responses in these tissues, insulitis has only been detected in one each of the AAb+ and T1D donors. General characteristics of donors tested are listed in **Table 1**.

Mechanisms of NK cell action in diabetes are not well understood, and phenotypic differences in NK cells residing in different tissues may confound the results reported to date (40). Increased expression of stimulatory receptors on NK cells has been reported in both diabetic mice (79) and humans (80), while others maintain that a lack of NK cell activation contributes to

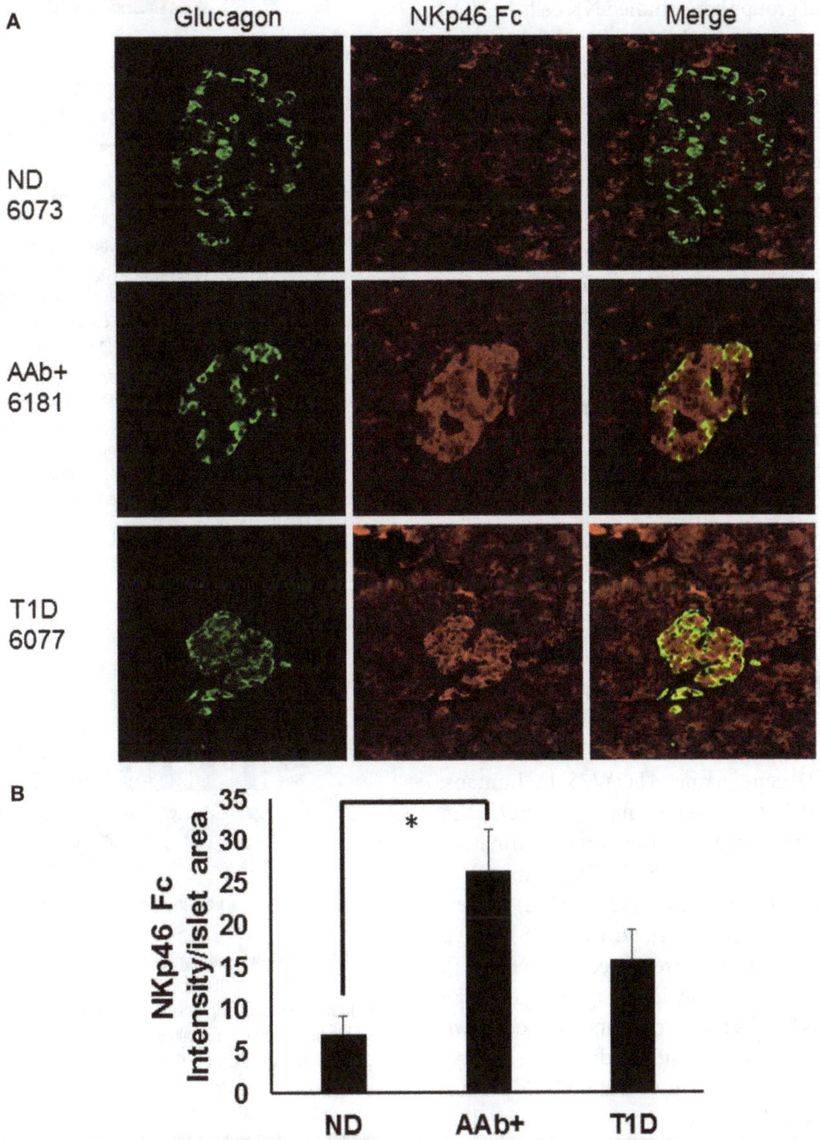

FIGURE 1 | Human islets express NKp46 *ligands*. **(A)** Representative images comparing donor pancreas tissues from Network for Pancreatic Organ Donors with Diabetes (nPOD) biorepository samples. Sections were stained with antibodies against glucagon (green) and the NKp46 Fc chimeric receptor (red). **(B)** Quantification of NKp46 Fc staining per islet area. Density of NKp46 Fc staining was determined for each islet area. Islets for each donor were assessed, and donors of the same group were averaged. $N = 2$ for non-diabetic (ND); $N = 3$ for both autoantibody positive (AAb+) and T1D. $^{*}p < 0.05$ by one-way ANOVA.

TABLE 1 | Donor profiles for NKp46 ligand staining.

nPOD case #	Donor type	Age	AAb+	Diabetes duration (years)	Insulitis
6048	ND	30	–	–	N
6073	ND	19.2	–	–	N
6151	AAb+	30	GADA	–	N
6181	AAb+	31.9	GADA	–	N
6197	AAb+	22	GADA, IA2A	–	Y
6077	T1D	32.9	mIAA	18	N
6083	T1D	15.2	mIAA	11	N
6088	T1D	31.2	mIAA, GADA, IA2A, ZnT8	5	Y

diabetes development (10, 68, 73, 81). This could be due in part to the type of analysis, as genomic studies do not always translate to protein expression. Several groups have studied NK cells in NOD mice. Both found that murine pancreatic NK cells exhibit a different phenotype from those found in the spleen and lymph nodes and have increased proliferative capacity (56, 82); however, there is not a consensus on levels of IFN-γ production, as one indicates lower levels *ex vivo*, but normal levels *in vivo* (82). Depletion of NK1.1$^+$ cells in NOD.NK1.1 congenic mice did not significantly affect disease onset, but the depletion protocol also removed NK/T cells (82). These tissue-specific phenotypic differences may also alter the detectability of the NK cells residing within the human pancreas using standard methodologies, but this has not yet been studied in humans. NOD mice have been shown to have a defect in IL-15 production, which contributes to NK cell dysfunction (68). IL-15 is required for NK cell maturation, and although NOD mice are not completely IL-15 deficient, they do show impaired NK cell development. Taken in concert with other systemic alterations in the NOD strain, the impact of this IL-15 defect has not been fully explored. As mentioned previously, NK cells functionally adjust to the absence of IL-15 by responding to IL-12 and IL-18 in order to produce IFN-γ (83), and by responding to pathogenic stimuli in the presence of IL-12 (69).

THE PROINFLAMMATORY MEDIATOR, 12-LO, IN T1D

12-Lipoxygenase [(12-LO) gene name *ALOX12S* in humans; 12/15-lipoxygenase (12/15-LO), gene name *Alox15* in mice] converts arachidonic acid to the proinflammatory 12(S)-hydroxyeicosatetraenoic acid (12(S)-HETE) through a 12-S-hydroperoxy-eicosatetraenoic acid (12-HPETE) intermediate (84, 85). IL-12 signaling downstream of 12(S)-HETE production (86, 87) activates STAT4 [reviewed in Ref. (88)], contributing to additional inflammation. IL-12 signaling through STAT4 strongly activates NK cells and T cells and is also known to be a strong contributor to autoimmune conditions in general [reviewed in Refs. (89, 90)]. In addition to T1D, 12/15-LO has been implicated in many inflammatory processes, including cancers (91, 92), asthma (93), and Type 2 diabetes (94).

Several lines of evidence indicate a critical role for 12/15-LO in the pathogenesis of T1D. It has been shown that deletion of STAT4 signaling molecules, which are downstream of 12/15-LO activation, in NOD mice protects the NOD strain from

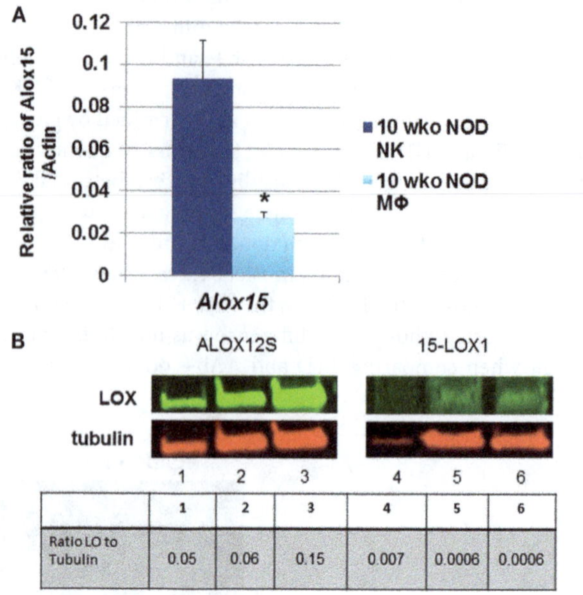

FIGURE 2 | Natural killer (NK) cells express 12/15-lipoxygenase (12/15-LO). **(A)** Murine non-obese diabetic (NOD) natural killer cells express Alox15. mRNA levels of the *Alox15* gene were tested in NK cells from NOD mice. These levels were compared to thioglycollate-induced peritoneal macrophages from 10-week-old NOD mice using the relative ratio of *Alox15/Actb*. *$p < 0.05$ using a two-tailed Student's *t*-test to compare NK vs. macrophages in age-matched NOD mice, $n = 6$ mice per group. **(B)** 12-Lipoxygenase (12-LO) protein expression in human NK92 cells. The human NK92 cell line was tested for protein expression of 12-LO by western blotting. ALOX12S expression was most abundant in the cell line, which is the most abundant form found in human islets. Lanes 1 and 4 are nuclear proteins from the two pooled NK92 samples; lanes 2 and 5 are cytoplasmic proteins from one NK92 sample; lanes 3 and 6 are cytoplasmic proteins from different NK92 samples.

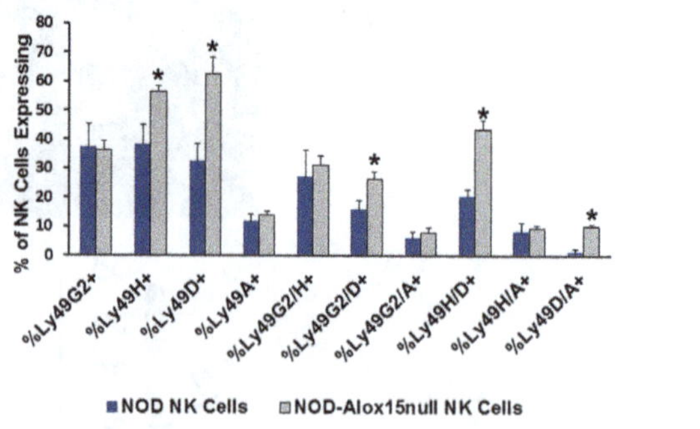

FIGURE 3 | Pancreatic lymph node natural killer (NK) cell expression of NK cell markers. Ly49 receptors determine which targets NK cells recognize and respond to during interactions with potential targets. Several of the expression patterns are altered in the absence of *Alox15*, with *Alox15^{null}* cells expressing higher proportions of the activating Ly49 receptors [*$p < 0.05$ using a two-tailed Student's *t*-test to compare receptor expression in non-obese diabetic (NOD) vs. NOD-*Alox15^{null}* NK cells for each receptor or receptor pair]. $n = 4$ mice/group.

developing T1D (95). Subsequently, we published that the NOD mouse line congenic for the global *Alox15* (NOD-*Alox15^{null}*) deletion is >98% protected from developing spontaneous

T1D (61). This line boasts a narrow congenic region delineated through extensive microsatellite mapping, and shows significantly reduced disease incidence (~2%). To understand the origin of the protection seen in these mice, wild-type NOD mice were tested for their expression 12/15-LO in islets, macrophages, and lymphocytes. Islets and macrophages expressed the enzyme in appreciable amounts, while lymphocytes had either low or undetectable amounts (96). Additionally, *Alox15^null^* mice have been shown to express decreased levels of IL-12 (96) and IL-18 (97), which are cytokines that contribute to NK cell IFN-γ production (83). Since publication, this strain has been shipped to additional vivaria and maintained this phenotype. Subsequent studies of human islets have also indicated 12-LO expression under inflamed conditions (98, 99), which feeds into the detrimental cycle of inflammation.

Natural killer cell expression of 12/15-LO has not been extensively studied, although historical data suggest that NK cells expressed a member of the lipoxygenase family (100). Using more modern information and methods, we discovered that both mouse and the human NK92 cell line express 12/15-LO and 12-LO, respectively (**Figure 2**). Surprisingly, this expression of 12/15-LO in freshly isolated NOD mouse NK cells is significantly higher (3.3-fold more) than that seen in thioglycollate-induced NOD macrophages (61, 96). Since NK cells are closely related to T cells, we expected that expression levels would be similar to those seen in T cells, which is almost undetectable (96). While

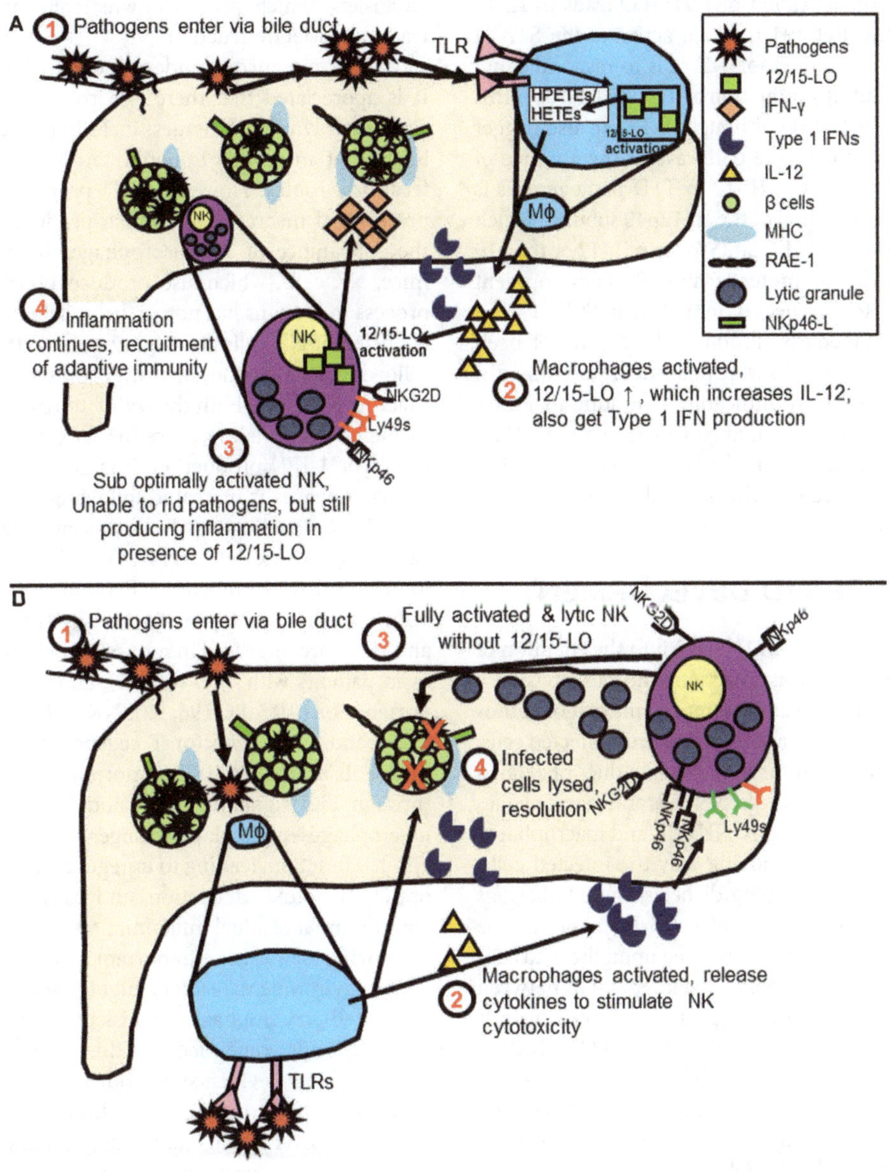

FIGURE 4 | (A) Model of natural killer (NK) cell activation leading to type 1 diabetes (T1D) in the presence of 12/15-lipoxygenase (12/15-LO) following virus infection. IL-12 production stimulates NK interferon-gamma (IFN-γ) response, feeds cycle of 12/15-LO activation and inflammation. **(B)** Model of NK cell activation in absence of 12/15-lipoxygenase following virus infection. NK cells respond to macrophage T1 IFN production following TLR signaling by using lytic mechanisms to rid virus-infected cells. Reduced inflammation prevents T1D development.

investigating the downstream effects of 12/15-LO expression in our NOD-*Alox15*^{null} mice, we found that the pancreatic lymph node NK cells of the NOD-*Alox15*^{null} mice had an increased percentage of NK cells expressing activating markers (**Figure 3**), which are similar phenotypically to peripheral blood NK cells from ND human controls (10). Taken together, it appears that activation of 12/15-LO, which leads to increased IL-12 levels (96), increases the inflammatory nature of the NK cells, presumably through the 12/15-LO pathway. We are currently testing whether NK cells are better able to resolve infections without contributing to the chronic inflammatory milieu in the absence of 12/15-LO.

Several additional lines of evidence suggest that NK cells are strongly influenced by 12/15-LO activity and that they have the capacity to play an important role in the development of diabetes. As mentioned above, activation of 12/15-LO leads to IL-12 production [reviewed in Ref. (94)], which activates the STAT4 signaling cascade that is required for NK cells to respond functionally (101–103), including production of IFN-γ (104, 105). This combination can exacerbate T1D, although IL-12 can also trigger the activation of different cytokine pathways in the absence of IFN-γ (106). The involvement of IL-12 in T1D pathogenesis is not without controversy. Deletion of the IL-12p40 subunit, which can heterodimerize with either IL-12p35 to form IL-12 or the p19 subunit to form IL-23, did not protect against T1D development (107). This may be due to the effect of inhibiting both IL-12 and IL-23 generation simultaneously, although IL-23 had not been discovered at the time these results were published. Subsequently, the same group published work indicating that administration of exogenous IL-12 exacerbated diabetes development (106). Importantly, when key molecules in the 12/15-LO pathway (i.e., 12/15-LO or STAT4), upstream of IL-12, are disrupted in NOD mice, diabetes is prevented (61, 95).

A NEW MODEL OF T1D DEVELOPMENT

By bringing NK cell expression of 12/15-LO into the equation of diabetes initiation following virus infection, one can envision a model in which duodenal NK cells encounter some sort of pathogen- or virus-infected cells, such as Coxsackievirus-infected cells. As the pathogen is transmitted through the bile duct or related vasculature on the way to the pancreas, NK cells and macrophages are alerted. Under normal conditions, NK cells and macrophages quickly dispense of the virus, removing only the infected cells. In a patient susceptible to developing diabetes, the interactions are altered, perhaps due to activation of 12/15-LO either by the virus directly or due to increased stress placed upon the beta cells upon infection (19). This leads to abnormal interactions between the innate immune cells with islets expressing NK cell ligands and prevents the resolution of the infection. 12/15-LO activation is known to feed into a vicious cycle of chronic inflammation, which in this instance, may be perpetuated by macrophages and NK cells (shown graphically in **Figure 4**). As mentioned earlier, in individuals with susceptible HLA haplotypes, or in mice (in was left out inadvertently) with susceptible MHC haplotypes, chronic inflammation signals the diabetogenic T cells to join the fight. This leads to significant islet destruction. Both HLA Class I and II molecules strongly influence the T cell responses in humans, as they dictate the ability of the T cells to recognize and react to autoantigens during the T cell development process, as well as in the periphery (108). This autoreactivity can be precipitated by stress placed on the islets, perhaps due to inflammatory processes. Such stress may lead to HLA Class II-mediated recognition of hybrid insulin (109) or posttranslationally modified (110) peptides by CD4^{+} T cells, thereby breaking peripheral tolerance to neoantigens and furthering the disease progression.

CONCLUSION

We have hypothesized that activation of NK cell 12/15-LO (or 12-LO, *ALOX12*, in humans) contributes to T1D initiation by affecting the normal innate immune interplay between NK cells and islets, which primes downstream autoimmune responses leading to islet destruction.

At best, our current understanding of T1D initiation is murky. It is appreciated that there is a role for cells of the mucosal-associated lymphoid tissues, including NK cells, and it is quite likely that infectious initiation of T1D would occur through fecal-oral routes. However, T1D progression also requires the presence of macrophages, which produce 12/15-LO. Following the appearance of the macrophages in the pancreas of NOD mice, NK cells, which also produce 12/15-LO, are found. This process in humans has not yet been delineated, and, therefore, it is unclear if NK cells are migrating from the gut to the pancreas following an infection, or if they are recruited by other means. Macrophages have both the ability to respond to virus infections through TLR signaling, as well as activate NK cells through IL-12 and Type 1 IFN production. It is known that IL-12 production in macrophages is increased following 12/15-LO activation and that IL-12 signaling can feedback into the 12/15-LO signaling cascade (84). NK cell 12/15-LO is then a target for activation following IL-12 stimulation. IL-12, in concert with IL-18, is also known to drive IFN-γ production by NK cells (83). Both IL-12 and IL-18 are increased in mouse models of T1D (67, 96), as well as in patients with T1D (65, 66), and both are increased in the presence of 12/15-LO (96, 97). NK cell-derived IFN-γ could aid in expanding the effector T cell population (111). Conversely, in the absence of 12/15-LO, normal IL-12 levels [as generated through TLR signaling (112)] and Type 1 IFNs from activated macrophages might play a stronger role in influencing pancreatic NK cell function, leading to upregulation of activating receptors, optimal cytotoxic activation, and clearance of viral pathogens with minimal residual inflammation.

Moving forward, it is important to understand mechanisms by which environmental factors might spark the activation of 12-LO in NK cells, macrophages, and islets, leading to the development of T1D. While some pieces of this puzzle remain to be placed, there is striking evidence that our hypothesis and model is possible. Many of the remaining questions can be answered in part by the use of novel global and conditional knock-outs of 12/15-LO on the NOD background in experiments with Coxsackievirus infections. By understanding the order in which these events occur, we will be better able to design selective therapies that might prevent the disease development and progression without resorting to global immunosuppression.

METHODS

Mice

Female NOD/ShiLtJ (NOD) mice were ordered from Jackson Laboratory (Bar Harbor, ME, USA); global NOD-*Alox15^{null}* mice (bred on-site at EVMS) were housed in SPF conditions and treated in accordance with the AAALAC and IACUC guidelines at the Eastern Virginia Medical Center. Mice were euthanized by asphyxiation with CO_2. Blood glucose levels were assessed following euthanasia at 4 and 10 weeks of age. Spleens, lymph nodes, and islets were removed.

Cell Isolations

Natural killer cells were isolated from spleen using cell isolation kits from Stem Cell Technologies (Vancouver, BC, Canada) per the manufacturer's instructions. Purity of the isolated populations was assessed by flow cytometry (see below) after staining with antibodies against cell surface markers including anti-CD3, anti-CD19, anti-NKp46, and anti-CD11b. Cells were generally 85–90% pure.

Flow Cytometry

Cells isolated from the pancreatic draining lymph nodes of NOD and NOD-*Alox15^{null}* mice at 10 weeks of age were stained with antibodies against cell surface markers for T (CD3), B (CD19), and NK cells (NKp46, Ly49A, Ly49G2, Ly49D, Ly49H). Gates were determined by using fluorescence minus one controls. All antibodies were purchased from Biolegend (San Diego, CA, USA).

qRT-PCR

mRNA was isolated from indicated cells and tissues using the RNeasy Kit from QIAgen (Germantown, MD, USA), and used to generate cDNA for use in qRT-PCR assays as described (96). 12/15-LO expression in mouse cells was assessed by a SYBR green protocol, and compared to a newly available *Alox15* Taqman probe (Thermofisher Scientific, Waltham, MA, USA). Expression was tested in two independent experiments using five mice per group for each experiment.

Western Blotting

Cell lysates from the NK92 human NK cell line was used as a source of proteins to measure level human 12-LO levels using the Odyssey LI-COR system (Lincoln, NE, USA) as previously described (61). Nuclear and cytosolic proteins were fractionated and tested separately. Duplicate samples were stained with antibodies recognizing tubulin, ALOX12S, and ALOX15-1.

Immunofluorescence

Formalin-fixed, paraffin-embedded tissues sections from human pancreas tissues (obtained through nPOD) were stained as described with antibodies to glucagon (DAKO, Copenhagen, Denmark), and the NKp46 Ligand (using the NKp46 Fc chimera, R&D Systems, Minneapolis, MN, USA) as described previously (48), with a modification using tyramide amplification (Perkin Elmer, Waltham, MA, USA) to amplify NKp46 Fc staining. Islet area was determined, and the intensity of NKp46 Fc staining within the islet area was calculated using NIH Image J. Data are expressed as density of NKp46 Fc staining per islet area for ND, autoantibody positive, and T1D donor ($n = 3$ donors per group), which is calculated with the following equation: [Integrated density − (area of selected cell × mean fluorescence of background readings)]/total islet area = average fluorescence per islet.

Statistical Procedures

Statistically significant differences were determined by the use of Student's *t*-test where appropriate, or ANOVA followed by *post hoc* testing. Significant differences in all cases were determined by $p < 0.05$.

AUTHOR CONTRIBUTIONS

MM conceived the hypothesis outlined. MS and MM wrote the manuscript. MM, LG, and MS contributed to experimental design and data analysis. MS and LG critically reviewed the manuscript prior to submission.

ACKNOWLEDGMENTS

The authors wish to acknowledge the support of the Network for Pancreatic Organ Donors with Diabetes (nPOD), including Irina Kusmartseva. Additionally, this work was supported by a Junior Faculty Award from the American Diabetes Association (ADA#7-11-JF-33) and the Helmsley Charitable Trust George S. Eisenbarth nPOD Award for Team Science (#2015PG-TID052-668894).

REFERENCES

1. Ziegler A-G, Nepom GT. Prediction and pathogenesis in type 1 diabetes. *Immunity* (2010) 32:468–78. doi:10.1016/j.immuni.2010.03.018
2. Howson JMM, Walker NM, Clayton D, Todd JA, Type 1 Diabetes Genetics Consortium. Confirmation of HLA class II independent type 1 diabetes associations in the major histocompatibility complex including HLA-B and HLA-A. *Diabetes Obes Metab* (2009) 11:31–45. doi:10.1111/j.1463-1326.2008.01001.x
3. Noble JA, Erlich HA. Genetics of type 1 diabetes. *Cold Spring Harb Perspect Med.* (2012) 2:a007732. doi:10.1101/cshperspect.a007732
4. Abbas AK, Lichtman AH, Pillai S. Basic immunology: functions and disorders of the immune system. *Basic Immunol* (2012):303–5. doi:10.1007/978-1-62703-589-7_1
5. Morris MA, Satin-Smith M. Type 1 diabetes mellitus: is a cure in sight? In: Khardori R, Ullal J, Lieb DC, editors. *Diabetes Mellitus – Clinical Focus Series in Endocrinology*. Jaypee Brothers Medical Publishing (in press).

6. Størling J, Pociot F. Type 1 diabetes candidate genes linked to pancreatic islet cell inflammation and beta-cell apoptosis. *Genes (Basel)* (2017) 8:1–12. doi:10.3390/genes8020072
7. Waugh K, Snell-Bergeon J, Michels A, Dong F, Steck AK, Frohnert BI, et al. Increased inflammation is associated with islet autoimmunity and type 1 diabetes in the Diabetes Autoimmunity Study in the Young (DAISY). *PLoS One* (2017) 12:e0174840. doi:10.1371/journal.pone.0174840
8. Kracht MJ, van Lummel M, Nikolic T, Joosten AM, Laban S, van der Slik AR, et al. Autoimmunity against a defective ribosomal insulin gene product in type 1 diabetes. *Nat Med* (2017) 23:501–7. doi:10.1038/nm.4289
9. Tersey SA, Nishiki Y, Templin AT, Cabrera SM, Stull ND, Colvin SC, et al. Islet β-cell endoplasmic reticulum stress precedes the onset of type 1 diabetes in the nonobese diabetic mouse model. *Diabetes* (2012) 61:818–27. doi:10.2337/db11-1293
10. Qin H, Lee IF, Panagiotopoulos C, Wang X, Chu AD, Utz PJ, et al. Natural killer cells from children with type 1 diabetes have defects in NKG2D-dependent function and signaling. *Diabetes* (2011) 60:857–66. doi:10.2337/db09-1706
11. Gamble DR, Taylor KW. Seasonal incidence of diabetes mellitus. *Br Med J* (1969) 3:631–3. doi:10.1136/bmj.3.5671.631
12. Gamble DR, Kinsley ML, FitzGerald MG, Bolton R, Taylor KW. Viral antibodies in diabetes mellitus. *Br Med J* (1969) 3:627–30. doi:10.1136/bmj.3.5671.627
13. Horwitz MS, Bradley LM, Harbertson J, Krahl T, Lee J, Sarvetnick N. Diabetes induced by *Coxsackie virus*: initiation by bystander damage and not molecular mimicry. *Nat Med* (1998) 4:781–5. doi:10.1038/nm0798-781
14. Lincez PJ, Shanina I, Horwitz MS. Reduced expression of the MDA5 gene IFIH1 prevents autoimmune diabetes. *Diabetes* (2015) 64:2184–93. doi:10.2337/db14-1223
15. McCall KD, Thuma JR, Courreges MC, Benencia F, James CB, Malgor R, et al. Toll-like receptor 3 is critical for coxsackievirus B4-induced type 1 diabetes in female nod mice. *Endocrinology* (2015) 156:453–61. doi:10.1210/en.2013-2006
16. Richer MJ, Lavallée DJ, Shanina I, Horwitz MS. Toll-like receptor 3 signalling on macrophages is required for survival following coxsackievirus B4 infection. *PLoS One* (2009) 4:e4127.doi:10.1371/journal.pone.0004127
17. Davydova B, Härkönen T, Kaialainen S, Hovi T, Vaarala O, Roivainen M. Coxsackievirus immunization delays onset of diabetes in non-obese diabetic mice. *J Med Virol* (2003) 69:510–20. doi:10.1002/jmv.10339
18. Serreze DV, Wasserfall C, Ottendorfer EW, Stalvey M, Pierce MA, Gauntt C, et al. Diabetes acceleration or prevention by a coxsackievirus B4 infection: critical requirements for both interleukin-4 and gamma interferon. *J Virol* (2005) 79:1045–52. doi:10.1128/JVI.79.2.1045-1052.2005
19. Gallagher GR, Brehm MA, Finberg RW, Barton BA, Shultz LD, Greiner DL, et al. Viral infection of engrafted human islets leads to diabetes. *Diabetes* (2015) 64:1358–69. doi:10.2337/db14-1020
20. Laiho JE, Oikarinen M, Richardson SJ, Frisk G, Nyalwidhe J, Burch TC, et al. Relative sensitivity of immunohistochemistry, multiple reaction monitoring mass spectrometry, in situ hybridization and PCR to detect Coxsackievirus B1 in A549 cells. *J Clin Virol* (2016) 77:21–8. doi:10.1016/j.jcv.2016.01.015
21. Hyöty H. Viruses in type 1 diabetes. *Pediatr Diabetes* (2016) 17(Suppl 22):56–64. doi:10.1111/pedi.12370
22. Honkanen H, Oikarinen S, Nurminen N, Laitinen OH, Huhtala H, Lehtonen J, et al. Detection of enteroviruses in stools precedes islet autoimmunity by several months: possible evidence for slowly operating mechanisms in virus-induced autoimmunity. *Diabetologia* (2017) 60:424–31. doi:10.1007/s00125-016-4177-z
23. Krogvold L, Edwin B, Buanes T, Frisk G, Skog O, Anagandula M, et al. Detection of a low-grade enteroviral infection in the islets of langerhans of living patients newly diagnosed with type 1 diabetes. *Diabetes* (2015) 64:1682–7. doi:10.2337/db14-1370
24. Richardson SJ, Willcox A, Bone AJ, Foulis AK, Morgan NG. The prevalence of enteroviral capsid protein vp1 immunostaining in pancreatic islets in human type 1 diabetes. *Diabetologia* (2009) 52:1143–51. doi:10.1007/s00125-009-1276-0
25. Robinson CM, Pfeiffer JK. Viruses and the microbiota. *Annu Rev Virol* (2014) 1:55–69. doi:10.1146/annurev-virology-031413-085550
26. Pellegrini S, Sordi V, Bolla AM, Saita D, Ferrarese R, Canducci F, et al. Duodenal mucosa of patients with type 1 diabetes shows distinctive inflammatory profile and microbiota. *J Clin Endocrinol Metab* (2017) 102:1468–77. doi:10.1210/jc.2016-3222
27. Oikarinen M, Tauriainen S, Oikarinen S, Honkanen T, Collin P, Rantala I, et al. Type 1 diabetes is associated with enterovirus infection in gut mucosa. *Diabetes* (2012) 61:687–91. doi:10.2337/db11-1157
28. Laitinen OH, Honkanen H, Pakkanen O, Oikarinen S, Hankaniemi MM, Huhtala H, et al. Coxsackievirus B1 is associated with induction of β-cells autoimmunity that portends type 1 diabetes. *Diabetes* (2014) 63:446–55. doi:10.2337/db13-0619
29. Hodik M, Anagandula M, Fuxe J, Krogvold L, Dahl-Jørgensen K, Hyöty H, et al. Coxsackie–adenovirus receptor expression is enhanced in pancreas from patients with type 1 diabetes. *BMJ Open Diabetes Res Care* (2016) 4:e000219. doi:10.1136/bmjdrc-2016-000219
30. Ylipaasto P, Klingel K, Lindberg AM, Otonkoski T, Kandolf R, Hovi T, et al. Enterovirus infection in human pancreatic islet cells, islet tropism in vivo and receptor involvement in cultured islet beta cells. *Diabetologia* (2004) 47:225–39. doi:10.1007/s00125-003-1297-z
31. Marré ML, Profozich JL, Coneybeer JT, Geng X, Bertera S, Ford MJ, et al. Inherent ER stress in pancreatic islet β cells causes self-recognition by autoreactive T cells in type 1 diabetes. *J Autoimmun* (2016) 72:33–46. doi:10.1016/j.jaut.2016.04.009
32. Richardson SJ, Rodriguez-Calvo T, Gerling IC, Mathews CE, Kaddis JS, Russell MA, et al. Islet cell hyperexpression of HLA class I antigens: a defining feature in type 1 diabetes. *Diabetologia* (2016) 59:2448–58. doi:10.1007/s00125-016-4067-4
33. Padgett LE, Broniowska KA, Hansen PA, Corbett JA, Tse HM. The role of reactive oxygen species and proinflammatory cytokines in type 1 diabetes pathogenesis. *Ann N Y Acad Sci* (2013) 1281:16–35. doi:10.1111/j.1749-6632.2012.06826.x
34. Fallahi P, Corrado A, Di Domenicantonio A, Frenzilli G, Antonelli A, Ferrari SM. CXCR3, CXCR5, CXCR6, and CXCR7 in diabetes. *Curr Drug Targets* (2016) 17:515–9. doi:10.2174/1389450115666141229153949
35. Driver JP, Racine JJ, Ye C, Lamont DJ, Newby BN, Leeth CM, et al. Interferon-γ limits diabetogenic CD8+ T-cell effector responses in type 1 diabetes. *Diabetes* (2017) 66:710–21. doi:10.2337/db16-0846
36. Hultgren B, Huang X, Dybdal N, Stewart TA. Genetic absence of gamma-interferon delays but does not prevent diabetes in NOD mice. *Diabetes* (1996) 45:812–7. doi:10.2337/diab.45.6.812
37. Wang B, André I, Gonzalez A, Katz JD, Aguet M, Benoist C, et al. Interferon-gamma impacts at multiple points during the progression of autoimmune diabetes. *Proc Natl Acad Sci U S A* (1997) 94:13844–9. doi:10.1073/pnas.94.25.13844
38. Angelo LS, Banerjee PP, Monaco-Shawver L, Rosen JB, Makedonas G, Forbes LR, et al. Practical NK cell phenotyping and variability in healthy adults. *Immunol Res* (2015) 62:341–56. doi:10.1007/s12026-015-8664-y
39. Marçais A, Viel S, Grau M, Henry T, Marvel J, Walzer T. Regulation of mouse NK cell development and function by cytokines. *Front Immunol* (2013) 4:1–4. doi:10.3389/fimmu.2013.00450
40. Zhang C, Tian Z. NK cell subsets in autoimmune diseases. *J Autoimmun* (2017) 83:22–30. doi:10.1016/j.jaut.2017.02.005
41. Reefman E, Kay JG, Wood SM, Offenhäuser C, Brown DL, Roy S, et al. Cytokine secretion is distinct from secretion of cytotoxic granules in NK cells. *J Immunol* (2010) 184:4852–62. doi:10.4049/jimmunol.0803954
42. Spits H, Lanier LL. Natural killer or dendritic: what's in a name? *Immunity* (2007) 26:11–6. doi:10.1016/j.immuni.2007.01.004
43. Homann D, Jahreis A, Wolfe T, Hughes A, Coon B, van Stipdonk MJ, et al. CD40L blockade prevents autoimmune diabetes by induction of bitypic NK/DC regulatory cells. *Immunity* (2002) 16:403–15. doi:10.1016/S1074-7613(02)00290-X
44. Hanna J, Gonen-Gross T, Fitchett J, Rowe T, Daniels M, Arnon TI, et al. Novel APC-like properties of human NK cells directly regulate T cell activation. *J Clin Invest* (2004) 114:1612–23. doi:10.1172/JCI22787
45. Ljunggren HG, Kärre K. In search of the 'missing self': MHC molecules and NK cell recognition. *Immunol Today* (1990) 11:237–44. doi:10.1016/0167-5699(90)90097-S
46. Seliger B, Ritz U, Ferrone S. Molecular mechanisms of HLA class I antigen abnormalities following viral infection and transformation. *Int J Cancer* (2006) 118:129–38. doi:10.1002/ijc.21312
47. Foulis A, Farquharson M, Meager A. Immunoreactive α-interferon in insulin-secreting β cells in type 1 diabetes mellitus. *Lancet* (1987) 2(8573):1423–7. doi:10.1016/S0140-6736(87)91128-7

48. Mandelboim O, Lieberman N, Lev M, Paul L, Arnon TI, Bushkin Y, et al. Recognition of haemagglutinins on virus-infected cells by NKp46 activates lysis by human NK cells. *Nature* (2001) 409:1055–60. doi:10.1038/35059110
49. Magri G, Muntasell A, Romo N, Sáez-Borderías A, Pende D, Geraghty DE, et al. NKp46 and DNAM-1 NK cell receptors drive the response to human cytomegalovirus infected myeloid dendritic cells overcoming viral immune evasion strategies. *Blood* (2011) 117:848–56. doi:10.1182/blood-2010-08-301374
50. Pegram HJ, Andrews DM, Smyth MJ, Darcy PK, Kershaw MH. Activating and inhibitory receptors of natural killer cells. *Immunol Cell Biol* (2011) 89:216–24. doi:10.1038/icb.2010.78
51. Flodström M, Maday A, Balakrishna D, Cleary MM, Yoshimura A, Sarvetnick N. Target cell defense prevents the development of diabetes after viral infection. *Nat Immunol* (2002) 3:373–82. doi:10.1038/ni771
52. Morris MA, Ley K. Trafficking of natural killer cells. *Curr Mol Med* (2004) 4:431–8. doi:10.2174/1566524043360609
53. Pang G, Buret A, Batey RT, Chen QY, Couch L, Cripps A, et al. Morphological, phenotypic and functional characteristics of a pure population of CD56+ CD16- CD3- large granular lymphocytes generated from human duodenal mucosa. *Immunology* (1993) 79:498–505.
54. Eiras P, Leon F, Camarero C, Lombardia M, Roldan E, Bootello A, et al. Intestinal intraepithelial lymphocytes contain a CD3- CD7+ subset expressing natural killer markers and a singular pattern of adhesion molecules. *Scand J Immunol* (2000) 52:1–6. doi:10.1046/j.1365-3083.2000.00761.x
55. Ivanova D, Krempels R, Ryfe J, Weitzman K, Stephenson D, Gigley JP. NK cells in mucosal defense against infection. *Biomed Res Int* (2014) 2014:413982. doi:10.1155/2014/413982
56. Brauner H, Elemans M, Lemos S, Broberger C, Holmberg D, Flodström-Tullberg M, et al. Distinct phenotype and function of NK cells in the pancreas of nonobese diabetic mice. *J Immunol* (2010) 184:2272–80. doi:10.4049/jimmunol.0804358
57. Willcox A, Richardson SJ, Bone AJ, Foulis AK, Morgan NG. Analysis of islet inflammation in human type 1 diabetes. *Clin Exp Immunol* (2009) 155:173–81. doi:10.1111/j.1365-2249.2008.03860.x
58. Dotta F, Censini S, van Halteren AG, Marselli L, Masini M, Dionisi S, et al. Coxsackie B4 virus infection of β cells and natural killer cell insulitis in recent-onset type 1 diabetic patients. *Proc Natl Acad Sci U S A* (2007) 104:5115–20. doi:10.1073/pnas.0700442104
59. Campbell-Thompson M, Fu A, Kaddis JS, Wasserfall C, Schatz DA, Pugliese A, et al. Insulitis and β-cell mass in the natural history of type 1 diabetes. *Diabetes* (2016) 65:719–31. doi:10.2337/db15-0779
60. Ishigaki K, Kochi Y, Suzuki A, Tsuchida Y, Tsuchiya H, Sumitomo S, et al. Polygenic burdens on cell-specific pathways underlie the risk of rheumatoid arthritis. *Nat Genet* (2017) 49(7):1120–5. doi:10.1038/ng.3885
61. McDuffie M, Maybee NA, Keller SR, Stevens BK, Garmey JC, Morris MA, et al. Nonobese diabetic (NOD) mice congenic for a targeted deletion of 12/15-lipoxygenase are protected from autoimmune diabetes. *Diabetes* (2008) 57:199–208. doi:10.2337/db07-0830
62. Jansen A, Homo-Delarche F, Hooijkaas H, Leenen PJ, Dardenne M, Drexhage HA. Immunohistochemical characterization of monocytes-macrophages and dendritic cells involved in the initiation of the insulitis and beta-cell destruction in NOD mice. *Diabetes* (1994) 43:667–75. doi:10.2337/diab.43.5.667
63. Gur C, Porgador A, Elboim M, Gazit R, Mizrahi S, Stern-Ginossar N, et al. The activating receptor NKp46 is essential for the development of type 1 diabetes. *Nat Immunol* (2010) 11:121–8. doi:10.1038/ni.1834
64. Zhang C, Zhang J, Niu J, Zhou Z, Zhang J, Tian Z. Interleukin-12 improves cytotoxicity of natural killer cells via upregulated expression of NKG2D. *Hum Immunol* (2008) 69:490–500. doi:10.1016/j.humimm.2008.06.004
65. Ryba-Stanislawowska M, Rybarczyk-Kapturska K, Mysliwiec M, Mysliwska J. Elevated levels of serum IL-12 and IL-18 are associated with lower frequencies of CD4(+)CD25 (high)FOXP3 (+) regulatory t cells in young patients with type 1 diabetes. *Inflammation* (2014) 37:1513–20. doi:10.1007/s10753-014-9878-1
66. Altinova AE, Yetkin I, Akbay E, Bukan N, Arslan M. Serum IL-18 levels in patients with type 1 diabetes: relations to metabolic control and microvascular complications. *Cytokine* (2008) 42:217–21. doi:10.1016/j.cyto.2008.02.006
67. Frigerio S, Holländer GA, Zumsteg U. Functional IL-18 is produced by primary pancreatic mouse islets and NIT-1 beta cells and participates in the progression towards destructive insulitis. *Horm Res* (2002) 57:94–104.
68. Suwanai H, Wilcox MA, Mathis D, Benoist C. A defective Il15 allele underlies the deficiency in natural killer cell activity in nonobese diabetic mice. *Proc Natl Acad Sci U S A* (2010) 107:9305–10. doi:10.1073/pnas.1004492107
69. Sun JC, Ma A, Lanier LL. Cutting edge: IL-15-independent NK cell response to mouse cytomegalovirus infection. *J Immunol* (2009) 183:2911–4. doi:10.4049/jimmunol.0901872
70. Lieberman LA, Villegas EN, Hunter CA. Interleukin-15-deficient mice develop protective immunity to Toxoplasma gondii. *Infect Immun* (2004) 72:6729–32. doi:10.1128/IAI.72.11.6729-6732.2004
71. Poggi A, Zocchi MR. Antigen presenting cells and stromal cells trigger human natural killer lymphocytes to autoreactivity: evidence for the involvement of natural cytotoxicity receptors (NCR) and NKG2D. *Clin Dev Immunol* (2006) 13:325–36. doi:10.1080/17402520600578194
72. Ogasawara K, Hamerman JA, Ehrlich LR, Bour-Jordan H, Santamaria P, Bluestone JA, et al. NKG2D blockade prevents autoimmune diabetes in NOD mice. *Immunity* (2004) 20:757–67. doi:10.1016/j.immuni.2004.05.008
73. Ogasawara K, Hamerman JA, Hsin H, Chikuma S, Bour-Jordan H, Chen T, et al. Impairment of NK cell function by NKG2D modulation in NOD mice. *Immunity* (2003) 18:41–51. doi:10.1016/S1074-7613(02)00505-8
74. Maier LM, Howlett SK, Rainbow KM, Clark J, Howson JM, Todd JA, et al. NKG2D-RAE-1 receptor-ligand variation does not account for the NK cell defect in nonobese diabetic mice. *J Immunol* (2008) 181:7073–80. doi:10.4049/jimmunol.181.10.7073
75. Foster CE, Colonna M, Sun PD. Crystal structure of the human natural killer (NK) cell activating receptor NKp46 reveals structural relationship to other leukocyte receptor complex immunoreceptors. *J Biol Chem* (2003) 278:46081–6. doi:10.1074/jbc.M308491200
76. Ponassi M, Cantoni C, Biassoni R, Conte R, Spallarossa A, Pesce A, et al. Structure of the human NK cell triggering receptor NKp46 ectodomain. *Biochem Biophys Res Commun* (2003) 309:317–23. doi:10.1016/j.bbrc.2003.08.007
77. Rahier J, Goebbels RM, Henquin JC. Cellular composition of the human diabetic pancreas. *Diabetologia* (1983) 24:366–71. doi:10.1007/BF00251826
78. Stefan Y, Orci L, Malaisse-Lagae F, Perrelet A, Patel Y, Unger RH. Quantitation of endocrine cell content in the pancreas of nondiabetic and diabetic humans. *Diabetes* (1982) 31:694–700. doi:10.2337/diab.31.8.694
79. Belanger S, Tai L-H, Anderson SK, Makrigiannis AP. Ly49 cluster sequence analysis in a mouse model of diabetes: an expanded repertoire of activating receptors in the NOD genome. *Genes Immun* (2008) 9:509–21. doi:10.1038/gene.2008.43
80. van der Slik AR, Koeleman BP, Verduijn W, Bruining GJ, Roep BO, Giphart MJ. KIR in type 1 diabetes: disparate distribution of activating and inhibitory natural killer cell receptors in patients versus HLA-matched control subjects. *Diabetes* (2003) 52:2639–42. doi:10.2337/diabetes.52.10.2639
81. Rodacki M, Svoren B, Butty V, Besse W, Laffel L, Benoist C, et al. Altered natural killer cells in type 1 diabetic patients. *Diabetes* (2007) 56:177–85. doi:10.2337/db06-0493
82. Beilke JN, Meagher CT, Hosiawa K, Champsaur M, Bluestone JA, Lanier LL. NK cells are not required for spontaneous autoimmune diabetes in NOD mice. *PLoS One* (2012) 7:e36011. doi:10.1371/journal.pone.0036011
83. Keppel MP, Saucier N, Mah AY, Vogel TP, Cooper MA. Activation-specific metabolic requirements for NK Cell IFN-γ production. *J Immunol* (2015) 194:1954–62. doi:10.4049/jimmunol.1402099
84. Dobrian AD, Lieb DC, Cole BK, Taylor-Fishwick DA, Chakrabarti SK, Nadler JL. Functional and pathological roles of the 12- and 15-lipoxygenases. *Prog Lipid Res* (2011) 50:115–31. doi:10.1016/j.plipres.2010.10.005
85. Kuhn H, O'Donnell VB. Inflammation and immune regulation by 12/15-lipoxygenases. *Prog Lipid Res* (2006) 45:334–56. doi:10.1016/j.plipres.2006.02.003
86. Cole BK, Kuhn NS, Green-Mitchell SM, Leone KA, Raab RM, Nadler JL, et al. 12/15-Lipoxygenase signaling in the endoplasmic reticulum stress response. *Am J Physiol Endocrinol Metab* (2012) 302:E654–65. doi:10.1152/ajpendo.00373.2011

87. Dioszeghy V, Rosas M, Maskrey BH, Colmont C, Topley N, Chaitidis P, et al. 12/15-Lipoxygenase regulates the inflammatory response to bacterial products in vivo. *J Immunol* (2008) 181:6514–24. doi:10.4049/jimmunol.181.9.6514
88. Liang Y, Pan H-F, Ye D-Q. Therapeutic potential of STAT4 in autoimmunity. *Expert Opin Ther Targets* (2014) 18:945–60. doi:10.1517/13543776.2014.971754
89. Nepom GT, Ehlers M, Mandrup-Poulsen T. Anti-cytokine therapies in T1D: concepts and strategies. *Clin Immunol* (2013) 149:279–85. doi:10.1016/j.clim.2013.02.003
90. Pope RM, Shahrara S. Possible roles of IL-12-family cytokines in rheumatoid arthritis. *Nat Rev Rheumatol* (2013) 9:252–6. doi:10.1038/nrrheum.2012.170
91. Gondek T, Szajewski M, Szefel J, Aleksandrowicz-Wrona E, Skrzypczak-Jankun E, Jankun J, et al. Evaluation of 12-lipoxygenase (12-LOX) and plasminogen activator inhibitor 1 (pai-1) as prognostic markers in prostate cancer. *Biomed Res Int* (2014) 2014:102478. doi:10.1155/2014/102478
92. Kang KH, Ling TY, Liou HH, Huang YK, Hour MJ, Liou HC, et al. Enhancement role of host 12/15-lipoxygenase in melanoma progression. *Eur J Cancer* (2013) 49:2747–59. doi:10.1016/j.ejca.2013.03.030
93. Mabalirajan U, Rehman R, Ahmad T, Kumar S, Leishangthem GD, Singh S, et al. 12/15-lipoxygenase expressed in non-epithelial cells causes airway epithelial injury in asthma. *Sci Rep* (2013) 3:1540. doi:10.1038/srep01540
94. Imai Y, Dobrian AD, Weaver JR, Butcher MJ, Cole BK, Galkina EV, et al. Interaction between cytokines and inflammatory cells in islet dysfunction, insulin resistance and vascular disease. *Diabetes Obes Metab* (2013) 15:117–29. doi:10.1111/dom.12161
95. Yang Z, Chen M, Ellett JD, Fialkow LB, Carter JD, McDuffie M, et al. Autoimmune diabetes is blocked in Stat4-deficient mice. *J Autoimmun* (2004) 22:191–200. doi:10.1016/j.jaut.2003.08.006
96. Green-Mitchell SM, Tersey SA, Cole BK, Ma K, Kuhn NS, Cunningham TD, et al. Deletion of 12/15-lipoxygenase alters macrophage and islet function in NOD-Alox15null mice, leading to protection against type 1 diabetes development. *PLoS One* (2013) 8:e56763. doi:10.1371/journal.pone.0056763
97. Martínez-Clemente M, Ferré N, Titos E, Horrillo R, González-Périz A, Morán-Salvador E, et al. Disruption of the 12/15-lipoxygenase gene (Alox15) protects hyperlipidemic mice from nonalcoholic fatty liver disease. *Hepatology* (2010) 52:1980–91. doi:10.1002/hep.23928
98. Ma K, Nunemaker CS, Wu R, Chakrabarti SK, Taylor-Fishwick DA, Nadler JL. 12-Lipoxygenase products reduce insulin secretion and {beta}-cell viability in human islets. *J Clin Endocrinol Metab* (2010) 95:887–93. doi:10.1210/jc.2009-1102
99. Grzesik WJ, Nadler JL, Machida Y, Nadler JL, Imai Y, Morris MA. Expression pattern of 12-lipoxygenase in human islets with type 1 diabetes and type 2 diabetes. *J Clin Endocrinol Metab* (2015) 100:E387–95. doi:10.1210/jc.2014-3630
100. Leung KH, Ip MM, Koren HS. Regulation of human natural killing. IV. Role of lipoxygenase in regulation of natural killing activity. *Scand J Immunol* (1986) 24(4):371–80. doi:10.1111/j.1365-3083.1986.tb02124.x
101. Lee S-H, Fragoso MF, Biron CA. Cutting edge: a novel mechanism bridging innate and adaptive immunity: IL-12 induction of CD25 to form high-affinity IL-2 receptors on NK cells. *J Immunol* (2012) 189:2712–6. doi:10.4049/jimmunol.1201528
102. Chang HC, Lewis D, Tung CY, Han L, Henriquez SM, Voiles L, et al. Soypeptide lunasin in cytokine immunotherapy for lymphoma. *Cancer Immunol Immunother* (2014) 63:283–95. doi:10.1007/s00262-013-1513-8
103. Sun JC, Madera S, Bezman NA, Beilke JN, Kaplan MH, Lanier LL. Proinflammatory cytokine signaling required for the generation of natural killer cell memory. *J Exp Med* (2012) 209:947–54. doi:10.1084/jem.20111760
104. Duluc D, Tan F, Scotet M, Blanchard S, Frémaux I, Garo E, et al. PolyI:C plus IL-2 or IL-12 induce IFN-gamma production by human NK cells via autocrine IFN-beta. *Eur J Immunol* (2009) 39:2877–84. doi:10.1002/eji.200838610
105. Jaime-Ramirez AC, Mundy-Bosse BL, Kondadasula S, Jones NB, Roda JM, Mani A, et al. IL-12 enhances the antitumor actions of trastuzumab via NK cell IFN- production. *J Immunol* (2011) 186:3401–9. doi:10.4049/jimmunol.1000328
106. Trembleau S, Penna G, Bosi E, Mortara A, Gately MK, Adorini L. Interleukin 12 administration induces T helper type 1 cells and accelerates autoimmune diabetes in NOD mice. *J Exp Med* (1995) 181:817–21. doi:10.1084/jem.181.2.817
107. Trembleau S, Penna G, Gregori S, Chapman HD, Serreze DV, Magram J, et al. Pancreas-infiltrating Th1 cells and diabetes develop in IL-12-deficient nonobese diabetic mice. *J Immunol* (1999) 163:2960–8.
108. Tsai S, Santamaria P. MHC class II polymorphisms, autoreactive T-cells, and autoimmunity. *Front Immunol* (2013) 4(321):1–7. doi:10.3389/fimmu.2013.00321
109. Delong T, Wiles TA, Baker RL, Bradley B, Barbour G, Reisdorph R, et al. Pathogenic CD4 T cells in type 1 diabetes recognize epitopes formed by peptide fusion. *Science* (2016) 351:711–4. doi:10.1126/science.aad2791
110. Marré ML, James EA, Piganelli JD. β cell ER stress and the implications for immunogenicity in type 1 diabetes. *Front Cell Dev Biol* (2015) 3:67. doi:10.3389/fcell.2015.00067
111. Cook KD, Waggoner SN, Whitmire JK. NK cells and their ability to modulate T cells during virus infections. *Crit Rev Immunol* (2014) 34:359–88. doi:10.1615/CritRevImmunol.2014010604
112. Ma X, Yan W, Zheng H, Du Q, Zhang L, Ban Y, et al. Regulation of IL-10 and IL-12 production and function in macrophages and dendritic cells [version 1; referees: 3 approved]. *F1000Res* (2015) 4(F1000 Faculty Rev):1465. doi:10.12688/f1000research.7010.1

5

Mapping T Cell Responses to Native and Neo-Islet Antigen Epitopes in at Risk and Type 1 Diabetes Subjects

Sefina Arif, Irma Pujol-Autonell, Yogesh Kamra, Evangelia Williams, Norkhairin Yusuf, Clara Domingo-Vila, Yasaman Shahrabi, Emily Pollock, Leena Khatri, Mark Peakman, Timothy Tree and Anna Lorenc*

Department of Immunobiology, King's College London, Guy's Hospital, London, United Kingdom

***Correspondence:**
Sefina Arif
Sefina.arif@kcl.ac.uk

Aims: Recent studies highlight the potentially important role of neoepitopes in breaking immune tolerance in type 1 diabetes. T cell reactivity to these neoepitopes has been reported, but how this response compares quantitatively and phenotypically with previous reports on native epitopes is not known. Thus, an understanding of the relationship between native and neoepitopes and their role as tolerance breakers or disease drivers in type 1 diabetes is required. We set out to compare T cell reactivity and phenotype against a panel of neo- and native islet autoantigenic epitopes to examine how this relates to stages of type 1 diabetes development.

Methods: Fifty-four subjects comprising patients with T1D, and autoantibody-positive unaffected family members were tested against a panel of neo- and native epitopes by ELISPOT (IFN-γ, IL-10, and IL-17). A further subset of two patients was analyzed by Single Cell Immune Profiling (RNAseq and TCR α/β) after stimulation with pools of native and neoepitope peptides.

Results: T cell responses to native and neoepitopes were present in patients with type 1 diabetes and at-risk subjects, and overall, there were no significant differences in the frequency, magnitude, or phenotype between the two sets of peptide stimuli. Single cell RNAseq on responder T cells revealed a similar profile in T1D patients stimulated with either neo- or native epitopes. A pro-inflammatory gene expression profile (TNF-α, IFN-γ) was dominant in both native and neoepitope stimulated T cells. TCRs with identical clonotypes were found in T cell responding to both native and neoepitopes.

Conclusion/Interpretation: These data suggest that in peripheral blood, T cell responses to both native and neoepitopes are similar in terms of frequency and phenotype in patients with type 1 diabetes and high-risk unaffected family members. Furthermore, using a combination of transcriptomic and clonotypic analyses, albeit using a limited panel of peptides, we show that neoepitopes are comparable to native epitopes currently in use for immune-monitoring studies.

Keywords: neoepitopes, T cells, cytokines, T cell receptor, genes, type 1 diabetes, autoantibody, transcriptome

INTRODUCTION

Type 1 diabetes arises as a result of immune-mediated loss of β cell mass and function. A lack of self-tolerance against islet autoantigens facilitates this destruction; one of the hallmarks of type 1 diabetes pathogenesis is the autoantigen-specific clonal expansion of T cells (1). Upon stimulation with peptides of islet autoantigens, these T cells respond and secrete cytokines such as interferon-γ, IL-10, and IL-17 which can be measured in subjects with type 1 diabetes and used to illustrate the heterogeneity of the disease (2–4) Furthermore, T cell responses elicited against peptides of proinsulin distinguish age-related heterogeneity in type 1 diabetes pathogenesis (4). Previous studies have suggested that T cell epitopes such as proinsulin peptide C13–32 elicit pro-inflammatory responses in approximately 70% of patients (4), and responses to this epitope can also be detected in autoantibody-positive unaffected family members (3).

Recent studies have highlighted the role of the β cell in orchestrating its own sustained attrition and demise by enabling a repertoire of non-germline encoded "neoepitopes" previously not encountered by the immune system (5).

Neoepitopes in T1D can be generated through several mechanisms including post-translational modification of peptides, for example *via* enzymatic deamidation or citrullination which can augment binding to HLA molecules and boost T cell responses (6); alternative RNA-splicing results in proteins being encoded from an alternative open reading frame (7) and peptide fusion of islet-derived peptides (8). Peptide fusion is a post-translational modification in which peptide fragments of proteins such as proinsulin are modified through fusion with peptides from other secretory granule proteins resulting in novel peptidic species termed hybrid insulin peptides (HIPs).

The fact that neoepitope specific T cells have been isolated from the islets of subjects with type 1 diabetes after death (8, 9) has provided a strong implication that these antigenic drivers and T cells directed against them could be relevant to disease pathology.

Similarly, T cell reactivity to neoepitopes such as modified glucose-regulated protein 78 (GRP78), HIPS and post-translationally modified GAD peptides has been demonstrated in the peripheral blood of subjects with type 1 diabetes and is observed in a greater frequency in these individuals compared to healthy donors (10–12).

In some cases, reactivity to neoepitopes has been shown to be more enhanced than that directed to the native epitopes (10, 12); for example, CD4 T cells directed against citrullinated GRP78 elicited T cell responses at a greater frequency in patients compared to the native epitope. Thus, growing evidence suggests that neoepitopes are relevant in type 1 diabetes pathology, but whether these are germane to the pathological response, are early drivers of disease or arise secondarily, and whether they serve as biomarkers remain issues to be addressed.

It is not clear how T cell responses to native and neoepitopes interlink and indeed which comes first; hence, an understanding of the relationship between native and neoepitopes and their role as tolerance breakers or disease drivers in type 1 diabetes is required. In order to gain this knowledge, both sets of epitopes need to be tested in parallel on the same patient cohorts.

In this study, we set out to evaluate T cell response to neoepitopes and established native epitopes in patients with type 1 diabetes and high-risk autoantibody-positive non-diabetic subjects to determine whether an epitope hierarchy exists. We then proceed to analyze T cells responding to native and neoepitopes at the single cell level and compare TCR usage to help address the phenotypic, transcriptomic, and clonal nature of the responses.

METHODS

Subjects

Blood was obtained from 54 subjects, 41 of whom had type 1 diabetes, and 13 subjects comprised of autoantibody-positive unaffected family members (UFMs); both groups consisted of children (≤16 years of age) and adults (≥16 years of age). In the type 1 diabetes group there were 14 participants in the group comprising of children (disease duration <1.5 months; median age 11 years; nine males) and 27 in the adult group (disease duration <8 months; median age 24 years; 14 males). In the UFM, there were five children (median age 11; 5 males) and eight adults (median age 37; six males). Forty-six subjects were recruited through the INNODIA natural history study (13). HLA and autoantibody data on all the subjects are shown in **Table 1**.

In addition, to examine the immune signature at the single cell level using transcriptomics, we obtained 130–160 ml of blood from two of the subjects with type 1 diabetes described above (two females, ages 30 and 34 years; duration of diabetes: 6 and 12 months) and identified as ND01 and ND02.

Ethical approval for this study was granted by the Ethics committee and institutional review board, and informed consent/assent was obtained from all subjects enrolled or their guardians.

Detection of β-Cell-Specific CD4+ T Cells by Cytokine ELISPOT

Peptides representing native proinsulin epitopes (PIPs) or neoepitopes: hybrid insulin peptides (HIPs) (PIPs: C13–32; C19-A3; C22-A5, and HIPs: C peptide-IAPP1; C peptide-IAPP2; C peptide-NPY) were synthesized and purified by high-performance liquid chromatography (Thermo Hybaid, Germany).

Interferon-γ (IFN-γ), interleukin-17A (IL-17A), and IL-10 production by CD4+ T cells was detected by enzyme-linked immunospot (ELISPOT) assay, performed as described previously (2, 4), in triplicate for each peptide. Briefly, fresh PBMCs supplemented with peptide were dispensed into 48-well plates at a density of 3×10^6 in 0.5 ml RPMI-1640 supplemented with antibiotics (TC medium; Life Technologies Ltd.) and 10% human AB serum (Sigma, Dorset, United Kingdom) and incubated at 37°C to a final concentration of 10 µg/ml. Control

TABLE 1 | HLA and autoantibody status of subjects with type 1 diabetes and unaffected family members (UFM).

Subject	HLA-DR/DQ				AUTOANTIBODIES			
	DR4+	**DQ8+**	**DR3+**	**DQ2+**	**IAA**	**GADA**	**IA2A**	**ZnT8A**
ND01	N	N	Y	Y	NEG	POS	NEG	POS
ND02	Y	Y	Y	Y	POS	NEG	NEG	NEG
ND03	Y	Y	N	N	N/A	N/A	N/A	N/A
ND04	N	N	Y	Y	N/A	N/A	N/A	N/A
ND05	N	N	Y	Y	POS	POS	POS	POS
ND06	N	N	Y	Y	POS	POS	POS	POS
ND07	N	N	Y	Y	POS	POS	POS	NEG
ND08	N	N	N	N	POS	POS	POS	POS
ND09	N	N	N	N	POS	NEG	NEG	NEG
ND10	N	N	N	N	NEG	NEG	NEG	NEG
ND11	N	N	Y	Y	POS	POS	POS	POS
ND12	N	N	N	N	POS	NEG	POS	POS
ND13	N	N	N	N	POS	POS	POS	NEG
ND14	N	N	N	N	POS	NEG	NEG	POS
ND15	N	N	Y	Y	NEG	POS	POS	POS
ND16	N	N	N	N	POS	POS	POS	POS
ND17	Y	N	N	N	NEG	POS	POS	POS
ND18	Y	Y	N	N	POS	POS	POS	POS
ND19	Y	Y	N	N	POS	NEG	POS	POS
ND20	Y	Y	Y	Y	POS	POS	POS	POS
ND21	Y	Y	Y	Y	POS	POS	POS	POS
ND22	Y	Y	Y	Y	NEG	POS	NEG	POS
ND23	Y	Y	N	N	POS	POS	NEG	POS
ND24	Y	Y	Y	Y	NEG	NEG	NEG	NEG
ND25	Y	Y	Y	Y	NEG	POS	NEG	NEG
ND26	Y	Y	Y	Y	POS	NEG	NEG	NEG
ND27	Y	Y	Y	Y	POS	POS	NEG	NEG
ND28	Y	N	N	N	POS	POS	NEG	POS
ND29	Y	Y	Y	Y	NEG	POS	NEG	POS
ND30	Y	N	N	N	POS	NEG	NEG	NEG
ND31	Y	Y	N	N	POS	NEG	POS	NEG
ND32	Y	Y	N	N	POS	POS	POS	NEG
ND33	Y	Y	Y	Y	POS	POS	POS	POS
ND34	Y	Y	Y	Y	NEG	POS	POS	POS
ND35	Y	Y	Y	Y	POS	POS	POS	POS
ND36	N	N	Y	Y	NEG	POS	POS	NEG
ND37	Y	Y	N	N	NEG	POS	NEG	NEG
ND38	Y	Y	N	N	N/A	POS	POS	POS
ND39	Y	Y	N	N	N/A	POS	POS	NEG
ND40	Y	Y	N	N	N/A	POS	POS	N/A
ND41	Y	Y	Y	Y	N/A	GAD	NEG	N/A
UFM01	N	N	N	N	NEG	POS	NEG	NEG
UFM02	Y	Y	N	N	POS	NEG	NEG	NEG
UFM03	N	N	Y	Y	NEG	NEG	POS	NEG
UFM04	N	N	Y	Y	NEG	POS	POS	POS
UFM05	N	N	Y	Y	NEG	POS	NEG	NEG
UFM06	Y	Y	N	N	POS	NEG	NEG	NEG
UFM07	N	N	Y	Y	NEG	POS	NEG	NEG
UFM08	Y	Y	N	N	NEG	POS	NEG	NEG
UFM09	Y	Y	N	N	POS	NEG	NEG	NEG
UFM10	N	N	Y	Y	POS	NEG	NEG	NEG
UFM11	N	N	Y	Y	POS	POS	POS	POS
UFM12	N/A	N/A	N/A	N/A	NEG	POS	NEG	NEG
UFM13	N	N	Y	Y	NEG	POS	POS	POS

wells contained TC medium with an equivalent concentration of peptide diluent alone (DMSO). Pediacel, a penta-vaccine, was obtained from Sanofi Pasteur Ltd. (Guildford, U.K.) and used at 1 µl/ml to examine anamnestic responses induced by vaccination or infection as previously described (4).

Pre-warmed TC medium/10% AB serum was added 24 h later, and 48 h after stimulation, cells were washed and resuspended in TC medium containing 10% human AB serum and brought to a concentration of 10^6/300 µl; 100 µl was dispensed in triplicate into wells of 96-well ELISA plates

(Nunc Maxisorp; Merck Ltd., Poole, United Kingdom) pre-blocked with 1% BSA in PBS and precoated with monoclonal anti-IFN-γ, anti-IL-10, or anti-IL17 capture Ab (U-Cytech, Utrecht, The Netherlands). After capture at 37°C for 20–22 h, plates were washed in PBS/Tween 20, and spots developed according to the manufacturer's instructions. Plates were dried, and spots of 80–120 µm were counted in a BioReader 3000 (BioSys, Karben, Germany), and data were expressed as stimulation index (SI) values (mean spot number of test peptide/mean spot number of diluent). The SI takes account of background, spontaneous responsiveness in the negative control, and ROC plots can be used to assign cut-off values as described previously; SI values ≥3 was taken to indicate a positive response for IFN-γ and IL-10 and ≥2 for IL-17A.

We have previously demonstrated that CD4+ T cells elicit the responses to the native peptides used in this assay by showing that depleting CD4+ cells abolished the cytokine responses (14).

Isolation and Single Cell Transcriptional Profiling of β-Cell-Specific CD4+ T Cells

Peptides were pooled into two groups, those consisting of native epitopes in one and neoepitopes in the second group. The pools comprised of the three proinsulin peptides and included peptides of GAD (115–127 and 265–284) in the native group (pool 1) and deamidated and citrullinated versions of these in the neoepitopes pool [GAD 115–127 (120E) and GAD 265–284 (272cit.)] together with C-peptide IAPP1 and C-peptide-NPY peptides (pool 2); these were synthesized and purified by high-performance liquid chromatography (Thermo Hybaid, Germany). Each of the two experiments was conducted using blood obtained from two individuals with type 1 diabetes; PBMCs at 2 × 10^6/ml were added to 20 wells of a 48-well plate; pool 1 peptides were added at a final concentration of 10 µg/ml to each well; this was repeated for an additional 20 wells where pool 2 was added at a final concentration of 10 µg/ml. Pediacel was used as positive control, and 1 µl/ml was added to a well containing cells at 2 × 10^6/ml, and medium alone was used as a negative control. Anti-CD40 (Biolegend, clone G28.5, 303611) was added at a final concentration of 2 µg/ml to each well, and the cells were incubated for 18–20 h.

The cells were then harvested and washed with phosphate buffered saline (PBS). An antibody staining master mix consisting of anti-CD19 (M5E2, 561391), anti-CD3 (SK7, 641415), anti-CD4 (SK3, 345768), anti-CD45-RO (UCHL1, 337168), anti-CD95 (DX2, 561978), anti-CD154 (TRAP1, 555700), anti-CD69 (FN50, 555530) (BD Biosciences, Oxford, UK), and anti-CD27 [(O323, 302830) Biolegend, London UK] was prepared and spilt into five tubes. Anti-human Hashtag 1 (TotalSeqC 0251), anti-human Hashtag 2 (TotalSeqC 0252), anti-human Hashtag 3 (TotalSeqC 0253), anti-human Hashtag 4 (TotalSeqC 0254), and anti-human Hashtag 5 (TotalSeqC 0255) (Biolegend, London, UK) were added at a concentration of 0.1 µg/µl to each of the five tubes. The hashtags were used to barcode the samples as follows: patient 1 pool 1 (Hashtag 1); patient 1 pool 2 (Hashtag 2) patient 2 pool 1 (Hashtag 3); patient 2 pool 2 (Hashtag 4), and Pediacel (patients 1 and 2; Hashtag 5).

The hashtag barcoded cells were incubated for 20 min in the dark and washed three times in FACS buffer (PBS with 3% FCS and 2% human AB) (both from Sigma, UK). CD4+ T cells responding to stimulation were identified by co-expression of CD69, and CD154 were sorted into 35 µl PBS using a BD FACSAria III cytometer as previously described (15).

Sorted cells were characterized using the 10× Chromium Controller Single-cell Immune Profiling system which simultaneously defines gene expression and T cell receptor profiles from single cells in the same sample; this was conducted at the Genomics facility at Guy's and St Thomas' Biomedical Research Centre. Briefly, single-cell suspensions were used to generate full-length cDNA in gel beads (containing Unique Molecular identifiers—UMI) in an emulsion master mix from 5′ V1 chemistry. The cDNA was amplified and subsequently size selected at the clean-up stage: smaller fragments were separated and stored for feature-barcoding/cell-hashing library preparation and the large fragments for gene expression (GEX) and T cell VDJ according to the manufacturer's instructions.

The GEX libraries were enzymatically fragmented and indexed while the T cell library was first enriched [using Chromium Single Cell V(D) J Enrichment Kit, Human T Cell, PN-1000005] and then fragmented and indexed for further sequencing. All the three final indexed libraries (feature barcoded + GEX + VDJ) were diluted to 4 nM concentrations and then pooled together at a ratio of 1:4:1 (feature barcoded library: GEX library: VDJ library) before being sequenced at 10 pM on HisSeq Rapid flow cell using an Illumina's HiSeq2500 instrument.

Cell ranger software (version 4) was used for calculating 5′ genes, and VDJ sequence construction and downstream secondary analysis were performed using Loupe Cell Browser (version 3.1.1.) and Seurat_3.2.2 in R (version 4.0.3).

Cell Ranger output was filtered to remove doublets, genes expressed in less than four cells, cells expressing less than 700 genes, and cells with more than 10% counts from mitochondrial gene transcription. We also eliminated all MAIT cells (identified by their TCR alpha TRAV1-2) and cells with double TCRB as potential doublets and cells identified as contaminating non-T cells in the first round of clustering. We then mapped all the remaining cells to a PBMC reference (16) (**Supplementary Figure 1**) with symphony and harmony and excluded all cells which, according to the outcome of knnPredict() function, were not CD4 T cells. We also assigned T cell subtypes whenever possible. Barcodes of cells used for the downstream analysis are included in **Supplementary File 1**.

For clustering purposes, each of 10× runs was split by individual and reintegrated with Seurat to remove individual effects.

Dimension reduction (PCA, UMAP) and clustering were performed on this cleaned dataset with exclusion of TCR, mitochondrial genes, and ribosomal protein genes. UMAP was performed on first 30 PCA axes and with 50 neighbors. Clusters were determined by SNN algorithm, with resolution of 0.2. Gene expression between clusters was compared with FindConservedMarkers() function in Seurat by MAST, and top genes (all with adjusted p values in each individual <0.0005 and fold change >2) are shown in **Figure 4C**. Comparison of gene expression between native and neoepitope pools was also performed in Seurat with MAST, with each individual included as a latent variable (results included in **Supplementary Table 1**).

Original Cell Ranger-reported clonotypes require all TCRB and TCRA chains of two cells to be identical to pertain to the same clone; we assumed that two cells are from the same TCR clone if they shared both TCR chains and there was no conflict in their B chains (so if they shared identical TCRA and TCRB, or two TCRA when at least one of the cells did not have TCRB reported). TCR sequences were compared using three-point matches (V-CDR3-J) and TCR chains within our experiments and against external databases when the data was available.

Statistical Analysis

The proportion of individuals responding to individual peptides was compared using Fisher's exact test and one-way ANOVA. Responses to native and neoepitopes were compared using paired t-tests. Differential gene expression between clusters and in response to peptide pools was tested with MAST method as implemented in Seurat, with individual as a latent variable. Frequency of clonotypes was determined by dividing the number of clonotypes by the total number of cells.

Data Availability

A 10× data was submitted to Array Express (E-MTAB-10323).

RESULTS

Comparison of T Cell Responses to Neoepitopes and Native Epitopes in Type 1 Diabetes and Preclinical Subjects by Cytokine ELISPOT

We set out to compare the magnitude, prevalence, and phenotype of the T cells responding to native and neoepitopes derived from islet autoantigens in individuals with or at risk of developing clinical type 1 diabetes using a sensitive cytokine ELISPOT. We selected native peptides of proinsulin (PIPs), representing naturally processed and presented epitopes known to elicit CD4 responses in PBMC from individuals with type 1 diabetes (2–4) and hybrid insulin peptides (HIPs), known to activate CD4 T cells isolated from pancreatic islets from deceased organ donors with type 1 diabetes (8, 9).

Firstly, we compared responses to native and neoepitopes in all individuals (pre-clinical and clinical type 1 diabetes). As depicted in **Figure 1A** and **Supplementary Figures 2A–C**, all peptides stimulated responses for all three cytokines in at least a proportion of individuals tested. All the peptides show a similar overall level of stimulation. Responses to Pediacel were detected in all of the patients for all three cytokines (**Supplementary Figures 3** and **4**).

As it is possible that the hierarchy of epitope immunodominance may be influenced by the stage of disease, we separated the subjects into patients with type 1 diabetes and

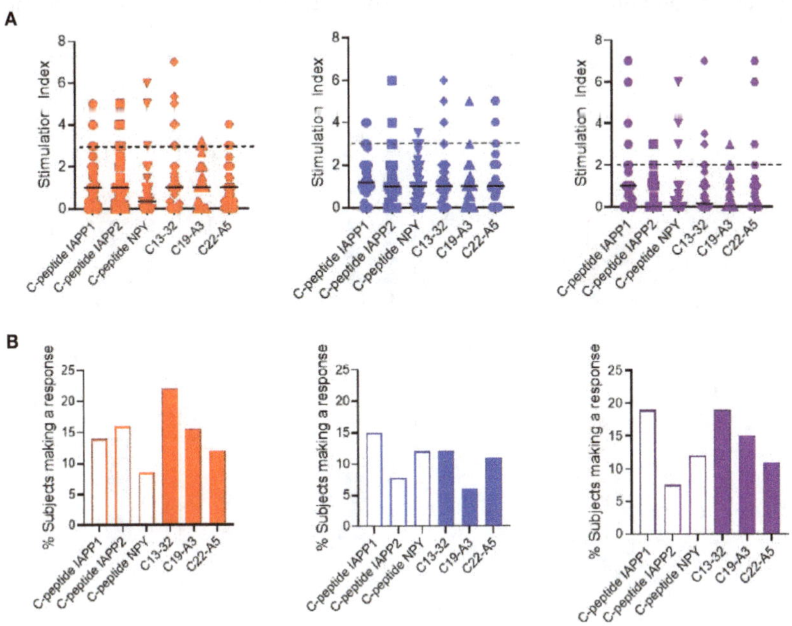

FIGURE 1 | Cytokine T cell responses were measured by ELISPOT, and data are expressed as SI [stimulation index (mean spot number of test peptide/mean spot number of diluent)]. **(A)** Magnitude of IFN-γ (red) IL-10 (blue) and IL-17 (purple) responses in preclinical and subjects with type 1 diabetes against neo- (C-peptide-IAPP1, C-peptide-IAPP2 and C-peptide-NPY) and native epitopes (C13–32, C19-A3, C22-A5). The dashed line represents the cut-off for positivity for the stimulation index (three for interferon-γ and IL-10 and two for IL-17). **(B)** Prevalence of IFN-γ (red) IL-10 (blue) and IL-17 (purple) responses measured by ELISPOT in preclinical and subjects with type 1 diabetes against individual peptides of neo- (open bars) and native (filled bars) epitopes.

those with preclinical disease. In subjects with type 1 diabetes, C-peptide-NPY elicits the highest interferon-γ response, C-peptide-IAPP2 the highest IL-10 and IL-17 responses were observed at a similar magnitude for C-peptide-IAPP1, C13-32, and C22-A5 (**Supplementary Figure 5A**). In preclinical subjects, C13–32 elicited the highest interferon-γ and IL-10 responses and C22-A5 the highest IL-17 response (**Supplementary Figure 6A**). However again, none of these differences reached statistical significance.

We have previously applied a ROC plot approach to establish criteria for defining a positive or negative response to individual peptide stimulation in cytokine ELISPOT assays (2, 4). We applied these criteria to the current data to determine the prevalence of positive responses in all the individuals tested and show that although there is a significant response to each peptide, there is no clear peptide immunodominance (**Figure 1B**). For interferon-γ responses, neoepitopes elicit a response in 8–14% of subjects and native epitopes in 12–22%. For IL-10, neoepitopes elicit a response in 8–15% of subjects and native epitopes in 6–12%, and finally IL-17 responses are present against 8–19% of neoepitopes and 11–19% of native epitopes.

Examining positive responses based on clinical group, in the subjects with type 1 diabetes, interferon-γ responses were observed in 6–16% against neoepitopes and 10–5% of native epitopes. IL-10 responses in 8–11% against neoepitopes and 0–12% of native epitopes and IL-17 against 10–26% of neoepitopes and 9–20% of native epitopes (**Supplementary Figure 5B**). In preclinical subjects, interferon-γ responses were observed against 8–23% of neoepitopes and 8–17% of native epitopes; IL-10 against 8–23% of neoepitopes and 8–31% of native epitopes, and no IL-17 responses were observed against neoepitopes and 8–15% subjects responded to native epitopes (**Supplementary Figure 6B**).

As responses to individual peptides were low, we pooled responses into two groups representing neo- or native epitopes and compared the magnitude of the response (**Figure 2A**) and the proportion of subjects mounting a positive response (**Figure 2B**). Although the overall magnitude of the response is similar, in terms of prevalence of positive responses, we observed a higher proportion of interferon-γ and IL-17 responses in response to native epitopes compared to neoepitopes (37 *vs.* 22% and 31 *vs.* 23% respectively). IL-10 responses were similar to both native and neoepitopes.

When segregating pooled responses by clinical group, the magnitude of response to neo- and native epitopes was similar in both groups (**Supplementary Figures 7A** and **8A**). Examining the proportion of individuals with a positive response, we observed that subjects with type 1 diabetes trended towards higher interferon-γ responses to native *vs.* neoepitopes (45 *vs* 36% respectively). In contrast, in preclinical subjects, IL-10 and IL-17 responses were more prevalent to native epitopes (85 *vs* 62% (IL-10) and 31 *vs* 8% (IL-17) while interferon-γ responses were similar to both neo- and native epitopes (54%) (**Supplementary Figures 7B** and **8B**).

Next, we compared the relative production of each cytokine stimulated by individual peptides to investigate if any single or group of epitopes led to a distinct polarization of the immune response.

When examining the magnitude of response, each peptide was capable of stimulating a range of cytokines in different individuals with no peptide clearly eliciting a stronger response to a particular cytokine (**Figure 3A**). However, when examining the proportion of individuals who mount a positive response, we note that C-peptide-IAPP2 trends towards increased stimulation of a

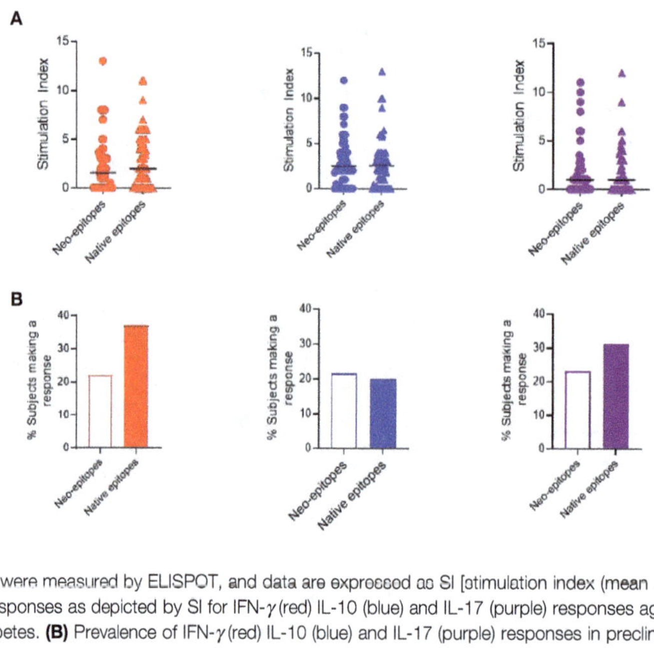

FIGURE 2 | Cytokine T cell responses were measured by ELISPOT, and data are expressed as SI [stimulation index (mean spot number of test peptide/mean spot number of diluent)]. **(A)** Magnitude of responses as depicted by SI for IFN-γ (red) IL-10 (blue) and IL-17 (purple) responses against pooled neo- and native epitopes in preclinical and subjects with type 1 diabetes. **(B)** Prevalence of IFN-γ (red) IL-10 (blue) and IL-17 (purple) responses in preclinical and subjects with type 1 diabetes against pooled peptides of neo- (open bars) and native (filled bars) epitopes.

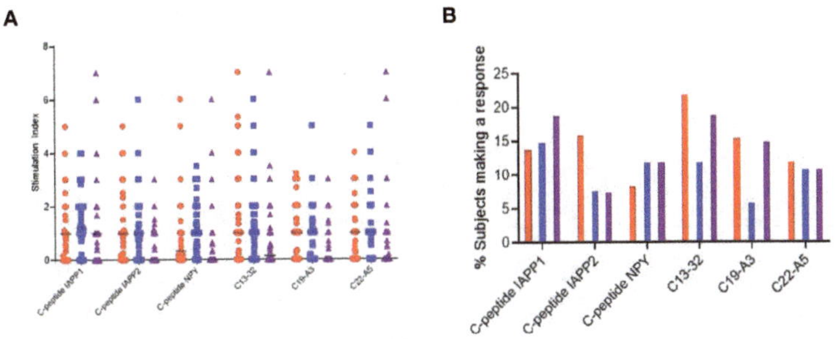

FIGURE 3 | Cytokine T cell responses were measured by ELISPOT, and data are expressed as SI [stimulation index (mean spot number of test peptide/mean spot number of diluent)]. **(A)** Magnitude of IFN-γ (red) IL-10 (blue) and IL-17 (purple) responses depicted as stimulation indices for individual peptides of neoepitopes (three on the left) and native (three on the right) in preclinical and subjects with type 1 diabetes. **(B)** Frequency of IFN-γ (red) IL-10 (blue) and IL-17 (purple) responses to individual peptides of neoepitopes (three on the left) and native (three on the right) in preclinical and subjects with type 1 diabetes.

significant IFN-γ response, C13-32 and C19-A3 trend towards increased IFN-γ and IL-17 compared to IL-10, whereas the remainder showed no particular polarization (**Figure 3B**).

All the peptides except C19-A3 elicited multiple cytokines: interferon-γ and IL10 were detected in 3.8% of patients. C-pep-IAPP1 was the only peptide to elicit IL-10 and IL-17 responses, and these were detected in 3.8% of patients; interferon-γ and IL17 responses were only detected in one patient (1.9%), and in one patient, responses to all three cytokines were observed.

Finally, we examined responses to native and neoepitopes specifically in children as we have previously reported that native proinsulin epitopes are preferentially targeted by interferon-γ producing T cells in this group (4). We show that 11/14 (79%) of children made a response to the native epitopes compared to 8/14 (57%) to neoepitopes ($p = 0.04$). Furthermore, despite the small numbers in the current study, we confirm that as reported previously, the native epitope C13–32 elicits interferon-γ response in more than 40% of children with type 1 diabetes (**Supplementary Figure 9A**). Indeed, two thirds of all interferon-γ responses in all the subjects are detected in children. An interferon-γ response is also seen against the native epitope, C19-A3; in contrast, the neoepitopes tend to elicit IL-17 responses albeit at a lower frequency. IL-10 responses were seen in preclinical subjects particularly to C-pep-IAAP1; however, the number of subjects here are small (**Supplementary Figure 9B**).

Although the native peptides were initially identified as being HLA-DR4 restricted, we now know that these promiscuous responses are observed in non-HLA DR4 individuals, and for both native and neoepitopes we observed responses in non-HLA DR4/DQ8 individuals (**Supplementary Table 3**).

Single Cell Transcriptional Profiling of CD4 T Cells Responding to Neo- and Native Epitopes

To further investigate the phenotype of neo- and native epitope-specific T cells, we conducted an unbiased transcriptional analysis including TCR clonotyping. Responding T cells were isolated based on CD154 and CD69 co-expression following brief *ex-vivo* culture with a pool of peptides representing native or neoepitopes and profiled using scRNA-seq *via* the 10× Genomics pipeline. As a positive control we used T cells activated by Pediacel from the same patients.

Data from donors were filtered and integrated as described in *Methods*, and cells were projected in two dimensions (UMAP). Data for subjects ND01 and ND02 are shown in **Figure 4A**. We performed cell clustering based on gene expression and independently inferred cell subtype by mapping to a reference PBMC dataset (16). The main clusters corresponded to memory CD4 and naïve T cells (**Figure 4B**). In concordance with this, cluster markers are genes preferentially expressed in memory (S100A10, S100A4, LGALS3) or naïve (FABP, SELL) cells (**Figure 4C**; there is also a very small cluster—cluster 3 which comprises of memory-like cells with expression of PLZF.

Cells from both individuals are similarly split between clusters, although ND01 has higher fraction of Tregs and ND02 more naïve cells (**Supplementary Figures 10A, B**).

We then compared cells stimulated with peptide pools in each subject (**Figure 4D**) and show that for each subject, the composition of native and neoepitope stimulated samples does not differ in reference-based assignment or clusters.

Importantly, T cells responded to native or neoepitopes co-cluster (**Figure 4E**) for each individual, implying no general distinction between the responding cells.

We explored this further by comparing gene expression profiles of cells stimulated with either neo- or native epitopes for both patients and found no significant differences in gene expression (**Supplementary Table 1**).

We then examined expression of selected pro-inflammatory genes including *IL-17A*, *IL-22*, *TNF-α*, *INF-γ*, and *IL-32* and anti-inflammatory genes *IL-4* and *IL-10* in cells stimulated with either neo- or native epitopes (**Figure 5A**). *IL-17A* expression was generally low, although expression was slightly higher in patient ND01; *IL-22* expression was greater than *IL-17A*; similarly, expression of this was higher in patient ND01; there were no differences in cells stimulated with either neo- or native epitopes. *TNF-α* and *INF-γ* expression was higher in patient

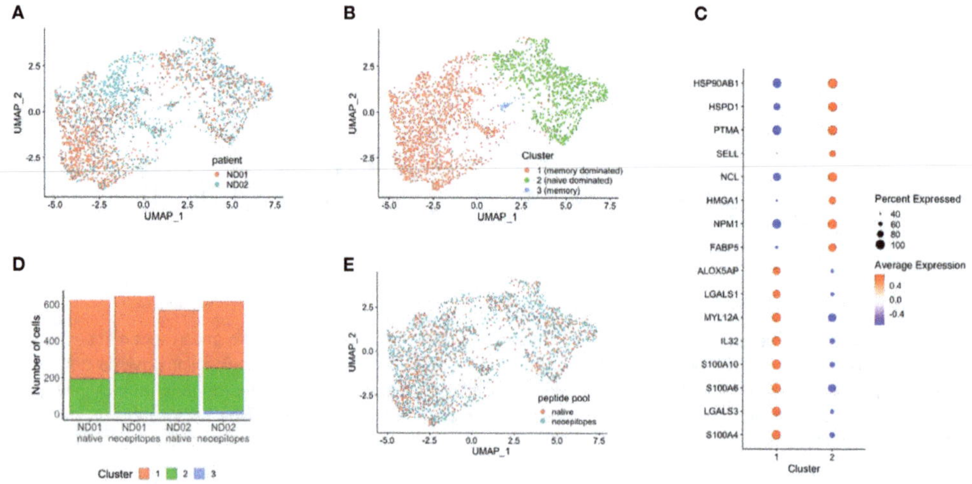

FIGURE 4 | PBMCs from subjects ND01 and ND02 were stimulated with native (proinsulin peptides: C13–32, C19-A3, C22-A5; GAD peptides: 115–125, 265–284) and neoepitopes [C-pep-IAPP1, C-pep-NPY, GAD 115-127 (120E), GAD 265-284 (272 cit)] and each patient/pool was labeled with a different hashtag as described in *Methods*. Antigen-responsive cells were identified by expression of CD154/CD69, and immune profiling was subsequently conducted on single cells. Cells from subjects **(A)** ND01 and ND02 separate into **(B)** three clusters (0–3) based on gene expression similarity. **(C)** Clusters differ by expression of memory and naïve cell specific genes. **(D)** Cells reacting to native and neoepitopes are similarly split between clusters and **(E)** have similar patterns of expression.

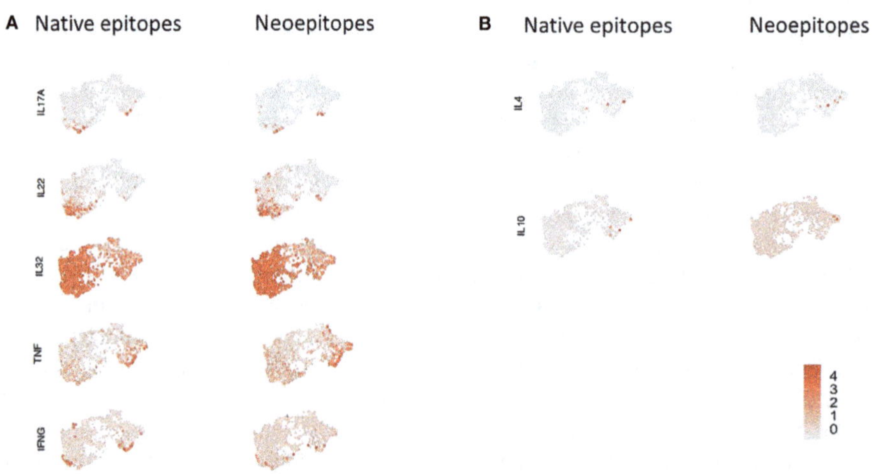

FIGURE 5 | PBMCs from subjects ND01 and ND02 were stimulated with native [proinsulin peptides: C13–32, C19-A3, C22-A5; GAD peptides: 115–125, 265–284) and neoepitopes (C-pep-IAPP1, C-pep- NPY, GAD 115-127 (120E), GAD 265-284 (272 cit)]. Antigen-responsive cells were identified by expression of CD154/CD69, and immune profiling was conducted on single cells. **(A)** Cells were stimulated with native (right) and neoepitopes (left), and gene expression (depicted in pink) of **(A)** *IL-17A, IL-22, IL-32, TNF-α,* and *IFN-γ* and **(B)** *IL-4* and *IL-10* was examined. Level of expression corresponds to greater intensity of color.

ND02, and expression in cells stimulated with either neo- or native epitopes was similar.

Interestingly, *IL-32* gene expression was by far the most extensive and present in both patients in response to both neo- and native epitope stimulated cells.

In contrast, expression of the anti-inflammatory cytokines (**Figure 5B**), *IL-4* and *IL-10* was undetectable in patient ND01 and very low in ND02 for both native and neoepitopes.

TCR Use of Cells Responding to Neo- and Native Epitopes

The Single Cell Immune Profiling system allows the synchronized identification of gene expression and T cell receptor profiles from single cells in the same sample. We used this approach to assess the number and profile of TCR clonotypes and determine whether any are shared between T cells stimulated with either neo- or native epitopes.

For patient set ND01/ND02 we identified 76 clonotypes shared between T cells responding to native and neoepitopes in subject ND01 and seven such clonotypes for ND02 (**Table 2**). Each of these TCR receptors was present in 2–30 cells, and again there was no preference towards either native or neoepitopes. Of the 76 clonotypes in ND01, four of the TCRB sequences (highlighted in red) corresponded to sequences in the JDRF npod database (http://clonesearch.jdrfnpod.org) where they were present in the pancreatic lymph nodes and spleen of both patients with type 1 diabetes and healthy controls (17) (**Table 2**). Representative data are shown in **Figure 6**.

For both sets of patients, stimulating T cell with native or neoepitopes did not lead to a preferential expansion of specific clonotypes shared between peptide pools.

Finally, we also investigated TCR clones that were expanded by one peptide pool only (**Supplementary Table 2**). Subject ND01 had identical number of clonotypes, with similar number of cells expanded to either native or neoepitope pools. In contrast, ND02 had more expanded clones in the native epitope pool compared to the neoepitope pool (eight *versus* one). Eight of the TCRB chains were also present in the JDRF npod database, where they were present in the pancreatic lymph nodes and spleen of both patients with type 1 diabetes and healthy controls at frequencies ranging from 0.0008 to 0.002% which is comparable to the 0.004–0.005% for both native and neoepitopes in the present study. Taken together, these data show the need for testing more patients to determine whether there is a quantitative difference in expanded clonotypes between native and neoepitopes.

DISCUSSION

In agreement with observations made by others we can detect T cell responsive to HIPs in PBMCs and that these cells respond with a range of cytokine production. We wanted to determine if they were present at a higher frequency or with a different phenotype to PIPS and demonstrated that this is not the case. Our findings contrast with those recently published by Mitchell et al. (18); however, we did not test all the HIPs that they used. It is possible that some HIPs elicit stronger responses than those we tested, but equally some PIPs may elicit stronger responses than the ones they tested—there was only one PIP in their panel and that differed in amino acid sequence to the three used in our panel. Moreover, in that study there was no difference between the negative control (no antigen) and B9-23 in either autoantibody-positive or autoantibody-negative individuals for either IFN-γor IL-10; for C10-24, they report very low reactivity too indicating that overall, they saw very low reactivity to native peptides in their study.

In the present study, through a detailed phenotypic analysis, we show that HIPs are not better than conventional islet epitopes in eliciting IFN-γ, IL-10, or IL-17 specific T cell responses in both patients with type 1 diabetes and high-risk unaffected family members. On the contrary, pro-inflammatory responses tend to be more frequent to islet epitopes when responses are measured collectively. Furthermore, in terms of epitope hierarchy, the native epitope, C13-32, elicits the most frequent IFN-γ and IL-10 responses in patients with type 1 diabetes and preclinical subjects respectively consistent with our previous studies (3, 4). This was confirmed in a subgroup analysis on children with type 1 diabetes where interferon-γresponses to all the PIPs including C13-32 were higher than those observed against HIPS despite comparable HLA-DR4 and HLA-DQ8 prevalence.

The three HIPs used here were selected based on two previous studies which described IFN-γ producing CD4 T cell clones specific for these HIPS isolated from islets of type 1 diabetes patients (8, 9).

During the course of this study, Baker et al., published data measuring IFN-γT cell responses by ELISPOT against a series of HIPs including the three used in the present study and showed minimal reactivity: C-peptide-IAAP1 elicited IFN-γ responses in 0/35 patients and both C-peptide-IAAP2 and C-peptide NPY in 1/35 patients each (3%) (11). In contrast, we detected reactivity in 16% of subjects with type 1 diabetes for C-peptide-IAAP1; reactivities to C-peptide-IAAP2 and C-peptide NPY were also higher than those reported by Baker et al. (14% and 6% respectively). We also show frequent IL-17 T cell responses to C-peptide-IAAP1 which suggests that this epitope may be relevant in type 1 diabetes as it elicits multiple cytokine reactivity.

Baker et al. also tested responses against the native Ins75–90 peptide and report reactivity in ~10% of patients; this peptide corresponds to Ins75–92 (C19-A3) which we have used not only in the present study but extensively in the past and reported reactivity in more than 50% of subjects with type 1 diabetes (4). Due to limitations in the volume of blood available, it was beyond the scope of this study to test a wider selection of peptides presented by overlapping HLAs, but the frequencies of DR4 and DQ8 were compatible (63% and 56% respectively). Furthermore, using a single peptide concentration for stimulation does not allow us to differentiate between higher and lower affinities of the native and neoepitopes for MHC.

These variations in frequency of responses can be attributed to differences in assay design; Baker et al. stimulated their cells for 96 h prior to transfer to anti-IFN-γ antibody coated plates whereas we stimulate for 48 h, and they also report a much higher background response which could be due to differences in the serum/media used, during cell transfer to the anti-IFN-γ coated plate and the longer incubation time. The fact that cytokine responses to Pediacel were detected in all the subjects does validate the robustness of the ELISPOT assay used in the current study.

The lack of phenotypic differences in T cells responding to either native or neoepitopes is further substantiated by the Single Cell Immune-Profiling data which detects subtle differences in gene expression. Intriguingly, when focusing on pro-inflammatory cytokines, we noted that IL-32 expression was very high in patients responding to both native and neoepitopes. This ubiquitous expression could be because of culture conditions, but it is unlikely as its expression is dependent on stimulation (19). A potential role for IL-32 in type 1 diabetes

TABLE 2 | T cell clonotypes shared amongst native and neoepitopes.

Patient Set & Clonotype	Subject	TRA	TRB	Cells' native epitopes	Cells Neo-epitopes
ND01/ND02 1	ND01	CALISGGGADGLTF	CSVGSQPQHF	21	11
ND01/ND02 4	ND01	CAAINAGNNRKLIW	CAWNKKKGLTYNEQFF	5	5
ND01/ND02 5	ND01	CATDAMNSNYQLIW	CASTTGPQNEKLFF	2	7
ND01/ND02 9	ND01	CAVGTGTASKLTF	CASSTTSLSSYEQYF	4	2
ND01/ND02 12	ND01	CAVSTGGGNKLTF	CSARLGAQNTGELFF	4	3
ND01/ND02 13	ND01	CAVPRSGNTGKLIF	CASSLPGVTNYGYTF	3	4
ND01/ND02 20	ND01	CAANMYALNF	CASSPGQGANTGELFF	4	2
ND01/ND02 21	ND01	CAGIQGAQKLVF	CASSFIAGGPSDTQYF	1	1
ND01/ND02 27	ND01	CILRDSGATNKLIF	CAAGQPNTGELFF	3	3
ND01/ND02 273	ND01	CAVPDQTGANNLFF	CASSTHRVNAEAFF	1	1
ND01/ND02 276	ND01	CALMNQGGKLIF	CSVEDPDSRTDTQYF	1	1
ND01/ND02 19	ND01	CAVISNTGKLIF	CASSRGQGAEKLFF	3	2
ND01/ND02 23	ND01	CATDPWSGANSKLTF	CASGFTGGYNEQFF	3	1
ND01/ND02 230	ND01	CASSGGSYIPTF	CASSLGRGASTEAFF	1	1
ND01/ND02 234	ND01	CVARRGGGGNKLTF	CASSPGTGQETQYF	1	1
ND01/ND02 2351/3227	ND01	CAVRSNQAGTALIF	CASSAAGASSYEQYF	1	1
		CAVGGNTNAGKSTF			
		CAVRSNQAGTALIF	CASSAAGASSYEQYF		
ND01/ND02 28	ND01	CLVGDISTSGTYKYIF	CASRHARQPQHF	3	2
ND01/ND02 287	ND01	CAGSGTMNYGGSQGNLIF	CASSGQGGGNTEAFF	1	1
ND01/ND02 30	ND01	CVVTGYNNNDMRF	CAIREGYGYTF	2	3
ND01/ND02 37	ND01	CAGPDMDSNYQLIW	CASRYRGGSGRELFF	2	3
ND01/ND02 38	ND01	CAFIWGSSNTGKLIF	CASRRGQANYGYTF	2	1
ND01/ND02 48	ND01	CILARSGAGSYQLTF	CASSYFGRGTDTQYF	3	2
ND01/ND02 18	ND01	CVVNTVTGGGNKLTF	CASSLRGPYGYTF	2	2
ND01/ND02 22	ND01	CAVRIQGAQKLVF	CASSYSEVYNEQFF	2	2
ND01/ND02 26	ND01	CALSASKIIF	CASSLSRESNQPQHF	1	1
ND01/ND02 263	ND01	CALSDRPGSARQLTF	CSASPTPQVGGTEAFF	1	1
ND01/ND02 264	ND01	CALPLSKTGANNLFF	CASSSTGGYEQYF	1	1
ND01/ND02 221	ND01	CALRSGANSKLTF	CASSLSLAPSDEQFF	1	1
ND01/ND02 2297/6	ND01	CAVSDTGGFKTIF	CATSETGKYQETQYF	4	5
		CAVGPAGTGGFKTIF	CATSETGKYQETQYF		
		CAVSDTGGFKTIF			
ND01/ND02 29	ND01	CAVNPGNTPLVF	CSARDDRTAAEAFF	3	1
ND01/ND02 31/42	ND01	CAVADSNYQLIW	CASSSLTGGLYNEQFF	4	5
		CAVSYTGGGNKLTF			
		CAVSYTGGGNKLTF	CASSSLTGGLYNEQFF		
ND01/ND02 32	ND01	CAVRDGGTGGFKTIF	CASSLGAQYTGELFF	1	1
ND01/ND02 33	ND01	CAAPLKTSYDKVIF	CASSLDRGVQPQHF	2	2
ND01/ND02 335	ND01	CAVEDGGNDYKLSF	CASSAGTGRHTDTQYF	1	1
		CAVVPPFTGGGNKLTF			
ND01/ND02 349	ND01	CALSEARDAGNMLTF	CSARGQGVATSNQPQHF	1	1
ND01/ND02 319	ND01	CLVGDIRGGGYQKVTF	CSVEVDRAGTEAFF	1	1
ND01/ND02 43	ND01	CAASGWGSARQLTF	CASSYRAPGDNSPLHF	2	2
ND01/ND02 47	ND01	CALKAAGNKLTF	CASAGEHTGELFF	3	1
ND01/ND02 49	ND01	CAPRGNDYKLSF	CSAIDNTDTQYF	2	2
ND01/ND02 53	ND01	CAVDAAGNKLTF	CASSADILLREQYF	3	1
ND01/ND02 54	ND01	CAAGGATNKLIF	CASSPRALENTEAFF	1	1
ND01/ND02 57	ND01	CAVSNQAGTALIF	CASSLRGTGGYTF	1	1
ND01/ND02 58	ND01	CALSENTNAGKSTF	CSAQGGGDTEAFF	1	2
ND01/ND02 62	ND01	CALSRTGYSTLTF	CASVVLGNTEAFF	3	1
ND01/ND02 69	ND01	CAVFTGGFKTIF	CATSVRGDYNEQFF	2	2
ND01/ND02 11	ND01	CAVYHAGNMLTFT	CASSTGTGGYEQYF	1	2
ND01/ND02 113	ND01	CAGAGGSYIPTF	CASSPGGPVGNTIYF	1	1
ND01/ND02 116	ND01	CAMRKGDYKLSF	CASSAGRGSDYGYTF	1	1
		CAVLGGGGFKTIF			
ND01/ND02 117	ND01	CAASAIKYGGSQGNLIF	CASSQDTASGAYEQYF	1	1
ND01/ND02 140	ND01	CAASAALQTGANNLFF	CASSLGQGAEAFF	2	1
ND01/ND02 142	ND01	CALTSRGGFGNVLHC	CSAREGAGANVLTF	2	1
ND01/ND02 151	ND01	CAVKEVDSSYKLIF	CASSTGTGAEMNTEAFF	1	1
ND01/ND02 153	ND01	CARGNNDYKLSF	CASSATLQGGGYTF	1	1

(Continued)

TABLE 2 | Continued

Patient Set & Clonotype	Subject	TRA	TRB	Cells' native epitopes	Cells Neo-epitopes
ND01/ND02 1584/52	ND01	CILRDAFGNEKLTF	CSARRDLGNQPQHF	2	1
		CILRDAFGNEKLTF	CSARRDLGNQPQHF		
		CAGHNNAGNMLTF			
ND01/ND02 247	ND01	CAAMNTGGFKTIF	CASSELSSGRNNEQFF	1	1
ND01/ND02 248	ND01	CAVGAGYGGATNKLIF	CASSRGVTEAFF	1	1
ND01/ND02 257	ND01	CALMNTGFQKLVF	CASSFGLRQGGRVGEEYF	1	1
		CSLRYSGAGSYQLTF			
ND01/ND02 1878/44	ND01	CASQRGSQGNLIF	CASSSGLAGGLEQYF	1	1
		CALNTGTASKLTF			
		CALNTGTASKLTF	CASSSGLAGGLEQYF		
ND01/ND02 190	ND01	CALRDTGGFKTIF	CASSAGTGGLFGELFF	1	1
ND01/ND02 199	ND01	CAVASNTGKLIF	CSVEDSGNTIYF	1	1
ND01/ND02 205	ND01	CALSSQGTYKYIF	CASSETGRGIEQYF	1	1
		CAGVFMRF			
ND01/ND02 207	ND01	CATHASGGSYIPTF	CASKNQGTYGYTF	1	1
ND01/ND02 209	ND01	CAVGIAGNTPLVF	CASSPSWDFHGYTF	1	1
ND01/ND02 64	ND01	CAVPNQAGTALIF	CASSQRGTYEQYF	2	1
ND01/ND02 65	ND01	CATDTSYTGANSKLTF	CASSRILTSGNRGVTQYF	2	1
ND01/ND02 67	ND01	CAVGVSGNTPLVF	CASSVLSGGETQYF	1	2
ND01/ND02 75	ND01	CVVSDRDTGFQKLVF	CASSVAGSVSDTQYF	2	1
ND01/ND02 77	ND01	CALISGGGADGLTF		1	1
ND01/ND02 78	ND01	CVVGDFGNEKLTF	CASSLVQAYYSGNTIYF	2	1
ND01/ND02 79	ND01	CALSGGGSARQLTF	CASSSSLRRFNYGYTF	2	1
ND01/ND02 82	ND01	CAFRGTGNQFYF	CASSITGTTYEQYF	1	2
ND01/ND02 83	ND01	CAGRSGGYQKVTF	CSVERRGGDTQYF	1	2
ND01/ND02 91	ND01	CAVIPMNSGYSTLTF	CASSPRPQGQSYNEQFF	2	1
ND01/ND02 92	ND01	CAVGPWGNEKLTF	CASSLDSKPEAFF	2	1
ND01/ND02 94	ND01	CAASLGAGSYQLTF	CSARGAGGLTYEQYF	1	2
ND01/ND02 98	ND01	CAASIRSGTYKYIF	CASSLRLTGGNNEQFF	2	1
ND01/ND02 99	ND01	CAANDQTGANNLFF	CASRKAGGPYEQYF	1	2
ND01/ND02	ND02	CASSPQGGSEKLVF	CASSFFRGRNTEAFF	1	2
ND01/ND02 8	ND02	CAVYSGNTPLVF	CASKAQGPGNTIYF	3	7
ND01/ND02 81	ND02	CAVGQQGGSEKLVF	CASRSPRDRNTEAFF	2	2
ND01/ND02 194	ND02	CAASRDTGFQKLVF	CASSRTGRTDQPQHF	1	1
ND01/ND02 196	ND02	CAMREGPNDYKLSF	CSARDFLRLAGGEETQYF	1	1
ND01/ND02 200	ND02	CAVGTQGGSEKLVF	CASRSNRDRNTEAFF	1	1
ND01/ND02 362	ND02	CIVGYSTLTF	CASSLARLVAGGDNEQFF	1	1

Sequences highlighted in red correspond to those listed in the JDRF npod TCR database.

has been suggested in two recent studies describing gene upregulation in pancreatic β cells (20) and the detection of *IL32* transcripts preceding the onset of autoantibodies in type 1 diabetes (21). IL-32 has been implicated in inflammatory bowel disease (IBD) and rheumatoid arthritis (RA) (22) where it is thought to orchestrate a panoply of other cytokines; indeed, in RA, IL-32 participates in the interplay with IL-17 in disease pathogenesis by amplifying inflammation in the synovium (23). Based on these data and previous studies on the role of IL-17 in T1D (2, 24), the elevated expression of IL-32 described in the present study warrants further investigation, and future studies will address whether IL-32 is produced by T cell stimulated with islet autoantigenic peptides. Overall, the lack of differences in gene expression and the similarity in composition of cells within clusters further substantiate that there is no difference in T cells responding to native or neoepitopes.

Finally, we were able to assess the number and profile of clonotypes present in immune response upon stimulation. Further evidence of the lack of distinction between T cells responding to native compared to neoepitopes comes from the T cell clonotype data which shows no preferential expansion of clonotypes. For this part of the study the T cells were stimulated with native peptide pools consisting of proinsulin and GAD or neoepitope peptide pools consisting of HIPs and modified GAD epitopes. There is very little sequence homology between the proinsulin and hybrid insulin peptides in the native and neoepitopes pools, whereas there is only one amino acid difference between the two GAD epitopes (deamidation and citrullination) in the two pools thus implying that the shared clonotypes must be targeting one of the GAD peptides. This is supported by the fact that clonotype 1 in patient ND03 has the TCRB chain sequence: CASSPATGGSSYNEQFF which has been previously identified in T cells stimulated with GAD (25).

Interestingly, four of the shared clonotypes in the current study have TCRB sequences found in the nPOD TCR database where they are present in the pancreatic lymph nodes and spleens of patients with type 1 diabetes. The shared TCR clonotypes between cells stimulated by the native and neoepitope pools suggest a lineage relationship between cells recognizing the two types of epitopes, although the specificity of

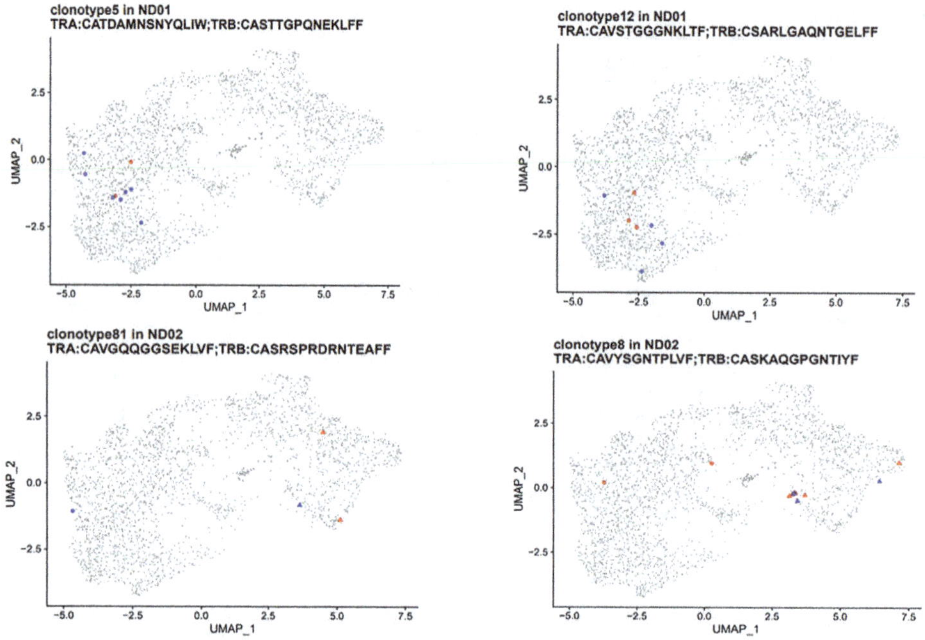

FIGURE 6 | PBMCs from subjects with type 1 diabetes were stimulated with native [proinsulin peptides: C13–32, C19-A3, C22-A5; GAD peptides: 115–25, 265–284) and neoepitopes (C-pep-IAPP1, C-pep-NPY, GAD 115–127 (120E), GAD 265–284 (272 cit)]. Antigen-responsive cells were identified by and sorted on expression of CD154/CD69. Immune profiling was conducted on single cells from which cDNA was synthesized, followed by library construction and sequencing as described in *Methods*. TCR clonotypes (both α and β chains) were examined in patients ND01 (top panel) and ND02 (bottom panel). T cells responding to native epitopes are shown in red and those responding to neoepitopes are shown in blue. Clusters are marked by point shapes (circle, triangle, and square).

these clonotypes has not been demonstrated. TCRs unique to either native or neoepitopes were also detected, but the specificity is not known. Future work will address the exact specificity of the epitope by transducing the TCR sequences into immortalized TCR–/– cell lines such as Jurkat cells and screening the relevant peptides.

We were only able to test two patients in the single Cell Immune profiling system, and our peptide panel for both native and neoepitopes had to be limited as we were constrained in the volume of blood available especially from juvenile subjects—this is a potential weakness in the study; however, the Immune Profiling data can be regarded as exploratory and can be used to guide future studies.

In summary, neoepitopes in T1D have a significant role in type 1 diabetes pathology; however, as the list of potential targets grows there is an even more pressing need to appraise and validate these epitopes and determine whether any have biomarker potential. By using a combination of phenotypic, transcriptomic, and clonotypic analyses we show that as it stands, neoepitopes are comparable to the native epitopes currently in use for immuno-monitoring studies.

AUTHOR CONTRIBUTIONS

SA designed and performed experiments, analyzed data, and wrote the manuscript. IP-A designed experiments and analyzed the data, YK, EW, NY, CD-V, YS, EP, and LK performed experiments and analyzed data. AL analyzed data and reviewed the manuscript. SA and MP designed research studies. SA and MP conceived ideas and reviewed the manuscript. SA and MP oversaw research. TT reviewed and edited the manuscript. MP is the guarantor of this work and, as such, had full access to all the data in the study and takes responsibility for the integrity of the data and the accuracy of the data analysis. All authors contributed to the article and approved the submitted version.

REFERENCES

1. In't Veld P. Insulitis in Human Type 1 Diabetes: The Quest for an Elusive Lesion. *Islets* (2011) 3(4):131–8. doi: 10.4161/isl.3.4.15728
2. Arif S, Moore F, Marks K, Bouckenooghe T, Dayan CM, Planas R, et al. Peripheral and Islet Interleukin-17 Pathway Activation Characterizes Human Autoimmune Diabetes and Promotes Cytokine-Mediated Beta-Cell Death. *Diabetes* (2011) 60(8):2112–9. doi: 10.2337/db10-1643
3. Arif S, Leete P, Nguyen V, Marks K, Nor NM, Estorninho M, et al. Blood and Islet Phenotypes Indicate Immunological Heterogeneity in Type 1 Diabetes. *Diabetes* (2014) 63(11):3835–45. doi: 10.2337/db14-0365
4. Arif S, Gibson VB, Nguyen V, Bingley PJ, Todd JA, Guy C, et al. Beta-Cell Specific T-Lymphocyte Response has a Distinct Inflammatory Phenotype in Children With Type 1 Diabetes Compared With Adults. *Diabetes Med* (2017) 34(3):419–25. doi: 10.1111/dme.13153
5. Soleimanpour SA, Stoffers DA. The Pancreatic Beta Cell and Type 1 Diabetes:

Innocent Bystander or Active Participant? *Trends Endocrinol Metab* (2013) 24 (7):324–31. doi: 10.1016/j.tem.2013.03.005

6. McGinty JW, Marre ML, Bajzik V, Piganelli JD, James EA. T Cell Epitopes and Post-Translationally Modified Epitopes in Type 1 Diabetes. *Curr Diabetes Rep* (2015) 15(11):90. doi: 10.1007/s11892-015-0657-7
7. Gonzalez-Duque S, Azoury ME, Colli ML, Afonso G, Turatsinze JV, Nigi L, et al. Conventional and Neo-Antigenic Peptides Presented by Beta Cells Are Targeted by Circulating Naive Cd8+ T Cells in Type 1 Diabetic and Healthy Donors. *Cell Metab* (2018) 28(6):946–60.e6. doi: 10.1016/j.cmet.2018.07.007
8. Delong T, Wiles TA, Baker RL, Bradley B, Barbour G, Reisdorph R, et al. Pathogenic CD4 T Cells in Type 1 Diabetes Recognize Epitopes Formed by Peptide Fusion. *Science* (2016) 351(6274):711–4. doi: 10.1126/science.aad2791
9. Babon JA, DeNicola ME, Blodgett DM, Crevecoeur I, Buttrick TS, Maehr R, et al. Analysis of Self-Antigen Specificity of Islet-Infiltrating T Cells From Human Donors With Type 1 Diabetes. *Nat Med* (2016) 22(12):1482–7. doi: 10.1038/nm.4203
10. Buitinga M, Callebaut A, Marques Camara Sodre F, Crevecoeur I, Blahnik-Fagan G, Yang ML, et al. Inflammation-Induced Citrullinated Glucose-Regulated Protein 78 Elicits Immune Responses in Human Type 1 Diabetes. *Diabetes* (2018) 67(11):2337–48. doi: 10.2337/db18-0295
11. Baker RL, Rihanek M, Hohenstein AC, Nakayama M, Michels A, Gottlieb PA, et al. Hybrid Insulin Peptides Are Autoantigens in Type 1 Diabetes. *Diabetes* (2019) 68(9):1830–40. doi: 10.2337/db19-0128
12. McGinty JW, Chow IT, Greenbaum C, Odegard J, Kwok WW, James EA. Recognition of Posttranslationally Modified GAD65 Epitopes in Subjects With Type 1 Diabetes. *Diabetes* (2014) 63(9):3033–40. doi: 10.2337/db13-1952
13. Mathieu C, Lahesmaa R, Bonifacio E, Achenbach P, Tree T. Immunological Biomarkers for the Development and Progression of Type 1 Diabetes. *Diabetologia* (2018) 61(11):2252–8. doi: 10.1007/s00125-018-4726-8
14. Arif S, Tree TI, Astill TP, Tremble JM, Bishop AJ, Dayan CM, et al. Autoreactive T Cell Responses Show Proinflammatory Polarization in Diabetes But a Regulatory Phenotype in Health. *J Clin Invest* (2004) 113 (3):451–63. doi: 10.1172/JCI19585
15. Gomez-Tourino I, Kamra Y, Baptista R, Lorenc A, Peakman M. T Cell Receptor Beta-Chains Display Abnormal Shortening and Repertoire Sharing in Type 1 Diabetes. *Nat Commun* (2017) 8(1):1792. doi: 10.1038/s41467-017-01925-2
16. Kang JB, Nathan A, Millard N, Rumker L, Moody DB, Korsunsky I, et al. Efficient and Precise Single-Cell Reference Atlas Mapping With Symphony. *bioRxiv* (2020) 2020:11.18.389189. doi: 10.1101/2020.11.18.389189
17. Seay HR, Yusko E, Rothweiler SJ, Zhang L, Posgai AL, Campbell-Thompson M, et al. Tissue Distribution and Clonal Diversity of the T and B Cell Repertoire in Type 1 Diabetes. *JCI Insight* (2016) 1(20):e88242. doi: 10.1172/jci.insight.88242
18. Mitchell AM, Alkanani AA, McDaniel KA, Pyle L, Waugh K, Steck AK, et al. T-Cell Responses to Hybrid Insulin Peptides Prior to Type 1 Diabetes Development. *Proc Natl Acad Sci USA* (2021) 118(6):e2019129118. doi: 10.1073/pnas.2019129118
19. Hong JT, Son DJ, Lee CK, Yoon DY, Lee DH, Park MH. Interleukin 32, Inflammation and Cancer. *Pharmacol Ther* (2017) 174:127–37. doi: 10.1016/j.pharmthera.2017.02.025
20. Safari-Alighiarloo N, Taghizadeh M, Mohammad Tabatabaei S, Namaki S, Rezaei-Tavirani M. Identification of Common Key Genes and Pathways Between Type 1 Diabetes and Multiple Sclerosis Using Transcriptome and Interactome Analysis. *Endocrine* (2020) 68(1):81–92. doi: 10.1007/s12020-019-02181-8
21. Kallionpaa H, Somani J, Tuomela S, Ullah U, de Albuquerque R, Lonnberg T, et al. Early Detection of Peripheral Blood Cell Signature in Children Developing Beta-Cell Autoimmunity at a Young Age. *Diabetes* (2019) 68 (10):2024–34. doi: 10.2337/db19-0287
22. de Albuquerque R, Komsi E, Starskaia I, Ullah U, Lahesmaa R. The Role of Interleukin-32 in Autoimmunity. *Scand J Immunol* (2020) 93:e13012. doi: 10.1111/sji.13012
23. Moon YM, Yoon BY, Her YM, Oh HJ, Lee JS, Kim KW, et al. Il-32 and IL-17 Interact and Have the Potential to Aggravate Osteoclastogenesis in Rheumatoid Arthritis. *Arthritis Res Ther* (2012) 14(6):R246. doi: 10.1186/ar4089
24. Abdel-Moneim A, Bakery HH, Allam G. The Potential Pathogenic Role of IL-17/Th17 Cells in Both Type 1 and Type 2 Diabetes Mellitus. *BioMed Pharmacother* (2018) 101:287–92. doi: 10.1016/j.biopha.2018.02.103
25. Eugster A, Lindner A, Catani M, Heninger AK, Dahl A, Klemroth S, et al. High Diversity in the TCR Repertoire of GAD65 Autoantigen-Specific Human CD4+ T Cells. *J Immunol* (2015) 194(6):2531–8. doi: 10.4049/jimmunol.1403031

6

Innate Viral Receptor Signaling Determines Type 1 Diabetes Onset

*Zachary J. Morse and Marc S. Horwitz**

Department of Microbiology and Immunology, University of British Columbia, Vancouver, BC, Canada

Correspondence:
Marc S. Horwitz
mhorwitz@mail.ubc.ca

Heritable susceptibility of the autoimmune disorder, type 1 diabetes (T1D), only partially equates for the incidence of the disease. Significant evidence attributes several environmental stressors, such as vitamin D deficiency, gut microbiome, dietary antigens, and most notably virus infections in triggering the onset of T1D in these genetically susceptible individuals. Extensive epidemiological and clinical studies have provided credibility to this causal relationship. Infection by the enterovirus, coxsackievirus B, has been closely associated with onset of T1D and is considered a significant etiological agent for disease induction. Recognition of viral antigens *via* innate pathogen-recognition receptors induce inflammatory events which contribute to autoreactivity of pancreatic self-antigens and ultimately the destruction of insulin-secreting beta cells. The activation of these specific innate pathways and expression of inflammatory molecules, including type I and III interferon, prime the immune system to elicit either a protective regulatory response or a diabetogenic effector response. Therefore, sensing of viral antigens by retinoic acid-inducible gene I-like receptors and toll-like receptors may be detrimental to inducing autoreactivity initiated by viral stress and resulting in T1D.

Keywords: type 1 diabetes, autoimmunity, innate immunity, toll-like receptors, RIG-I-like receptors, MDA5, type I and III interferon, coxsackievirus B

INTRODUCTION

Characterized by the destruction of the insulin-secreting beta cells of the pancreas and subsequent loss of blood glucose regulation, type 1 diabetes (T1D) is an autoimmune disorder whose onset is triggered by a combination of both genetic and environmental factors. Virus infections, vitamin D deficiency, dietary antigens, and disruption in the gut microbiota all have been implicated in eliciting T1D development in genetically susceptible individuals (1–4). Significant evidence suggests a strong causal association between genes involved in host–virus interactions and susceptibility to

---

Abbreviations: CVB, coxsackievirus B; DC, dendritic cell; dsRNA, double-stranded RNA; GWAS, genome-wide association studies; IFIH1, interferon induced with helicase C domain 1; IFN, interferon; IFNAR, type I interferon receptor; IFNλR, type III interferon receptor; IRF7, interferon regulatory factor 7; LCMV, lymphocytic choriomeningitis virus; MDA5, melanoma differentiation-associated protein 5; MYD88, myeloid differentiation primary response gene 88; NOD mice, non-obese diabetic mice; pDC, plasmacytoid dendritic cell; poly I:C, polyinosinic:polycytidylic acid; PRR, pattern-recognition receptor; RA, rheumatoid arthritis; RIG-I, retinoic acid-inducible gene I; RLR, RIG-I-like receptors; SLE, systemic lupus erythematosus; SNP, single nucleotide polymorphism; ssRNA, single-stranded RNA; T1D, type 1 diabetes; TLR, toll-like receptor; T_{REG}, regulatory T cell; VP1, viral protein 1.

T1D. Using genome-wide association studies (GWAS), single nucleotide polymorphisms (SNPs) and gene variants conferring risk for T1D have been identified in multiple sites including the *interferon induced with helicase C domain 1* (*IFIH1*), *HLA class II*, *CTLA-4*, *insulin*, and *PTPN22* genes (5–7). The precise mechanisms leading to a loss of self-tolerance experienced in T1D are not adequately understood. Virus-mediated activation of T1D has been proposed to be caused by several different processes including direct islet infection, increased exposure to self-antigens which may have been previously sequestered, bystander activation, and molecular mimicry (8, 9).

Natural drift of genetic predisposition cannot adequately explain why the incidence of T1D has increased approximately 1.8% annually from 2002 to 2012 worldwide (10, 11). The concordance rate for T1D among monozygotic twins is about 35% by age 60, signifying significant contributions from environmental factors ultimately leads to the onset of autoimmunity (12). Indeed, epidemiological evidence indicates a link between virus infections and development of T1D as well as multiple other autoimmune disorders, including multiple sclerosis (MS), systemic lupus erythematosus (SLE), and rheumatoid arthritis (RA). Studies have demonstrated geographical and seasonal differences, as well as disease outbreaks, correlate with increased incidence of T1D (11, 13–17).

Upon virus infection, initial innate sensing likely primes genetically susceptible or protected individuals for an effector or regulatory immunological response, respectively (18). Therefore, signaling from pattern-recognition receptors (PRRs) that identify pathogen-associated molecular patterns (PAMPs) associated with certain viruses could determine whether infection will promote T1D induction. The production of interferon (IFN) from this PRR–PAMP interaction is a prominent immunological response for defense of virus infections. All three types of IFN, type I (IFN-α, -β, -ε, -κ, and -ω), type II (IFN-γ), and type III (IFN-λ1, -2, -3, and -4), stimulate the production of pro-inflammatory molecules from the interferon-stimulated genes (ISGs) to induce a strong antiviral state to prevent spreading of the infection to surrounding cells and also to establish an adaptive immune response (19, 20). Accordingly, alterations in signaling stemming from PRR activation represent the foundational mechanisms leading to T1D development by producing an IFN signature which is conducive for autoimmunity.

INNATE VIRAL RECEPTORS

Genome-wide association studies indicate heritable differences in viral receptors and their related genes influence T1D susceptibility. Functional diversity of innate PRRs due to genetic variants may push the immune homeostasis toward an imbalance between pathogen hypersusceptibility and autoimmunity. In conjunction with an inherent variation, several different viruses have been implicated in causing inappropriate responses leading to T1D (4, 21). Among these viral candidates, enteroviruses such as coxsackievirus B (CVB) have been the most notable etiological agent attributed to T1D (22–24).

Dependent on the signals received from PRRs, innate immune cells including dendritic cells (DCs) macrophages, monocytes, natural killer cells and innate lymphoid cells can contribute to establishing either an effector inflammatory response or a more tolerogenic response by secreting cytokines, chemokines, and through priming of naïve T cells. While cross-reactivity of lymphocytes due to homology between viral and endogenous antigens and have been proposed in the establishment of T1D, non-specific immune stimulation causing persistent and low-grade inflammation are more likely underlaying the cause of pathogen-induced triggering of autoimmunity (25). The scale of an immune response is reliant on tightly regulated activation and inhibitory signals which may tip into an exaggerated or improper response causing the loss of self-tolerance (26).

Innate immunity and PRRs represent the first line of defense to coordinate the immune system for pathogen clearance and sets the stage for ensuing cellular and molecular pathway activation. The initial inflammatory state established with innate recognition of viral products induces beta cell damage and is then followed by apoptotic events and an effector T lymphocyte response killing the beta cells. Therefore, placing emphasis on the PRRs is critical for understanding the pathogenesis of autoimmune diabetes. There are three primary families of PRRs involved in detecting viral products: toll-like receptors (TLRs), retinoic acid-inducible gene I (RIG-I)-like receptors (RLRs), and nucleotide oligomerization domain-like receptors (27). Summarized in **Figure 1**, this review will focus on the contribution of RLRs and TLRs to T1D following engagement with their respective viral PAMPs.

RLRs IN T1D

The RLR family consists of RIG-I, melanoma differentiation-associated protein 5 (MDA5), and Laboratory of Genetics and Physiology 2 (LGP2), which are cytosolic receptors that recognize pieces of viral RNA from picornaviruses, flaviviruses, and paramyxoviruses (28). RLRs primarily bind viral replication intermediates [i.e., double-stranded RNA (dsRNA)] in infected cells and promote recruitment of transcription factors and adaptor molecules to restrict virus replication and prevent spread to other cells. Among a diverse range of effects, activation of MDA5 and RIG-I induce a potent type I and III IFN expression which go on to stimulate antiviral gene expression and increase antigen presentation (29, 30). LGP2 can bind short pieces of dsRNA and acts as a negative regulator for both RIG-I and MDA5; however, it lacks N-terminal caspase activation and recruitment domains necessary for signaling (31).

Expressed from the *IFIH1* gene, MDA5 is a cytosolic helicase which binds long viral dsRNA to induce a type I and III IFN response (18, 32). MDA5 has been identified as an important part of the host immune response to CVB and is necessary for preventing early replication of the virus and potentiating tissue damage (33). Various SNPs in the *IFIH1* gene have been found to confer either greater or reduced susceptibility for the onset of T1D (7). These SNPs likely alter the expression and activation of MDA5 when challenged with pathogenic stress. The A946T

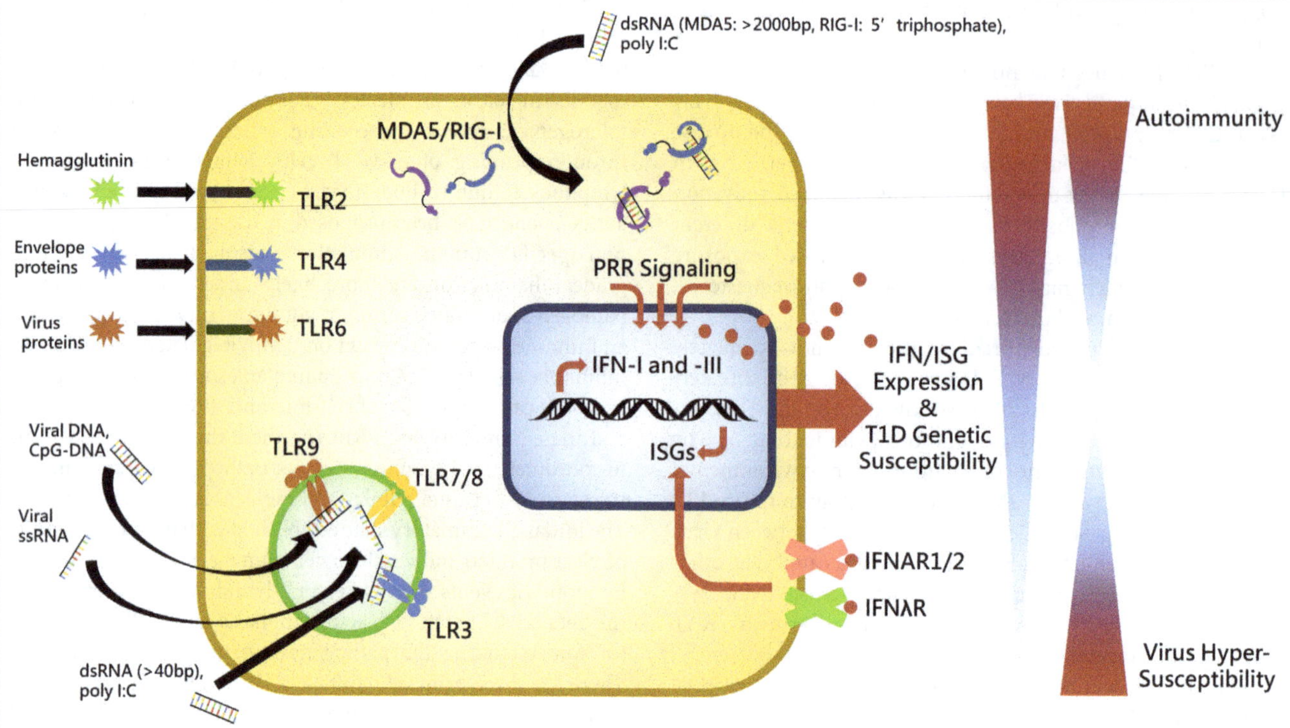

FIGURE 1 | Summary of toll-like receptor (TLR)- and RIG-I-like receptors virus-associated ligands and the relationship between interferon (IFN) expression, genetic susceptibility, and autoimmunity. Upon ligand binding, cytosolic MDA5 and RIG-I receptors induce activation of the adaptor molecule, VISA (also called MAVS, IPS1, and CARDIF), endosomally located toll-like receptor 3 (TLR3) recruits TRIF (also known as TICAM), and TLR2, -4, -6, -7, -8, and -9 interact with myeloid differentiation primary response protein 88 (MYD88) in order to provide IFN expression stimulation in the cell nucleus. IFN induces expression of various interferon-stimulated genes (ISGs) which perform positive feedback on IFN genes. IFN is released from the cell to establish an antiviral state in surrounding cells and act in an autocrine and paracrine manner by binding to its cell surface receptors, IFNAR1/2 and IFNλR. Individuals exhibiting heightened genetic susceptibility to type I diabetes (T1D) can have increased basal and pathogen-elicited expression of IFN causing the immune system to skew toward a self-reactive state. Conversely, significantly diminished IFN expression would render a host unable to mount a proper response to virus infection. Thus balance of receptor stimulation between autoimmunity and virus hypersusceptibility is tightly regulated and pathogenic stimuli which exacerbates inflammation in genetically susceptible individuals may result in loss of tolerance.

(rs1990760) mutation in *IFIH1* has been implicated in the development of multiple autoimmune diseases, including T1D, SLE, and MS (34, 35). Individuals which exhibit loss-of-function SNPs on even a single allele in RLR genes including E627* and I923V in MDA5 generally benefit from protection to T1D (35, 36). Hyperexpression or constitutive activation of MDA5 by mutagenesis has been shown to promote development of type I interferonopathies including SLE and Aicardi-Goutières syndrome (37–39). Diabetic patients which are heterozygous for the A946T SNP have a more robust ISG expression and immune response to CVB challenge when compared to healthy controls, potentially signifying an enhanced ability to promote IFN and ISG signal transduction during infection (40, 41). Accordingly, mutations in *IFIH1* causing gain-of-function are associated with hyperexpression of both IFN-I and -III (32, 39). Gorman et al. recently found that mice homozygous for the 946T variant as well as mice simultaneously exhibiting two *IFHI1* risk alleles (843R and 946T) have increased basal activation of *IFIH1*-related genes, enhanced protection from encephalomyocarditis virus infection, increased incidence of autoimmunity, and are inherently more sensitive to self RNA ligands (42). These mutations conferring T1D risk may be altering the homeostatic intensity of inflammatory molecule expression and/or the kinetics of target binding and activation—causing ligands to produce more potent or prolonged IFN responses. For example, the E627* mutation in MDA5 causes loss of a portion of the protein's C-terminal region and consequently forfeiture of dsRNA ligand binding (36). The A946T risk variant is also associated with heightened sensitivity to IFN-α in SLE patients so this mutation may allow receptors to become more easily activated (43). This evidence supports the notion that pathogen-mediated T1D is likely similar to the described type I interferonopathy disorders.

Our lab has previously exhibited the importance of MDA5 signaling by demonstrating reduced expression of the receptor can be protective for T1D. Non-obese diabetic (NOD) mice which were heterozygous for a null *IFIH1* allele (MDA5$^{+/-}$) and expressed roughly half as much MDA5 as wild-type NOD mice were shown to have decreased incidence of spontaneous disease

(18). More importantly, upon CVB4 infection, these heterozygous mice were completely protected from diabetes onset while about 50% of homozygous NOD mice carrying a full complement of *IFIH1* developed T1D within 7 days of infection. MDA5 knockout mice were also completely protected from spontaneous T1D onset; however, they were highly susceptible to virus. Compared to homozygous mice, the $MDA5^{+/-}$ mice displayed a specific type I IFN response characterized by a large spike in IFN-β occurring three days post-infection. It appears this particular IFN signature provides a succinct signal from IFN-β that is sufficient to clear the virus without inducing autoimmunity. Furthermore, $MDA5^{+/-}$ mice had decreased $CD4^+$ and $CD8^+$ effector T cells as well as a robust $CD4^+CD25^+Foxp3^+$ regulatory T cells (T_{REG}) response that suppressed IFN-γ-producing $CD4^+$ T cells, thereby preventing T1D.

TLRs IN T1D

Toll-like receptors are broadly expressed PRRs in both immune and non-immune cells which detect microbial- and viral-associated PAMPs (44). Upon recognition of pathogenic and/or foreign material, TLRs influence a number of immunologic mechanisms including activation and maturation of antigen-presenting cells (APCs), antibody production, downregulating T_{REG} responses, and inducing a pro-inflammatory environment through secretion of various cytokines and chemokines (45). Each of the TLRs may be stimulated with endogenous DNA or RNA antigens produced during cell death that may be a result of virus infection (46). However, those specifically recognizing viral-associated ligands: toll-like receptor 3 (TLR3), TLR7, TLR8, and TLR9 (and to a lesser extent TLR2, TLR4, and TLR6), have all been implicated in having a role in the diabetogenic potential of certain viruses (45, 47).

Toll-Like Receptor 3

Binding short pieces of dsRNA, TLR3 is an endosomal receptor heavily expressed in classical DCs and a variety of epithelial cells (47). Unlike all other TLRs, TLR3 is MYD88-independent and instead utilizes the adaptor molecule TRIF for signal transduction following activation (44). The dsRNA mimetic polyinosinic:polycytidylic (poly I:C) is recognized by TLR3 and has been shown in various mouse studies to either protect or induce and increase severity of T1D depending on dose and administration (48–50). NOD mice deficient for TLR3 have high mortality from CVB4 infections and the few that survive develop T1D (51). However, in some instances, TLR3-KO NOD mice can show less severe insulitis as well as some reduced susceptibility to T1D induction following CVB4 infection, but experience no difference in spontaneous disease development (52). TLR3 signaling within resident macrophages is critical for antiviral host defense to CVB4 as well as altering marginal zone B cell composition in NOD mice (50, 51). This indicates that enhanced TLR3 activation may participate in T1D development as a result of virus infection. Certain polymorphisms in the *TLR3* gene have shown to be associated with increased risk of T1D and more aggressive pathology (rs3775291 and rs13126816) while others impart protection (rs5743313 and rs11721827) (53).

Toll-Like Receptors 7 and 8

Expressed in the endosome, TLR7 and TLR8 recognize single-stranded RNA (ssRNA) while TLR9 is typically activated by binding unmethylated CpG DNA ligands from DNA viruses and microbial pathogens (54). TLR9-KO NOD mice have significantly lower rates of spontaneous diabetes, reduced activation of diabetogenic $CD8^+$ cytotoxic T cells (CTLs), and elevated expression of the immunosuppressive marker CD73, particularly on T_{REG} cells (55–57). Thus, activation of TLR9 induces a less tolerogenic immunological state that contributes to the pathogenesis and acceleration of T1D.

Using rat insulin promoter mice expressing lymphocytic choriomeningitis virus glycoprotein (LCMV-GP), researchers have shown that LCMV infection produced IFN-α *via* stimulation of TLR3 and TLR7; this in turn increased the expression of MHC class I molecules in the insulin-secreting beta cells of the pancreas (58). This mechanism, where TLR-mediated expression of IFN-α upregulates MHC-I in the islets, was shown to be vital for the diabetogenic potential of LCMV and subsequent progression toward an overt autoreactive response. LCMV-GP-specific CTLs in the pancreas were unable to cause disease without hyperexpression of MHC-I (58). Stimulation of TLR7 in conjunction with CD40 activation of DCs can induce diabetogenic CTLs in the pancreatic lymph nodes of NOD mice to promote onset of autoimmunity (59). Even the repeated topical administration of a TLR7 agonist, imiquimod, is sufficient to promote T1D development while inhibition using IRS661 can significantly decrease onset (59). TLR7 signaling in plasmacytoid DCs (pDCs) primes B and T cell activation *via* IFN-I secretion in rotavirus infections; however, inhibition of TLR7 is able to block this process from occurring and prevent acceleration of T1D following infection (60). The role of TLR7 and TLR8 in promoting autoimmunity has also been indicated in CVB3-induced self-reactivity toward myocardial tissue (61).

Environmental Inducers of TLRs

Previously, therapeutics for T1D prevention and treatment in the past have been primarily aimed at modifying or suppressing the adaptive immunity. Today, a shift in perspective of clinical methodology points toward targeting innate components to tolerize early pathogen-stimulated mechanisms as an effective strategy. Bednar and colleagues demonstrated that a TLR4-agonist monoclonal antibody, TLR4–MD-2, was able to halt and reverse fulminant T1D by inducing APC tolerance to pathogen in NOD mice (62). TLR4 is typically activated by lipopolysaccharides and other microbial products; however, envelope proteins from viruses including CVB can also stimulate its activation (63). Although it is uncertain whether CVB interaction with TLR4 is involved in T1D.

The natural route of enteroviral infection is through the gut, where the biodiversity of bacteria, viruses, fungi, and other microorganisms are significant mediators of immune homeostasis and autoimmunity (64). Accordingly, stimulation of the innate immunity and signaling on the mucosal surfaces from environmental pathogens could be detrimental to T1D onset. All TLRs other than TLR3 use the adaptor molecule MYD88 for signal transduction. Deletion of MyD88 in specific pathogen-free NOD mice confers resistance to diabetes (65). T1D resistance through loss of MYD88 is attributed to disruption in the gut flora since these MYD88-KO mice develop autoimmunity when housed in germ-free facilities (65). A "balanced signal hypothesis" has been suggested where microbiota-derived stimulation of TLR4 signaling through the adaptor molecule, TRIF, provides a tolerogenic effect on T1D pathogenesis, while TLR2 signaling promotes diabetogenesis (66). Commensal virus communities likely contribute similarly to innate stimulation through PRR recognition of viral ligands. A recent study has determined the intestinal virome is significantly altered prior to onset of autoimmunity in T1D-susceptible children (67). The overall diversity of the gut virome is reduced preceding disease development and certain viruses, such as *Circoviridae* and various bacteriophages, are significantly associated with either negative or positive T1D risk (67). This signifies a complex host–microbiome–virome relationship contributes to T1D and further studies are necessary to understand how these interactions alter disease and inflammation to skew genetically susceptible individuals toward either a protective or disease-causing state.

T1D DISPLAYS INTERFERONOPATHY-LIKE QUALITIES

Type I IFN

Pattern-recognition receptor activation and signaling remain the predominant inducer for IFN signatures that can protect as well as portend onset of not only T1D, but are also typical of rheumatic disorders such as SLE and RA (68, 69). The synergistic effects of type I and III IFNs are significant mediators for the adaptive immune system that promote lymphocyte maturation and mediate antigen presentation (19, 70). Accordingly, the IFN expression elicited by PRR activation is essential to autoimmune development. As such, it has been proposed that virus infections including CVB may be inducing localized interferonopathy-like characteristics within the islet microenvironment to trigger autoreactivity (71). Islets from patients recently experiencing onset of T1D exhibit heightened expression of certain ISGs in the islet and peri-islet regions in a manner which is similar to islets infected with virus (72). Knocking out the type I IFN receptor (IFNAR) in the T1D-susceptible rat strain, LEW.1WR1, protects from T1D, reduces insulitis, and delays onset following poly I:C or virus challenge (73). Originating with PRR stimulation, aberrant activation of pDCs and genetic mutations in the IFN signaling pathway likely contribute to the IFN signature evident in T1D induction (74).

Transient upregulation of type I IFN can be seen in genetically predisposed children preceding the seroconversion of T1D-related autoantibodies (75). Nearly all cells produce and respond to type I IFN; however, pDCs secrete a considerable amount of systemic IFN-α. Indeed, the secretion of IFN-α through TLR7- and TLR9-stimulated pDCs in the PLN of NOD mice is critical for onset of T1D (76). Blocking IFN-α signaling through IFNAR1 of young NOD mice (2–3 weeks old) significantly delays onset and incidence of diabetes as well as promote secretion of immunoregulatory cytokines, IL-4 and IL-10, in splenic $CD4^+$ T cells (76). Treating human islet cells with IFN-α *in vitro* triggers endoplasmic reticulum stress which disrupts insulin production by hindering the conversion of proinsulin to insulin signifying a potential mechanism by which IFN-α may be prompting development of T1D (77). Using a neutralizing antibody against IFN-α or using a specific agonist for S1PR1, an immune regulatory receptor which mediates IFN-α autoamplification, protects T1D onset in a *Rip*-LCMV mouse model by limiting the infiltration of autoreactive T cells into the islets and by inducing expression of tolerogenic receptor genes, such as *Pdcd1*, *Lag3*, *Ctla4*, *Tigit*, and *Btla* (78). This immunomodulation is able to prevent the autoreactive T cells from harming the insulin-secreting beta cells thus preserving the glucoregulatory function of the pancreas. Accordingly, the progression from prediabetes to full-onset disease requires signaling from IFN-α.

The transcription factor, interferon regulatory factor 7 (IRF7), is constitutively expressed in pDCs and is expressed in most other cells upon IFNAR activation (79). IRF7 is involved in signal transduction from MYD88-dependant endosomal TLRs (TLR7, TLR8, and TLR9) as well as RLRs to trigger IFN gene expression. A study by Hienig et al. used rat tissues to elucidate the IRF7-driven inflammatory network (IDIN) to relate that genetic mapping with known viral response genes and disease GWAS (80). It was determined that an rs9585056 SNP (on chromosome 13q32), located in the orthologous human genes controlling IDIN, was significantly associated with susceptibility to T1D and promoted expression of the IRF7-driven signaling network. Similar to gain-of-function mutations in *IFIH1*, this type of genetic predisposition would cause vigorous antiviral engagement resulting in an IFN and immune response which may be more pathogenic than the actual virus.

Type III IFN

While all nucleated cells respond to type I IFN, the type III IFN receptor (IFNλR) is primarily only expressed on pDCs and epithelial cells including pancreatic islet cells. Type III IFNs bind to the IFNλR consisting of dimer of IFNLR1 and IL10R2 domains. There is significant overlap in signaling pathways and activation between IFN-III and IFN-I; however, non-redundant roles for IFN-III in host antiviral responses exist (70, 81). Islets from humans exhibiting a protective *IFHI1* rs1990760 (946A/T) polymorphism produce an increased IFN-III response following CVB3 infection, likely through IRF-1 signaling, when compared to individuals with a risk-associated genotype (946T/T) (32). It is uncertain whether this additional expression of IFN-λ has protective qualities or whether it is simply a compensatory mechanism for lower IFN-I signaling from MDA5. However, IFN-λ-treated DCs are able to promote the specific proliferation of T_{REG} cells *in vitro* and IFN-λ treatment has been exhibited to improve pathology of RA in mice by reducing inflammatory neutrophils (82, 83). Collectively, this signifies IFN-III may be contributing to diabetes pathogenesis and should be further studied.

TIMING IS IMPORTANT FOR THE VIRAL ETIOLOGY OF T1D

Acute versus Persistent Infections

With regards to T1D induction, it is unclear whether virus infections are being sustained or acute infections are initiating mechanisms which go on unregulated even after viral clearance. If the virus becomes persistent, remnants of the infection linger within tissue-specific microenvironments to provide continuous stimulation of innate receptors to produce chronic inflammation as illustrated in **Figure 2**. Some picornaviruses such as Theiler's murine encephalomyelitis virus have been shown to persist in certain tissues to provide sufficient inflammation to drive autoimmunity (84). Conversely, acute infections may be priming the host and establishing events which direct an autoreactive effector response. Initial infections may be activating pathways which proceed with incessant positive feedback likely due to genetic differences which result in functional variations in innate compsonents, receptor activation/deactivation, and/or signaling pathway elements.

Coxsackievirus B is a positive sense ssRNA virus with a tropism for the pancreas, heart, and liver; however, it does not appear to establish cytolytic infections of pancreatic beta cells (85). Rather, CVB is likely promoting a pro-inflammatory environment within the pancreas to elicit autoimmunity (86). Infecting human islets with CVB3 induces potent expression of type I and III IFN, MDA5, RIG-I, and TLR3 along with a variety of inflammatory cytokines (32). Clinical evidence suggests some individuals who develop a loss of tolerance against insulin early in life (1–3 years) have an impaired capacity to mount a sufficient defense against the enterovirus viral capsid protein, viral protein 1 (VP1), that may cause an inability to sufficiently clear CVB following infection (87). Correspondingly, persistent pancreatic cell CVB4 infections have been shown to induce epigenetic changes by promoting production of dysregulated microRNAs targeting T1D risk genes (88).

Prolonged viral infections may be providing sustained activation of PRR signaling for the expression of IFN-I, IFN-III, and inflammatory cytokines, leading to a robust lymphocyte response and induction of autoimmunity. Low-grade enterovirus infections have been demonstrated to be established and maintained within the pancreatic islets of patients recently experiencing onset of T1D (3–9 weeks prior) but rarely in healthy controls (89). Persistent enteroviral presence has also been detected in the gut mucosa of T1D patients, however, viral genomes seem to be maintained in the absence of viral protein expression or production of infective particles (90). It is not clear whether defective replication is allowing production of the viral genes without assembly of virus particles or if virus components are simply persisting in the tissue after infections. However, conformational differences and modification of viral PAMPS may be dictating innate signaling. Stem-loop structures in long dsRNA are preferentially recognized by MDA5, while 5′ di- or triphosphate motifs on dsRNA are sensed by RIG-I (28, 91). Deletion or alterations

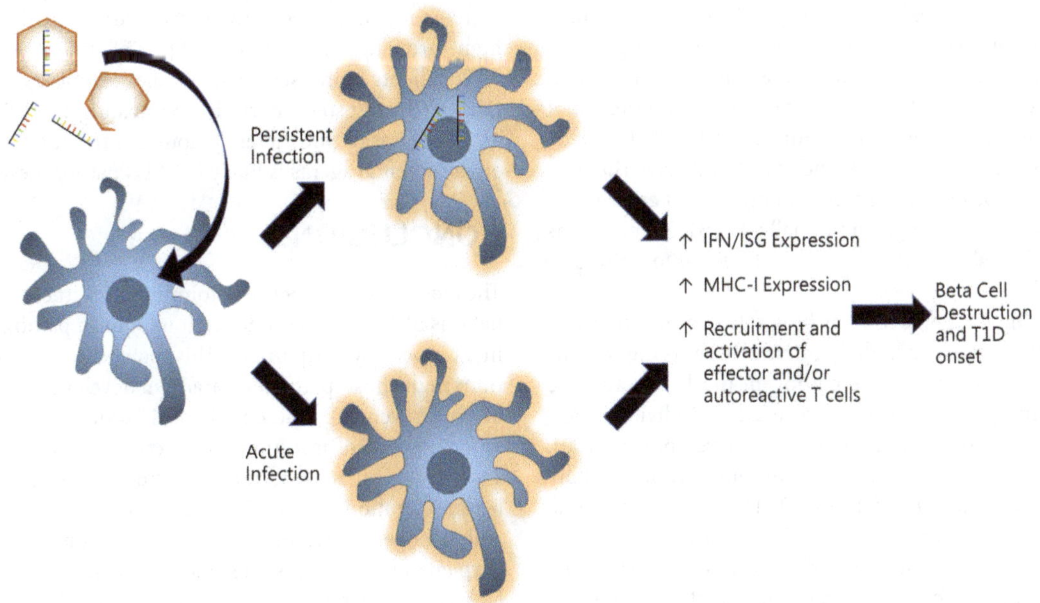

FIGURE 2 | Model for persistent versus acute infections in pancreas for promoting type I diabetes (T1D). Virus infections induce proinflammatory signaling in resident and infiltrating antigen-presenting cells of the pancreas. Persistent infections whereby viral products including enteroviral 5′ terminally deleted double-stranded RNA are maintained in tissue microenvironments to produce low-grade inflammatory signaling. Alternatively, acute infections may result in unregulated positive feedback mechanisms which produce chronic inflammation even after the virus is cleared.

in the structural composition of viral genomic PAMPs may be altering innate receptor signaling. CVB is known to persist in myocardial tissues following naturally occurring deletion of 5′ end terminal genomic sequences resulting in reduced virus replication and loss of cytopathicity (92–94). A recent study has shown that 5′ terminally deficient CVB persists also in the pancreas of NOD mice for at least several weeks following an acute wave of infection (95). The 5′ end of the CVB genome includes a cloverleaf-like tertiary structure which may be favorably sensed by MDA5; however, it is unknown exactly how innate sensing is affected with these terminal deleted viruses. Persistence of modulated enteroviruses may be providing sustained innate activation for prolonged inflammatory responses in and/or around the islets that result in the loss of self-tolerance in T1D. Alternatively, loss of structurally relevant motifs for RLR sensing may actually render receptors like MDA5 unable to bind the modified dsRNA ligands.

Temporal Determinants of T1D-Related Virus Infections

A systematic review compiling and analyzing clinical studies over approximately the last two decades, found that individuals had about 10 times higher odds of having enterovirus infections before or during onset of diabetes or prediabetes when compared to controls (24). Patients experiencing fulminant T1D directly following suspected enterovirus infection had strong expression of MDA, RIG-I, and VP1 in the islets when compared to T1D and non-diabetic control patients (96). Furthermore, mononuclear cells which infiltrate the pancreata of patients experiencing fulminant T1D had high expression of TLR3 and TLR4 (96). A recent study by Laitinen et al. screening systematically collected blood samples from birth through seroconversion for T1D-related autoantibodies and progression to clinical T1D, found that children were at higher T1D risk if infected with CVB1 (97). However, the patient was protected if exposed to either CVB3 or CVB6 prior to CVB1. Phylogenetic similarity between CVB1, CVB3, and CVB6 indicates the possibility that cross-protection between highly related enterovirus serotypes may be occurring. Additionally, CVB1 infection has been often followed by the appearance of islet autoantibodies about 6 months later (98, 99).

Characterizing temporal relationships between infection and autoimmunity onset are incredibly intricate due to the incredibly multifactorial nature of the pathogen, the hosts, and the disease. The timing of pathogen exposure and an individual's age likely has crucial impact on immunological development (100). It was recently determined that weaning pups from a colony of NOD mice with low incidence of T1D in a "diabetogenic environment" (i.e., with a colony of NOD mice with high T1D incidence) is able to transfer rates of diabetes development by adapting similar gut microbiota and promoting development of B cells in the mesenteric lymph nodes which are inherently more easily activated (101). This transmittance is only evident when the mice are weaned together, as this environmental exposure does not affect rate of diabetes onset when mice are co-housed starting at 3 weeks of age. Mustonen et al. performed a clinical analysis among children with HLA-dependent T1D genetic risk (exhibited DR3-DQ2 and/or DR4-DQ8 haplotypes) in Finland, Estonia, and Russian Karelia to determine disease trends in T1D susceptibility (102). Children who exhibited seroconversion of T1D-related autoantibodies had their first infection earlier and overall had more infections in the first year of their lives especially in the respiratory tract. Furthermore, those which progressed to T1D had twice as many infections in the first 3 years of their lives than non-diabetic children. It can be questioned, however, whether inherent susceptibility to T1D also confers lower tolerance to pathogens or whether the children experienced onset of T1D due to stress of the frequency of infections they experienced. A report from The Environmental Determinants of Diabetes in the Young study has confirmed that young children experiencing recent respiratory infections withstand a heightened risk of developing T1D-related autoimmunity; however, more work is necessary to determine specific viral agents present in the preceding months before autoantibody seroconversion (103).

While enteroviruses remain the most likely candidate for T1D onset, numerous other viruses have been shown to have roles in promoting or protecting T1D (104). Links between many viruses, however, seem to be more circumstantial and less evident. For instance, a study was performed examining the spatio-temporal exposure of viruses using geographical disease incidence rates in France and relating that data with mapping of T1D patient residences and the timing of the patients' T1D onset (105). This analysis indicates a positive correlation between summer diarrhea and influenza-like infections at 1–3 years of age with eventual development of T1D while there was negative relationship between varicella. Additionally, evidence suggests autoreactivity in NOD mice may be induced as a consequence of an immunological response against endogenous retrovirus-secreted microvesicles in the islets (106). Recently, a study using high-throughput proteomic profiling of antibodies in new-onset T1D patients found serum antibodies exhibit a significant reactivity against Epstein–Barr virus viral antigens (107). Ultimately, a multifactorial and heterogenous contribution from multiple environmental agents is likely for T1D pathogenesis.

CONCLUSION

The increased incidence of autoimmunity witnessed in developed nations likely signifies a deleterious shift in pathogenic environment especially early in life. This may be due to modern alterations in the host–pathogen paradigm developed over milleniums of co-evolvement. Epidemiological studies have not indicated an emergence of infections that could adequately explain such a significant increase in autoimmunity. Thus, it is likely caused by an alteration in how individuals respond to environmental and pathogenic stressors. One rationalization for this change, the "hygiene hypothesis," states that a reduction in pathogenic and environmental antigen exposure particularly during development has caused the immune system to produce over-exaggerated responses resulting in increased rates of autoimmunity. Decreased interaction with typical environmental antigens has fostered inexperience by innate host receptors, causing over-sensitization and improper stimulation of inflammatory pathways.

Environmental induction of T1D *via* viral infection may essentially require a "perfect storm" of immune reactivity where genetic susceptibility allows PRR signaling to render a target organ susceptible to attack by self-reactive lymphocytes. A balance of signaling by different receptors including RLRs and TLRs is providing opposing forces to simultaneously promote and inhibit autoimmunity and certain environmental stressors may be sufficient to tip that balance toward autoimmunity by inducing pro-inflammatory signaling. Ultimately, the timing, pathogenesis, and target site of infection influences the likelihood of antigen-non-specific bystander activation of autoreactive B and T cells. Understanding these pathways may hold a high degree of therapeutic potential to block onset of autoimmunity by mediating antigen exposure, developing relevant vaccines, and managing molecular pathogenesis mechanisms which confer disease development.

AUTHOR CONTRIBUTIONS

ZM and MH conceptualized, wrote, and edited the manuscript. ZM created the figures.

ACKNOWLEDGMENTS

The authors would like to thank Dr. Michelle Krakowski, Isobel C. Mouat, and Virginie S. E. Jean-Baptiste for their critical reviewing of this manuscript.

REFERENCES

1. Aw W, Fukuda S. Understanding the role of the gut ecosystem in diabetes mellitus. *J Diabetes Investig* (2017). doi:10.1111/jdi.12673
2. Knip M, Simell O. Environmental triggers of type 1 diabetes. *Cold Spring Harb Perspect Med* (2012) 2:a007690. doi:10.1101/cshperspect.a007690
3. Knip M, Veijola R, Virtanen SM, Hyöty H, Vaarala O, Akerblom HK. Environmental triggers and determinants of type 1 diabetes. *Diabetes* (2005) 54(Suppl 2):S125–36. doi:10.2337/diabetes.54.suppl_2.S125
4. van der Werf N, Kroese FGM, Rozing J, Hillebrands J-L. Viral infections as potential triggers of type 1 diabetes. *Diabetes Metab Res Rev* (2007) 23:169–83. doi:10.1002/dmrr.695
5. Bakay M, Pandey R, Hakonarson H. Genes involved in type 1 diabetes: an update. *Genes (Basel)* (2013) 4:499–521. doi:10.3390/genes4030499
6. Pociot F, Kaur S, Nielsen LB. Effects of the genome on immune regulation in type 1 diabetes. *Pediatr Diabetes* (2016) 17:37–42. doi:10.1111/pedi.12336
7. Smyth DJ, Cooper JD, Bailey R, Field S, Burren O, Smink LJ, et al. A genome-wide association study of nonsynonymous SNPs identifies a type 1 diabetes locus in the interferon-induced helicase (IFIH1) region. *Nat Genet* (2006) 38:617–9. doi:10.1038/ng1800
8. Coppieters KT, Boettler T, von Herrath M. Virus infections in type 1 diabetes. *Cold Spring Harb Perspect Med* (2012) 2:a007682. doi:10.1101/cshperspect.a007682
9. Massilamany C, Koenig A, Reddy J, Huber S, Buskiewicz I. Autoimmunity in picornavirus infections. *Curr Opin Virol* (2016) 16:8–14. doi:10.1016/j.coviro.2015.10.004
10. Ingelfinger JR, Jarcho JA. Increase in the incidence of diabetes and its implications. *N Engl J Med* (2017) 376:1473–4. doi:10.1056/NEJMe1616575
11. Long AE, Gillespie KM, Rokni S, Bingley PJ, Williams AJK. Rising incidence of type 1 diabetes is associated with altered immunophenotype at diagnosis. *Diabetes* (2012) 61:683–6. doi:10.2337/db11-0962
12. Redondo MJ, Jeffrey J, Fain PR, Eisenbarth GS, Orban T. Concordance for islet autoimmunity among monozygotic twins. *N Engl J Med* (2008) 359:2849–50. doi:10.1056/NEJMc0805398
13. DIAMOND Project Group. Incidence and trends of childhood type 1 diabetes worldwide 1990-1999. *Diabet Med* (2006) 23:857–66. doi:10.1111/j.1464-5491.2006.01925.x
14. EURODIAB ACE Study Group. Variation and trends in incidence of childhood diabetes in Europe. *Lancet* (2000) 355:873–6. doi:10.1016/S0140-6736(99)07125-1
15. Green A, Patterson CC; EURODIAB TIGER Study Group, Europe and Diabetes. Trends in the incidence of childhood-onset diabetes in Europe 1989-1998. *Diabetologia* (2001) 44(Suppl 3):B3–8. doi:10.1007/PL00002950
16. Oikarinen S, Tauriainen S, Hober D, Lucas B, Vazeou A, Sioofy-Khojine A, et al. Virus antibody survey in different European populations indicates risk association between coxsackievirus B1 and type 1 diabetes. *Diabetes* (2014) 63:655–62. doi:10.2337/db13-0620
17. Wagenknecht LE, Roseman JM, Herman WH. Increased incidence of insulin-dependent diabetes mellitus following an epidemic of coxsackievirus B5. *Am J Epidemiol* (1991) 133:1024–31. doi:10.1093/oxfordjournals.aje.a115811
18. Lincez PJ, Shanina I, Horwitz MS. Reduced expression of the MDA5 gene IFIH1 prevents autoimmune diabetes. *Diabetes* (2015) 64:2184–93. doi:10.2337/db14-1223
19. Mostafavi S, Yoshida H, Moodley D, LeBoité H, Rothamel K, Raj T, et al. Parsing the interferon transcriptional network and its disease associations. *Cell* (2016) 164:564–78. doi:10.1016/j.cell.2015.12.032
20. Schneider WM, Chevillotte MD, Rice CM. Interferon-stimulated genes: a complex web of host defenses. *Annu Rev Immunol* (2014) 32:513–45. doi:10.1146/annurev-immunol-032713-120231
21. Richardson SJ, Horwitz MS. Is type 1 diabetes "going viral"? *Diabetes* (2014) 63:2203–5. doi:10.2337/db14-0510
22. Andréoletti L, Hober D, Hober-Vandenberghe C, Belaich S, Vantyghem MC, Lefebvre J, et al. Detection of coxsackie B virus RNA sequences in whole blood samples from adult patients at the onset of type I diabetes mellitus. *J Med Virol* (1997) 52:121–7. doi:10.1002/(SICI)1096-9071(199706)52:2<121::AID-JMV1>3.0.CO;2-5
23. Sarmiento L, Cabrera-Rode E, Lekuleni L, Cuba I, Molina G, Fonseca M, et al. Occurrence of enterovirus RNA in serum of children with newly diagnosed type 1 diabetes and islet cell autoantibody-positive subjects in a population with a low incidence of type 1 diabetes. *Autoimmunity* (2007) 40:540–5. doi:10.1080/08916930701523429
24. Yeung W-CG, Rawlinson WD, Craig ME. Enterovirus infection and type 1 diabetes mellitus: systematic review and meta-analysis of observational molecular studies. *BMJ* (2011) 342:d35. doi:10.1136/bmj.d35
25. Roep BO, Hiemstra HS, Schloot NC, De Vries RRP, Chaudhuri A, Behan PO, et al. Molecular mimicry in type 1 diabetes: immune cross-reactivity between islet autoantigen and human cytomegalovirus but not coxsackie virus. *Ann N Y Acad Sci* (2002) 958:163–5. doi:10.1111/j.1749-6632.2002.tb02961.x
26. Quicke KM, Diamond MS, Suthar MS. Negative regulators of the RIG-I-like receptor signaling pathway. *Eur J Immunol* (2017) 47:615–28. doi:10.1002/eji.201646484
27. Thompson MR, Kaminski JJ, Kurt-Jones EA, Fitzgerald KA. Pattern recognition receptors and the innate immune response to viral infection. *Viruses* (2011) 3:920–40. doi:10.3390/v3060920
28. Yoneyama M, Onomoto K, Jogi M, Akaboshi T, Fujita T. Viral RNA detection by RIG-I-like receptors. *Curr Opin Immunol* (2015) 32:48–53. doi:10.1016/j.coi.2014.12.012
29. Loo Y-M, Gale M. Immune signaling by RIG-I-like receptors. *Immunity* (2011) 34:680–92. doi:10.1016/j.immuni.2011.05.003
30. Odendall C, Dixit E, Stavru F, Bierne H, Franz KM, Fiegen A, et al. Diverse intracellular pathogens activate Type III Interferon expression from peroxisomes. *Nat Immunol* (2014) 15:717–26. doi:10.1038/ni.2915
31. Komuro A, Horvath CM. RNA- and virus-independent inhibition of antiviral signaling by RNA helicase LGP2. *J Virol* (2006) 80:12332–42. doi:10.1128/JVI.01325-06

32. Domsgen E, Lind K, Kong L, Hühn MH, Rasool O, Kuppeveld F, et al. An IFIH1 gene polymorphism associated with risk for autoimmunity regulates canonical antiviral defence pathways in coxsackievirus infected human pancreatic islets. *Sci Rep* (2016) 6:39378. doi:10.1038/srep39378
33. Hühn MH, McCartney SA, Lind K, Svedin E, Colonna M, Flodström-Tullberg M. Melanoma differentiation-associated protein-5 (MDA-5) limits early viral replication but is not essential for the induction of type 1 interferons after coxsackievirus infection. *Virology* (2010) 401:42–8. doi:10.1016/j.virol.2010.02.010
34. Cen H, Wang W, Leng R-X, Wang T-Y, Pan H-F, Fan Y-G, et al. Association of IFIH1 rs1990760 polymorphism with susceptibility to autoimmune diseases: a meta-analysis. *Autoimmunity* (2013) 46:455–62. doi:10.3109/08916934.2013.796937
35. Nejentsev S, Walker N, Riches D, Egholm M, Todd JA. Rare variants of IFIH1, a gene implicated in antiviral responses, protect against type 1 diabetes. *Science* (2009) 324:387–9. doi:10.1126/science.1167728
36. Shigemoto T, Kageyama M, Hirai R, Zheng J, Yoneyama M, Fujita T. Identification of loss of function mutations in human genes encoding RIG-I and MDA5: implications for resistance to type I diabetes. *J Biol Chem* (2009) 284:13348–54. doi:10.1074/jbc.M809449200
37. Crampton SP, Deane JA, Feigenbaum L, Bolland S. IFIH1 gene dose effect reveals MDA5-mediated chronic type I IFN gene signature, viral resistance, and accelerated autoimmunity. *J Immunol* (2012) 1950(188):1451–9. doi:10.4049/jimmunol.1102705
38. Funabiki M, Kato H, Miyachi Y, Toki H, Motegi H, Inoue M, et al. Autoimmune disorders associated with gain of function of the intracellular sensor MDA5. *Immunity* (2014) 40:199–212. doi:10.1016/j.immuni.2013.12.014
39. Rice GI, del Toro Duany Y, Jenkinson EM, Forte GM, Anderson BH, Ariaudo G, et al. Gain-of-function mutations in IFIH1 cause a spectrum of human disease phenotypes associated with upregulated type I interferon signaling. *Nat Genet* (2014) 46:503–9. doi:10.1038/ng.2933
40. Downes K, Pekalski M, Angus KL, Hardy M, Nutland S, Smyth DJ, et al. Reduced expression of IFIH1 is protective for type 1 diabetes. *PLoS One* (2010) 5:e12646. doi:10.1371/journal.pone.0012646
41. Schulte BM, Gielen PR, Kers-Rebel ED, Prosser AC, Lind K, Flodström-Tullberg M, et al. Enterovirus exposure uniquely discriminates type 1 diabetes patients with a homozygous from a heterozygous melanoma differentiation-associated protein 5/interferon induced with helicase C domain 1 A946T genotype. *Viral Immunol* (2016) 29:389–97. doi:10.1089/vim.2015.0140
42. Gorman JA, Hundhausen C, Errett JS, Stone AE, Allenspach EJ, Ge Y, et al. The A946T variant of the RNA sensor IFIH1 mediates an interferon program that limits viral infection but increases the risk for autoimmunity. *Nat Immunol* (2017) 18:744–52. doi:10.1038/ni.3766
43. Robinson T, Kariuki SN, Franek BS, Kumabe M, Kumar AA, Badaracco M, et al. Autoimmune disease risk variant of IFIH1 is associated with increased sensitivity to IFN-α and serologic autoimmunity in lupus patients. *J Immunol* (2011) 1950(187):1298–303. doi:10.4049/jimmunol.1100857
44. Kawasaki T, Kawai T. Toll-like receptor signaling pathways. *Front Immunol* (2014) 5:461. doi:10.3389/fimmu.2014.00461
45. Kawai T, Akira S. The role of pattern-recognition receptors in innate immunity: update on toll-like receptors. *Nat Immunol* (2010) 11:373–84. doi:10.1038/ni.1863
46. Rifkin IR, Leadbetter EA, Busconi L, Viglianti G, Marshak-Rothstein A. Toll-like receptors, endogenous ligands, and systemic autoimmune disease. *Immunol Rev* (2005) 204:27–42. doi:10.1111/j.0105-2896.2005.00239.x
47. Akira S, Uematsu S, Takeuchi O. Pathogen recognition and innate immunity. *Cell* (2006) 124:783–801. doi:10.1016/j.cell.2006.02.015
48. Ewel CH, Sobel DO, Zeligs BJ, Bellanti JA. Poly I:C accelerates development of diabetes mellitus in diabetes-prone BB rat. *Diabetes* (1992) 41:1016–21. doi:10.2337/diab.41.8.1016
49. Moriyama H, Wen L, Abiru N, Liu E, Yu L, Miao D, et al. Induction and acceleration of insulitis/diabetes in mice with a viral mimic (polyinosinic-polycytidylic acid) and an insulin self-peptide. *Proc Natl Acad Sci U S A* (2002) 99:5539–44. doi:10.1073/pnas.082120099
50. Wilson CS, Elizer SK, Marshall AF, Stocks BT, Moore DJ. Regulation of B lymphocyte responses to toll-like receptor ligand binding during diabetes prevention in non-obese diabetic (NOD) mice. *J Diabetes* (2015) 8:120–31. doi:10.1111/1753-0407.12263
51. Richer MJ, Lavallée DJ, Shanina I, Horwitz MS. Toll-like receptor 3 signaling on macrophages is required for survival following coxsackievirus B4 infection. *PLoS One* (2009) 4:e4127. doi:10.1371/journal.pone.0004127
52. McCall KD, Thuma JR, Courreges MC, Benencia F, James CBL, Malgor R, et al. Toll-like receptor 3 is critical for coxsackievirus B4-induced type 1 diabetes in female NOD mice. *Endocrinology* (2015) 156:453–61. doi:10.1210/en.2013-2006
53. Assmann TS, de Almeida Brondani L, Bauer AC, Canani LH, Crispim D. Polymorphisms in the TLR3 gene are associated with risk for type 1 diabetes mellitus. *Eur J Endocrinol* (2014) 170:519–27. doi:10.1530/EJE-13-0963
54. Kumar H, Kawai T, Akira S. Pathogen recognition in the innate immune response. *Biochem J* (2009) 420:1–16. doi:10.1042/BJ20090272
55. Tai N, Wong FS, Wen L. TLR9 deficiency promotes CD73 expression in T cells and diabetes protection in nonobese diabetic mice. *J Immunol* (2013) 1950(191):2926–37. doi:10.4049/jimmunol.1300547
56. Wong FS, Hu C, Zhang L, Du W, Alexopoulou L, Flavell RA, et al. The role of toll-like receptors 3 and 9 in the development of autoimmune diabetes in NOD mice. *Ann N Y Acad Sci* (2008) 1150:146–8. doi:10.1196/annals.1447.039
57. Zhang Y, Lee AS, Shameli A, Geng X, Finegood D, Santamaria P, et al. TLR9 blockade inhibits activation of diabetogenic CD8+ T cells and delays autoimmune diabetes. *J Immunol* (2010) 1950(184):5645–53. doi:10.4049/jimmunol.0901814
58. Lang KS, Recher M, Junt T, Navarini AA, Harris NL, Freigang S, et al. Toll-like receptor engagement converts T-cell autoreactivity into overt autoimmune disease. *Nat Med* (2005) 11:138–45. doi:10.1038/nm1176
59. Lee AS, Ghoreishi M, Cheng WK, Chang T-YE, Zhang YQ, Dutz JP. Toll-like receptor 7 stimulation promotes autoimmune diabetes in the NOD mouse. *Diabetologia* (2011) 54:1407–16. doi:10.1007/s00125-011-2083-y
60. Pane JA, Webster NL, Coulson BS. Rotavirus activates lymphocytes from non-obese diabetic mice by triggering toll-like receptor 7 signaling and interferon production in plasmacytoid dendritic cells. *PLoS Pathog* (2014) 10:e1003998. doi:10.1371/journal.ppat.1003998
61. Triantafilou K, Orthopoulos G, Vakakis E, Ahmed MAE, Golenbock DT, Lepper PM, et al. Human cardiac inflammatory responses triggered by coxsackie B viruses are mainly toll-like receptor (TLR) 8-dependent. *Cell Microbiol* (2005) 7:1117–26. doi:10.1111/j.1462-5822.2005.00537.x
62. Bednar KJ, Tsukamoto H, Kachapati K, Ohta S, Wu Y, Katz JD, et al. Reversal of new-onset type 1 diabetes with an agonistic TLR4/MD-2 monoclonal antibody. *Diabetes* (2015) 64:3614–26. doi:10.2337/db14-1868
63. Triantafilou K, Triantafilou M. Coxsackievirus B4-induced cytokine production in pancreatic cells is mediated through toll-like receptor 4. *J Virol* (2004) 78:11313–20. doi:10.1128/JVI.78.20.11313-11320.2004
64. Filyk HA, Osborne LC. The multibiome: the intestinal ecosystem's influence on immune homeostasis, health, and disease. *EBioMedicine* (2016) 13:46–54. doi:10.1016/j.ebiom.2016.10.007
65. Wen L, Ley RE, Volchkov PY, Stranges PB, Avanesyan L, Stonebraker AC, et al. Innate immunity and intestinal microbiota in the development of type 1 diabetes. *Nature* (2008) 455:1109–13. doi:10.1038/nature07336
66. Burrows MP, Volchkov P, Kobayashi KS, Chervonsky AV. Microbiota regulates type 1 diabetes through toll-like receptors. *Proc Natl Acad Sci U S A* (2015) 112:9973–7. doi:10.1073/pnas.1508740112
67. Zhao G, Vatanen T, Droit L, Park A, Kostic AD, Poon TW, et al. Intestinal virome changes precede autoimmunity in type I diabetes-susceptible children. *Proc Natl Acad Sci U S A* (2017) 114:E6166–75. doi:10.1073/pnas.1706359114
68. Conigliaro P, Perricone C, Benson RA, Garside P, Brewer JM, Perricone R, et al. The type I IFN system in rheumatoid arthritis. *Autoimmunity* (2010) 43:220–5. doi:10.3109/08916930903510914
69. Crow MK. Type I interferon in the pathogenesis of lupus. *J Immunol* (2014) 1950(192):5459–68. doi:10.4049/jimmunol.1002795
70. Lazear HM, Nice TJ, Diamond MS. Interferon-λ: immune functions at barrier surfaces and beyond. *Immunity* (2015) 43:15–28. doi:10.1016/j.immuni.2015.07.001
71. Jean-Baptiste VSE, Xia C-Q, Clare-Salzler MJ, Horwitz MS. Type 1 diabetes and type 1 interferonopathies: localization of a type 1 common thread of virus infection in the pancreas. *EBioMedicine* (2017) 22:10–7. doi:10.1016/j.ebiom.2017.06.014
72. Lundberg M, Krogvold L, Kuric E, Dahl-Jørgensen K, Skog O. Expression of interferon-stimulated genes in insulitic pancreatic islets of patients recently diagnosed with type 1 diabetes. *Diabetes* (2016) 65:3104–10. doi:10.2337/db16-0616

73. Qaisar N, Lin S, Ryan G, Yang C, Oikemus SR, Brodsky MH, et al. A critical role for the type I interferon receptor in virus-induced autoimmune diabetes in rats. *Diabetes* (2017) 66:145–57. doi:10.2337/db16-0462
74. Xia C-Q, Peng R, Chernatynskaya AV, Yuan L, Carter C, Valentine J, et al. Increased IFN-α-producing plasmacytoid dendritic cells (pDCs) in human Th1-mediated type 1 diabetes: pDCs augment Th1 responses through IFN-α production. *J Immunol* (2014) 1950(193):1024–34. doi:10.4049/jimmunol.1303230
75. Ferreira RC, Guo H, Coulson RMR, Smyth DJ, Pekalski ML, Burren OS, et al. A type I interferon transcriptional signature precedes autoimmunity in children genetically at-risk of type 1 diabetes. *Diabetes* (2014) 63:2538–50. doi:10.2337/db13-1777
76. Li Q, Xu B, Michie SA, Rubins KH, Schreriber RD, McDevitt HO. Interferon-α initiates type 1 diabetes in nonobese diabetic mice. *Proc Natl Acad Sci U S A* (2008) 105:12439–44. doi:10.1073/pnas.0806439105
77. Lombardi A, Tomer Y. Interferon alpha impairs insulin production in human beta cells via endoplasmic reticulum stress. *J Autoimmun* (2017) 80:48–55. doi:10.1016/j.jaut.2017.02.002
78. Marro BS, Ware BC, Zak J, de la Torre JC, Rosen H, Oldstone MBA. Progression of type 1 diabetes from the prediabetic stage is controlled by interferon-α signaling. *Proc Natl Acad Sci U S A* (2017) 114:3708–13. doi:10.1073/pnas.1700878114
79. Honda K, Taniguchi T. IRFs: master regulators of signalling by toll-like receptors and cytosolic pattern-recognition receptors. *Nat Rev Immunol* (2006) 6:644–58. doi:10.1038/nri1900
80. Heinig M, Petretto E, Wallace C, Bottolo L, Rotival M, Lu H, et al. A trans-acting locus regulates an anti-viral expression network and type 1 diabetes risk. *Nature* (2010) 467:460–4. doi:10.1038/nature09386
81. Pott J, Mahlakõiv T, Mordstein M, Duerr CU, Michiels T, Stockinger S, et al. IFN-lambda determines the intestinal epithelial antiviral host defense. *Proc Natl Acad Sci U S A* (2011) 108:7944–9. doi:10.1073/pnas.1100552108
82. Blazek K, Eames HL, Weiss M, Byrne AJ, Perocheau D, Pease JE, et al. IFN-λ resolves inflammation via suppression of neutrophil infiltration and IL-1β production. *J Exp Med* (2015) 212:845–53. doi:10.1084/jem.20140995
83. Mennechet FJD, Uzé G. Interferon-λ-treated dendritic cells specifically induce proliferation of FOXP3-expressing suppressor T cells. *Blood* (2006) 107:4417–23. doi:10.1182/blood-2005-10-4129
84. Trottier M, Schlitt BP, Kung AY, Lipton HL. Transition from acute to persistent Theiler's virus infection requires active viral replication that drives proinflammatory cytokine expression and chronic demyelinating disease. *J Virol* (2004) 78:12480–8. doi:10.1128/JVI.78.22.12480-12488.2004
85. Dotta F, Censini S, van Halteren AGS, Marselli L, Masini M, Dionisi S, et al. Coxsackie B4 virus infection of beta cells and natural killer cell insulitis in recent-onset type 1 diabetic patients. *Proc Natl Acad Sci U S A* (2007) 104:5115–20. doi:10.1073/pnas.0700442104
86. Schulte BM, Lanke KHW, Piganelli JD, Kers-Rebel ED, Bottino R, Trucco M, et al. Cytokine and chemokine production by human pancreatic islets upon enterovirus infection. *Diabetes* (2012) 61:2030–6. doi:10.2337/db11-1547
87. Ashton MP, Eugster A, Walther D, Daehling N, Riethausen S, Kuehn D, et al. Incomplete immune response to coxsackie B viruses associates with early autoimmunity against insulin. *Sci Rep* (2016) 6:32899. doi:10.1038/srep32899
88. Engelmann I, Alidjinou EK, Bertin A, Bossu J, Villenet C, Figeac M, et al. Persistent coxsackievirus B4 infection induces microRNA dysregulation in human pancreatic cells. *Cell Mol Life Sci* (2017) 74(20):3851–61. doi:10.1007/s00018-017-2567-0
89. Krogvold L, Edwin B, Buanes T, Frisk G, Skog O, Anagandula M, et al. Detection of a low-grade enteroviral infection in the islets of Langerhans of living patients newly diagnosed with type 1 diabetes. *Diabetes* (2015) 64:1682–7. doi:10.2337/db14-1370
90. Oikarinen M, Tauriainen S, Oikarinen S, Honkanen T, Collin P, Rantala I, et al. Type 1 diabetes is associated with enterovirus infection in gut mucosa. *Diabetes* (2012) 61:687–91. doi:10.2337/db11-1157
91. Wu B, Peisley A, Richards C, Yao H, Zeng X, Lin C, et al. Structural basis for dsRNA recognition, filament formation, and antiviral signal activation by MDA5. *Cell* (2013) 152:276–89. doi:10.1016/j.cell.2012.11.048
92. Bouin A, Nguyen Y, Wehbe M, Renois F, Fornes P, Bani-Sadr F, et al. Major persistent 5′ terminally deleted coxsackievirus B3 populations in human endomyocardial tissues. *Emerg Infect Dis* (2016) 22:1488–90. doi:10.3201/eid2208.160186
93. Kim K-S, Tracy S, Tapprich W, Bailey J, Lee C-K, Kim K, et al. 5'-Terminal deletions occur in coxsackievirus B3 during replication in murine hearts and cardiac myocyte cultures and correlate with encapsidation of negative-strand viral RNA. *J Virol* (2005) 79:7024–41. doi:10.1128/JVI.79.11.7024-7041.2005
94. Lévêque N, Garcia M, Bouin A, Nguyen JHC, Tran GP, Andreoletti L, et al. Functional consequences of RNA 5' terminal deletions on coxsackievirus B3 RNA replication and ribonucleoprotein complex formation. *J Virol* (2017). doi:10.1128/JVI.00423-17
95. Tracy S, Smithee S, Alhazmi A, Chapman N. Coxsackievirus can persist in murine pancreas by deletion of 5' terminal genomic sequences. *J Med Virol* (2015) 87:240–7. doi:10.1002/jmv.24039
96. Aida K, Nishida Y, Tanaka S, Maruyama T, Shimada A, Awata T, et al. RIG-I- and MDA5-initiated innate immunity linked with adaptive immunity accelerates beta-cell death in fulminant type 1 diabetes. *Diabetes* (2011) 60:884–9. doi:10.2337/db10-0795
97. Laitinen OH, Honkanen H, Pakkanen O, Oikarinen S, Hankaniemi MM, Huhtala H, et al. Coxsackievirus B1 is associated with induction of β-cell autoimmunity that portends type 1 diabetes. *Diabetes* (2014) 63:446–55. doi:10.2337/db13-0619
98. Oikarinen S, Martiskainen M, Tauriainen S, Huhtala H, Ilonen J, Veijola R, et al. Enterovirus RNA in blood is linked to the development of type 1 diabetes. *Diabetes* (2011) 60:276–9. doi:10.2337/db10-0186
99. Stene LC, Oikarinen S, Hyöty H, Barriga KJ, Norris JM, Klingensmith G, et al. Enterovirus infection and progression from islet autoimmunity to type 1 diabetes: the Diabetes and Autoimmunity Study in the Young (DAISY). *Diabetes* (2010) 59:3174–80. doi:10.2337/db10-0866
100. Hiltunen M, Hyöty H, Knip M, Ilonen J, Reijonen H, Vähäsalo P, et al. Islet cell antibody seroconversion in children is temporally associated with enterovirus infections. Childhood Diabetes in Finland (DiMe) Study Group. *J Infect Dis* (1997) 175:554–60. doi:10.1093/infdis/175.3.554
101. De Riva A, Wållberg M, Ronchi F, Coulson R, Sage A, Thorne L, et al. Regulation of type 1 diabetes development and B-cell activation in nonobese diabetic mice by early life exposure to a diabetogenic environment. *PLoS One* (2017) 12:e0181964. doi:10.1371/journal.pone.0181964
102. Mustonen N, Siljander H, Peet A, Tillmann V, Härkönen T, Ilonen J, et al. Early childhood infections precede development of beta-cell autoimmunity and type 1 diabetes in children with HLA-conferred disease risk. *Pediatr Diabetes* (2017). doi:10.1111/pedi.12547
103. Lönnrot M, Lynch KF, Elding Larsson H, Lernmark Å, Rewers MJ, Törn C, et al. Respiratory infections are temporally associated with initiation of type 1 diabetes autoimmunity: the TEDDY study. *Diabetologia* (2017) 60:1931–40. doi:10.1007/s00125-017-4365-5
104. Rodriguez-Calvo T, von Herrath MG. Enterovirus infection and type 1 diabetes: closing in on a link? *Diabetes* (2015) 64:1503–5. doi:10.2337/db14-1931
105. Bougnères P, Le Fur S; Isis-Diab Collaborative Group, Valtat S, Kamatani Y, Lathrop M, et al. Using spatio-temporal surveillance data to test the infectious environment of children before type 1 diabetes diagnosis. *PLoS One* (2017) 12:e0170658. doi:10.1371/journal.pone.0170658
106. Bashratyan R, Regn D, Rahman MJ, Marquardt K, Fink E, Hu W-Y, et al. Type 1 diabetes pathogenesis is modulated by spontaneous autoimmune responses to endogenous retrovirus antigens in NOD mice. *Eur J Immunol* (2017) 47:575–84. doi:10.1002/eji.201646755
107. Bian X, Wallstrom G, Davis A, Wang J, Park J, Throop A, et al. Immunoproteomic profiling of antiviral antibodies in new-onset type 1 diabetes using protein arrays. *Diabetes* (2016) 65:285–96. doi:10.2337/db15-0179

7

Neutrophil Extracellular Traps Caused by Gut Leakage Trigger the Autoimmune Response in Non-Obese Diabetic Mice

Qi You[1†], Yiming Shen[1†], Yiling Wu[1], Yuyan Li[2], Chang Liu[2], Fengjie Huang[1], Harvest F. Gu[3] and Jie Wu[1*]*

[1] College of Life Science and Technology, China Pharmaceutical University, Nanjing, China, [2] State Key Laboratory of Natural Medicines, China Pharmaceutical University, Nanjing, China, [3] Center for Pathophysiology, School of Basic Medicine and Clinical Pharmacy, China Pharmaceutical University, Nanjing, China

***Correspondence:**
Jie Wu
wujie@cpu.edu.cn
Harvest F. Gu
feng.gu@cpu.edu.cn

[†]These authors have contributed equally to this work

Increased formation of neutrophil extracellular traps (NETs) is associated with gut leakage in type 1 diabetes (T1D). To explore the mechanism of how enteropathy exacerbated by NETs triggers pancreatic autoimmunity in T1D, we carried out a correlation analysis for NET formation with gut barrier functions and autoimmunity in nonobese diabetic (NOD) mice. Inducing chronic colitis or knocking out of peptidyl arginine deiminase type 4 (PAD4) in NOD mice were used to further study the effect of NET formation on the progression of T1D. Microbial alterations in Deferribacteres and Proteobacteria, along with the loss of gut barrier function, were found to be associated with increased endotoxin and abnormal formation of NETs in NOD mice. Both DSS-induced colitis and knockout of PAD4 in NOD mice indicated that PAD4-dependent NET formation was involved in the aggravation of gut barrier dysfunction, the production of autoantibodies, and the activation of enteric autoimmune T cells, which then migrated to pancreatic lymph nodes (PLNs) and caused self-damage. The current study thus provides evidence that PAD4-dependent NET formation is engaged in leaky gut triggering pancreatic autoimmunity and suggests that either degradation of NETs or inhibition of NET formation may be helpful for innovative therapeutic interventions in T1D.

Keywords: autoimmunity, gut barrier function, neutrophil extracellular traps, peptidyl arginine deiminase type 4, type 1 diabetes

INTRODUCTION

Type 1 diabetes (T1D) is a chronic autoimmune disease characterized by insulin-producing pancreatic beta cells destroyed by autoreactive T cells (1, 2). Adequate evidence has been provided to confirm the leaky gut-affecting pancreas pathogenic theory. For instance, the development of clinical diabetes in patients and preclinical models (diabetes-prone rats) of T1D is often preceded by increased intestinal permeability (1, 2). It has been proposed that the loss of gut barrier function caused by enteric infections (3), commensal microbiota dysbiosis (4, 5), dietary antigen exposure, and local inflammation (6) could lead to the uncontrolled invasion of bacterial components, followed by the generation of islet-reactive CD4- or CD8-positive T cells (7) in gut-associated lymphoid tissue (GALT), and these cells possess PLN homing abilities and ultimately induce insulitis (8–10). However, in this process, the transition from innate immunity to adaptive immunity after losing gut barrier integrity has rarely been mentioned.

Neutrophils are essential innate immune cells in the recognition and elimination of invasive pathogens (11), and their contribution to the pathogenesis of T1D was demonstrated in NOD mice, in which neutrophils infiltrated the pancreas and could form NETs (12). In line with this finding, in T1D patients, a reduced circulating neutrophil number was accompanied by the rise of neutrophils or NETs in their pancreas (13, 14). Our previous clinical study suggested that NET formation is increased in new-onset T1D patients compared with healthy controls (15). Parackova et al. have recently indicated that NET-induced dendritic cell activation led to Th1 polarization in T1D patients (16). As a special way of capturing invasive bacteria, NETs contain abundant cytosolic proteins, especially those with post-translational modifications, such as PAD4 that drives citrullination, which is an important potential source of self-antigens to promote the loss of immune tolerance and autoimmunity (17) and increase the generation of antineutrophil cytoplasmic antibodies (ANCAs) (18) and anti-cyclic citrullinated peptide antibodies (ACPAs) (19). Masses of self-DNA sprayed in this process were proven to be capable of activating plasmacytoid dendritic cells (pDCs) or monocytes through cGAS-STING and triggering proinflammatory cytokines to drive autoimmune pathology in T1D patients (20). In addition, B cells activated by self-DNA produce an anti-dsDNA antibody to trigger an autoimmune response (21).

We recently reported that degradation of NETs in the gut of NOD mice by nuclease production due to recombinant *Lactococcus lactis* could protect against T1D development (22). In the current study, we aimed to investigate whether NETs participation in the T1D progression is triggered by gut leakage. First, we verified the correlation between abnormal NET formation and gut leakage in preclinical models of autoimmune T1D. Then we investigated whether aggravated gut leakage induced by 2% dextran sulfate sodium (DSS) could increase NET formation and accelerate T1D occurrence in NOD mice accordingly. Finally, we examined whether decreased NET formation and improved gut barrier function could alleviate T1D progression in PAD4 knockout mice. Thereby, data from the current study may reveal that NET mediator roles in the progression of T1D are triggered by intestinal barrier breakage and associated with both cell-mediated immunity and humoral immunity.

METHODS AND MATERIALS

Animals

Both NOD/LtJ and BALB/c mice were female and purchased from Huafukang Bioscience Co., Inc. (Beijing, China). PAD4-/- mice with the NOD/LtJ background were purchased from Animal Model Research Center of Nanjing University (Nanjing, China). All mice were maintained under specific pathogen-free conditions in Animal Laboratory Center of China Pharmaceutical University (CPU, Nanjing, China). Animal care and all experimental methods were performed following the relevant guidelines and regulations and approved by the local ethics committee in CPU.

Induction of Chronic DSS Colitis

A solution of 2% (wt/vol) DSS (molecular weight: 36,000–50,000 Da; MP Biomedicals, Solon, USA) was orally administered to 4-week-old NOD/LtJ mice in drinking water for three cycles of 7 days at intervals of 2 weeks before the mice were at 13 weeks old and an additional three cycles of 7 days at intervals of 1 week afterward.

Neutrophil Isolation and NETs Assay

Spleen neutrophils were isolated with Percoll (Solarbio, Beijing, China) gradients as described (23). NETs assay was performed as protocols published (24). Neutrophils were resuspended in RPMI-1640 containing 5-10% FBS and plated at 5×10^5 cells per well in 24-well plates (Thermo Fisher, Massachusetts, US). After incubation for 0.5-1 h, the cells were stimulated with PMA (8 μM, MedChemExpress, New Jersey, USA), ionomycin (10 μM, MedChemExpress, New Jersey, USA) or fecal microbiota (2×10^7 CFU), and the neutrophils were incubated for an additional 3 h to form NETs. Cells were stained with SYTOX green (1:1000, KeyGEN BioTech, Nanjing, China) for NETs quantification or, in some experiments, fixed in 2% paraformaldehyde, permeabilized, blocked, and stained with anti-H3cit (1:1000, Abcam, cat. no. ab5103) and anti-rabbit secondary antibodies (1:200, Servicebio, Wuhan, China). Images were acquired on an Axiovert 200 M wide-field fluorescence microscope (Nikon) with a coupled camera. The percentages of H3cit high cells and NETs were determined from five or six nonoverlapping fields per well, and the average was taken from 2-3 biological repetitions in every experiment.

Mononuclear Cell Isolation and Co-Culture With NETs

First, spleen mononuclear cells were isolated using Percoll (Solarbio, Beijing, China) gradients as described (25). After stimulating 5×10^5 neutrophils with or without ionomycin *in vitro*, the culture medium was carefully removed, the NETs/neutrophils were washed slightly 2-3 times by RPMI-1640 (10% FBS) and resuspended in 300 μL RPMI-1640 containing 5-10% FBS. NETs/neutrophils were then added to wells containing 5×10^6 mononuclear cells in 500 μL culture medium and co-cultured for 7 days, with medium added every two days.

Min6 Cell Culture and *In Vitro* Lymphocyte Cell Migration Assay

Min6 beta cells (CL-0674, Procell Life Science&Technology Co., Ltd. Wuhan, China) were cultured with RPMI-1640 (10% FBS, 50 mM β-mercaptoethanol) for 24 h (authentication and no mycoplasma contamination reports were provided by the supplier), and Min6 cell-containing medium was transferred to the bottom of 24-well Boyden chambers (NEST, Wuxi, China) for an additional 12 h of culture. A total of 1×10^5 lymphocyte cells was seeded onto the porous permeable membrane in the upper chambers. After 12-14 h, the migrated cells in the bottom chamber were collected and counted.

Diabetes Incidence

Diabetes was weekly monitored by measuring blood glucose levels with a Boshilong blood glucose meter (Houmeide Biotechnology, Taipei, China). After two consecutive blood glucose measurements ≥13.8 mmol/L, the mice were then considered to be diabetic.

16S rRNA Microbiota Analysis

Total genomic DNA from samples was extracted by using the CTAB/SDS (Sangon Biotech, Shanghai, China) method. 16S rRNA genes were amplified using barcoded sample-specific primers: 16S V4-V5: 515F-907R. All PCRs were carried out in 30 µL reactions with 15 µL of Phusion® High-Fidelity PCR Master Mix (New England Biolabs (Beijing) LTD, Beijing, China), 0.2 µM forward and reverse primers, and approximately 10 ng template DNA. Thermal cycling consisted of initial denaturation at 98°C for 1 min, followed by 30 cycles of denaturation at 98°C for 10 s, annealing at 50°C for 30 s, and elongation at 72°C for 60 s. Finally, samples were held at 72°C for 5 min. Amplicons were loaded onto a 2% agarose gel, and samples with bright main strips between 400-450 bp were chosen for further experiments. PCR products were mixed in equidensity ratios. Then, the mixed PCR products were purified with a Gene JET Gel Extraction Kit (Thermo Scientific, Waltham, USA). Sequencing libraries were generated using the NEB Next ® UltraTM DNA Library Prep Kit for Illumina (New England Biolabs (Beijing) LTD, Beijing, China) following the manufacturer's recommendations, and index codes were added. The library quality was assessed on the Qubit@ 2.0 Fluorometer (Thermo Scientific, Waltham, USA) and Agilent Bioanalyzer 2100 system (Agilent Technologies, Beijing, China). Finally, the library was sequenced on an Illumina MiSeq platform (Illumina, San Diego, USA), and 250 bp/300 bp paired-end reads were generated. Paired-end reads were assigned to each sample according to the unique barcodes, and sequence analysis was performed by the UPARSE software package using the UPARSE-OTU and UPARSE-OTU ref algorithms.

Histopathological Analysis and Immunofluorescence

The pancreas and colon were fixed in 4% paraformaldehyde and embedded in paraffin (Servicebo, Wuhan, China). To assess histopathological signs of diabetes, consecutive sections (4 µm) were then stained with hematoxylinand eosin (H&E, Sangon Biotech, Shanghai, China) and scored for insulitis, in which 0 stood for no infiltration, 1 stood for periinsulitis, 2 stood for infiltration covering approximately half of the islet, 3 stood for infiltration covering approximately 75% of the islet and 4 stood for full insulitis. For colon sections, after H&E staining, three independent parameters were determined: the depth of injury (scores 0, 1, 2 and 3 for none, mucosal, mucosal/submucosal and transmural, respectively), muscle layer thickness, and the ratio of villus height/crypt depth. Sections were also stained with PAD4 (Proteintech, Wuhan, China), Ly6G (Servicebio, Wuhan, China), H3cit (Abcam) and insulin (Servicebio, Wuhan, China) and subsequent fluorescein-labeled secondary antibodies to display NET formation or insulin production. Histological staining of mucins and calculation of mucus thickness were conducted according to previous descriptions (26).

NET-Associated Biomarkers and T1D Autoantibody Detection

Serum samples and pancreas tissue homogenates were all stored at -80°C and thawed at 4°C for 20 min before testing. Circulating NE, MPO, PAD4, ACPA, dsDNA-Ab, IAA, ZnT8A, IA2A and GADA were measured individually by commercial enzyme-linked immunosorbent assay (ELISA) kits, according to the manufacturer's protocols (Tongwei Biotech, Shanghai, China). Absorbance was measured using a multifunction microporous plate detector (Spark, Tecan Group Ltd, Männedorf, Switzerland). For the detection of ANCAs in serum, first, NET formation operated just like the methods "Neutrophil isolation and NETs assay" showed. Then, the supernatant was discharged carefully by slow suction and micrococcal nuclease (1 U/mL, Solarbio, Beijing, China) was added to digest NETs at 37°C for 20 min followed by 5 mM EDTA to stop the nuclease activity. The supernatant was collected and centrifuged to eliminate cell debris. The total cytoplasmic content was diluted 1:300 in buffer (0.1 M Na2CO3, 0.1 M NaHCO3, pH=9.6) and incubated at 4°C overnight in 96-well plates. After blocking with 5% BSA (37°C, 2 h), the serum samples were diluted 1:200 in 5% BSA and incubated at 37°C for 2 h. After washing with PBST (PBS containing 0.5% Tween 20), HRP-conjugated goat anti-mouse IgG (1:3000, Servicebio, Wuhan, China) was added and incubated at 37°C for 1 h. TMB was added to all wells (Beyotime Biotechnology, Shanghai, China), and the samples were incubated in the dark for 30 min at 37°C, then 2 M H2SO4 was used to stop the reaction. The absorbance at 450 nm was measured using a multifunction microporous plate detector (Spark, Tecan Group Ltd, Männedorf, Switzerland). To assess cf-DNA levels *in vivo*, the PICOGREEN®, Quant-iT™ dsDNA Assay Kit (Thermo Fisher, Massachusetts, US) was used according to the manufacturer's protocols. To detect circulating H3cit levels, anti-H3cit (1:1000, Abcam) and anti-H3 (1:3000, Proteintech, Wuhan, China) were diluted in buffer and followed the routines mentioned above.

LPS Detection in Serum

Serum samples were all stored at -80°C and thawed at 4°C for 20 min before testing. LPS was measured individually by commercial ELISA kits, according to the manufacturer's protocols (Tongwei Biotech, Shanghai, China). Absorbance was measured using a multifunction microporous plate detector (Spark, Tecan Group Ltd, Männedorf, Switzerland).

Cross-Reaction of Insulin Autoantibody (IAA) With NETs Associated Auto-Antigens

Lysed NETs (1:300) or insulin (1:200, Yuanye, Shanghai, China, 1 mg/ml) was diluted in buffer (0.1 M Na2CO3, 0.1 M NaHCO3, pH=9.6) and incubated at 4°C overnight in 96-well plates.

After blocking these two plates with 5% BSA (37°C, 2 h), the serum samples were diluted 1:200 in 5% BSA and incubated with NET protein at 37°C for 2 h. Another uncoated plate was also blocked with 5% BSA (37°C, 2 h) and then incubated with the same diluted samples at the same time. Next, all samples from NET-coated plates or uncoated plates were collected and added to insulin-coated plates, followed by 2 h of incubation at 37°C. After subsequent routines, the differences in absorbance were compared between pretreated subjects and untreated subjects of the same sample. The cross-reaction ratio $=(OD_{(uncoated+insulin)} - OD_{(NET\ protein+insulin)})/OD_{(uncoated+insulin)}$

Western Blotting

Pancreatic samples were snap-frozen and homogenized in RIPA buffer (Sangon Biotech, Shanghai, China) on ice. After centrifugation at 12000 rpm for 10 min at 4°C, the protein content of the supernatant was mixed with loading buffer. An equal amount of protein per sample was resolved on gradient gels (15% Tris-glycine gels) and electroblotted on PVDF membranes, which were then incubated with primary antibodies (rabbit polyclonal anti-H3cit, Abcam; rabbit polyclonal anti-GAPDH, Servicebo) at 4°C overnight and subsequently with appropriate HRP-conjugated secondary antibodies (Servicebo, Wuhan, China) for 1 h at room temperature. The blots were developed with enhanced chemiluminescence substrate (Sangon Biotech, Shanghai, China). Blots were quantified using ImageJ software.

In Vivo Permeability Assay

Intestinal permeability was determined by FITC-dextran assay as previously described (8). First, 20 mL/kg of body weight PBS containing 20 mg/mL FITC-conjugated dextran (FITC-dextran; molecular mass, 4.4 kDa; FD4, Sigma-Aldrich) was administered to each mouse by oral gavage. Three hours later, blood was collected in anticoagulant tubes and centrifuged to obtain the plasma (4000 rpm, 5 min at 4°C). Then, 50 ml of plasma was added to a 96-well microplate. The concentration of fluorescein was determined by a multifunction microporous plate detector (Spark, Tecan Group Ltd, Männedorf, Switzerland) with an excitation wavelength of 485 nm and an emission wavelength of 530 nm using serially diluted samples of the FITC-dextran marker as the standard.

Oral Glucose Tolerance Test

Nondiabetic mice in each group (n=8) were selected for the oral glucose tolerance test (OGTT). After 12 h of fasting overnight, the basal blood glucose was detected, followed by oral administration of glucose solution (2g/kg). Then, the blood glucose was monitored at the following time points: 15 min, 30 min, 60 min and 90 min.

Flow Cytometry

Analysis Single-cell suspensions from pancreatic lymph nodes (PLNs), mesenteric lymph nodes (MLNs), spleens and cultured cells were resuspended in staining buffer containing PBS and 1% FBS, stained with monoclonal antibodies against surface markers, fixed and permeabilized using the BD Cytofix/Cytoperm kit, and finally stained for intracellular transcription factors. The following antibodies were used: FITC anti-mouse CD4 (RM4-5; BD), APC anti-mouse CD25 (PC61; BioLegend), PE-cy7 anti-mouse ROR-γt (B2D; Invitrogen), APC anti-mouse T-bet (4B10; BioLegend), APC anti-mouse GATA-3 (16E10A2; BioLegend), Alexa Fluor 647 anti-mouse FoxP3 (MF23; BD), and APC anti-mouse α4β7 (DATK32; Proteintech).

RNA Isolation and RT-qPCR

Immediately after the mice were sacrificed, the colon and pancreas were cut into pieces and placed in 500 μL RNA storage preserving fluid (Tiangen Biotech Beijing CO., LTD), followed by storage at -80°C. After homogenization in 500 μL TRIzol reagent (Sangon Biotech, Shanghai, China), the RNA was extracted by adding 100 μL of chloroform and precipitating the aqueous phase with 200 μL of isopropanol. cDNA was synthesized using HiFi Script cDNA Synthesis Kit (Sangon Biotech, Shanghai, China). RT-qPCR analyses were conducted to quantitate the relative mRNA expression using Ultra SYBR Mixture (Sangon Biotech, Shanghai, China). The primer sequences are shown in the **Supplemental Table 1**. Gene expression was normalized using GAPDH as the reference gene. To analyze the relative fold change, we employed the $2^{-\triangle\triangle CT}$ method.

Statistical Analysis

SPSS 22.0 software (SPSS, Chicago, USA) was used for statistical analysis. The statistical significance of differences between two or more samples was calculated by an unpaired two-tailed Student's t test or one ANOVA test. Correlations were analyzed by the Spearman correlation test. The cumulative diabetes incidence was calculated using Kaplan–Meier estimation, whereas the statistical significance was evaluated by the log-rank test. All data are presented as means ± SEM, and P<0.05 was used to indicate a statistically significant difference.

RESULTS

Abnormal NET Formation Correlated With Loss of the Gut Barrier and Alterations in the Gut Microbiota in NOD Mice Before T1D Onset

Previous studies have mentioned that NOD mice exhibit prominently increased gut permeability compared to BALB/c mice at approximately 10-12 weeks old (8), and invasive microbes are indispensable for islet-reactive T cell action (27). However, little is known about the microbial changes at this time. Hence, we first conducted microbial analysis in NOD mice at four different stages (**Supplementary Figure 1A**). Interestingly, the abundance of Deferribacteres or Proteobacteria in NOD mice after 12 weeks was increased sharply when compared with mice before 12 weeks (**Supplementary Figure 1B**), and principal coordinates analysis (PCOA) exhibited the significant difference between the two groups (**Supplementary Figure 1C**). Moreover, we discovered that two gram-negative bacterial families, Desulfovibrionaceae and Deferribacteraceae, displayed significant augmentation, while the other two families, Muribaculaceae and Lactobacillaceae, which are short-chain fatty acid producers, were markedly reduced in NOD mice after 12 weeks (**Supplementary Figures 1D, E**). The increased abundance of Desulfovibrionaceae, an essential endotoxin producer, was in line with the increased endotoxin/ lipopolysaccharide (LPS) level in the serum of NOD mice after 12 weeks of age (**Figure 1E**), which indicated a high risk of subsequently abnormal neutrophil-forming NETs in NOD mice. Then, an ionomycin stimulation experiment confirmed this finding and showed that neutrophils in NOD mice were easier to form NETs *in vitro* when compared with BALB/c mice, and diabetic NOD mice released more NETs compared to prediabetic mice (**Figures 1A, B**). In line with this, the circulating levels of NET biomarkers, such as cf-DNA and H3cit in NOD mice exhibited obvious differences from BALB/c. The serum concentrations of cf-DNA (**Figure 1C**) were higher in NOD mice at all times, and highly significant increases in H3cit and LPS was observed in NOD mice at 10-12 weeks of age compared with 4-6 weeks of age (**Figures 1D, E**). More importantly, the strong correlation between LPS and H3cit only in NOD mice (**Figure 1F**) but not BALB/c mice (**Figure 1G**) suggested that the loss of gut barrier function and the invasion of booming gram-negative bacteria led to the abnormal generation of NETs before T1D onset, which could be a potential pathogenic factor.

In addition to verifying increased intestinal permeability (**Figure 1H**), obvious histological lesions, higher gut damage

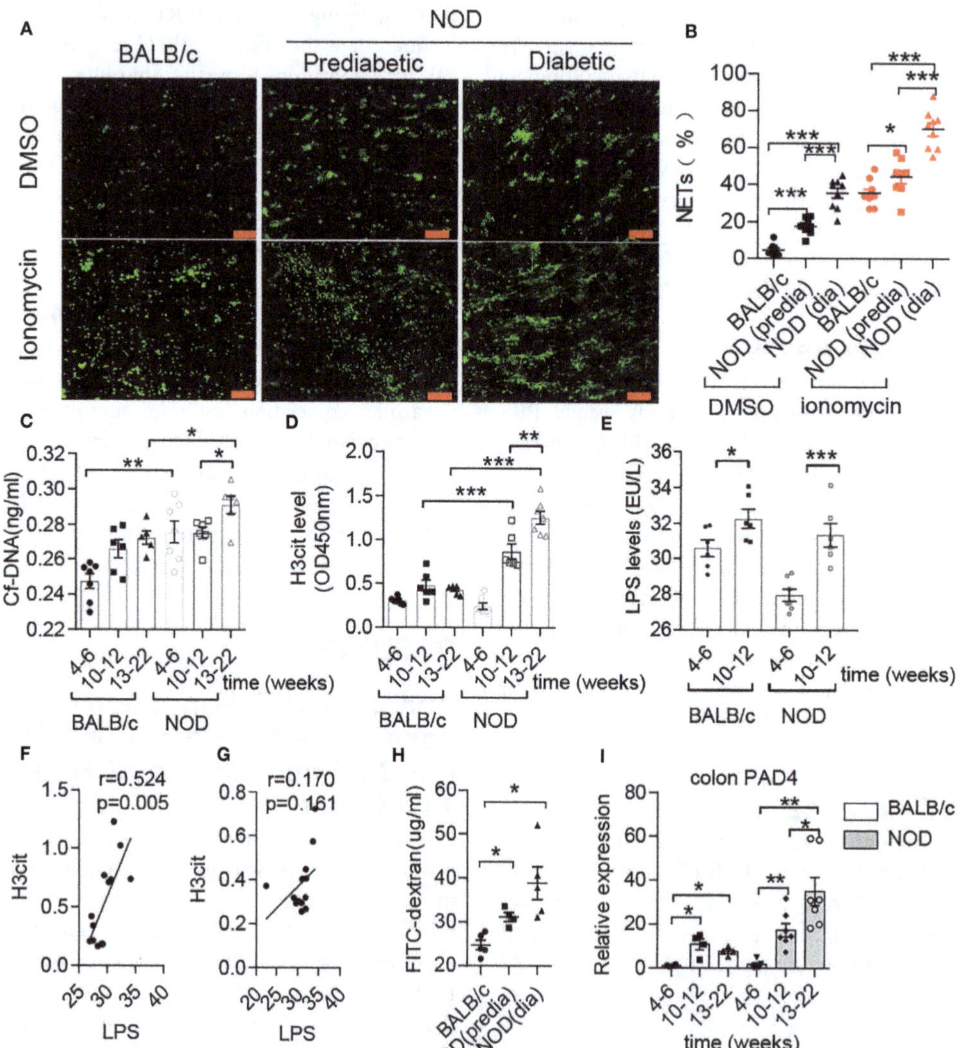

FIGURE 1 | Abnormal NET formation correlated with increased LPS levels in NOD mice. **(A, B)** NET formation ability in NOD mice *vs.* BALB/c mice (n= 4). NET quantification was conducted twice for each mouse. Circulating levels of cf-DNA **(C)**, H3cit **(D)** and LPS **(E)** in NOD mice *vs.* BALB/c mice at different ages (n= 5-7). Spearman correlation analysis of H3cit **(F, G)** with LPS in NOD mice (n= 13) compared with BALB/c mice (n= 13). **(H)** FITC-dextran *in vivo* permeability assay in female BALB/c and NOD mice (n= 5). **(I)** RT-qPCR analysis of PAD4 in colons from NOD (n= 7, respectively, at different ages) and BALB/c mice (n= 4, respectively, at different ages). The scale bars indicate 100 μm **(A)**. Data are shown as the mean ± SEM. *P < 0.05, **P < 0.01, and ***P < 0.001.

scores and lower villus height/crypt depth ratios located in the colon of NOD mice after 10-12 weeks of age (**Supplementary Figures 2A, B**), we further observed the increased inflammatory cytokines IL-1β, IL-17 and TNF-α in colons of NOD mice (**Supplementary Figure 2C**). In contrast to BALB/c mice, continuously increased mRNA expression of PAD4 was detected in the NOD colon at different weeks (**Figure 1I**). Taken together, these results demonstrated that NET formation correlated with gut leakage and alterations in the gut microbiota in NOD mice.

NETs Caused Cellular Immunity and Humoral Immunity in NOD Mice

Increased Th1 and Th17 and decreased Treg were observed in MLNs of NOD mice compared with BALB/c mice after 12 weeks of age (**Supplementary Figures 2D, E**) as similar to the previous report (8). The latest clinical research on T1D patients has demonstrated that NETs can polarize naïve T cells to Th1 cells by activating pDCs (16). In addition, numerous studies on autoimmune diseases have also shown the role of NETs in inducing immune dysfunction (17). However, no clues have been found to test this process in NOD mice thus far. Therefore, we isolated neutrophils from diabetic NOD mice and stimulated them with ionomycin to form NETs *in vitro*, followed by coculture with autologous spleen mononuclear cells. The proliferation of memory Th1 and Th17 cells indicated that NETs in NOD mice possess the capacity to activate proinflammatory T cells, which could trigger beta cells destruction and autoimmune diabetes (**Figures 2A, B**). We then tested the migration capacity of lymphocytes from the MLN in NOD mice. Neutrophils from the spleen were stimulated to form NETs *in vitro* and then cocultured with autologous lymphocytes from MLNs. The results of the transwell migration assay showed that more lymphocytes could migrate to the insulinoma cell line MIN6 *in vitro* (**Figure 2C**). Taken together, these findings indicated that enteric lymphocytes could be activated by NETs and possessed a stronger response to beta cells.

As reported in other autoimmune diseases, such as arthritis, lupus and vasculitis, ANCAs, ACPAs or anti-dsDNA antibodies play critical roles in self-destruction. ANCA levels in serum were also elevated in NOD mice after 12 weeks of age (**Figure 2D**) compared with BALB/c mice of the same age. Moreover, ACPA was sharply increased at disease onset in NOD mice but not in BALB/c mice (**Figure 2E**). To explore whether the components of NETs and insulin shared common epitopes, the cross-reaction was performed, and the results showed that NET-associated autoantibodies could indeed cross-react with insulin at a ratio of 10-20% (**Figure 2F**). Pretreatment with the components of NETs led to a significantly lower serum level of IAA in NOD mice but not in BALB/c mice after 12 weeks of age.

DSS Triggered Increased NET Formation and Accelerated the Course of T1D

A previous report has shown that DSS-induced chronic colitis could trigger 60% BDC2.5XNOD mice developing T1D (8). In the current study, we performed similar methods for inducing loss of the gut barrier integrity through six administrations of DSS from 4 weeks old in NOD/LtJ to explore whether increased NET formation plays crosstalk roles between invasive commensal microbiota and the abnormal activation of autoimmunity. The chronic colitis was successfully induced by 2% DSS in NOD mice. During modeling, the body weight of mice decreased, and the disease activity index score significantly increased (**Figure 3A**). Increased LPS levels in the circulation and the elevated mRNA expression of NE, MPO, PAD4 and cathelicidin antimicrobial peptide (CAMP) in the colon in DSS-treated mice (**Figures 3B, C**), manifested abnormal generation of NETs after DSS treatment. Furthermore, we observed more neutrophil infiltration and H3cit catalyzed by PAD4 existed in severely damaged areas (**Figure 3D**). In line with this, the serum levels of PAD4, NE and MPO also increased significantly in DSS-treated mice (**Figure 3E**). Moreover, the neutrophils were easier to form NETs *in vitro* after DSS administration (**Figure 3F**).

After DSS treatment, the progression of T1D disease in NOD mice was obviously accelerated. In detail, T1D onset in DSS-induced colitis NOD mice started at 8 weeks old and reached maximum morbidity at 18 weeks, which was four weeks earlier than in the control group (**Figure 4A**). In addition, a significant increase in morbidity occurred at approximately 14 weeks old, just after the fourth DSS treatment. DSS-induced colitis aggravation of islet inflammation was observed in both prediabetic and diabetic NOD mice (**Figure 4B**). Subsequently, we detected phenotypes of T helper cells in the spleen, MLN and PLN of the DSS-treated group in comparison to the control group. We found that after DSS induction, the ratio of Th1/Th2 cells in the PLN increased significantly in NOD mice (**Figure 4C**), while there was little difference in the ratio of Th17/Treg cells between the two groups (**Figure 4D**). Accordingly, the mRNA expression levels of effector inflammatory cytokines of Th1 cells, such as TNF-α and IFN-γ, were increased in the pancreas (**Figure 4E**). In addition, higher circulating levels of autoantibodies such as zinc transporter 8 protein antibody (ZnT8A) and insulinoma-associated antigen 2 antibody (IA2A) in the DSS-treated group showed greater humoral autoimmunity after gut damage (**Figure 4F**). In addition, DSS treatment doubly strengthened the cross-reaction of NET-associated autoantibodies with insulin (**Figure 4G**). Moreover, increased H3cit was discovered in the pancreas (**Supplementary Figure 3A**) in accordance with increased PAD4 levels, which could trigger the activation of autoreactive T cells (28, 29) and the generation of autoantibodies and would be another powerful explanation for the aggravation of T1D after DSS-treatment.

PAD4 Knockout Diminished NET Formation in NOD Mice

Considering that PAD4 is essential for NET formation (30) and the generation of citrullinated protein *in vivo*, PAD4 knock out NOD mice were used to investigate whether it is possible to affect T1D development. Above all, we isolated neutrophils from

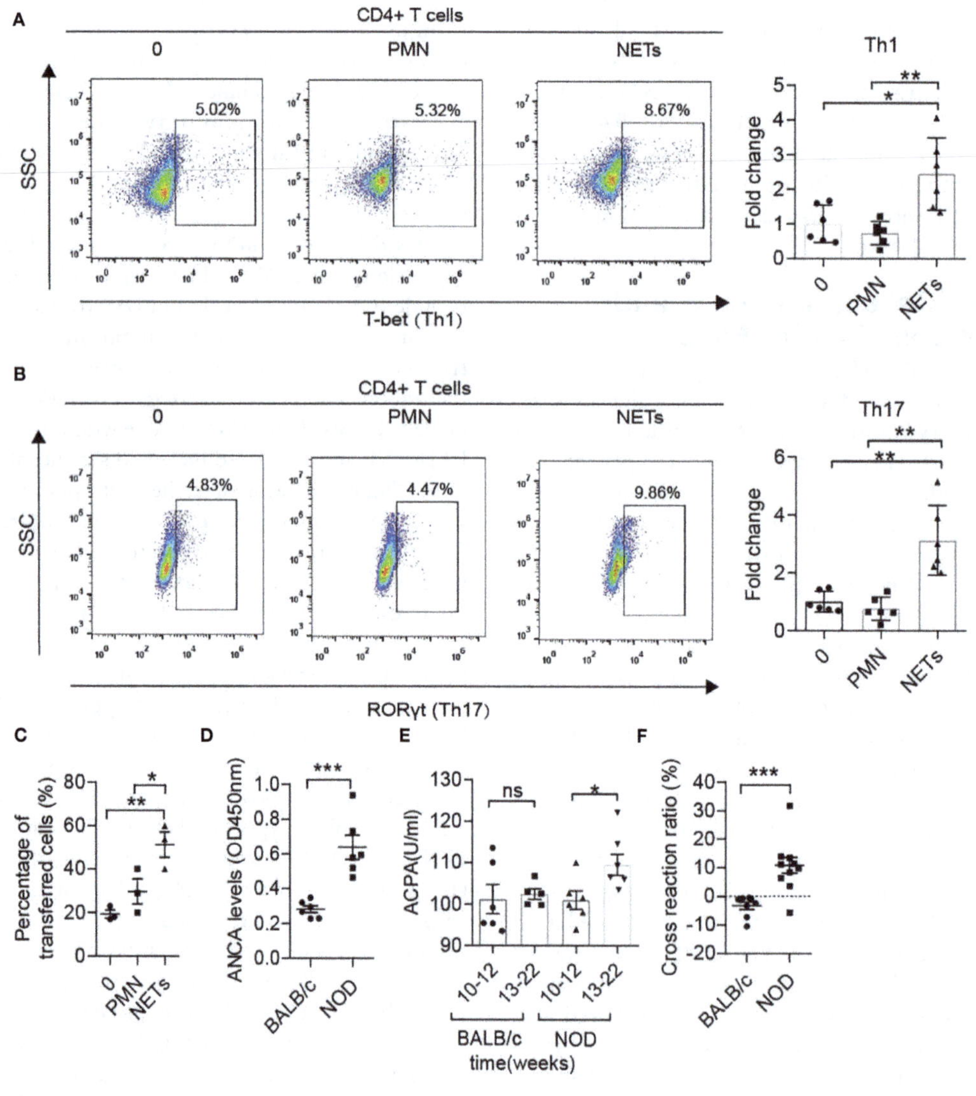

FIGURE 2 | The roles of NETs in the autoimmunity of NOD mice. **(A, B)** NETs triggered the proliferation of memory Th1 and Th17 cells from spleen mononuclear cells in diabetic NOD mice *in vitro* (n= 6). **(C)** The Transwell system showed the migration capacity of lymphocyte cells from the MLN in diabetic NOD mice (n= 3). **(D)** Increased ANCA was detected in NOD mice in comparison with BALB/c mice after 12 weeks of age (n= 6). Serum levels of ACPA **(E)** in NOD mice *vs.* BALB/c mice at different ages (n= 6). **(F)** Cross-reaction of IAA with NET-associated autoantigens in NOD mice (n= 10) but not BALB/c mice (n= 8) after 12 weeks of age. Data are shown as the mean ± SEM. $^{ns}P > 0.05$, $^{*}P < 0.05$, $^{**}P < 0.01$, and $^{***}P < 0.001$.

PAD4-/- mice and PAD4+/+ mice to test their ability to form NETs under different stimulation conditions *in vitro* (**Supplementary Figure 4A**). The results came out that neutrophils from PAD4-/- mice indeed exhibited a lower ability to form NETs, especially when stimulated by ionomycin and microbes, which was reflected by the lower percentage of H3cit+ neutrophils and NETs (**Supplementary Figures 4B, C**), as well as the decreased serum levels of H3cit and NE in PAD4-/- mice (**Supplementary Figure 4D**). Furthermore, the ACPA also decreased in PAD4-/- mice (**Supplementary Figure 4E**). These results suggested that the activation of humoral autoimmunity to citrullinated proteins or other components of NETs were decreased to some extent by PAD4 knockout in NOD mice.

Blocking NET Formation Improved Gut Barrier Function and Alleviated the Development of T1D

Recently, several studies have demonstrated that PAD4 inhibitor (31) or DNase I treatment could effectively achieve remission in NETs inducing colitis (32, 33). Therefore, we compared the barrier function and NET formation in the colon and enteric autoimmune T cells in PAD4-/- mice *vs.* WT mice. In PAD4 KO mice, recovery of gut barrier function was reflected at a decrease in gut permeability through FITC-dextran permeability assay (**Figure 5A**). The thinner muscle layer, higher villus height/crypt depth ratio (**Figure 5B**), higher mucus generation (**Figure 5C**), increased tight junction protein gene expression (MUC2,

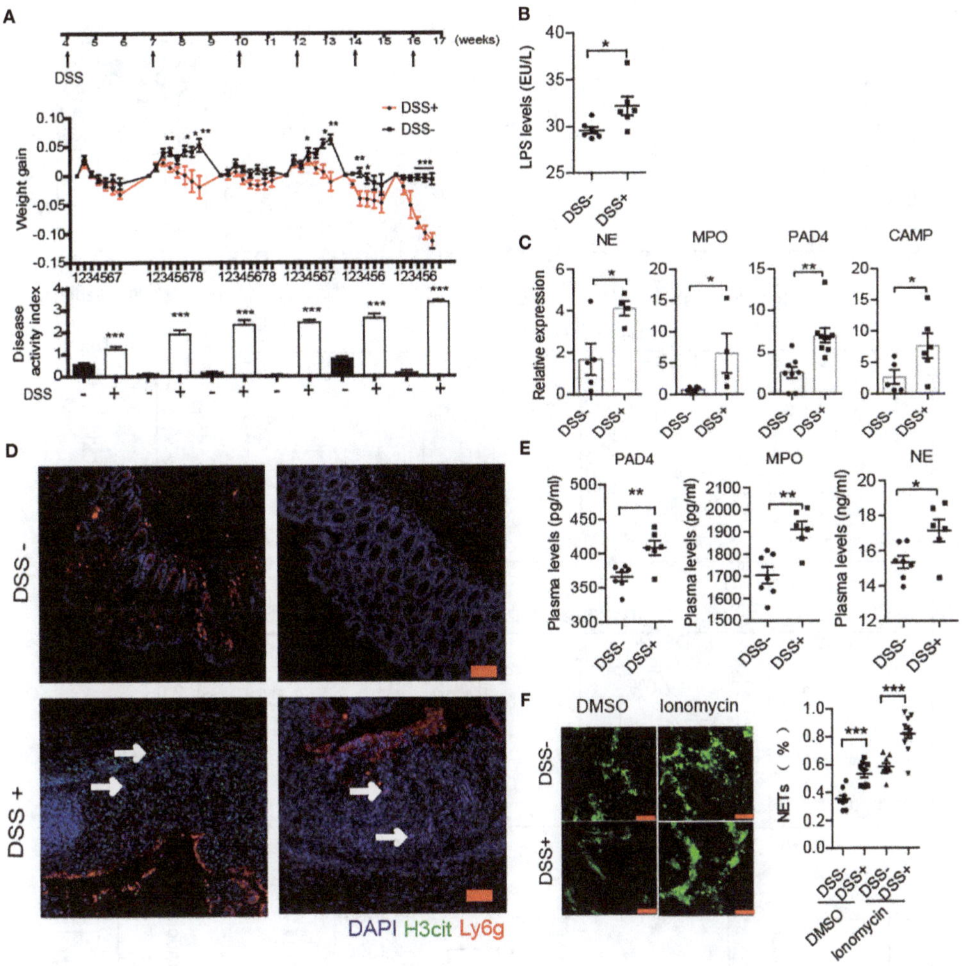

FIGURE 3 | DSS treatment triggered increased NET formation in NOD mice. **(A)** Six administrations of DSS induced chronic colitis in control (n= 14) and DSS-induced colitis NOD mice (n= 19). **(B)** Increased circulating LPS levels in DSS- induced colitis NOD mice (n= 6). **(C)** Elevated expression of NE, MPO, CAMP and PAD4 were found in colon homogenates of DSS-induced colitis NOD mice *vs.* control mice. **(D)** Immunofluorescent staining of Ly6G, H3cit and PAD4 in colon sections of DSS-induced colitis NOD *vs.* control mice. **(E)** Increased circulating NET biomarker levels in DSS-induced colitis NOD (n= 6) compared with the control mice (n= 7). **(F)** DSS administration enhanced neutrophils' capability of forming NETs *in vitro* (thrice NET quantification per mouse, n= 3). The scale bars indicate 50 μm **(D)** and 100 μm **(F)**. Data are shown as the mean ± SEM. *P < 0.05, **P < 0.01, and ***P < 0.001.

claudin1, cadherin1 and ZO-1) (**Figure 5D**) and claudin1 protein expression (**Supplementary Figure 3B**) in the colon also indicated recovery of the intestinal tract barrier. In addition, knockout of PAD4 resulted in lower levels of colon peroxidase activity (**Figure 5E**). Then, we focused on whether NET deficiency due to PAD4 knockout could alter the balance of T cell subsets. As expected, the ratios of Th1/Th2 (**Figure 5G**) and Th17/Treg (**Figure 5H**) cells in the MLN declined in KO mice at approximately 12 weeks of age. The mRNA expression levels of Th1 cytokines, such as TNF-α and IFN-γ, and Th17 cytokines, such as IL-17, were decreased in the colon of KO mice (**Figure 5F**).

Interestingly, we also found fewer Th1/Th17 cells in the PLN of KO mice at approximately 10-12 weeks of age (**Figures 6A, B**). The KO mice displayed better glucose tolerance and lower morbidity than WT mice (**Figures 6C, D**). More importantly, the serum levels of autoantibodies such as glutamic acid decarboxylase antibody (GADA) or IA2A decreased in KO mice (**Figure 6E**). In line with this, HE staining showed less inflammation in the pancreas of KO mice, which confirmed the alleviation of autoimmunity after PAD4 knockout (**Figure 6F**). To further verify the hypothesis that NETs mediate the loss of the gut barrier and activation of autoimmune T cells, we orally administered 2.5% DSS to both KO and WT mice for 7 days to destroy the intestinal barrier function. The results showed that the expression of IFN-γ in the pancreas was significantly higher in WT mice but not KO mice (**Supplementary Figure 5A**) after colitis induction. In addition, the migration capacity of enteric lymphocytes in KO mice after DSS treatment to MIN6 cells *in vitro* was weaker than that in WT mice with colitis (**Supplementary Figure 5B**). Most importantly, we observed a significant increase in enteric CD4+ T cells (integrin α4β7

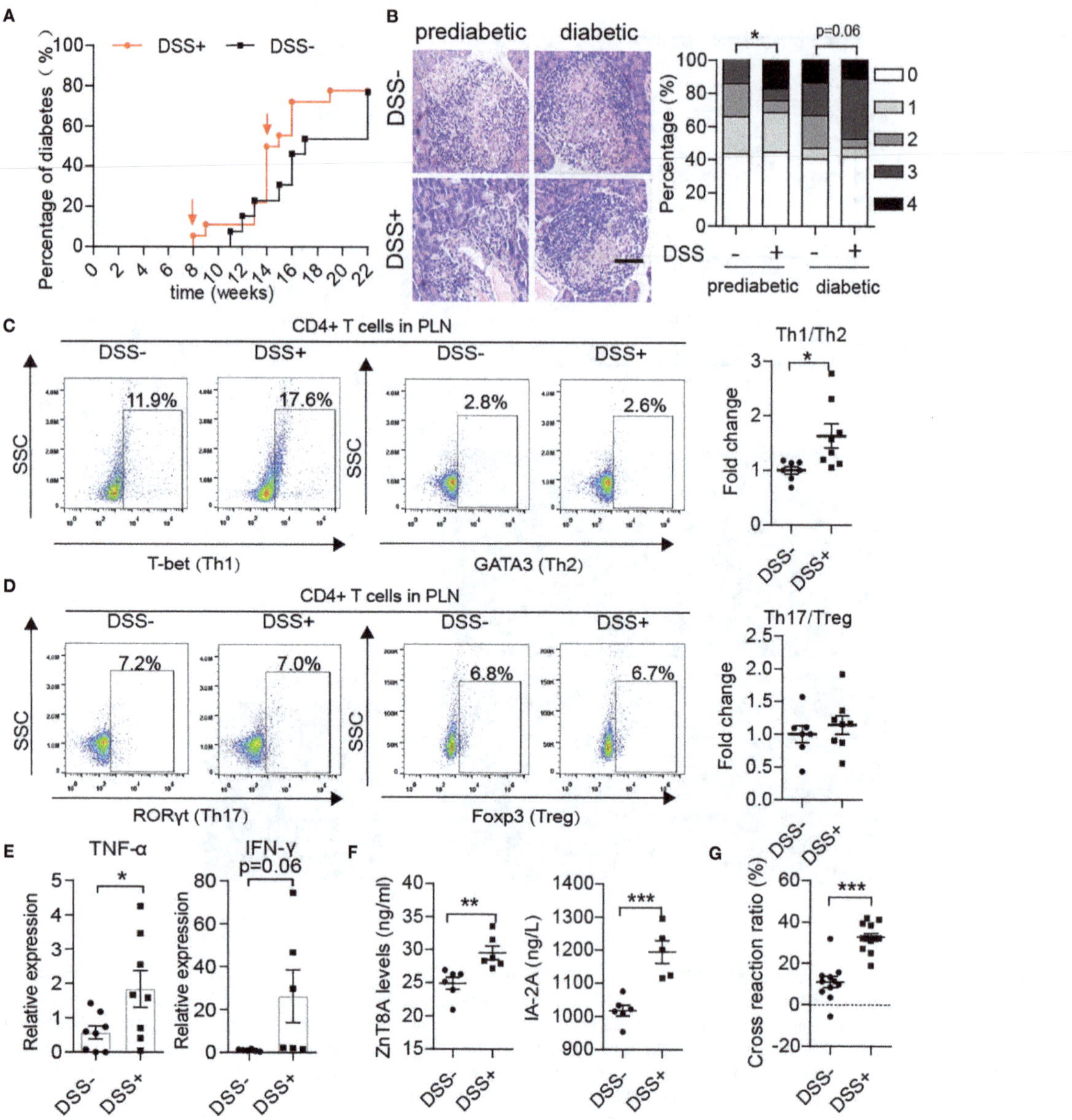

FIGURE 4 | DSS treatment aggravated autoimmunity in NOD mice and accelerated the course of type 1 diabetes. **(A)** Incidence of autoimmune diabetes in control (n= 14) and DSS-induced colitis NOD mice (n= 19). **(B)** HE staining of pancreatic tissue and insulitis scores showed more mononuclear cell infiltration in DSS-colitis NOD mice than in control mice at the prediabetic and diabetic stages, respectively (n= 6). **(C, D)** Representative flow cytometry plots (left) and bar graphs with mean percentages ± SEM (right) of Th1 and Th17 within PLN of control and DSS-induced colitis NOD mice (two independent experiments; n= 3-4 mice per group). **(E)** RT-qPCR analysis of cytokine genes encoding TNF-α and IFN-γ on tissue homogenates from the pancreas of DSS-induced colitis NOD mice and the control (n= 6-8). **(F)** Detection of circulating T1D-associated autoantibodies (ZnT8-ab, IA-2A) in DSS-induced colitis NOD mice and the control (n= 6). **(G)** Cross-reaction of IAA with NET-associated autoantigens in DSS-induced colitis NOD mice (n= 12) *vs.* control mice (n= 11). The scale bars indicate 200 μm **(B)**. Data are shown as the mean ± SEM. *P < 0.05, **P < 0.01, and ***P < 0.001.

positive) (**Supplementary Figure 5C**), especially Th17 and Th1 cells (**Supplementary Figures 5D, E**) in the PLNs of WT mice but not KO mice with colitis. Meanwhile, the expression of integrin α4/β7 showed the same differences in the pancreas (**Supplementary Figure 5F**). Overall, our data demonstrated that NET deficiency prevents autoimmune T cells from traveling from GALT to the PLN to cause pancreatic beta cells destruction.

DISCUSSION

Accumulating evidence has demonstrated that gut barrier dysfunction and commensal microbial disorders could be critical pathogenic factors triggering T1D (34). However, knowledge of how gut leakage and invasive gut microbes in T1D patients or animal models promote beta cells

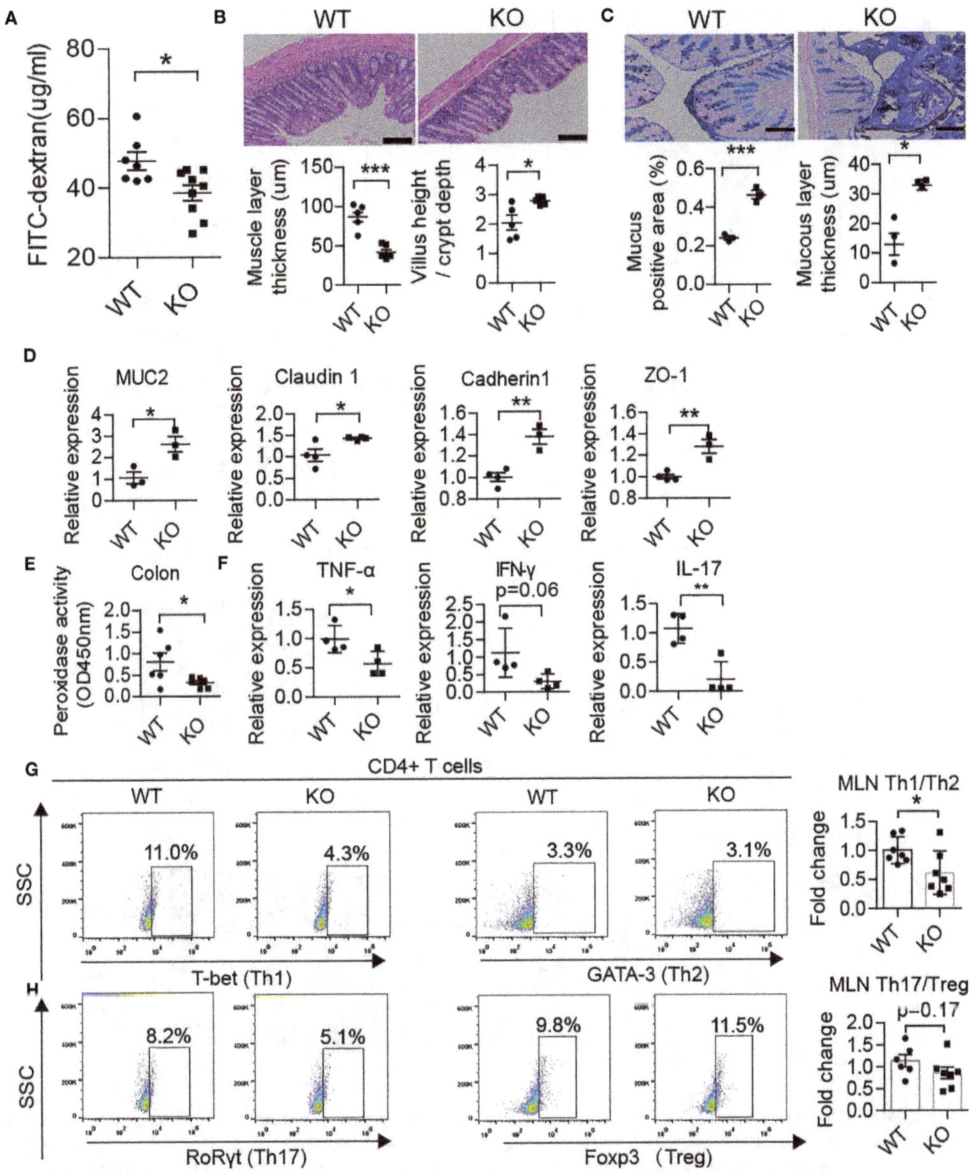

FIGURE 5 | PAD4 knockout improved gut barrier function. **(A)** FITC-dextran *in vivo* permeability assay in female WT (n= 7) and KO mice (n= 9). **(B)** HE staining of colon tissue and muscle layer thickness and the ratio of the villus height/crypt depth in female WT and KO mice (n= 5). **(C)** AB-PAS staining of colon tissue and the percentage of the positive area or mucous layer thickness in female WT (n= 3) and KO mice (n= 3). **(D)** RT-qPCR analysis of genes encoding MUC2, claudin 1, cadherin1 and ZO-1 in tissue homogenates from the colon of WT (n= 4) and KO mice (n= 3). **(E)** Decreased peroxidase activity in colon homogenates of KO mice (n= 6) compared with WT mice (n= 5). **(F)** RT-qPCR analysis of genes encoding TNF-α, IFN-γ and IL-17 in tissue homogenates from the colon of WT and KO mice (n= 4). Representative flow cytometry plots (bottom) and bar graph with mean percentages ± SEM (top) of Th1 and Th2 cells and their ratio **(G)** and Th17 and Treg cells and their ratio **(H)** within the MLN of WT and KO mice (two independent experiments; n= 6-7 mice per group). PAD4-/- or PAD4+/+ mice were all after 10-12 weeks old **(A–H)**. The scale bars indicate 100 μm **(B, C)**. Data are shown as the mean ± SEM. *P < 0.05, **P < 0.01, and ***P < 0.001.

autoimmunity is still limited. In the current study, we have demonstrated that excessive NET formation caused by gut leakage may be one critical factor link between innate and adaptive immune responses.

In general, susceptible individuals, chronic enteric infections first activate the innate immune response and subsequently trigger autoimmunity (35). A previous clinical observation has shown that LPS exposure arising primarily from Bacteroides precludes early immune education and contributes to the development of T1D (36). Our previous clinical study has demonstrated that circulating LPS concentration is elevated in new-onset T1D patients, while the increased internal LPS levels are relate to the changes of bacteria from Deferribacteres or Proteobacteria in NOD mice after the development of diabetes, which usually

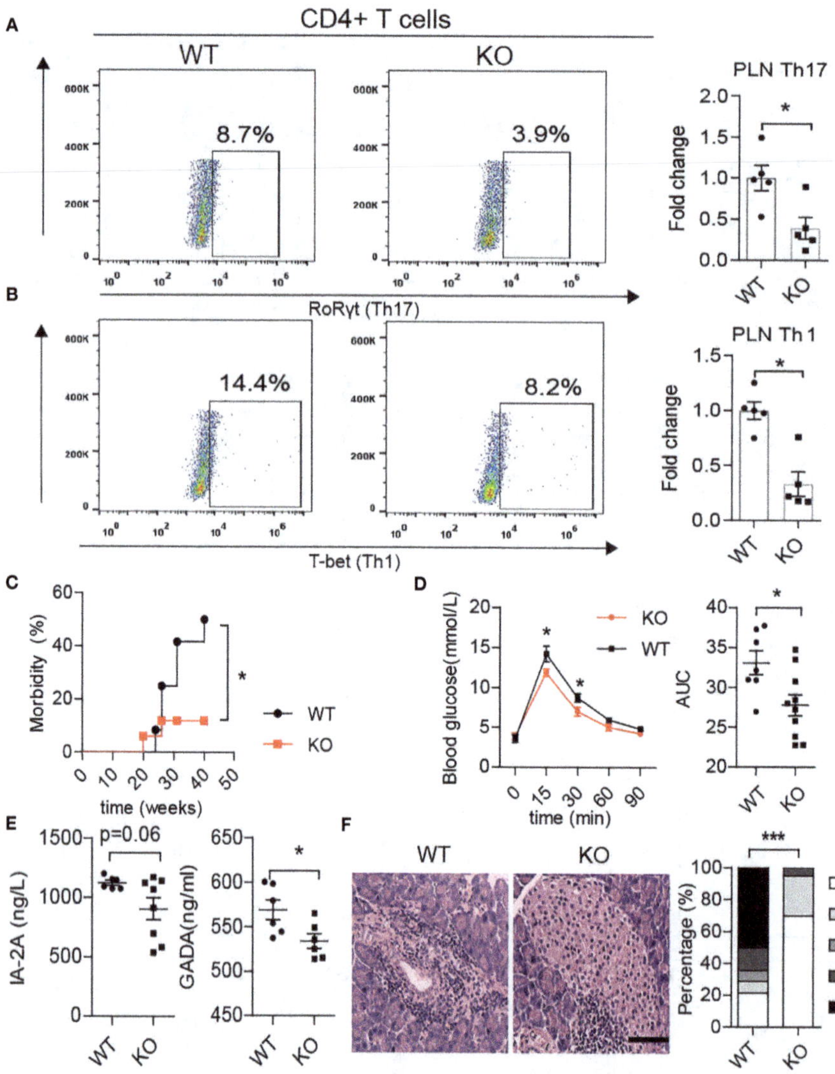

FIGURE 6 | PAD4 knockout alleviated the development of T1D in NOD mice. Representative flow cytometry plots and bar graphs with mean percentages ± SEM of Th17 **(A)** and Th1 **(B)** cells within the PLN of WT and KO mice (n= 5 mice per group). **(C)** Incidence of autoimmune diabetes in WT (n= 12) and KO mice (n=15). **(D)** OGTT of nondiabetic WT (n= 7) and KO mice (n= 10). **(E)** Serum levels of IA2 and GADA autoantibodies in WT *vs.* KO mice (n= 6-8). **(F)** HE staining of pancreatic tissue and insulitis score showing more mononuclear cells infiltration in WT mice than in KO mice (n= 3). PAD4-/- or PAD4+/+ mice were all after 12 weeks old **(A–F)**. The scale bars indicate 200 μm **(F)**. Data are shown as the mean ± SEM. *P < 0.05 and ***P < 0.001.

appears over 12 weeks of age. Similar to the previous study, neutrophils in NOD mice in the current study were also liable to form NETs and resulted in abnormal oscillation of the circulating levels of cf-DNA, H3cit and PAD4 at the prediabetic or diabetic stage compared with BALB/c mice of the same age. Importantly, a strong positive correlation between LPS and these biomarkers of NETs was found, which suggested that invasive gram-negative bacteria were potent in triggering NET formation *in vivo* after gut barrier disruption. Furthermore, we found that neutrophil infiltration and NET formation was increased in the leaky gut of NOD mice but not in BALB/c mice.

DNA and cellular contents released by NETs can be taken up by DCs (37) and can effectively induce the polarization of naïve T cells to Th1 and Th17 cells (38, 39). In the current study, we demonstrated for the first time that the population of memory inflammatory T cells were increased in mononuclear cells after coculturing with autologous NETs in NOD mice. Furthermore, after stimulation with NETs, enteric lymphocyte cells from MLNs exhibited a stronger migration ability to mouse insulinoma cells, which suggested the role of NETs in promoting self-islet reactive immune cell generation in GALT of NOD mice. In addition, increased NET-associated autoantibodies and the cross-reaction of IAA with NET contents in NOD mice revealed that NETs could trigger autoimmune processes in this T1D animal model.

The pathogenic role of NETs in DSS-induced colitis has been widely proven (32, 40), and PAD4 plays critical role in this process (41). In the current study, our induction of chronic colitis in NOD mice also proved that gut leakage occurred together with the increased NET formation *in vivo*. Thereby, we observed aggravation of autoimmunity or insulitis and a stronger cross-reaction of IAA with NET contents in DSS-induced colitis mice, as well as the acceleration of T1D development, which suggested that the higher the exposure of NETs *in vivo*, the more serious the self-damage. According to the recent reports, PAD4-deficient mice may hardly generate NETs *in vivo* and barely affect other functions of neutrophils (30, 42, 43). Moreover, compared to healthy controls, neutrophils from T1D patients tended to form NETs after ionomycin stimulation (24), which indicated that PAD4-dependent NETs might contribute to the disease. When we knocked out PAD4 in NOD mice, neutrophils' ability to generate NETs was found to decrease significantly. Interestingly, the recovery of gut barrier function and a reduction in autoimmune T cells were also found in our PAD4-deficient mice, in terms of fewer autoimmune Th1/Th17 cells in the PLN or autoantibodies and milder insulitis, which resulted in lower disease incidence and better glucose tolerance. The heterodimeric integrin $\alpha4\beta7$ expressed on T cells, specifies the recruitment of T cells to the intestinal mucosa upon its interaction with its ligand (26). In this study, a prominent increase in integrin $\alpha4\beta7$-positive T cells in PLNs was discovered in WT but not in KO mice after DSS administration, in line with the elevated expression of integrin $\alpha4\beta7$ in the pancreas. The data indicated that the improvement of gut barrier function and suppression of gut inflammation through affecting PAD4-dependent NET formation could control T1D development, which enriched the previous gut-affecting pancreas theory. Taking together, we have represented a schematic diagram to explain this mechanism in **Figure 7**.

In conclusion, the current study provides evidence that PAD4-dependent NET formation plays an essential mediating role in the

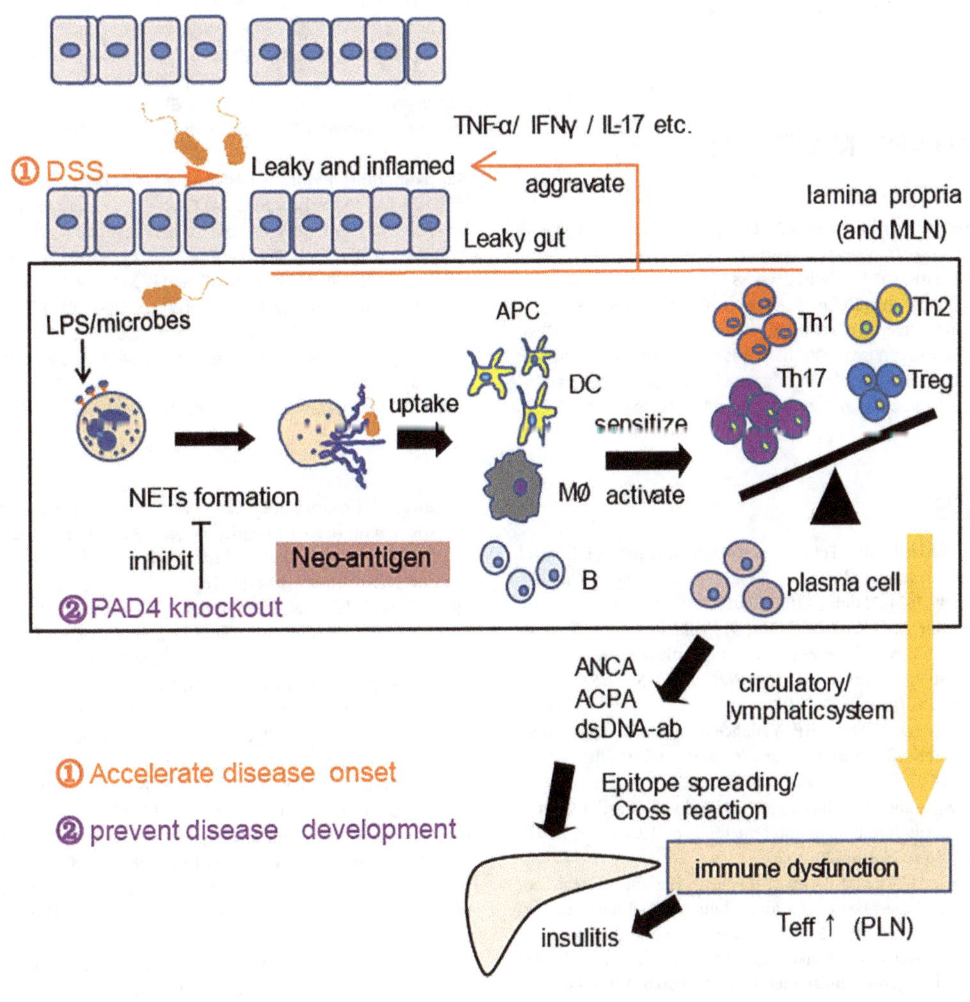

FIGURE 7 | A proposed mechanism for NET to mediate gut leakage, triggering T1D by activating the autoimmune response in NOD mice. Abnormal NET formation caused by gut barrier dysfunction and abnormal microbiota could trigger the activation of autoimmune responses and ultimately induce islet destruction. DSS treatment worsens the situation and accelerates disease onset, while PAD4 deficiency leading to a decrease of NET formation results in restoring gut barrier integrity and showing the potential of T1D prevention.

gut-pancreas axis by modulating the migration of enteric autoimmune T cells and activating autoantibodies, suggesting that clearing abnormal NETs in the gut with nuclease or blocking NET formation with PAD4 inhibitors may be a new therapy approach for T1D prevention and treatment.

AUTHOR CONTRIBUTIONS

JW conceived the study. QY and YW designed and performed experiments, analyzed experimental data, and prepared the manuscript. YS contributed to the cells experiment. JW, YL, CL, and FH supervised the research. JW, HG, and YS interpreted the data and revised the manuscript. QY and YS contributed equally to this work. All authors contributed to the article and approved the submitted version.

ACKNOWLEDGMENTS

The English language of this article was edited by American Journal Experts.

SUPPLEMENTARY MATERIAL

Supplementary Figure 1 | Commensal microbial disorders in NOD mice after 12 weeks of age. **(A)** Phylum-level phylogenetic classification of 16S rRNA frequencies in the fecal pellets of NOD/LtJ mice at 4, 8 and 12 weeks old and at the disease onset stage (n=5-6). Relative abundance of *Deferribacteres* and *Proteobacteria* **(B)**, microbial principal coordinate analysis **(C)** and 16S sequencing comparisons **(D)** in NOD/LtJ mice before 12 weeks of age *vs.* after 12 weeks of age. The bacterial families shown represent those found to be significantly different in the pairwise comparison. **(E)** Relative abundance of *Desulfovibrionaceae* and *Deferribacteraceae* in NOD/LtJ mice at 4 and 12 weeks old and at the disease onset stage. $^{*}P < 0.05$, $^{**}P < 0.01$, and $^{***}P < 0.001$.

Supplementary Figure 2 | Gut barrier dysfunction and autoimmune disorders in NOD mice compared with BALB/c mice. **(A)** Hematoxylin and eosin staining of colon tissue in female BALB/c and NOD mice. **(B)** Muscle layer thickness, gut damage score and the ratio of villus height/crypt depth in female BALB/c and NOD mice (n=3). **(C)** RT-qPCR analysis of cytokine genes encoding TNF-α, interleukin-1β (IL-1β) and IL-17A in tissue homogenates from the colons of NOD and BALB/c mice (n=5-7). Flow cytometry shows the bar graph with mean percentages ± SEM of Th17 **(D)**, Th1 **(E)** and Treg **(F)** cells within the MLNs of NOD and BALB/c mice (two independent experiments, n=3 each group every time). BALB/c and NOD mice were all after 12 weeks old **(A–C)**. The scale bars indicate 100 μm **(A)**. Data are shown as the mean ± SEM. $^{*}P < 0.05$ and $^{***}P < 0.001$.

Supplementary Figure 3 | Western blotting analysis of h3cit in pancreas and Claudin1 in colons. **(A)** Western blotting analysis of h3cit from pancreas homogenates in DSS-colitis NOD mice (n=8) and the control (n=6). **(B)** Western blotting analysis of claudin 1 from colon tissue of WT and KO mice (n=3). Data are shown as the mean ± SEM. $^{*}P < 0.05$.

Supplementary Figure 4 | PAD4 knockout diminished neutrophil NET formation. **(A)** Detection of neutrophils from $PAD4^{-/-}$ or $PAD4^{+/+}$ mice (n= 3), forming NETs under different stimulation conditions [DMSO, ionomycin (10 μM), PMA (8 μM), fecal microbes ($2*10^7$)] *in vitro*. The percentage of cells that were hypercitrullinated at histone H3 **(B)** and produced NETs **(C)** in neutrophils was calculated (three quantifications for each mouse). **(D)** Lower serum levels of NET biomarkers were detected in KO mice than in WT mice (n= 6-9). **(E)** Detection of CCPA in WT and KO mice (n=6). $PAD4^{-/-}$ or $PAD4^{+/+}$ mice were all after 10-12 weeks old **(A–E)**. The scale bars indicate 100 μm **(A)**. Data are shown as the mean ± SEM. $^{*}P < 0.05$ and $^{**}P < 0.01$.

Supplementary Figure 5 | PAD4 deficiency diminished enteric lymphocyte T cells traveling to the pancreas. **(A)** RT-qPCR analysis of cytokine genes encoding IFN-γ in tissue homogenates from the pancreas of WT and KO mice with or without DSS treatment (n=3-4). **(B)** The Transwell system shows the migration capacity of lymphocyte cells from MLNs in WT and KO mice with or without DSS treatment (n=3). The percentage and number of enteric $CD4^+$ T **(C)**, Th17 **(D)** and Th1 **(E)** cells in PLNs from WT and KO mice with or without DSS treatment (n=3). **(F)** RT-qPCR analysis of integrin α4/β7 in tissue homogenates of pancreas from WT and KO mice with or without DSS treatment (n=3-4). $PAD4^{-/-}$ or $PAD4^{+/+}$ mice were all after 10-12 weeks old **(A–F)**. Data are shown as the mean ± SEM. $^{*}P < 0.05$.

REFERENCES

1. Bosi E, Molteni L, Radaelli MG, Folini L, Fermo I, Bazzigaluppi E, et al. Increased Intestinal Permeability Precedes Clinical Onset of Type 1 Diabetes. *Diabetologia* (2006) 49:2824–7. doi: 10.1007/s00125-006-0465-3
2. Watts T, Berti I, Sapone A, Gerarduzzi T, Not T, Zielke R, et al. Role of the Intestinal Tight Junction Modulator Zonulin in the Pathogenesis of Type I Diabetes in BB Diabetic-Prone Rats. *Proc Natl Acad Sci USA* (2005) 102:2916–21. doi: 10.1073/pnas.0500178102
3. Lee AS, Gibson DL, Zhang Y, Sham HP, Vallance BA, Dutz JP. Gut Barrier Disruption by an Enteric Bacterial Pathogen Accelerates Insulitis in NOD Mice. *Diabetologia* (2010) 53:741–8. doi: 10.1007/s00125-009-1626-y
4. Giongo A, Gano KA, Crabb DB, Mukherjee N, Novelo LL, Casella G, et al. Toward Defining the Autoimmune Microbiome for Type 1 Diabetes. *ISME J* (2011) 5:82–91. doi: 10.1038/ismej.2010.92
5. de Goffau MC, Luopajarvi K, Knip M, Ilonen J, Ruohtula T, Harkonen T, et al. Fecal Microbiota Composition Differs Between Children With Beta-Cell Autoimmunity and Those Without. *Diabetes* (2013) 62:1238–44. doi: 10.2337/db12-0526
6. Honkanen J, Vuorela A, Muthas D, Orivuori L, Luopajärvi K, Tejesvi MVG, et al. Fungal Dysbiosis and Intestinal Inflammation in Children With Beta-Cell Autoimmunity. *Front Immunol* (2020) 11:468. doi: 10.3389/fimmu.2020.00468
7. Brown EM, Kenny DJ, Xavier RJ. Gut Microbiota Regulation of T Cells During Inflammation and Autoimmunity. *Annu Rev Immunol* (2019) 37:599–624. doi: 10.1146/annurev-immunol-042718-041841
8. Sorini C, Cosorich I, Lo Conte M, De Giorgi L, Facciotti F, Luciano R, et al. Loss of Gut Barrier Integrity Triggers Activation of Islet-Reactive T Cells and Autoimmune Diabetes. *Proc Natl Acad Sci USA* (2019) 116:15140–9. doi: 10.1073/pnas.1814558116
9. Jaakkola I, Jalkanen S, Hanninen A. Diabetogenic T Cells are Primed Both in Pancreatic and Gut-Associated Lymph Nodes in NOD Mice. *Eur J Immunol* (2003) 33:3255–64. doi: 10.1002/eji.200324405
10. Turley SJ, Lee JW, Dutton-Swain N, Mathis D, Benoist C. Endocrine Self and Gut non-Self Intersect in the Pancreatic Lymph Nodes. *Proc Natl Acad Sci USA* (2005) 102:17729–33. doi: 10.1073/pnas.0509006102
11. Honda M, Kubes P. Neutrophils and Neutrophil Extracellular Traps in the Liver and Gastrointestinal System. *Nat Rev Gastroenterol Hepatol* (2018) 15:206–21. doi: 10.1038/nrgastro.2017.183
12. Diana J, Simoni Y, Furio L, Beaudoin L, Agerberth B, Barrat F, et al. Crosstalk Between Neutrophils, B-1a Cells and Plasmacytoid Dendritic Cells Initiates Autoimmune Diabetes. *Nat Med* (2013) 19:65–73. doi: 10.1038/nm.3042
13. Vecchio F, Lo Buono N, Stabilini A, Nigi L, Dufort MJ, Geyer S, et al. Abnormal Neutrophil Signature in the Blood and Pancreas of Presymptomatic and Symptomatic Type 1 Diabetes. *JCI Insight* (2018) 3: e122146. doi: 10.1172/jci.insight.122146
14. Valle A, Giamporcaro GM, Scavini M, Stabilini A, Grogan P, Bianconi E, et al. Reduction of Circulating Neutrophils Precedes and Accompanies Type 1 Diabetes. *Diabetes* (2013) 62:2072–7. doi: 10.2337/db12-1345

15. You Q, He DM, Shu GF, Cao B, Xia YQ, Xing Y, et al. Increased Formation of Neutrophil Extracellular Traps is Associated With Gut Leakage in Patients With Type 1 But Not Type 2 Diabetes. *J Diabetes* (2019) 11:665–73. doi: 10.1111/1753-0407.12892
16. Parackova Z, Zentsova I, Vrabcova P, Klocperk A, Sumnik Z, Pruhova S, et al. Neutrophil Extracellular Trap Induced Dendritic Cell Activation Leads to Th1 Polarization in Type 1 Diabetes. *Front Immunol* (2020) 11:661. doi: 10.3389/fimmu.2020.00661
17. Papayannopoulos V. Neutrophil Extracellular Traps in Immunity and Disease. *Nat Rev Immunol* (2018) 18:134–47. doi: 10.1038/nri.2017.105
18. Nakazawa D, Masuda S, Tomaru U, Ishizu A. Pathogenesis and Therapeutic Interventions for ANCA-Associated Vasculitis. *Nat Rev Rheumatol* (2019) 15:91–101. doi: 10.1038/s41584-018-0145-y
19. Khandpur R, Carmona-Rivera C, Vivekanandan-Giri A, Gizinski A, Yalavarthi S, Knight JS, et al. NETs are a Source of Citrullinated Autoantigens and Stimulate Inflammatory Responses in Rheumatoid Arthritis. *Sci Transl Med* (2013) 5:178ra40. doi: 10.1126/scitranslmed.3005580
20. Zentsova I, Parackova Z, Kayserova J, Palova-Jelinkova L, Vrabcova P, Volfova N, et al. Monocytes Contribute to DNA Sensing Through the TBK1 Signaling Pathway in Type 1 Diabetes Patients. *J Autoimmun* (2019) 105:102294. doi: 10.1016/j.jaut.2019.06.005
21. Wang X, Xia Y. Anti-Double Stranded DNA Antibodies: Origin, Pathogenicity, and Targeted Therapies. *Front Immunol* (2019) 10:1667. doi: 10.3389/fimmu.2019.01667
22. Liang Y, Wang X, He D, You Q, Zhang T, Dong W, et al. Ameliorating Gut Microenvironment Through Staphylococcal Nuclease-Mediated Intestinal NETs Degradation for Prevention of Type 1 Diabetes in NOD Mice. *Life Sci* (2019) 221:301–10. doi: 10.1016/j.lfs.2019.02.034
23. Xue J, Zhao Z, Zhang L, Xue L, Shen S, Wen Y, et al. Neutrophil-Mediated Anticancer Drug Delivery for Suppression of Postoperative Malignant Glioma Recurrence. *Nat Nanotechnol* (2017) 12:692–700. doi: 10.1038/nnano.2017.54
24. Wong SL, Demers M, Martinod K, Gallant M, Wang Y, Goldfine AB, et al. Diabetes Primes Neutrophils to Undergo NETosis, Which Impairs Wound Healing. *Nat Med* (2015) 21:815–9. doi: 10.1038/nm.3887
25. Boxio R, Bossenmeyer-Pourié C, Steinckwich N, Dournon C, Nüsse O. Mouse Bone Marrow Contains Large Numbers of Functionally Competent Neutrophils. *J Leukoc Biol* (2004) 75:604–11. doi: 10.1189/jlb.0703340
26. Kempster SL, Kaser A. α4β7 Integrin: Beyond T Cell Trafficking. *Gut* (2014) 63:1377–9. doi: 10.1136/gutjnl-2013-305967
27. Mariño E, Richards JL, McLeod KH, Stanley D, Yap YA, Knight J, et al. Gut Microbial Metabolites Limit the Frequency of Autoimmune T Cells and Protect Against Type 1 Diabetes. *Nat Immunol* (2017) 18:552–62. doi: 10.1038/ni.3713
28. McGinty JW, Chow I-T, Greenbaum C, Odegard J, Kwok WW, James EA. Recognition of Posttranslationally Modified GAD65 Epitopes in Subjects With Type 1 Diabetes. *Diabetes* (2014) 63:3033–40. doi: 10.2337/db13-1952
29. James EA, Pietropaolo M, Mamula MJ. Immune Recognition of β-Cells: Neoepitopes as Key Players in the Loss of Tolerance. *Diabetes* (2018) 67:1035–42. doi: 10.2337/dbi17-0030
30. Martinod K, Fuchs TA, Zitomersky NL, Wong SL, Demers M, Gallant M, et al. PAD4-Deficiency Does Not Affect Bacteremia in Polymicrobial Sepsis and Ameliorates Endotoxemic Shock. *Blood* (2015) 125:1948–56. doi: 10.1182/blood-2014-07-587709
31. Zhang T, Mei Y, Dong W, Wang J, Huang F, Wu J. Evaluation of Protein Arginine Deiminase-4 Inhibitor in TNBS- Induced Colitis in Mice. *Int Immunopharmacol* (2020) 84:106583. doi: 10.1016/j.intimp.2020.106583
32. Li T, Wang C, Liu Y, Li B, Zhang W, Wang L, et al. Neutrophil Extracellular Traps Induce Intestinal Damage and Thrombotic Tendency in Inflammatory Bowel Disease. *J Crohns Colitis* (2020) 14:240–53. doi: 10.1093/ecco-jcc/jjz132
33. Lin EY-H, Lai H-J, Cheng Y-K, Leong K-Q, Cheng L-C, Chou Y-C, et al. Neutrophil Extracellular Traps Impair Intestinal Barrier Function During Experimental Colitis. *Biomedicines* (2020) 8:275. doi: 10.3390/biomedicines8080275
34. Pan L-L, Li B-B, Pan X-H, Sun J. Gut Microbiota in Pancreatic Diseases: Possible New Therapeutic Strategies. *Acta Pharmacol Sin* (2020) 42:1027–39. doi: 10.1038/s41401-020-00532-0
35. Torres-Aguilar H, Sosa-Luis SA, Aguilar-Ruiz SR. Infections as Triggers of Flares in Systemic Autoimmune Diseases: Novel Innate Immunity Mechanisms. *Curr Opin Rheumatol* (2019) 31:525–31. doi: 10.1097/BOR.0000000000000630
36. Vatanen T, Kostic AD, D'Hennezel E, Siljander H, Franzosa EA, Yassour M, et al. Variation in Microbiome LPS Immunogenicity Contributes to Autoimmunity in Humans. *Cell* (2016) 165:842–53. doi: 10.1016/j.cell.2016.04.007
37. Sangaletti S, Tripodo C, Chiodoni C, Guarnotta C, Cappetti B, Casalini P, et al. Neutrophil Extracellular Traps Mediate Transfer of Cytoplasmic Neutrophil Antigens to Myeloid Dendritic Cells Toward ANCA Induction and Associated Autoimmunity. *Blood* (2012) 120:3007–18. doi: 10.1182/blood-2012-03-416156
38. Zhang H, Qiu S-L, Tang Q-Y, Zhou X, Zhang J-Q, He Z-Y, et al. Erythromycin Suppresses Neutrophil Extracellular Traps in Smoking-Related Chronic Pulmonary Inflammation. *Cell Death Dis* (2019) 10:678. doi: 10.1038/s41419-019-1909-2
39. Qiu S-L, Zhang H, Tang Q-Y, Bai J, He Z-Y, Zhang J-Q, et al. Neutrophil Extracellular Traps Induced by Cigarette Smoke Activate Plasmacytoid Dendritic Cells. *Thorax* (2017) 72:1084–93. doi: 10.1136/thoraxjnl-2016-209887
40. Dinallo V, Marafini I, Di Fusco D, Laudisi F, Franzè E, Di Grazia A, et al. Neutrophil Extracellular Traps Sustain Inflammatory Signals in Ulcerative Colitis. *J Crohns Colitis* (2019) 13:772–84. doi: 10.1093/ecco-jcc/jjy215
41. Chumanevich AA, Causey CP, Knuckley BA, Jones JE, Poudyal D, Chumanevich AP, et al. Suppression of Colitis in Mice by Cl-Amidine: A Novel Peptidylarginine Deiminase Inhibitor. *Am J Physiol Gastrointest Liver Physiol* (2011) 300:G929–38. doi: 10.1152/ajpgi.00435.2010
42. Saha P, Yeoh BS, Xiao X, Golonka RM, Singh V, Wang Y, et al. PAD4-Dependent NETs Generation are Indispensable for Intestinal Clearance of Citrobacter Rodentium. *Mucosal Immunol* (2019) 12:761–71. doi: 10.1038/s41385-019-0139-3
43. Eghbalzadeh K, Georgi L, Louis T, Zhao H, Keser U, Weber C, et al. Compromised Anti-Inflammatory Action of Neutrophil Extracellular Traps in PAD4-Deficient Mice Contributes to Aggravated Acute Inflammation After Myocardial Infarction. *Front Immunol* (2019) 10:2313. doi: 10.3389/fimmu.2019.02313

8

The Role of NOD Mice in Type 1 Diabetes Research: Lessons from the Past and Recommendations for the Future

*Yi-Guang Chen[1], Clayton E. Mathews[2] and John P. Driver[3]**

[1] Department of Pediatrics, Medical College of Wisconsin, Milwaukee, WI, United States, [2] Department of Pathology, Immunology and Laboratory Medicine, College of Medicine, University of Florida, Gainesville, FL, United States, [3] Department of Animal Sciences, University of Florida, Gainesville, FL, United States

***Correspondence:**
John P. Driver
jdriver@ufl.edu*

For more than 35 years, the NOD mouse has been the primary animal model for studying autoimmune diabetes. During this time, striking similarities to the human disease have been uncovered. In both species, unusual polymorphisms in a major histocompatibility complex (MHC) class II molecule confer the most disease risk, disease is caused by perturbations by the same genes or different genes in the same biological pathways and that diabetes onset is preceded by the presence of circulating autoreactive T cells and autoantibodies that recognize many of the same islet antigens. However, the relevance of the NOD model is frequently challenged due to past failures translating therapies from NOD mice to humans and because the appearance of insulitis in mice and some patients is different. Nevertheless, the NOD mouse remains a pillar of autoimmune diabetes research for its usefulness as a preclinical model and because it provides access to invasive procedures as well as tissues that are rarely procured from patients or controls. The current article is focused on approaches to improve the NOD mouse by addressing reasons why immune therapies have failed to translate from mice to humans. We also propose new strategies for mixing and editing the NOD genome to improve the model in ways that will better advance our understanding of human diabetes. As proof of concept, we report that diabetes is completely suppressed in a knock-in NOD strain with a serine to aspartic acid substitution at position 57 in the MHC class II Aβ. This supports that similar non-aspartic acid substitutions at residue 57 of variants of the human class II HLA-DQβ homolog confer diabetes risk.

Keywords: NOD mouse, type 1 diabetes, preclinical, congenic, genetics, gene editing

INTRODUCTION

Since becoming available to the scientific community, the NOD mouse has been used extensively and has provided significant contributions to our mechanistic understanding of autoimmunity and type 1 diabetes (T1D). Indeed, the NOD mouse has been used to understand many facets of human T1D and has been the preferred model for invasive, preclinical/translational studies. While the NOD mouse has a number of critics, this model should be viewed as an important component of a comprehensive approach to understanding T1D. The NOD remains a standout model because it develops spontaneous T1D with genetic and environmental components that are relevant to the human disease. Further, as recent studies have demonstrated and as we describe below, new protocols to specifically modify single base pairs can generate loci that contain risk alleles that are orthologous to the human on the NOD background. Therefore, the NOD mouse remains a powerful and valuable implement in the investigator's toolbox.

A major strength of the NOD model is the existence of spontaneous autoimmunity and T1D. Similar to the human condition, NOD mice develop autoantibodies (1) and exhibit increases in circulating autoreactive T cells (2, 3) prior to the onset of T1D. The β cell antigens that are targeted are also similar between these species (4). However, in the NOD mouse, the initiating antigen appears to be insulin (1), whereas in human T1D it is thought to result from several initiating antigens (5, 6). These autoimmune phenotypes are followed by the onset of hyperglycemia (7). A progressive loss of β cell function is present in both human and NOD mice suggesting similarities in β cell loss or dysfunction. While hyperglycemia in NOD females and males begins close to 12 and 15 weeks of age, respectively (8), immune infiltration into the pancreatic islets, insulitis, begins much earlier. Pathogenic T cells have been isolated from the islets of 5-week-old NOD mice (9). By 12 weeks of age, insulitis is present throughout the pancreas of NOD mice. A dissimilarity of the diabetes when comparing human and NOD mice is the appearance of insulitis. Studies from the nPOD bio-repository have been critical in defining insulitis in humans where this pathogenic lesion is less severe and less frequent than what can be observed in NOD mice (10). This may result from the fact that the autoimmunity in parental NOD mice is very aggressive and disease onset occurs over an abbreviated timeline (weeks) compared to the decidedly more attenuated onset in humans (i.e., years after the appearance of autoantibodies). Insulitis and T1D incidence in NOD mice can be reduced through genetic modification. While hundreds of variant NOD mice have been made that represent less intense forms of T1D, the idea of improving the NOD as a model for human T1D by decreasing the potency of the autoimmune response remains largely unexplored. The potential of this strategy is discussed below.

Genetics play a significant role in autoimmunity and important similarities exist when equating T1D-risk loci in human and NOD mice. The disease is polygenic in both species with over 50 loci linked to risk in human and NOD diabetes (11). However, a single locus is responsible for the majority of the risk: major histocompatibility complex (MHC) class II. Early papers were critical in establishing that NOD mice encode a T1D-risk MHC haplotype that has important resemblances to the HLA risk alleles in human. Since these publications, genetic and biochemical studies have linked risk to amino acid residue 57. The high-risk DQ2 and DQ8 alleles of human as well as the A^{g7} molecule of the NOD have small polar amino acids substituted for an aspartic acid at position 57. The importance of this amino acid substitution is discussed in detail by Bettini and Bettini in this issue of *Frontiers in Endocrinology* (Co-published in the same edition of FiE). The genetic variations that impart risk in HLA/MHC arise from single-nucleotide polymorphisms that change the amino acid sequence. Similarly, other genes such as *Ctla4* and *mt-Nd2* are linked to risk in both humans and NOD mice. A single leucine to methionine substitution in *mt-Nd2* as well as the human homolog, *mt-ND2*, provides β cells with enhanced resistance to autoimmune destruction (12, 13). While HLA/MHC and *mt-ND2*/*mt-Nd2* represent genes with protein and biochemical differences, these non-synonymous changes in T1D are more the exception than the rule. Only seven of the >50 single-nucleotide polymorphisms associated with T1D arise in coding regions (14). The polymorphism in *Ctla4* of NOD mice results in altered splicing. While the polymorphism in *CTLA4* is not in an identical location, the risk variant is similarly associated with altered splicing of CTLA4 (15–17). Therefore, genes such as *CTLA4* can be modeled in the NOD mouse to aid in understanding the role of non-coding genetic variation in pathogenesis of T1D. Recent advances in genetic editing have further promoted the use of NOD to understand how specific SNPs can affect protein function. Editing of the NOD genome has been used to swap T1D risk or resistance alleles allowing for the role of specific SNPs, such in MHC Class II (described below) or *Ptpn22* (18), in the regulation of autoimmunity to be identified.

Another concept that holds true across species is that T1D onset results from the sum of the genetic parts. In human subjects, T1D risk increases as the haplotype of an individual contains more credible T1D susceptibility SNPs (19, 20). Similarly, by subtracting risk loci from the NOD genome through backcrossing or genetic modification, T1D risk can be altered (11). As discussed in detail below, the NOD represents a powerful tool to study epistasis.

In the current review, we highlight past contributions NOD mice have made to T1D research and outline strategies to better utilize this model in future. Included is an overview of NOD mouse's track record as a preclinical model for developing T1D therapies and a discussion about the impact NOD congenic mice have made to understanding the genetic basis of T1D. Also discussed is a strategy to develop panels of NOD congenic mice from existing congenic stocks to better mimic the spectrum of human autoimmune diabetes subtypes. Finally, we summarize existing and emerging technologies for editing the NOD genome that should greatly enhance the NOD mouse as a research tool, especially for identifying genes that contribute to T1D development.

PRECLINICAL PERFORMANCE OF THE NOD MOUSE

While the NOD mouse has proved useful in many preclinical research areas, significant tension has arisen over the performance of this mouse strain in bench-to-bedside efforts due to a failure to translate therapies developed in the NOD model to humans. The NOD model has been used for at least 30 years to identify agents or protocols that delay, prevent, or reverse disease. In general, investigators apply three approaches: early prevention (treatment is initiated at 3–4 weeks of age), late prevention (begin treatment at 10–12 weeks of age), or intervention after onset of T1D (reversal). Most preclinical successes in NOD have come in early prevention, where a wide array of agents or protocols can block disease. It should be noted that in most cases the impact of the drug/agent under investigation on autoimmunity (i.e., insulin autoantibodies or the presence of β cell reactive T cells) was not assessed. Further, many of these have seen little to no confirmation by independent laboratories. A recent NIH funded effort to confirm the effects of specific agents was unsuccessful at repeating the majority of the successes that were previously published (21). Late prevention represents a modality that is similar to trials established in humans where autoantibody positive individuals are identified and enrolled, such as the Diabetes Prevention Trial 1 or the recent oral insulin trial (22–24). To date, there has been a failure to translate late prevention successes in the NOD to prevention of human T1D.

At time of writing, very few therapies have resulted in T1D reversal in new-onset NOD mice and fewer still in NOD mice with established disease. Of the agents that have shown benefit, anti-CD3, and the combination of antithymocyte globulin (ATG) and granulocyte-colony stimulating factor (G-CSF) have been used in clinical trials. Preclinical studies using these modalities demonstrated an ability to reverse T1D in 39% of NOD females after onset (25). Multicenter preclinical efforts using anti-CD3 produced similar results, with less than 50% of the treated NOD mice exhibiting long-term T1D reversal (26). The rates of T1D reversal were significantly different when comparing sites, where anti-CD3 efficacy ranged from 10 to 80% among the four locations. Similarly, trials with anti-CD3 resulted in a minority of patients responding to therapy (i.e., preservation of c-peptide responses), yet none of the efforts with anti-CD3 resulted in insulin-free status for the patients (27–29). Likewise, use of ATG + G-CSF in a small multicenter clinical trial (25 total patients: 17 receiving ATG + G-CSF and 8 placebo) established that this combination did not induce T1D-remission but was effective in preventing erosion of β cell function 12 months after treatment (30). The 2-year data for ATG + G-CSF were less promising. At 24 months only 50% of the individuals who received therapy had preservation of β cell function (31). This is similar to the ATG + G-CSF reversal rates in NOD mice (32).

These data provide caution for moving agents forward for clinical trials that have been developed using NOD mice. A recent paper in Science Translational Medicine (33) has called for standards in clinical diagnosis as well as timing of therapy initiation in NOD mice. In preclinical studies, it is well established that NOD mice should be treated immediately after onset of T1D for maximal therapeutic response. Most groups have now established protocols for checking mice every other day for T1D onset allowing for initiation of therapy as soon as 1 day after diagnosis (21, 27, 28). In humans, trials enroll participants much more slowly and this delay in therapeutic administration likely postpones protection of the β cell mass allowing for further β cell loss. Additionally, it is clear that prior to agents or protocols moving to clinical trial there must be independent replication. The lack of a systematic understanding of T1D in the NOD and humans also impacts success. Comprehensive studies in comparative immunology and endocrinology are needed to mechanistically detail T1D reversal in NOD mice.

ROLE OF NOD CONGENIC MICE IN T1D GENETICS

Since researchers first started mapping *insulin-dependent diabetes (Idd)* loci by outcrossing NOD mice to mouse strains that do not develop T1D [i.e., C57BL/6 (B6), C57BL/10 (B10), NOR, and C3H], considerable effort has been spent creating recombinant congenic mouse strains to delineate genetic intervals containing diabetes loci and identifying the genes within each interval that are responsible for T1D susceptibility or protection. Several regions have been refined through the generation of subcongenic stocks that encode different subregions of the original confidence interval. These strains have revealed how several of the original *Idd* regions are composed of multiple susceptibility and/or resistance alleles. Notable examples include *Idd3* that was dissected into *Idd3, Idd10, Idd17,* and *Idd18* (34–37), *Idd5* that was dissected into *Idd5.1, Idd5.2, Idd5.3,* and *Idd5.4* (38–41), and *Idd9* that was dissected into *Idd9.1, Idd9.2, Idd9.3, Idd9.4,* and *Idd9.5* (42–46). While many of the dominant *Idd* regions are now well delineated, relatively few of their underlying genes have been firmly established. This is because validation has been technically challenging, in large part because even small *Idd* intervals often contain large numbers of candidate genes. Slow progress in improving candidate gene identification has led to reduced support for large-scale mouse genetic studies, forcing many in the field to decommission their congenic stocks. A new generation of genetic tools discussed in Section "Strategies for Improving Candidate Gene Identification" may reverse the fortunes of some of these strains. Nevertheless, even without discovering the causative genes, congenic mice have provided valuable insight about the genetic causes of human T1D that no other resource could have delivered. Some of their most important contributions are described below.

Epistasis and Gene–Gene Interactions

Intercrossing congenic stocks has revealed that an individual's disease risk is ultimately determined by the interactive effect of multiple *Idd* resistance and susceptibility loci. The challenge of disentangling these complex networks was taken up by a few courageous groups who, over decades, have detailed how different combinations of disease resistance and susceptibility loci modulate diabetes and various disease sub-phenotypes on the autoimmune-permissive NOD background. The advantage of this approach is that eliminating genetic variability between *Idd* loci allows for the detection of gene-masking and gene–gene interaction effects that are normally concealed in conventional genetic association studies with human subjects as well as mouse studies involving F2 and backcross one generation for segregation analysis (47).

There are several examples of how interactions between individual *Idd* susceptibility and resistance alleles gives rise to graded levels of diabetes on the NOD background (48–51). Among the best characterized is the interplay between the *Idd3* and *Idd5* congenic intervals from C57 strains when introgressed into the NOD genome. Combining *Idd3* and *Idd5* confers almost complete protection from T1D and insulitis on the NOD background (38). Yet, combining *Idd3* with individual *Idd5* subloci results in a spectrum of diabetes protective effects [reviewed elsewhere (11, 47, 52)]. At one end of the spectrum, *Idd3/Idd5.1* NOD mice were found not more protected against T1D than *Idd3* mice (41). Hunter et al. posited that the lack of protection in NOD-*Idd3/Idd5.1* mice may result from T1D resistance alleles at *Idd3* increasing the expression of CTLA-4 on the surface of $CD4^+$ and $CD8^+$ T cells that may render higher levels of inhibitory ligand-independent CTLA-4 induced by protective alleles at *Idd5.1/Ctla-4* somewhat redundant (41, 53). On the other end of the spectrum, *Idd3/Idd5.1/Idd5.3* and *Idd3/Idd5.3* recombinant congenic strains were found to exhibit T1D resistance equal to NOD-*Idd3/Idd5* mice. The lack of T1D initiation in the presence of severe insulitis observed in the *Idd3/Idd5.1/Idd5.3* and *Idd3/Idd5.3* strains indicates that the interaction between *Idd5.2/Nramp1* and *Idd3* is not important for T1D protection, but does contribute to the marked reduction in insulitis (41, 54). Continued studies of these strains will provide models to address the knowledge gap in additive and synergistic genetic effects.

Gene–gene interactions also exist among the various *Idd5* subregions, including between *Idd5.1* and *Idd5.4*. *Idd5.4* encodes a B10-derived susceptibility allele without a known responsible gene product. *Idd5.4* significantly accelerates T1D in the presence of *Idd5.2* and *Idd5.3*, but has no impact on disease if *Idd5.1* is also present (41). This suggests that *Idd5.4* can neutralize the protective effects of *Idd5.2* and *Idd5.3* and that *Idd5.4* is in turn masked by the protective effects of *Idd5.1*. A plausible explanation for this phenomenon is that immune events regulated by the B10-derived susceptibility allele at *Idd5.4* are counteracted by *Idd5.1/CTLA-4* signaling in one or more cell types. Similar masking effects have been detected among other congenic regions including between *Idd19* and *Idd6* on Chr.6 (49), *Idd19* and *Idd20* on Chr.6 (51), *Idd21.2* and *Idd21.1* on Chr.18 (50), and *Idd14* and *Idd31* on Chr.13 (55).

Evidence for epistatic interactions in humans include a study by Winkler et al. that genotyped 12 non-HLA susceptibility genes (*ERBB3, PTPN2, IFIH1, PTPN22, CLEC16A, CD25, CTLA4, SH2B3, IL2, IL18RAP, IL10,* and *COBL*) in high-risk HLA positive children of parents with T1D that were prospectively followed from birth to the development of autoantibodies and disease (19). An analysis was performed to determine the combinations of genes that most accurately predicted T1D development. The results showed that T1D progression in high-risk HLA carriers was best predicted by a collection of 8 genes (*ERBB3, IFIH1, PTPN22, CLEC16A, CTLA4, SH2B3, IL18RAP,* and *COBL*) rather than all 12 SNPs. These results suggest the presence of gene–gene interactions that mask the effect of individual diabetes susceptibility alleles. Another study searched for interactions between 38 T1D-associated non-HLA loci and different HLA class II genotypes in a large collection of T1D samples (20). It was found that SNPs within two T1D-associated genes, *PTPN22* and *CTLA4*, alter the predicted diabetes risk of various HLA haplotypes, partly confirming earlier reports that the effect of a susceptibility allele at *PTPN22* is greater in individuals expressing low-risk than high-risk HLA class II genotypes (56–58). These and other GWAS studies show how some T1D genes but not others are strongly influenced by gene-gene interactions and masking effects.

Cellular Expression of Diabetes-Associated Genes

Congenic mice offer a powerful tool to determine how different T1D genes modulate diabetogenic immune responses within specific cell types, which cannot easily be accomplished by experimentation with human samples. Previous studies have used a variety of adoptive transfer or bone marrow chimerism methods to observe that T1D genetics regulate immune dysfunction. A good illustration is the use of the B6, B10, or NOR derived *Idd9/Idd11* resistance locus to inhibit diabetes. One set of studies found that complex genetic interactions within *Idd9/11* regulate how B cells contribute to disease by engrafting syngeneic bone marrow and B cells purified from different Chr. 4 subcongenic donors into lethally irradiated B cell-deficient and diabetes-resistant NOD.*IgH*^{null} mice (59, 60). Diabetes development was then monitored to determine if B cells expressing separate subcongenic intervals from the NOR strain protected recipient mice from T1D compared to standard NOD B cells. The results established that at least four adjacent intervals interactively contribute to how diabetogenic B cells become tolerized or cause T1D, including processes that increase the efficiency of B cell anergy or B cell hyperresponsiveness to B cell receptor stimulation.

We used a similar strategy to show that genes within the *Idd9/11* locus control pathogenic CD4 T cells responses in T1D (61). Lethally irradiated CD4-deficient NOD.*CD4*^{null} mice were reconstituted with syngeneic bone marrow and $CD4^+$ T cells isolated from NOD.NOR-(*D4Mit31-D4Mit310*)/DvsJ: (NOD-*Idd9/11*^{NOR}) NOD mice congenic for NOR genome on Chr. 4. In this system, transfer of $CD4^+$ T cells isolated from NOD-*Idd9/11*^{NOR} mice caused less diabetes than $CD4^+$ T cells isolated from NOD. It was also shown that $CD4^+$ T cells from BDC2.5 TCR transgenic mice have a reduced capacity to transfer T1D to immunodeficient NOD.CB17-*Prkdc*^{scid} (NOD-*Scid*) mice when they express protective alleles at *Idd9* (62). Hamilton-Williams et al. found that $CD4^+$ T cells that express protective B10 alleles at *Idd9.2* and *Idd9.3* suppress the expansion of diabetogenic $CD8^+$ T cells (63). Their approach involved reconstituting NOD-*Scid* mice with purified $CD4^+$ T cells from NOD or NOD.*Idd9* congenic mice co-transferred with CD4-depleted spleen and lymph node cells from NOD donors. After reconstitution, mice were infected with a vaccinia virus encoding the H-2K^d-restricted IGRP$_{206-214}$ epitope to measure the expansion of CD8 T cells specific for the islet antigen IGRP. High and low frequencies of IGRP-specific CD8 T cells were detected in mice, respectively, reconstituted with NOD and NOD.*Idd9* CD4 T cells indicating that *Idd9* protective alleles restore tolerance to islet IGRP through CD4 T cells.

Other cell types besides B cells and conventional $CD4^+$ T cells have been found to regulate diabetes through *Idd9*. Regulatory T cells (Tregs) expressing B10-derived *Idd9.1* genes have significantly higher suppressive activity than Tregs from standard NOD mice (64). The *Idd9.1* sub-locus has also been reported to increase the capacity for DCs to engage and potentiate natural killer T cells, which are required for *Idd9*-mediated diabetes protection (65). Reciprocal transfers of NOD and NOD.*Idd9* congenic mouse spleen and lymph node cells into NOD-*Scid* and NOD.*Idd9-Scid* recipients identified that non-lymphoid cells possess some component of *Idd9* protection (63). Another finding was that transplanted islets from NOD-*Idd9* mice are more resistant to destruction by CD8$^+$ T cells, suggesting that an element of *Idd9*-mediated T1D protection maps to insulin-producing β cells (66).

Studies dissecting the effects of *Idd9* and other T1D loci have demonstrated that diabetogenic immune responses develop from a complex interplay of genes in multiple cell types. Further, evidence suggests that different cell types can be affected by a single diabetes locus/gene with sometimes opposing effects on disease. Determining how individual *Idd* loci contribute to T1D by affecting immunoregulatory pathways in specific cells offers a useful strategy for identifying the genes underlying these regions.

Genetic Control of Insulitis

Congenic mice have revealed that non-MHC *Idd* loci can be separated into two classes; one that supports T1D by modulating the virulence of insulitis and/or the intrinsic resistance of β cells to cytotoxic stress, and a second class that supports T1D by regulating diabetogenic immune responses before insulitis occurs (67). In the first class, replacement of individual NOD susceptibility loci with resistance alleles from non-diabetes prone strains reduces the incidence of T1D but has no quantifiable effect on insulitis at the gross histological level compared to NOD mice of the same age. *Idd* loci that fall into this category include *Idd9* where introgression of B10-derived resistance alleles did not alter the cellular composition of insulitis. Instead this locus changed the pathogenic properties of leukocytes that accumulated in islets and shifted cytokine production from IFNγ and TNFα to an IL-4 response (43). The overlapped B6-derived *Idd11* interval also reduces the pathogenic effects of β cell-specific lymphocytes in islet infiltrates without affecting the overall amount of insulitis (44). Another example is *Idd6* where C3H-derived resistance alleles confer protection against T1D but not islet infiltration. However, subtle differences exist in the invading leukocyte populations including that CD4$^+$ T cells and B cells are slightly reduced, which is counterbalanced by an increase in non-lymphoid cells such as macrophages and dendritic cells (68).

Disease protection is highly variable among the second class of non-MHC *Idd* loci where resistance alleles protect against both T1D and insulitis. Some regions including *Idd10/18*, *Idd16*, and *Idd21* cause a mild reduction in pancreatic infiltration but only during the early phases of insulitis (34, 50, 69, 70). Most of these loci confer relatively modest protection against T1D. In contrast, loci such as *Idd3* and *Idd5* that each provide substantial diabetes protection also cause a considerable delay in insulitis, although almost all NOD.*Idd3* and NOD.*Idd5* congenic mice eventually develop significant islet infiltration (34, 38). Other *Idd* loci, including *Idd4* and *Idd13*, appear to change the distribution rather than the amount of insulitis (71, 72). NOD mice expressing either of these loci develop non-destructive peri-ductal infiltrates where invading cells remain mostly confined to the peri-islet zone until well after the age most NOD mice develop diabetes. As discussed above, none of the non-MHC *Idd* loci that block insulitis and T1D are sufficient on their own to substantially reduce islet inflammation. However, almost complete protection can be achieved when individual regions are combined, indicating that genetic interactions exist between specific loci that confer greater protection against islet inflammation than the collective effects of each separate region.

Together, these findings suggest that insulitis among patients is also under complex genetic control and that, in some people, combinations of T1D genes could cause high levels of non-destructive islet inflammation long before the onset of overt disease. In contrast, the degree of insulitis may correlate closely with progression to overt diabetes in patients that carry T1D genes that give rise to more virulent forms of insulitis.

MODELING THE GENETIC DIVERSITY OF HUMAN T1D

A major criticism of the NOD mouse has been that this model represents the equivalent of a single human case of T1D. Consequently, immune modulation protocols developed in the NOD mouse could be limited to a few subtypes of the human disease, which may partially explain why some interventions that have shown promise in NOD mice fail to preserve β cell function in patients (73). Better predictions from mouse models might be possible if future treatment protocols were screened using multicenter efforts with heterogeneous populations of NOD-derived mice to mimic the genetic variation among patients. Such a strategy could employ a panel of NOD-related recombinant congenic strains carrying different combinations *Idd* loci where each strain would express a unique set of genetic variants that give rise to a specific subtype of T1D (41). This is analogous to the different subtypes of T1D that arise in patients from various segregating combinations of susceptibility and resistance alleles. The potential of this strategy is that therapies capable of inhibiting diabetes across a panel of congenic strains are more likely to be successful in genetically heterogeneous humans. There are also advantages to finding treatments that only work in congenic mice with specific combinations of *Idd* loci, including that this could provide valuable information about the cellular and molecular mechanisms through which an immune modulation treatment affects disease. It may also help to identify specific subsets of patients that have less or more potential for responding to a particular immune therapy.

Choosing which congenic mice to include in a future drug testing panel presents a challenge because of the large number of *Idd* loci it is possible to combine. It is logical that strain selection should consider the nature of the immune modulation protocol being tested. For therapies like probiotic treatment and immune suppression protocols, where the mode of action is poorly understood or where multiple cell types and molecular pathways are involved, it may be best to test mice with a diverse array of congenic intervals designed to emulate the genetic variation in human T1D. Some of the NOD-related congenic stocks described in the Section "Epistasis and Gene–Gene Interaction" may be suitable candidates, especially those that develop NOD-like levels of T1D due to introgression of susceptibility loci from non-NOD mouse strains. A more targeted panel could be employed for therapies known to act through particular cellular or molecular pathways. For instance, immune modulation protocols designed to enhance

Tregs, such as low-dose IL-2 and combined ATG + G-CSF therapy, could be tested on congenic mice expressing different allelic variants of *Idd3*, *Idd6*, *Idd9.1*, and *Idd9.3* that each separately affect the suppressive properties of Tregs (64, 68, 74, 75). Another example is antigen-specific immunotherapy where autoantigens could be screened in NOD congenic mice expressing different variants of *Il2/Il21* (*Idd3*) (74, 76), *B2m* (*Idd13*) (72), and *Ptpn22* (*Idd18.2*) (77) that, respectively, modulate T cell activation/effector function, peptide presentation, and TCR signaling. All of these factors contribute to the fate of self-reactive T cells that encounter autoantigen and may affect the outcome of autoantigen immunotherapy.

An obvious drawback to testing diabetes therapies using congenic mouse panels is the additional time and resources involved. Even so, the investment is worthwhile if therapies that are ineffectual in humans could be recognized before progressing to clinical trials. An example of how testing the appropriate NOD congenic strain might have produced a different result to standard NOD mice and predicted the failure of a T1D treatment is low-dose IL-2 therapy, which increases the frequency of Tregs but has not been able to produce positive effects on diabetes in patients (78). A chief reason that this treatment advanced to clinical trials is that low levels of IL-2 potently suppresses T1D development and reverses recent onset T1D in NOD mice, presumably by enhancing Treg function and/or development (79). However, it is possible that NOD mice are particularly sensitive to this type of immune modulation because this strain carries a variant of *Il2* that reduces IL-2 gene expression and Treg function (74). An interesting question is whether the outcome of IL-2 treatment would be different in NOD.*Idd3* mice that express the B6 variant of *Il2* and results in higher levels of *Il2* gene expression (74). The answer might address whether low-dose IL-2 therapy has potential for improving immune regulation and result in enhanced β cell function in patients without an IL2/IL2R signaling deficiency. This is important because it is still unclear whether defects in the IL2/IL2R pathway play a significant role in most cases of human diabetes; although a gene variant of *IL2RA* (CD25) has been associated with T1D risk in people, it is protective but rare (80). Furthermore, the causative gene has yet to be identified for the chromosome 4q27 region containing *IL2* and *IL21* that is linked with T1D susceptibility (81).

Another limitation of testing T1D therapies with NOD congenic mice is that many *Idd* loci strongly suppress diabetes, which will require that some experiments be performed with large numbers of animals to achieve sufficient power. Indeed, only 10–20% of female NOD.*Idd3* mice develop T1D by 30 weeks of age (74, 76, 82). As mentioned above, the unique insights from congenic mice will often justify using strains with very low levels of disease. However, there is also potential to alter the genetic composition of congenic strains in ways that will increase the rate of diabetes. For instance, it may be feasible to use NOD mice heterozygous instead of homozygous for the *Idd3* locus, which develop 40% diabetes (76). These mice still produce more IL-2 than standard NOD mice and would presumably be less sensitive to IL-2 therapy. Another strategy could be to breed T1D-resistant congenic strains with NOD mice carrying congenic intervals that accelerate diabetes. For example, NOD.*Idd3* could be crossed to NOD mice carrying B6 alleles at *Idd18.2/Ptpn22* that are more diabetogenic than the corresponding NOD alleles (77).

STRATEGIES FOR IMPROVING CANDIDATE GENE IDENTIFICATION

Although genetic studies using inbred mice are costly because of the large number of mice required, they remain a powerful method of detecting rare T1D susceptibility alleles that are impractical to identify through GWAS analyses, which require tens or hundreds of thousands of human subjects (83, 84). Thus, for the reasons outlined above, the question is not whether pursuing the identity of T1D susceptibility and resistance alleles is worthwhile, but rather how to make this process more efficient by employing a comprehensive approach that utilized both human and mouse systems. Considerable encouragement comes from a new generation of genetic tools that may circumvent many of the most intractable obstacles that traditionally limited the identification of *Idd* candidate genes. Some of these are described in the following sections in the order of their development.

RNA Interference (RNAi)

RNA interference has proven useful for manipulating gene expression in NOD mice without introducing genetic contamination from other strains. This approach is based on a well-established transgenesis methodology that entails the direct introduction of short hairpin RNA (shRNA) containing constructs into NOD zygotes by viral transduction (85, 86). The shRNA-containing constructs are designed to silence genes that impact T1D. shRNA is a sequence of RNA that contains a tight hairpin turn. This structure is cleaved by intracellular machinery into small interfering RNA that knocks down any mRNA bearing a complementary sequence (87). Several companies are developing viral libraries that produce shRNA that integrate into the host genome and ensure stable gene silencing after integration. The silencing cassette can be incorporated into many different types of vectors, including lentiviral, adenoviral, or retroviral vectors. Using the NOD model, RNAi has already provided valuable insight into how expression of the T1D candidate genes *IL17* (88), *PTPN22* (89), *CTLA4* (90), *CLEC16A* (91), *RGS1* (92), and *Slc11a1* (*Nramp1*) (93) contribute to diabetes development. It is conceivable that T1D susceptibility genes can regulate disease progression in an age-dependent manner. Establishment of inducible RNAi has also enabled temporal control of target gene knockdown to determine their functions at different stages of disease progression (94).

Zinc Finger Nuclease (ZFN)

Zinc finger nucleases are fusion proteins containing a sequence-specific DNA-binding zinc finger domain and a nuclease domain (95, 96). Engineered ZFNs specifically recognize and bind a defined target gene sequence within the nucleus of a cell and introduce a double-strand break (DSB) (97, 98). The cellular DNA repair machinery fixes these breaks, most frequently *via* the non-homologous end joining (NHEJ) mechanism resulting in small deletions or insertions of the gene sequence (few to hundreds of base pairs) and disruption (knockout) of the target gene (97, 98). Injected as synthetic mRNAs, ZFNs typically work at the one-cell fertilized embryo stage, resulting in single-step, whole animal gene disruption, and infrequent mosaics (99). More precise genetic engineering can be achieved as well because a DSB also stimulates DNA repair *via* homology-directed repair (HDR) mechanism if a homologous DNA template is co-introduced into the cell (100). Because ZFN-mediated genetic manipulation can be done directly in NOD embryos, the resulting knock-in or knockout can be generated on a pure NOD genetic background. Thus, it eliminates carryover of closely linked passenger DNA that occurs when the induced mutation is introduced in non-NOD embryonic stem cells (129 or B6) and then the targeted allele is backcrossed onto NOD. This is particularly concerning when targeting genes within known *Idd* regions. To study the role of the *Idd9.3* candidate gene *Tnfrsf9* (encoding CD137/4-1BB), we used ZFN to disrupt this gene directly in NOD embryos (101). The NOD allele of CD137 is hypofunctional when compared to the B10 protein that is expressed within the *Idd9.3* congenic strain (102). Thus, it was thought that T1D development would be accelerated in the absence of CD137. Surprisingly, CD137-deficient NOD mice were less susceptible to T1D, indicating that this co-stimulatory molecule has a diabetogenic role. This conclusion could not have been made with certainty if CD137-deficient NOD mice were created by backcrossing the previously reported knockout alleles generated using 129 embryonic stem cells. We further established an important role of CD137 in promoting the accumulation of β cell autoreactive $CD8^+$ T cells (103). In addition, CD137 had a diabetes protective function when expressed in $CD4^+$ T cells, likely due to the immunosuppressive activity of soluble CD137 produced by Tregs (103).

As discussed earlier, the $H2^{g7}$ haplotype is essential for T1D development in NOD mice. A key component of the diabetogenic $H2^{g7}$ haplotype is the unique Ab^{g7} allele. The Ab^{g7} allele includes five nucleotide polymorphisms resulting in the conversion of two usually conserved proline and aspartic acid residues at positions 56 and 57 to histidine and serine (104). Significantly, the non-aspartic acid substitutions at residue 57 also characterize diabetogenic variants of the human class II HLA-DQβ homolog, such as DQ8 (105). While transgenic analyses have shown both histidine and serine, respectively, at positions 56 and 57 amino acid residues of $A\beta^{g7}$ to be important for T1D progression in NOD mice (106–108), their diabetogenic function has not been tested under a more physiological condition. To further study the role of amino acid residue at position 57 in $A\beta^{g7}$, we created a knock-in NOD strain by replacing the serine with an aspartic acid ($A\beta^{g7}$-S57D). This was achieved by co-injecting Ab^{g7}-specific ZFN coding mRNA and a plasmid construct for HDR into one-cell fertilized NOD embryos, which were subsequently transferred into pseudopregnant mothers, and live-born pups were screened for founders. We successfully established a knock-in NOD stock (formal name: NOD/ShiLtJ-*H2-Ab1*^{em2Ygch}/Ygch) with the precise 3 base pair alteration resulting an aspartic acid at position 57 in the MHC class II Aβ chain. The knock-in allele was confirmed at both the genomic DNA and cDNA levels. We used two different antibody clones (AMS-32.1 and 10-3.6) to determine if MHC class II expression was altered in NOD.$Ab^{g7\text{-}S57D}$ mice. The expression level of MHC class II on B cells and dendritic cells was found to be comparable in wild-type NOD and NOD.$Ab^{g7\text{-}S57D}$ mice when 10-3.6 was used to stain their splenocytes (**Figure 1** and not shown). Interestingly, the level of MHC class II staining was found to be lower on B cells and dendritic cells from NOD.$Ab^{g7\text{-}S57D}$ than those from wild-type NOD mice when AMS-32.1 was used (**Figure 1** and not shown). These results indicate that the aspartic

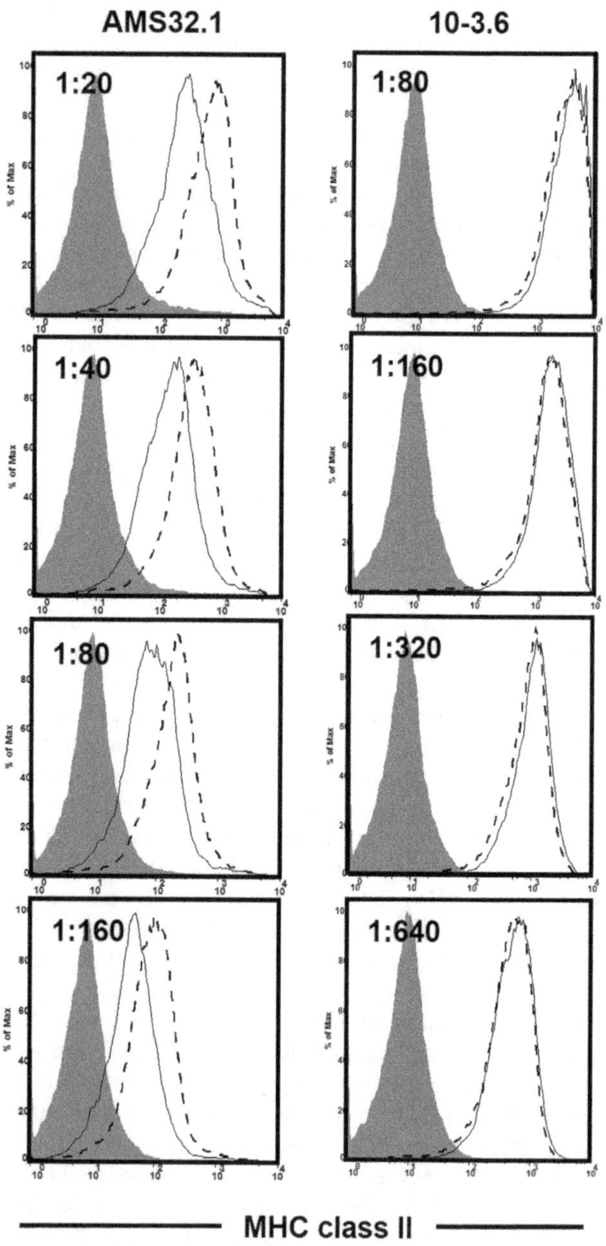

FIGURE 1 | Differential staining of the major histocompatibility complex (MHC) class II molecule in wild-type NOD and NOD.$Ab^{g7\text{-}S57D}$ mice. Total splenocytes were stained with anti-CD11c, anti-CD19, and the indicated I-Ab antibody clone at different titers. Shown is the I-Ab staining on B cells ($CD19^+$ $CD11c^-$) of NOD (dashed line) and NOD.$Ab^{g7\text{-}S57D}$ (solid line) mice. The shaded area is the negative control staining using splenocytes isolated from I-Ab deficient NOD mice (NOD/ShiLtJ-*H2-Ab1*^{em1Ygch}/J, JAX stock no. 027057). Similar results were obtained in two independent experiments.

acid substitution at position 57 in the Aβ chain alters the binding of AMS-32.1, presumably due to a conformational change of the antibody-binding epitope. Strikingly, diabetes development was completely suppressed in homozygous NOD.*Ab*$^{g7\text{-}S57D}$ mice (**Figure 2**), confirming the importance of the aspartic acid residue at position 57 of the Aβ chain in T1D. The availability of this novel strain will allow studies aimed to understand how diabetogenic MHC class II molecules select and activate β-cell autoreactive CD4 T cells.

Clustered Regularly Interspaced Short Palindromic Repeat (CRISPR) and CRISPR-Associated Protein 9 (Cas9)

Due to its high efficiency, the CRISPR/Cas9 system has become the top choice when considering gene targeting in a variety of animal models. Similar to ZFN mediated mutagenesis, CRISPR/Cas9 also introduces a DSB, followed by repair through NHEJ and HDR dependent mechanisms (109). Cas9 nuclease is recruited to a specific DNA sequence by a single-guide RNA that can be easily designed using publically available online tools (109). Several groups, including ours, have successfully used the CRISPR/Cas9 approach to disrupt genes directly on a pure NOD genetic background (18, 110–112). The importance of affinity maturation processes of B cells (class switch recombination and somatic mutation) for T1D development in NOD mice was demonstrated by ablation of the activation-induced cytidine deaminase gene (*Aicda*) (111). It was recently shown that IL-2 can indirectly enhance FOXP3 expression through downregulating the level of *Flicr*, a long non-coding RNA (112). The function of Tregs is impaired in NOD mice partly due to reduced IL-2 production by activated T cells in this strain (74). Deletion of *Flicr* decreased accumulation of FOXP3^{low} Tregs in pancreatic islets and suppressed T1D in NOD mice, likely by enhancing the stability and function of Tregs (112). *Ptpn22* has also been targeted in NOD mice using the CRISPR/Cas9 system (18). A nonsynonymous single nucleotide polymorphism resulting in an amino acid substitution (R620W) in human PTPN22 has been linked to numerous autoimmune diseases, including T1D (113).

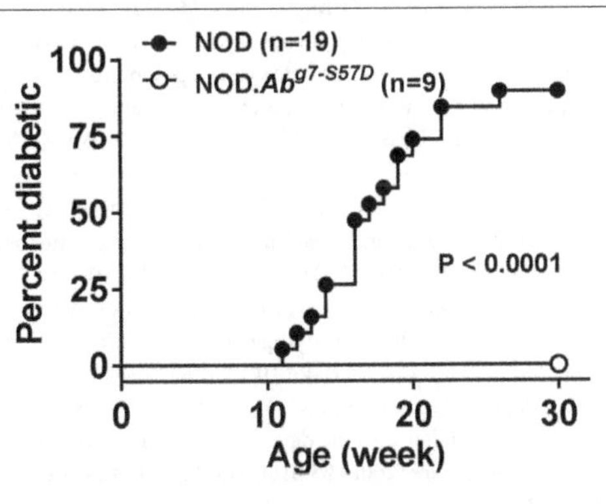

FIGURE 2 | NOD.*Ab*$^{g7\text{-}S57D}$ mice are completely resistant to type 1 diabetes. NOD and NOD.*Ab*$^{g7\text{-}S57D}$ mice were monitored for diabetes development weekly for 30 weeks by testing urine glucose. Diabetes onset was defined by two consecutive readings of >250 mg/dl.

Ptpn22 has been identified as a top candidate gene for the *Idd18.2* region in NOD mice. To further study the role of PTPN22 in T1D, the Sherman laboratory generated a *Ptpn22* knockout NOD mice as well as a knockin strain that has the R619W amino substitution to mimic the human variant (18). *Ptpn22* knockout NOD females developed more rapid onset of T1D (18). Similarly, NOD females expressing the *Ptpn22* KI allele (encoding 619W) also developed accelerated T1D (18), providing direct evidence to support the diabetogenic function of this variant.

Testing Human T1D Candidate Genes in NOD Mice

As noted above, the NOD mouse has been criticized for its usefulness as an animal model for human T1D, largely due to disappointing outcomes of clinical trials based on agents that showed therapeutic and/or preventive effects for mouse diabetes. The increased availability of human samples allowing direct examination of pancreata and lymphoid tissues isolated from organ donors at different stages of T1D progression has further decreased the enthusiasm of the NOD model (114). However, it remains a challenge to identify and to mechanistically study T1D susceptibility genes in human. The effect of a single gene on a phenotype is more difficult to detect due to heterogeneity in humans. Many genetic variations associated with T1D have a low phenotypic impact that overlaps when comparing carriers and non-carriers. In addition, human studies are mostly association in nature and strategies that allow investigators to directly analyze the diabetogenic function of a single SNP alone or in combination are limited. The CRISPR/Cas9 system makes it possible to engineer isogenic cell systems that can be used to specifically address the role of a SNP in gene expression and function (115). When combined with the ability to generate patient-derived iPSC and the advance of *in vitro* differentiation of iPSC into insulin-producing β-cells and hematopoietic stem cells, it may be possible to test the function of a SNP in cell types relevant to T1D (116, 117). However, these studies are not likely to overcome the difficulty to understand the course from altered gene expression/function to T1D development, which can only be dissected with *in vivo* experimental systems as disease progression is a consequence of combined effects that a variant elicits in different cell types in a time-dependent fashion. Combinational approaches using both mouse and human experimental systems are thus required to have a comprehensive understanding of the genetic control in T1D. The ability of nuclease based technology to efficiently and precisely modify the genome directly in NOD mice has opened a new door for current and future T1D genetic studies using this model.

Because T1D is a complex disease influenced by a large number of genes and ill-defined environmental factors, the NOD mouse remains an ideal animal model that provides a disease susceptible genetic background to test the diabetogenic function of a human candidate gene. For this reason, we have used both ZFNs and CRISPR/Cas9 systems to target mouse orthologs of human T1D candidate genes nominated by GWAS. As discussed above, the availability of the nuclease based technologies made it possible to do a relatively small scale but focused screening for genes that can regulate T1D progression in NOD mice. We have successfully targeted more than 40 genes directly in NOD mice. While these studies are still ongoing, the results obtained from this screening will allow us to provide additional evidence to support their roles in human T1D and prioritize them for future mechanistic studies. The eventual goal is to identify a pathway that could be pharmaceutically targeted for clinical translation.

CONCLUSION REMARKS

Despite some shortcomings, NOD mice and NOD-derived recombinant congenic strains provide many advantages for T1D research. As discussed above, the NOD mouse continues to be an important tool for dissecting the genetic control of T1D. As will be discussed below, we also describe T1D research areas where NOD mice and related strains can provide critical information in the next decade.

Previous studies have generated NOD mice transgenically expressing HLA class I and II molecules associated with human T1D (118–121). While HLA class II molecules in NOD mice are not able to promote T1D, expression of the HLA A2.1 allele accelerates diabetes development, providing a model for identifying peptides targeted by A2.1-restricted CD8^{+} T cells and for testing antigen-specific immunotherapy (122, 123). When combined with various versions of the severe immunodeficient NOD mice (e.g., NSG mice), expression of HLA class I or II molecules in the absence of murine counterparts provides a superior host for primary human T cells and hematopoietic stem cell-derived immune system (124). NSG mice that also express high-risk HLA class I or II molecules have been transplanted with human peripheral blood mononuclear cells or β-cell autoreactive T-cell clones/lines isolated from T1D patients to test the diabetogenic potential of the presumably pathogenic effectors (125–127). Although much progress has been made, overt diabetes has not been observed in HLA class I or II expressing NSG mice transfused with human T cells in various settings. The eventual goal is to reconstitute a T1D prone human immune system that targets β cells derived from the same subject in a mouse for studying "human" T1D. Recent advance in differentiating human iPS cells into functional insulin-producing β-cells and hematopoietic stem cells has brought us one step closer to this goal (116, 117).

Gut microbiome has emerged as an important component that modulates the progression of T1D in both humans and NOD mice (128–134). Longitudinal studies in humans showed that alteration of the diversity and species of gut microbiota preceded T1D onset (133). Studies in NOD mice have shown that manipulation of gut microbiota by means of antibiotics, fecal transfer, or co-housing can either suppress or promote diabetes development (128, 135–138). Collectively, these studies demonstrate that the NOD mouse can provide an excellent experimental platform for understanding the roles of gut microbiota in T1D. Recent studies also suggest that T1D modulation by gut microbiota is not likely to be caused by a single species but rather due to the balance of diverse species within the bacterial community. While it remains to be tested, experiments that utilize germ-free NOD mice reconstituted with fecal samples from T1D patients, at risk individuals, and healthy subjects may provide some information regarding the "good" and "bad" gut bacterial community. This knowledge can then be used to develop methods to alter the gut microbiota for T1D prevention and set the foundation for future clinical trials.

AUTHOR CONTRIBUTIONS

All authors listed have made a substantial, direct, and intellectual contribution to the work and approved it for publication.

REFERENCES

1. Melanitou E, Devendra D, Liu E, Miao D, Eisenbarth GS. Early and quantal (by litter) expression of insulin autoantibodies in the nonobese diabetic mice predict early diabetes onset. *J Immunol* (2004) 173:6603–10. doi:10.4049/jimmunol.173.11.6603
2. You S, Belghith M, Cobbold S, Alyanakian MA, Gouarin C, Barriot S, et al. Autoimmune diabetes onset results from qualitative rather than quantitative age-dependent changes in pathogenic T-cells. *Diabetes* (2005) 54:1415–22. doi:10.2337/diabetes.54.5.1415
3. Gregori S, Giarratana N, Smiroldo S, Adorini L. Dynamics of pathogenic and suppressor T cells in autoimmune diabetes development. *J Immunol* (2003) 171:4040–7. doi:10.4049/jimmunol.171.8.4040
4. Pugliese A. Autoreactive T cells in type 1 diabetes. *J Clin Invest* (2017) 127:2881–91. doi:10.1172/JCI94549
5. Regnell SE, Lernmark Å. Early prediction of autoimmune (type 1) diabetes. *Diabetologia* (2017) 60:1370–81. doi:10.1007/s00125-017-4308-1
6. Wester A, Skärstrand H, Lind A, Ramelius A, Carlsson A, Cedervall E, et al. An increased diagnostic sensitivity of truncated GAD65 autoantibodies in type 1 diabetes may be related to HLA-DQ8. *Diabetes* (2017) 66:735–40. doi:10.2337/db16-0891
7. Katsarou A, Gudbjörnsdottir S, Rawshani A, Dabelea D, Bonifacio E, Anderson BJ, et al. Type 1 diabetes mellitus. *Nat Rev Dis Primers* (2017) 3:17016. doi:10.1038/nrdp.2017.16
8. Mathews CE, Xue S, Posgai A, Lightfoot YL, Li X, Lin A, et al. Acute versus progressive onset of diabetes in NOD mice: potential implications for therapeutic interventions in type 1 diabetes. *Diabetes* (2015) 64:3885–90. doi:10.2337/db15-0449
9. DiLorenzo TP, Graser RT, Ono T, Christianson GJ, Chapman HD, Roopenian DC, et al. Major histocompatibility complex class I-restricted T cells are required for all but the end stages of diabetes development in nonobese diabetic mice and use a prevalent T cell receptor alpha chain gene rearrangement. *Proc Natl Acad Sci U S A* (1998) 95:12538–43. doi:10.1073/pnas.95.21.12538
10. Campbell-Thompson M, Fu A, Kaddis JS, Wasserfall C, Schatz DA, Pugliese A, et al. Insulitis and β-cell mass in the natural history of type 1 diabetes. *Diabetes* (2016) 65:719–31. doi:10.2337/db15-0779
11. Driver JP, Chen YG, Mathews CE. Comparative genetics: synergizing human and NOD mouse studies for identifying genetic causation of type 1 diabetes. *Rev Diabet Stud* (2012) 9:169–87. doi:10.1900/RDS.2012.9.169
12. Uchigata Y, Okada T, Gong JS, Yamada Y, Iwamoto Y, Tanaka M. A mitochondrial genotype associated with the development of autoimmune-related type 1 diabetes. *Diabetes Care* (2002) 25:2106. doi:10.2337/diacare.25.11.2106
13. Mathews CE, Leiter EH, Spirina O, Bykhovskaya Y, Gusdon AM, Ringquist S, et al. mt-Nd2 Allele of the ALR/Lt mouse confers resistance against both chemically induced and autoimmune diabetes. *Diabetologia* (2005) 48:261–7. doi:10.1007/s00125-004-1644-8

14. Onengut-Gumuscu S, Chen WM, Burren O, Cooper NJ, Quinlan AR, Mychaleckyj JC, et al. Fine mapping of type 1 diabetes susceptibility loci and evidence for colocalization of causal variants with lymphoid gene enhancers. *Nat Genet* (2015) 47:381–6. doi:10.1038/ng.3245
15. Vijayakrishnan L, Slavik JM, Illes Z, Greenwald RJ, Rainbow D, Greve B, et al. An autoimmune disease-associated CTLA-4 splice variant lacking the B7 binding domain signals negatively in T cells. *Immunity* (2004) 20:563–75. doi:10.1016/S1074-7613(04)00110-4
16. Ueda H, Howson JM, Esposito L, Heward J, Snook H, Chamberlain G, et al. Association of the T-cell regulatory gene CTLA4 with susceptibility to autoimmune disease. *Nature* (2003) 423:506–11. doi:10.1038/nature01621
17. Araki M, Chung D, Liu S, Rainbow DB, Chamberlain G, Garner V, et al. Genetic evidence that the differential expression of the ligand-independent isoform of CTLA-4 is the molecular basis of the Idd5.1 type 1 diabetes region in nonobese diabetic mice. *J Immunol* (2009) 183:5146–57. doi:10.4049/jimmunol.0802610
18. Lin X, Pelletier S, Gingras S, Rigaud S, Maine CJ, Marquardt K, et al. CRISPR-Cas9-mediated modification of the NOD mouse genome with Ptpn22R619W mutation increases autoimmune diabetes. *Diabetes* (2016) 65:2134–8. doi:10.2337/db16-0061
19. Winkler C, Krumsiek J, Lempainen J, Achenbach P, Grallert H, Giannopoulou E, et al. A strategy for combining minor genetic susceptibility genes to improve prediction of disease in type 1 diabetes. *Genes Immun* (2012) 13:549–55. doi:10.1038/gene.2012.36
20. Howson JM, Cooper JD, Smyth DJ, Walker NM, Stevens H, She JX, et al. Evidence of gene-gene interaction and age-at-diagnosis effects in type 1 diabetes. *Diabetes* (2012) 61:3012–7. doi:10.2337/db11-1694
21. Grant CW, Moran-Paul CM, Duclos SK, Guberski DL, Arreaza-Rubín G, Spain LM. Testing agents for prevention or reversal of type 1 diabetes in rodents. *PLoS One* (2013) 8:e72989. doi:10.1371/journal.pone.0072989
22. Diabetes Prevention Trial-Type 1 Diabetes Study Group. Effects of insulin in relatives of patients with type 1 diabetes mellitus. *N Engl J Med* (2002) 346:1685–91. doi:10.1056/NEJMoa012350
23. Skyler JS, Krischer JP, Wolfsdorf J, Cowie C, Palmer JP, Greenbaum C, et al. Effects of oral insulin in relatives of patients with type 1 diabetes: the diabetes prevention trial – type 1. *Diabetes Care* (2005) 28:1068–76. doi:10.2337/diacare.28.5.1068
24. Näntö-Salonen K, Kupila A, Simell S, Siljander H, Salonsaari T, Hekkala A, et al. Nasal insulin to prevent type 1 diabetes in children with HLA genotypes and autoantibodies conferring increased risk of disease: a double-blind, randomised controlled trial. *Lancet* (2008) 372:1746–55. doi:10.1016/S0140-6736(08)61309-4
25. Sherry NA, Chen W, Kushner JA, Glandt M, Tang Q, Tsai S, et al. Exendin-4 improves reversal of diabetes in NOD mice treated with anti-CD3 monoclonal antibody by enhancing recovery of beta-cells. *Endocrinology* (2007) 148:5136–44. doi:10.1210/en.2007-0358
26. Gill RG, Pagni PP, Kupfer T, Wasserfall CH, Deng S, Posgai A, et al. A preclinical consortium approach for assessing the efficacy of combined anti-CD3 plus IL-1 blockade in reversing new-onset autoimmune diabetes in NOD mice. *Diabetes* (2016) 65:1310–6. doi:10.2337/db15-0492
27. Herold KC, Gitelman SE, Masharani U, Hagopian W, Bisikirska B, Donaldson D, et al. A single course of anti-CD3 monoclonal antibody hOKT3gamma1(Ala-Ala) results in improvement in C-peptide responses and clinical parameters for at least 2 years after onset of type 1 diabetes. *Diabetes* (2005) 54:1763–9. doi:10.2337/diabetes.54.6.1763
28. Herold KC, Hagopian W, Auger JA, Poumian-Ruiz E, Taylor L, Donaldson D, et al. Anti-CD3 monoclonal antibody in new-onset type 1 diabetes mellitus. *N Engl J Med* (2002) 346:1692–8. doi:10.1056/NEJMoa012864
29. Keymeulen B, Vandemeulebroucke E, Ziegler AG, Mathieu C, Kaufman L, Hale G, et al. Insulin needs after CD3-antibody therapy in new-onset type 1 diabetes. *N Engl J Med* (2005) 352:2598–608. doi:10.1056/NEJMoa043980
30. Haller MJ, Gitelman SE, Gottlieb PA, Michels AW, Rosenthal SM, Shuster JJ, et al. Anti-thymocyte globulin/G-CSF treatment preserves β cell function in patients with established type 1 diabetes. *J Clin Invest* (2015) 125:448–55. doi:10.1172/JCI78492
31. Haller MJ, Gitelman SE, Gottlieb PA, Michels AW, Perry DJ, Schultz AR, et al. Antithymocyte globulin plus G-CSF combination therapy leads to sustained immunomodulatory and metabolic effects in a subset of responders with established type 1 diabetes. *Diabetes* (2016) 65:3765–75. doi:10.2337/db16-0823
32. Xue S, Posgai A, Wasserfall C, Myhr C, Campbell-Thompson M, Mathews CE, et al. Combination therapy reverses hyperglycemia in NOD mice with established type 1 diabetes. *Diabetes* (2015) 64:3873–84. doi:10.2337/db15-0164
33. Atkinson MA. Evaluating preclinical efficacy. *Sci Transl Med* (2011) 3:96cm22. doi:10.1126/scitranslmed.3002757
34. Wicker LS, Todd JA, Prins JB, Podolin PL, Renjilian RJ, Peterson LB. Resistance alleles at two non-major histocompatibility complex-linked insulin-dependent diabetes loci on chromosome 3, Idd3 and Idd10, protect nonobese diabetic mice from diabetes. *J Exp Med* (1994) 180:1705–13. doi:10.1084/jem.180.5.1705
35. Lord CJ, Bohlander SK, Hopes EA, Montague CT, Hill NJ, Prins JB, et al. Mapping the diabetes polygene Idd3 on mouse chromosome 3 by use of novel congenic strains. *Mamm Genome* (1995) 6:563–70. doi:10.1007/BF00352359
36. Podolin PL, Denny P, Lord CJ, Hill NJ, Todd JA, Peterson LB, et al. Congenic mapping of the insulin-dependent diabetes (Idd) gene, Idd10, localizes two genes mediating the Idd10 effect and eliminates the candidate Fcgr1. *J Immunol* (1997) 159:1835–43.
37. Todd JA, Aitman TJ, Cornall RJ, Ghosh S, Hall JR, Hearne CM, et al. Genetic analysis of autoimmune type 1 diabetes mellitus in mice. *Nature* (1991) 351:542–7. doi:10.1038/351542a0
38. Hill NJ, Lyons PA, Armitage N, Todd JA, Wicker LS, Peterson LB. NOD Idd5 locus controls insulitis and diabetes and overlaps the orthologous CTLA4/IDDM12 and NRAMP1 loci in humans. *Diabetes* (2000) 49:1744–7. doi:10.2337/diabetes.49.10.1744
39. Cornall RJ, Prins JB, Todd JA, Pressey A, DeLarato NH, Wicker LS, et al. Type 1 diabetes in mice is linked to the interleukin-1 receptor and Lsh/Ity/Bcg genes on chromosome 1. *Nature* (1991) 353:262–5. doi:10.1038/353262a0
40. Garchon HJ, Bedossa P, Eloy L, Bach JF. Identification and mapping to chromosome 1 of a susceptibility locus for periinsulitis in non-obese diabetic mice. *Nature* (1991) 353:260–2. doi:10.1038/353260a0
41. Hunter K, Rainbow D, Plagnol V, Todd JA, Peterson LB, Wicker LS. Interactions between Idd5.1/Ctla4 and other type 1 diabetes genes. *J Immunol* (2007) 179:8341–9. doi:10.4049/jimmunol.179.12.8341
42. Rodrigues NR, Cornall RJ, Chandler P, Simpson E, Wicker LS, Peterson LB, et al. Mapping of an insulin-dependent diabetes locus, Idd9, in NOD mice to chromosome 4. *Mamm Genome* (1994) 5:167–70. doi:10.1007/BF00352349
43. Lyons PA, Hancock WW, Denny P, Lord CJ, Hill NJ, Armitage N, et al. The NOD Idd9 genetic interval influences the pathogenicity of insulitis and contains molecular variants of Cd30, Tnfr2, and Cd137. *Immunity* (2000) 13:107–15. doi:10.1016/S1074-7613(00)00012-1
44. Brodnicki TC, McClive P, Couper S, Morahan G. Localization of Idd11 using NOD congenic mouse strains: elimination of Slc9a1 as a candidate gene. *Immunogenetics* (2000) 51:37–41. doi:10.1007/s002510050006
45. Hamilton-Williams EE, Rainbow DB, Cheung J, Christensen M, Lyons PA, Peterson LB, et al. Fine mapping of type 1 diabetes regions Idd9.1 and Idd9.2 reveals genetic complexity. *Mamm Genome* (2013) 24:358–75. doi:10.1007/s00335-013-9466-y
46. Lin B, Ciecko AE, MacKinney E, Serreze DV, Chen YG. Congenic mapping identifies a novel Idd9 subregion regulating type 1 diabetes in NOD mice. *Immunogenetics* (2017) 69:193–8. doi:10.1007/s00251-016-0957-3
47. Ridgway WM, Peterson LB, Todd JA, Rainbow DB, Healy B, Burren OS, et al. Gene-gene interactions in the NOD mouse model of type 1 diabetes. *Adv Immunol* (2008) 100:151–75. doi:10.1016/S0065-2776(08)00806-7
48. Fraser HI, Dendrou CA, Healy B, Rainbow DB, Howlett S, Smink LJ, et al. Nonobese diabetic congenic strain analysis of autoimmune diabetes reveals genetic complexity of the Idd18 locus and identifies Vav3 as a candidate gene. *J Immunol* (2010) 184:5075–84. doi:10.4049/jimmunol.0903734
49. Morin J, Boitard C, Vallois D, Avner P, Rogner UC. Mapping of the murine type 1 diabetes locus Idd20 by genetic interaction. *Mamm Genome* (2006) 17:1105–12. doi:10.1007/s00335-006-0076-9
50. Hollis-Moffatt JE, Hook SM, Merriman TR. Colocalization of mouse auto-

immune diabetes loci Idd21.1 and Idd21.2 with IDDM6 (human) and Iddm3 (rat). *Diabetes* (2005) 54:2820–5. doi:10.2337/diabetes.54.9.2820
51. Rogner UC, Boitard C, Morin J, Melanitou E, Avner P. Three loci on mouse chromosome 6 influence onset and final incidence of type I diabetes in NOD.C3H congenic strains. *Genomics* (2001) 74:163–71. doi:10.1006/geno.2001.6508
52. Driver JP, Serreze DV, Chen YG. Mouse models for the study of autoimmune type 1 diabetes: a NOD to similarities and differences to human disease. *Semin Immunopathol* (2011) 33:67–87. doi:10.1007/s00281-010-0204-1
53. Lundholm M, Motta V, Löfgren-Burström A, Duarte N, Bergman ML, Mayans S, et al. Defective induction of CTLA-4 in the NOD mouse is controlled by the NOD allele of Idd3/IL-2 and a novel locus (Ctex) telomeric on chromosome 1. *Diabetes* (2006) 55:538–44. doi:10.2337/diabetes.55.02.06.db05-1240
54. Lin X, Hamilton-Williams EE, Rainbow DB, Hunter KM, Dai YD, Cheung J, et al. Genetic interactions among Idd3, Idd5.1, Idd5.2, and Idd5.3 protective loci in the nonobese diabetic mouse model of type 1 diabetes. *J Immunol* (2013) 190:3109–20. doi:10.4049/jimmunol.1203422
55. Wang N, Elso CM, Mackin L, Mannering SI, Strugnell RA, Wijburg OL, et al. Congenic mice reveal genetic epistasis and overlapping disease loci for autoimmune diabetes and listeriosis. *Immunogenetics* (2014) 66:501–6. doi:10.1007/s00251-014-0782-5
56. Hermann R, Lipponen K, Kiviniemi M, Kakko T, Veijola R, Simell O, et al. Lymphoid tyrosine phosphatase (LYP/PTPN22) Arg620Trp variant regulates insulin autoimmunity and progression to type 1 diabetes. *Diabetologia* (2006) 49:1198–208. doi:10.1007/s00125-006-0225-4
57. Smyth DJ, Cooper JD, Howson JM, Walker NM, Plagnol V, Stevens H, et al. PTPN22 Trp620 explains the association of chromosome 1p13 with type 1 diabetes and shows a statistical interaction with HLA class II genotypes. *Diabetes* (2008) 57:1730–7. doi:10.2337/db07-1131
58. Steck AK, Liu SY, McFann K, Barriga KJ, Babu SR, Eisenbarth GS, et al. Association of the PTPN22/LYP gene with type 1 diabetes. *Pediatr Diabetes* (2006) 7:274–8. doi:10.1111/j.1399-5448.2006.00202.x
59. Stolp J, Chen YG, Cox SL, Henck V, Zhang W, Tsaih SW, et al. Subcongenic analyses reveal complex interactions between distal chromosome 4 genes controlling diabetogenic B cells and CD4 T cells in nonobese diabetic mice. *J Immunol* (2012) 189:1406–17. doi:10.4049/jimmunol.1200120
60. Silveira PA, Chapman HD, Stolp J, Johnson E, Cox SL, Hunter K, et al. Genes within the Idd5 and Idd9/11 diabetes susceptibility loci affect the pathogenic activity of B cells in nonobese diabetic mice. *J Immunol* (2006) 177:7033–41. doi:10.4049/jimmunol.177.10.7033
61. Chen YG, Scheuplein F, Osborne MA, Tsaih SW, Chapman HD, Serreze DV. Idd9/11 genetic locus regulates diabetogenic activity of CD4 T-cells in nonobese diabetic (NOD) mice. *Diabetes* (2008) 57:3273–80. doi:10.2337/db08-0767
62. Waldner H, Sobel RA, Price N, Kuchroo VK. The autoimmune diabetes locus Idd9 regulates development of type 1 diabetes by affecting the homing of islet-specific T cells. *J Immunol* (2006) 176:5455–62. doi:10.4049/jimmunol.176.9.5455
63. Hamilton-Williams EE, Wong SB, Martinez X, Rainbow DB, Hunter KM, Wicker LS, et al. Idd9.2 and Idd9.3 protective alleles function in CD4+ T-cells and nonlymphoid cells to prevent expansion of pathogenic islet-specific CD8+ T-cells. *Diabetes* (2010) 59:1478–86. doi:10.2337/db09-1801
64. Yamanouchi J, Puertas MC, Verdaguer J, Lyons PA, Rainbow DB, Chamberlain G, et al. Idd9.1 locus controls the suppressive activity of FoxP3+CD4+CD25+ regulatory T-cells. *Diabetes* (2010) 59:272–81. doi:10.2337/db09-0648
65. Ueno A, Wang J, Cheng L, Im JS, Shi Y, Porcelli SA, et al. Enhanced early expansion and maturation of semi-invariant NK T cells inhibited autoimmune pathogenesis in congenic nonobese diabetic mice. *J Immunol* (2008) 181:6789–96. doi:10.4049/jimmunol.181.10.6789
66. Hill NJ, Stotland A, Solomon M, Secrest P, Getzoff E, Sarvetnick N. Resistance of the target islet tissue to autoimmune destruction contributes to genetic susceptibility in type 1 diabetes. *Biol Direct* (2007) 2:5. doi:10.1186/1745-6150-2-5
67. Ghosh S, Palmer SM, Rodrigues NR, Cordell HJ, Hearne CM, Cornall RJ, et al. Polygenic control of autoimmune diabetes in nonobese diabetic mice. *Nat Genet* (1993) 4:404–9. doi:10.1038/ng0893-404
68. Rogner UC, Lepault F, Gagnerault MC, Vallois D, Morin J, Avner P, et al. The diabetes type 1 locus Idd6 modulates activity of CD4+CD25+ regulatory T-cells. *Diabetes* (2006) 55:186–92. doi:10.2337/diabetes.55.01.06.db05-0598
69. Robles DT, Eisenbarth GS, Dailey NJ, Peterson LB, Wicker LS. Insulin autoantibodies are associated with islet inflammation but not always related to diabetes progression in NOD congenic mice. *Diabetes* (2003) 52:882–6. doi:10.2337/diabetes.52.3.882
70. Pomerleau DP, Bagley RJ, Serreze DV, Mathews CE, Leiter EH. Major histocompatibility complex-linked diabetes susceptibility in NOD/Lt mice: subcongenic analysis localizes a component of Idd16 at the H2-D end of the diabetogenic H2(g7) complex. *Diabetes* (2005) 54:1603–6. doi:10.2337/diabetes.54.5.1603
71. Grattan M, Mi QS, Meagher C, Delovitch TL. Congenic mapping of the diabetogenic locus Idd4 to a 5.2-cM region of chromosome 11 in NOD mice: identification of two potential candidate subloci. *Diabetes* (2002) 51:215–23. doi:10.2337/diabetes.51.1.215
72. Serreze DV, Bridgett M, Chapman HD, Chen E, Richard SD, Leiter EH. Subcongenic analysis of the Idd13 locus in NOD/Lt mice: evidence for several susceptibility genes including a possible diabetogenic role for beta 2-microglobulin. *J Immunol* (1998) 160:1472–8.
73. Reed JC, Herold KC. Thinking bedside at the bench: the NOD mouse model of T1DM. *Nat Rev Endocrinol* (2015) 11:308–14. doi:10.1038/nrendo.2014.236
74. Yamanouchi J, Rainbow D, Serra P, Howlett S, Hunter K, Garner VE, et al. Interleukin-2 gene variation impairs regulatory T cell function and causes autoimmunity. *Nat Genet* (2007) 39:329–37. doi:10.1038/ng1958
75. Kachapati K, Adams DE, Wu Y, Steward CA, Rainbow DB, Wicker LS, et al. The B10 Idd9.3 locus mediates accumulation of functionally superior CD137(+) regulatory T cells in the nonobese diabetic type 1 diabetes model. *J Immunol* (2012) 189:5001–15. doi:10.4049/jimmunol.1101013
76. McGuire HM, Vogelzang A, Hill N, Flodström-Tullberg M, Sprent J, King C. Loss of parity between IL-2 and IL-21 in the NOD Idd3 locus. *Proc Natl Acad Sci U S A* (2009) 106:19438–43. doi:10.1073/pnas.0903561106
77. Fraser HI, Howlett S, Clark J, Rainbow DB, Stanford SM, Wu DJ, et al. Ptpn22 and Cd2 variations are associated with altered protein expression and susceptibility to type 1 diabetes in nonobese diabetic mice. *J Immunol* (2015) 195:4841–52. doi:10.4049/jimmunol.1402654
78. Long SA, Rieck M, Sanda S, Bollyky JB, Samuels PL, Goland R, et al. Rapamycin/IL-2 combination therapy in patients with type 1 diabetes augments Tregs yet transiently impairs β-cell function. *Diabetes* (2012) 61:2340–8. doi:10.2337/db12-0049
79. Grinberg-Bleyer Y, Baeyens A, You S, Elhage R, Fourcade G, Gregoire S, et al. IL-2 reverses established type 1 diabetes in NOD mice by a local effect on pancreatic regulatory T cells. *J Exp Med* (2010) 207:1871–8. doi:10.1084/jem.20100209
80. Lowe CE, Cooper JD, Brusko T, Walker NM, Smyth DJ, Bailey R, et al. Large-scale genetic fine mapping and genotype-phenotype associations implicate polymorphism in the IL2RA region in type 1 diabetes. *Nat Genet* (2007) 39:1074–82. doi:10.1038/ng2102
81. Todd JA, Walker NM, Cooper JD, Smyth DJ, Downes K, Plagnol V, et al. Robust associations of four new chromosome regions from genome-wide analyses of type 1 diabetes. *Nat Genet* (2007) 39:857–64. doi:10.1038/ng2068
82. Lyons PA, Armitage N, Argentina F, Denny P, Hill NJ, Lord CJ, et al. Congenic mapping of the type 1 diabetes locus, Idd3, to a 780-kb region of mouse chromosome 3: identification of a candidate segment of ancestral DNA by haplotype mapping. *Genome Res* (2000) 10:446–53. doi:10.1101/gr.10.4.446
83. Barrett JC, Clayton DG, Concannon P, Akolkar B, Cooper JD, Erlich HA, et al. Genome-wide association study and meta-analysis find that over 40 loci affect risk of type 1 diabetes. *Nat Genet* (2009) 41(6):703–7. doi:10.1038/ng.381
84. Morahan G, Mehta M, James I, Chen WM, Akolkar B, Erlich HA, et al. Tests for genetic interactions in type 1 diabetes: linkage and stratification analyses of 4,422 affected sib-pairs. *Diabetes* (2011) 60:1030–40. doi:10.2337/db10-1195
85. Rubinson DA, Dillon CP, Kwiatkowski AV, Sievers C, Yang L, Kopinja J, et al. A lentivirus-based system to functionally silence genes in primary mammalian cells, stem cells and transgenic mice by RNA interference. *Nat Genet* (2003) 33:401–6. doi:10.1038/ng1117

86. Tiscornia G, Singer O, Ikawa M, Verma IM. A general method for gene knockdown in mice by using lentiviral vectors expressing small interfering RNA. *Proc Natl Acad Sci U S A* (2003) 100:1844–8. doi:10.1073/pnas.0437912100
87. Rao DD, Vorhies JS, Senzer N, Nemunaitis J. siRNA vs. shRNA: similarities and differences. *Adv Drug Deliv Rev* (2009) 61:746–59. doi:10.1016/j.addr.2009.04.004
88. Joseph J, Bittner S, Kaiser FM, Wiendl H, Kissler S. IL-17 silencing does not protect nonobese diabetic mice from autoimmune diabetes. *J Immunol* (2012) 188:216–21. doi:10.4049/jimmunol.1101215
89. Zheng P, Kissler S. PTPN22 silencing in the NOD model indicates the type 1 diabetes-associated allele is not a loss-of-function variant. *Diabetes* (2012) 62:896–904. doi:10.2337/db12-0929
90. Gerold KD, Zheng P, Rainbow DB, Zernecke A, Wicker LS, Kissler S. The soluble CTLA-4 splice variant protects from type 1 diabetes and potentiates regulatory T-cell function. *Diabetes* (2011) 60:1955–63. doi:10.2337/db11-0130
91. Schuster C, Gerold KD, Schober K, Probst L, Boerner K, Kim MJ, et al. The autoimmunity-associated gene CLEC16A modulates thymic epithelial cell autophagy and alters T cell selection. *Immunity* (2015) 42:942–52. doi:10.1016/j.immuni.2015.04.011
92. Caballero-Franco C, Kissler S. The autoimmunity-associated gene RGS1 affects the frequency of T follicular helper cells. *Genes Immun* (2016) 17:228–38. doi:10.1038/gene.2016.16
93. Kissler S, Stern P, Takahashi K, Hunter K, Peterson LB, Wicker LS. In vivo RNA interference demonstrates a role for Nramp1 in modifying susceptibility to type 1 diabetes. *Nat Genet* (2006) 38:479–83. doi:10.1038/ng1766
94. Nowakowska DJ, Kissler S. Ptpn22 modifies regulatory T cell homeostasis via GITR upregulation. *J Immunol* (2016) 196:2145–52. doi:10.4049/jimmunol.1501877
95. Jacob HJ, Lazar J, Dwinell MR, Moreno C, Geurts AM. Gene targeting in the rat: advances and opportunities. *Trends Genet* (2010) 26:510–8. doi:10.1016/j.tig.2010.08.006
96. Urnov FD, Rebar EJ, Holmes MC, Zhang HS, Gregory PD. Genome editing with engineered zinc finger nucleases. *Nat Rev Genet* (2010) 11:636–46. doi:10.1038/nrg2842
97. Geurts AM, Moreno C. Zinc-finger nucleases: new strategies to target the rat genome. *Clin Sci* (2010) 119:303–11. doi:10.1042/CS20100201
98. Geurts AM, Cost GJ, Remy S, Cui X, Tesson L, Usal C, et al. Generation of gene-specific mutated rats using zinc-finger nucleases. *Methods Mol Biol* (2010) 597:211–25. doi:10.1007/978-1-60327-389-3_15
99. Geurts AM, Cost GJ, Freyvert Y, Zeitler B, Miller JC, Choi VM, et al. Knockout rats via embryo microinjection of zinc-finger nucleases. *Science* (2009) 325:433. doi:10.1126/science.1172447
100. Cui X, Ji D, Fisher DA, Wu Y, Briner DM, Weinstein EJ. Targeted integration in rat and mouse embryos with zinc-finger nucleases. *Nat Biotechnol* (2011) 29:64–7. doi:10.1038/nbt.1731
101. Chen YG, Forsberg MH, Khaja S, Ciecko AE, Hessner MJ, Geurts AM. Gene targeting in NOD mouse embryos using zinc-finger nucleases. *Diabetes* (2014) 63:68–74. doi:10.2337/db13-0192
102. Cannons JL, Chamberlain G, Howson J, Smink LJ, Todd JA, Peterson LB, et al. Genetic and functional association of the immune signaling molecule 4-1BB (CD137/TNFRSF9) with type 1 diabetes. *J Autoimmun* (2005) 25:13–20. doi:10.1016/j.jaut.2005.04.007
103. Forsberg MH, Ciecko AE, Bednar KJ, Itoh A, Kachapati K, Ridgway WM, et al. CD137 plays both pathogenic and protective roles in Type 1 diabetes development in NOD mice. *J Immunol* (2017) 198:3857–68. doi:10.4049/jimmunol.1601851
104. Acha-Orbea H, McDevitt HO. The first external domain of the nonobese diabetic mouse class II I-A beta chain is unique. *Proc Natl Acad Sci U S A* (1987) 84:2435–9. doi:10.1073/pnas.84.8.2435
105. Todd JA, Acha-Orbea H, Bell JI, Chao N, Fronek Z, Jacob CO, et al. A molecular basis for MHC class II-associated autoimmunity. *Science* (1988) 240:1003–9. doi:10.1126/science.3368786
106. Lund T, O'Reilly L, Hutchings P, Kanagawa O, Simpson E, Gravely R, et al. Prevention of insulin-dependent diabetes mellitus in non-obese diabetic mice by transgenes encoding modified I-A beta-chain or normal I-E alpha-chain. *Nature* (1990) 345:727–9. doi:10.1038/345727a0
107. Quartey-Papafio R, Lund T, Chandler P, Picard J, Ozegbe P, Day S, et al. Aspartate at position 57 of nonobese diabetic I-Ag7 beta-chain diminishes the spontaneous incidence of insulin-dependent diabetes mellitus. *J Immunol* (1995) 154:5567–75.
108. Singer SM, Tisch R, Yang XD, Sytwu HK, Liblau R, McDevitt HO. Prevention of diabetes in NOD mice by a mutated I-Ab transgene. *Diabetes* (1998) 47:1570–7. doi:10.2337/diabetes.47.10.1570
109. Harrison MM, Jenkins BV, O'Connor-Giles KM, Wildonger J. A CRISPR view of development. *Genes Dev* (2014) 28:1859–72. doi:10.1101/gad.248252.114
110. Qin W, Dion SL, Kutny PM, Zhang Y, Cheng AW, Jillette NL, et al. Efficient CRISPR/Cas9-mediated genome editing in mice by Zygote electroporation of nuclease. *Genetics* (2015) 200:423–30. doi:10.1534/genetics.115.176594
111. Ratiu JJ, Racine JJ, Hasham MG, Wang Q, Branca JA, Chapman HD, et al. Genetic and small molecule disruption of the AID/RAD51 axis similarly protects nonobese diabetic mice from type 1 diabetes through expansion of regulatory B lymphocytes. *J Immunol* (2017) 198:4255–67. doi:10.4049/jimmunol.1700024
112. Zemmour D, Pratama A, Loughhead SM, Mathis D, Benoist C. Flicr, a long noncoding RNA, modulates Foxp3 expression and autoimmunity. *Proc Natl Acad Sci U S A* (2017) 114:E3472–80. doi:10.1073/pnas.1700946114
113. Bottini N, Peterson EJ. Tyrosine phosphatase PTPN22: multifunctional regulator of immune signaling, development, and disease. *Annu Rev Immunol* (2014) 32:83–119. doi:10.1146/annurev-immunol-032713-120249
114. Pugliese A, Yang M, Kusmarteva I, Heiple T, Vendrame F, Wasserfall C, et al. The juvenile diabetes research foundation network for pancreatic organ donors with diabetes (nPOD) program: goals, operational model and emerging findings. *Pediatr Diabetes* (2014) 15:1–9. doi:10.1111/pedi.12097
115. Wallet MA, Santostefano KE, Terada N, Brusko TM. Isogenic cellular systems model the impact of genetic risk variants in the pathogenesis of type 1 diabetes. *Front Endocrinol* (2017) 8:276. doi:10.3389/fendo.2017.00276
116. Millman JR, Xie C, Van Dervort A, Gurtler M, Pagliuca FW, Melton DA. Generation of stem cell-derived beta-cells from patients with type 1 diabetes. *Nat Commun* (2016) 7:11463. doi:10.1038/ncomms11463
117. Sugimura R, Jha DK, Han A, Soria-Valles C, da Rocha EL, Lu YF, et al. Haematopoietic stem and progenitor cells from human pluripotent stem cells. *Nature* (2017) 545:432–8. doi:10.1038/nature22370
118. Kudva YC, Rajagopalan G, Raju R, Abraham RS, Smart M, Hanson J, et al. Modulation of insulitis and type 1 diabetes by transgenic HLA-DR3 and DQ8 in NOD mice lacking endogenous MHC class II. *Hum Immunol* (2002) 63:987–99. doi:10.1016/S0198-8859(02)00435-4
119. Marron MP, Graser RT, Chapman HD, Serreze DV. Functional evidence for the mediation of diabetogenic T cell responses by HLA A2.1 MHC class I molecules through transgenic expression in NOD mice. *Proc Natl Acad Sci U S A* (2002) 99:13753–8. doi:10.1073/pnas.212221199
120. Elliott JF, Liu J, Yuan ZN, Bautista-Lopez N, Wallbank SL, Suzuki K, et al. Autoimmune cardiomyopathy and heart block develop spontaneously in HLA-DQ8 transgenic IAbeta knockout NOD mice. *Proc Natl Acad Sci U S A* (2003) 100:13447–52. doi:10.1073/pnas.2235552100
121. Antal Z, Baker JC, Smith C, Jarchum I, Babad J, Mukherjee G, et al. Beyond HLA-A*0201: new HLA-transgenic nonobese diabetic mouse models of type 1 diabetes identify the insulin C-peptide as a rich source of CD8+ T cell epitopes. *J Immunol* (2012) 188:5766–75. doi:10.4049/jimmunol.1102930
122. Takaki T, Marron MP, Mathews CE, Guttmann ST, Bottino R, Trucco M, et al. HLA-A*0201-restricted T cells from humanized NOD mice recognize autoantigens of potential clinical relevance to type 1 diabetes. *J Immunol* (2006) 176:3257–65. doi:10.4049/jimmunol.176.5.3257
123. Niens M, Grier AE, Marron M, Kay TW, Greiner DL, Serreze DV. Prevention of "humanized" diabetogenic CD8 T-cell responses in HLA-transgenic NOD mice by a multipeptide coupled-cell approach. *Diabetes* (2011) 60:1229–36. doi:10.2337/db10-1523
124. Shultz LD, Brehm MA, Garcia-Martinez JV, Greiner DL. Humanized mice for immune system investigation: progress, promise and challenges. *Nat Rev Immunol* (2012) 12:786–98. doi:10.1038/nri3311
125. Unger WW, Pearson T, Abreu JR, Laban S, van der Slik AR, der Kracht SM, et al. Islet-specific CTL cloned from a type 1 diabetes patient cause beta-cell destruction after engraftment into HLA-A2 transgenic NOD/scid/IL2RG null mice. *PLoS One* (2012) 7:e49213. doi:10.1371/journal.pone.0049213

126. Viehmann Milam AA, Maher SE, Gibson JA, Lebastchi J, Wen L, Ruddle NH, et al. A humanized mouse model of autoimmune insulitis. *Diabetes* (2014) 63:1712–24. doi:10.2337/db13-1141
127. Whitfield-Larry F, Young EF, Talmage G, Fudge E, Azam A, Patel S, et al. HLA-A2-matched peripheral blood mononuclear cells from type 1 diabetic patients, but not nondiabetic donors, transfer insulitis to NOD-scid/gammac(null)/HLA-A2 transgenic mice concurrent with the expansion of islet-specific CD8+ T cells. *Diabetes* (2011) 60:1726–33. doi:10.2337/db10-1287
128. Wen L, Ley RE, Volchkov PY, Stranges PB, Avanesyan L, Stonebraker AC, et al. Innate immunity and intestinal microbiota in the development of type 1 diabetes. *Nature* (2008) 455:1109–13. doi:10.1038/nature07336
129. Markle JG, Frank DN, Mortin-Toth S, Robertson CE, Feazel LM, Rolle-Kampczyk U, et al. Sex differences in the gut microbiome drive hormone-dependent regulation of autoimmunity. *Science* (2013) 339:1084–8. doi:10.1126/science.1233521
130. Yurkovetskiy L, Burrows M, Khan AA, Graham L, Volchkov P, Becker L, et al. Gender bias in autoimmunity is influenced by microbiota. *Immunity* (2013) 39:400–12. doi:10.1016/j.immuni.2013.08.013
131. Endesfelder D, zu Castell W, Ardissone A, Davis-Richardson AG, Achenbach P, Hagen M, et al. Compromised gut microbiota networks in children with anti-islet cell autoimmunity. *Diabetes* (2014) 63:2006–14. doi:10.2337/db13-1676
132. Alkanani AK, Hara N, Gottlieb PA, Ir D, Robertson CE, Wagner BD, et al. Alterations in intestinal microbiota correlate with susceptibility to type 1 diabetes. *Diabetes* (2015) 64:3510–20. doi:10.2337/db14-1847
133. Kostic AD, Gevers D, Siljander H, Vatanen T, Hyotylainen T, Hamalainen AM, et al. The dynamics of the human infant gut microbiome in development and in progression toward type 1 diabetes. *Cell Host Microbe* (2015) 17:260–73. doi:10.1016/j.chom.2015.01.001
134. Vatanen T, Kostic AD, d'Hennezel E, Siljander H, Franzosa EA, Yassour M, et al. Variation in microbiome LPS immunogenicity contributes to autoimmunity in humans. *Cell* (2016) 165:842–53. doi:10.1016/j.cell.2016.04.007
135. Hansen CH, Krych L, Nielsen DS, Vogensen FK, Hansen LH, Sorensen SJ, et al. Early life treatment with vancomycin propagates *Akkermansia muciniphila* and reduces diabetes incidence in the NOD mouse. *Diabetologia* (2012) 55:2285–94. doi:10.1007/s00125-012-2564-7
136. Peng J, Narasimhan S, Marchesi JR, Benson A, Wong FS, Wen L. Long term effect of gut microbiota transfer on diabetes development. *J Autoimmun* (2014) 53:85–94. doi:10.1016/j.jaut.2014.03.005
137. Candon S, Perez-Arroyo A, Marquet C, Valette F, Foray AP, Pelletier B, et al. Antibiotics in early life alter the gut microbiome and increase disease incidence in a spontaneous mouse model of autoimmune insulin-dependent diabetes. *PLoS One* (2015) 10:e0125448. doi:10.1371/journal.pone.0125448
138. Hu Y, Peng J, Tai N, Hu C, Zhang X, Wong FS, et al. Maternal antibiotic treatment protects offspring from diabetes development in nonobese diabetic mice by generation of tolerogenic APCs. *J Immunol* (2015) 195:4176–84. doi:10.4049/jimmunol.1500884

9

Overcoming Obstacles in the Development of Antigen-Specific Immunotherapies for Type 1 Diabetes

Ranjeny Thomas [1†], *José M. Carballido* [2†], *Johnna D. Wesley* [3†] *and Simi T. Ahmed* [4*†]

[1] *University of Queensland Diamantina Institute, Princess Alexandra Hospital, Woolloongabba, QLD, Australia,* [2] *Translational Medicine/Preclinical Safety, Novartis Institutes for Biomedical Research, Basel, Switzerland,* [3] *Type 1 Diabetes, Immunology, & Kidney Disease Research, Novo Nordisk Research Center Seattle, Inc., Seattle, WA, United States,* [4] *Strategic Partnerships, The New York Stem Cell Foundation Research Institute, New York, NY, United States*

Correspondence:
Simi T. Ahmed
sahmed@nyscf.org

†These authors have contributed equally to this work

Antigen-specific immunotherapy (ASI) holds great promise for type 1 diabetes (T1D). Preclinical success for this approach has been demonstrated *in vivo*, however, clinical translation is still pending. Reasons explaining the slow progress to approve ASI are complex and span all stages of research and development, in both academic and industry environments. The basic four hurdles comprise a lack of translatability of pre-clinical research to human trials; an absence of robust prognostic and predictive biomarkers for therapeutic outcome; a need for a clear regulatory path addressing ASI modalities; and the limited acceptance to develop therapies intervening at the pre-symptomatic stages of disease. The core theme to address these challenges is collaboration—early, transparent, and engaged interactions between academic labs, pharmaceutical research and clinical development teams, advocacy groups, and regulatory agencies to drive a fundamental shift in how we think and treat T1D.

Keywords: T1D, autoimmunity, immunotherapy, tolerance, precision medicine

INTRODUCTION

Type 1 diabetes (T1D) is an autoimmune disease characterized by T-cell-dependent immune destruction of insulin-producing beta-cells, leading to dysregulated glucose homeostasis. T1D is triggered by complex genetic and environmental factors, progressing from asymptomatic to autoantibody-positive to overt dysglycemia. Since the 1920s, people diagnosed with T1D have had few options beyond exogenous insulin therapy. While the ever-evolving insulin formulations and pump systems can provide automated dosing and monitoring, these only treat a symptom of the disease, not the underlying pathophysiology. This is underscored by the fact that individuals with T1D still have a reduced life expectancy compared to the general population (1) and are not relieved of their disease management.

Non-antigen-specific immunotherapies, including cytokine blockade, inhibition of T-cell co-stimulation, selective immune cell depletion, and induction of polyclonal regulatory T-cells, have targeted features of T1D-related autoimmunity, not the loss of self-tolerance (2). Although these immunotherapies have improved the management of some autoimmune diseases, none have been approved for T1D. We propose that, to achieve a significant clinical impact in T1D, we need antigen-specific immunotherapies (ASI) that work in the pre-dysglycemic stage into the early insulin-requiring period of disease, preventing and reverting overt disease manifestations. In addition, ASI might be beneficial to individuals with long-duration T1D who have residual beta-cell function (3–5). These therapies, possibly in combination with regenerative approaches, could restore glucose homeostasis by reducing the autoinflammatory pressure. ASI include various immunoregulatory formulations of proteins or peptides +/- adjuvants; plasmid-based therapies encoding multiple antigens +/- immune modulators; and antigen-presenting cell-based and engineered antigen-specific T-cell-based therapies [reviewed in (6, 7)] and some peptide, protein, and DNA-based ASI approaches have been tested in T1D [reviewed in (8)]. ASIs require a high safety profile concomitant with exquisite target/organ specificity that does not compromise host responses to pathogens or elevate cancer risks. ASIs have been challenging to develop, there has been limited clinical success, and none are approved for any autoimmune disease. The underlying challenges required to drive success are complex and involve aspects of the translatability of pre-clinical research; the lack of robust prognostic and predictive biomarkers reflecting the heterogeneity of T1D; and the hesitancy to develop treatments to intervene with the disease prior to clinical diabetes onset (**Figure 1**). Nevertheless, ASI hold such potential to transform the treatment and prevention of T1D that we believe we are at a pivotal moment to solve these challenges and progress towards solutions for prevention and cure.

KEY CHALLENGES

Translatability of Pre-Clinical Research

The identification of autoantigens driving T1D-specific B- and T-cell responses is rooted in human data, and further defined and evaluated in pre-clinical models [reviewed by (8, 9)]. However, pre-clinical studies evaluating the prognostic, diagnostic, and therapeutic relevance of T1D-associated autoantigens have often been conducted in the absence of a strong drug development context. As such, there is no consensus on the strategies required to demonstrate the efficacy of ASI. The learnings from animal models are limited; their translatability has been a challenge due to underlying MHC differences and the diversity of autoantigen responses in different models. Additionally, no animal model provides translatable insight into the many complications that occur over time in people with life-long T1D or into the long-term benefits of ASI.

Further, the development path of ASI may differ depending on the age range of the target population due to different requirements in antigens, therapeutic combinations, and administration frequencies. And finally, understanding the similarities and differences in the immune response and treatment of pediatric- versus adult-onset T1D is critical to the long-term success of ASI but challenging to model.

Lack of Robust Prognostic and Predictive Biomarkers Reflecting the Heterogeneity of T1D

Currently, islet autoantibodies are the only prognostic biomarker for T1D. Standard tests measure glutamic acid decarboxylase 65 (GAD), insulin (IAA), protein tyrosine phosphatase islet antigen-2, and zinc transporter 8-specific antibodies. Their appearance predicts that clinical disease is almost certain within one's lifetime; however, they do not predict the timing of an individual's progression to disease (10). Autoantibodies are a hallmark of T1D, regardless of the symptomatic manifestations, yet they are not causal or informative for

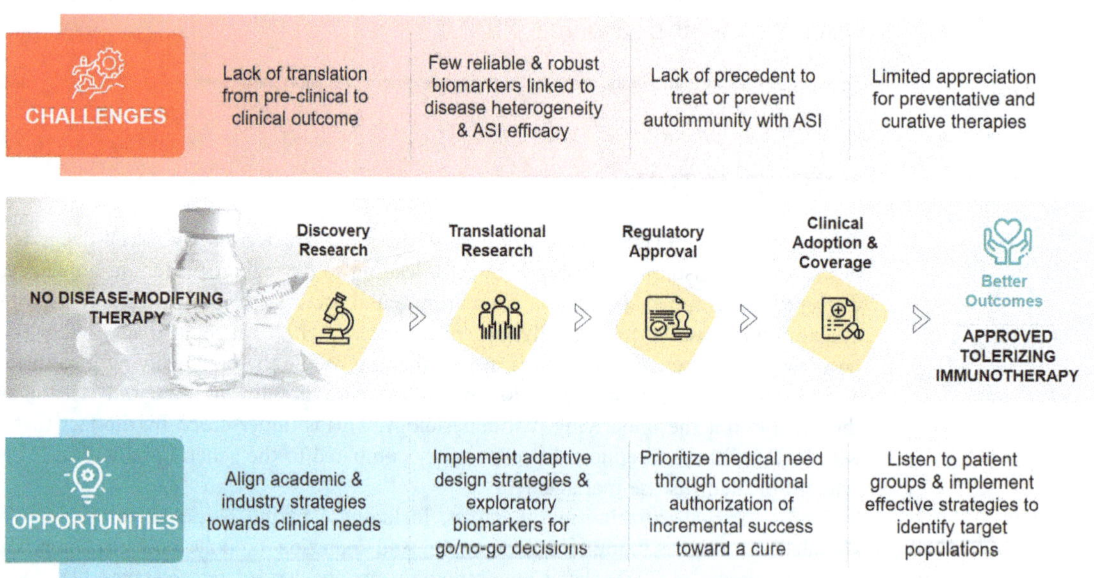

FIGURE 1 | Challenges and opportunities in the development of antigen-specific immunotherapies (ASIs) for T1D.

immediate therapeutic outcome. However, distinct T1D endotypes, driven by HLA-DRB1*03 or HLA-DRB1*04, have recently been associated with the selective appearance of GAD or IAA, respectively as the first detected autoantibody (11). These endotypes may impact the selection of tolerizing antigens and narrow patient selection for trials of peptide-based ASI, as suggested in recent trial reports (12, 13).

Autoantibody formation is preceded by pancreatic antigen-specific T-cell responses (14). However, autoreactive T-cell frequencies are highly variable in people with T1D and are also present in healthy subjects (15, 16). Though technology is rapidly advancing, especially for molecular assessment of T-cell repertoires, autoreactive T-cell-specific biomarkers suitable to predict efficacy of ASIs in T1D remain a significant roadblock. The lack of a biomarker toolkit to evaluate disease initiation and regression further challenges the design of efficient, rapid experimental studies or early clinical trials that could inform larger, phase 2 and 3 clinical trials. Although there are many reasons for this, the lack of access to the pancreas and limited data connecting peripheral immune biomarkers to beta-cell-related autoimmunity are key drivers. This challenge further hinders the identification of appropriate surrogate endpoints for clinical development of ASI in T1D (17). Ideally, predictive biomarkers for ASI should have high prognostic value for a positive clinical response outcome. For example, phenotypic changes in disease-related peripheral T cells or other surrogate markers should anticipate meaningful clinical outcomes such as reduced risk of clinical disease onset, delayed disease progression, partial or full remission, and/or reduced long-term complications (18). Without surrogate biomarkers, prevention trials may be prohibitively long (>10 years) and expensive and require that industry take on a higher risk of failure than is required with more conventional therapies. Moreover, the lack of method harmonization and of sufficient longitudinal samples to evaluate disease progression or treatment efficacy has hindered the development of a robust biomarker strategy to advance ASI for T1D.

Lack of Precedent for Treating Autoimmune Diseases With ASIs

T1D is a disease predominantly affecting children, with a notable pre-clinical asymptomatic period. The availability of life-saving insulin and more recent, novel closed loop delivery systems to treat dysglycemia has diminished the sense of urgency to find a cure or prevention for T1D. To date, no ASI approach has been approved for any autoimmune indication, and T1D is a difficult first indication in which to drive regulatory approval. ASI drug development and early phase trials are in progress in other diseases, including coeliac disease, pemphigus vulgaris, rheumatoid arthritis, and multiple sclerosis (19–21). Although it is tempting to speculate that achievements in these indications will facilitate the adoption of ASI for T1D, ASI approaches may not necessarily extrapolate from one disease to another, because antigens, disease-associated HLA, and disease mechanisms differ. Moreover, the lack of any approved disease-modifying therapy for T1D may add additional delays as there are no examples to follow.

Reluctance to Treat Prior to Overt Diabetes Onset

There are independent, notable challenges for ASIs when discussing and defining the target product profile for T1D —a key document that defines the characteristics of an innovative drug that addresses an unmet need. It seems there is agreement that intervention early in the disease carries the highest chance of success and several trials have been undertaken in people at risk of T1D, prior to overt disease (7). However, it is not broadly accepted that T1D starts earlier than the clinical diagnosis or that preventing further progression is more efficient than trying to reverse overt disease. This is compounded by the poor consensus among drug development teams regarding the desired impact of ASI on disease outcomes. For some, the goal is to permanently cure disease using tolerizing approaches in early disease stages e.g., prior to autoantibody development. For others, the goal is to establish 'functional tolerance' in pre-diagnosis (stage 2) or early onset to prevent further progression. Still others aspire to consolidate or combine ASI-induced immune tolerance with other immune-modulatory or beta-cell-preserving therapeutic strategies to quell fulminant disease. This lack of consensus is a challenge for drug developers, as this may lead to misaligned expectations of what a product might achieve in a clinical trial, with implications for trial design and outcome measures.

KEY OPPORTUNITIES

Improving Translation From Bench to Bedside

To further expand and de-risk findings from pre-clinical animal models, ASIs should be evaluated in physiologically relevant human platforms to provide greater mechanistic insight and to improve clinical translatability. With increasing access to humanized mouse models, compelling mechanism of action may be demonstrable for some ASIs, especially regarding HLA restriction of antigen and responding T cells (22). In such cases, investigational new drug (IND) applications may not need to include a demonstration of efficacy in a disease-relevant pre-clinical model (23). Furthermore, *ex vivo* tissue systems or organoids are becoming catalysts for the translation of ASIs, providing a bridge between pre-clinical and clinical studies. ASI-related researchers should take advantage of these biomimetic models whenever possible to test their therapeutic candidates. Importantly, these systems may allow assessment of drug responsiveness using representative tissue to understand disease heterogeneity. Although the availability of validated 3D systems that recapitulate *in vivo* tissue with accessible lymphatics and vascularization is not yet a reality, it is entirely plausible that the speed of technological progress will create such opportunities in the not-too-distant future.

Key learnings can be provided through small phase 0 and phase 1 clinical trials that include extensive immunologic analyses. These human studies are increasingly common (24), and may help further refine therapeutic tolerance restoration in individuals with autoimmune disease prior to embarking on large trials. However, it is critical that such small studies are clearly presented as hypothesis- or mechanism-generating, with insufficient power to define conclusive mechanism, and not as studies evaluating efficacy, to prevent over-interpretation of study results.

Early partnering between academia and industry and across public-private consortia should become the norm to accelerate preclinical drug development by integrating core academic and industry laboratories to enable generation of strong preclinical data packages. This partnering should help validate findings in multiple orthogonal animal models, allow for confidential vetting of leads, access to GMP-grade compounds for testing, evaluation of *in vivo* mechanisms and antigens in novel *ex vivo* systems, and create public-private project teams to guide development. Such teams would include clinical experts to de-risk therapeutic candidates effectively and early. Further, pharmaceutical companies should increasingly join forces with each other, and with smaller biotech companies, to co-develop ASI programs to share the risk and financial burden during early stages of T1D drug development. These partnerships could significantly lower costs and timelines, enabling all parties to reach go/no-go decisions that allow expansion or completion of partnerships at prespecified junctures. Similarly, central topics for development, such as positions on intellectual property rights, should be discussed and agreed upon early to establish clarity for downstream activities. For real progress to occur with ASI, collaborations during the ideation and development phases of drug development programs will be critical for clinical success.

Identifying and Developing Translational Biomarkers

The need for close collaboration between academic- and industry-based groups extends to the identification and development of ASI-relevant biomarkers. These partnerships should be initiated early in the pre-clinical phase, when ASI candidates and possible predictive biomarkers are being evaluated in animal studies and biomimetic *ex vivo* model systems. With recent technological advances, such as high dimensional mass cytometry, single-cell RNA sequencing, and T-cell receptor profiling, there are increasing numbers of composite measures that hold promise as biomarkers of progression or therapeutic effect [reviewed in (25)]. For example, detailed post-hoc analyses of peripheral immune cell samples from teplizumab and alefacept trials revealed a common "partial exhaustion" transcriptomic signature of antigen-specific $CD8^+$ T-cells (26, 27). Other recent studies have identified T-cell biomarkers associated with favorable prognosis close to T1D onset (28–30). Building on these tangible advancements, promising biomarkers and methods could be optimized for costs and feasibility to be applied in large, multi-center studies and validated for clinical trial use.

Much of the ongoing biomarker identification and development work for T1D has been done by academic consortia, like the Immune Tolerance Network and TrialNet, with access to relevant patient samples and a critical mass of expertise to establish clearer assay standards and procedures. This effort should be further enhanced through expanded, early collaboration involving pharmaceutical and biotechnology company partners. Increased early-stage public-private partnerships will help drive the validation and publication of robust and feasible biomarkers and assays that are subjected to industry-level rigor to refine their context of use, clarify their limitations, and to facilitate their inclusion in clinical trials in a harmonized and standardized fashion. Early successes will then enable testing of larger panels of biomarkers for broader use, such as in patient selection or stratification, that will be critical for future ASI development programs.

Clinical Trial and Approval Path for ASI in T1D

ASI development programs will strongly benefit from early identification of regulatory challenges and development of mitigation strategies. Consultation with clinicians, trial design experts, and statisticians should begin during late preclinical activities, and feedback from regulatory agencies must be solicited as early as possible to understand their requirements (e.g., trial design elements like sample size, outcome measures, primary and secondary endpoints, and safety outputs). These early interactions can also be an opportunity to inform regulatory colleagues on the disruptive potential of ASI to prevent or cure T1D. Importantly, clinical outcomes of ASI that extend beyond delaying onset and preserving functional beta cell mass (e.g., reduced hypoglycemic events, reduction in insulin needs, and acute or long-term complications), as well as other quality-of-life measures for the patient and their caregivers, should be discussed and captured comprehensively during clinical studies and/or in post-marketing efforts. Communication of cohesive, consistent messages from academic and industry stakeholders to regulators on the rationale and strategy guiding ASI development from preclinical to clinical testing, can be a vital catalyst for progress in this field.

Consumers (i.e., people who have or are at risk of T1D, caregivers, and clinicians) should be educated on the potential of ASIs to induce permanent change in the disease processes. A more deliberate inclusion of consumer stakeholders would be a welcome addition to academic and commercial discovery and development teams. This would involve their inclusion in grant applications, in preclinical development teams during IND package generation, within clinical study design discussions, and during evaluation of clinical study results.

Further, implementation of innovative trial designs for ASI can rapidly accelerate progress. This need is underscored by the collective outcomes from traditional disease-modifying monotherapy trials conducted in T1D to date, and by consistent feedback from clinical trial sponsors and investigators.

Moving to Curative and Prevention Therapies

ASI have the potential to provide solutions for multiple stages of T1D. ASI could be highly efficacious in early phases of disease, when there is limited autoimmunity, but ASI may also benefit people with long-term disease, especially those with residual beta-cell function. The ASI-mediated reduction of immune and metabolic stress on the beta cells could be sufficient and/or crucial, especially in combination with regenerative approaches, to restore quiescent beta-cell function. Applying the disease staging concepts of T1D could facilitate the identification of subjects who would benefit from immunotherapies intended to delay onset of or reverse T1D and to create a meaningful population health outcome (31). At-risk subjects have been successfully identified and enrolled in trials through clinical T1D consortia, such as TEDDY, TrialNet, ADDRESS, and INNODIA. Now, there is both a need and opportunity to identify large and diverse cohorts to participate in T1D trials. In fact, two general population screening programs have launched recently, one in a research setting (PLEDGE, https://research.sanfordhealth.org/fields-of-research/diabetes/pledge) and another at a patient community-level (T1Detect, https://www.jdrf.org/t1d-resources/t1detect/). Hopefully, they will pave the way for identifying at-risk subjects appropriate for clinical testing with disease-modifying therapies, including ASI.

ASI intervention should not be considered as a binary success-or-failure option in which accomplishments are compared to "one-and-done" therapies. The induction and maintenance of peripheral tolerance to pancreatic antigens may require regular therapeutic boosting in affected individuals. These could be very well received, provided they are safe, disease-specific, and patient friendly, e.g., they are administered sparsely and/or require non-invasive delivery options. Patient-focused organizations could increase discourse and information exchange amongst diverse stakeholders of the ASI development ecosystem by organizing workshops and interactive series that are designed to incentivize and facilitate drug development efforts. Such interactions could accelerate progress across the entire T1D immunotherapy field.

DISCUSSION

The abundance and speed of research witnessed during 2020 to fight COVID-19 forces us to consider whether comparable efforts could be achieved to effectively eliminate T1D. No specific remedies to fight SARS-CoV-2 infection existed before the December 2019 outbreak in Wuhan. However, the pandemic triggered an unprecedented worldwide effort to develop medicines to stop, treat, and prevent this infection. Immediate approaches aimed at repurposing existing drugs; then newly customized therapies, e.g., neutralizing monoclonal antibodies, proved more successful and, remarkably, SARS-CoV-2-specific vaccines were developed in record time (32). Interestingly, to date, there are >15 different COVID-19 vaccines authorized in different parts of the world including a few innovative options using completely novel technology platforms that could revolutionize vaccine development. The take-home message is that it is possible to develop innovative and efficacious solutions in a very short time.

The therapeutic options for T1D have seen minimal advancement in the past century, and the advances in the field have been restricted to incremental modifications of insulin formulations and delivery methods. Complementary to these treatments, the scientific community has explored a variety of "repurposing" options, mostly based on the use of non-specific immune modulators that have shown limited efficacy in clinical studies to-date (33). As in the case of COVID-19, it is time to understand the huge medical need associated with T1D and to make a concerted effort to develop curative solutions directed at the root cause of the disease: a breach in immune tolerance to pancreatic antigens. ASIs hold such potential and, like the new vaccines developed against SARS-CoV-2 infection, they promise a long-awaited transformative solution for the treatment and prevention of T1D.

AUTHOR CONTRIBUTIONS

RT, JC, JW, and SA all contributed equally to the ideation, writing, and reviewing of the manuscript. All authors contributed to the article and approved the submitted version.

ACKNOWLEDGMENTS

Figure 1 was conceived with inspiration from JDRF's mission statement and the strategic goals of the JDRF Disease-Modifying Therapies project area, which SA helped develop during her tenure at the Foundation.

REFERENCES

1. Huo L, Harding JL, Peeters A, Shaw JE, Magliano DJ. Life Expectancy of Type 1 Diabetic Patients During 1997-2010: a National Australian Registry-Based Cohort Study. *Diabetologia* (2016) 59:1177–85. doi: 10.1007/s00125-015-3857-4
2. Roep BO, Wheeler DCS, Peakman M. Antigen-Based Immune Modulation Therapy for Type 1 Diabetes: the Era of Precision Medicine. *Lancet Diabetes Endocrinol* (2019) 7:65–74. doi: 10.1016/S2213-8587(18)30109-8
3. Roep BO, Thomaidou S, van Tienhoven R, Zaldumbide A. Type 1 Diabetes Mellitus as a Disease of the Beta-Cell (do Not Blame the Immune System)? *Nat Rev Endocrinol* (2021) 17:150–61. doi: 10.1038/s41574-020-00443-4
4. Keenan HA, Sun JK, Levine J, Doria A, Aiello LP, Eisenbarth G, et al. Residual Insulin Production and Pancreatic Ss-Cell Turnover After 50 Years of Diabetes: Joslin Medalist Study. *Diabetes* (2010) 59:2846–53. doi: 10.2337/db10-0676
5. Oram RA, Sims EK, Evans-Molina C. Beta Cells in Type 1 Diabetes: Mass and Function; Sleeping or Dead? *Diabetologia* (2019) 62:567–77. doi: 10.1007/s00125-019-4822-4
6. Carballido JM, Santamaria P. Taming Autoimmunity: Translating Antigen-Specific Approaches to Induce Immune Tolerance. *J Exp Med* (2019) 216:247–50. doi: 10.1084/jem.20182287
7. Serra P, Santamaria P. Antigen-Specific Therapeutic Approaches for Autoimmunity. *Nat Biotechnol* (2019) 37:238–51. doi: 10.1038/s41587-019-0015-4
8. Loaiza Naranjo JD, Bergot AS, Buckle I, Hamilton-Williams EE. A Question of Tolerance-Antigen-Specific Immunotherapy for Type 1 Diabetes. *Curr Diabetes Rep* (2020) 20:70. doi: 10.1007/s11892-020-01363-3
9. Roep BO, Peakman M. Antigen Targets of Type 1 Diabetes Autoimmunity.

Cold Spring Harb Perspect Med (2012) 2:a007781. doi: 10.1101/cshperspect.a007781

10. Ziegler AG, Rewers M, Simell O, Simell T, Lempainen J, Steck A, et al. Seroconversion to Multiple Islet Autoantibodies and Risk of Progression to Diabetes in Children. *JAMA* (2013) 309:2473–9. doi: 10.1001/jama.2013.6285
11. Battaglia M, Ahmed S, Anderson MS, Atkinson MA, Becker D, Bingley PJ, et al. Introducing the Endotype Concept to Address the Challenge of Disease Heterogeneity in Type 1 Diabetes. *Diabetes Care* (2020) 43:5–12. doi: 10.2337/dc19-0880
12. Alhadj Ali M, Liu YF, Arif S, Tatovic D, Shariff H, Gibson VB, et al. Metabolic and Immune Effects of Immunotherapy With Proinsulin Peptide in Human New-Onset Type 1 Diabetes. *Sci Transl Med* (2017) 9:eaaf7779. doi: 10.1126/scitranslmed.aaf7779
13. Ludvigsson J, Sumnik Z, Pelikanova T, Nattero Chavez L, Lundberg E, Rica I, et al. Intralymphatic Glutamic Acid Decarboxylase With Vitamin D Supplementation in Recent-Onset Type 1 Diabetes: a Double-Blind, Randomized, Placebo-Controlled Phase IIb Trial. *Diabetes Care* (2021) 44:1–9. doi: 10.2337/dc21-0318
14. Heninger AK, Eugster A, Kuehn D, Buettner F, Kuhn M, Lindner A, et al. A Divergent Population of Autoantigen-Responsive CD4+ T Cells in Infants Prior to Beta Cell Autoimmunity. *Sci Transl Med* (2017) 9:eaaf8848. doi: 10.1126/scitranslmed.aaf8848
15. Skowera A, Ladell K, McLaren JE, Dolton G, Matthews KK, Gostick E, et al. Beta-Cell-Specific CD8 T Cell Phenotype in Type 1 Diabetes Reflects Chronic Autoantigen Exposure. *Diabetes* (2015) 64:916–25. doi: 10.2337/db14-0332
16. Yeo L, Woodwyk A, Sood S, Lorenc A, Eichmann M, Pujol-Autonell I, et al. Autoreactive T Effector Memory Differentiation Mirrors Beta Cell Function in Type 1 Diabetes. *J Clin Invest* (2018) 128:3460–74. doi: 10.1172/JCI120555
17. Musthaffa Y, Nel HJ, Ramnoruth N, Patel S, Hamilton-Williams EE, Harris M, et al. Optimization of a Method to Detect Autoantigen-Specific T-Cell Responses in Type 1 Diabetes. *Front Immunol* (2020) 11:587469. doi: 10.3389/fimmu.2020.587469
18. Ahmed S, Cerosaletti K, James E, Long SA, Mannering S, Speake C, et al. Standardizing T-Cell Biomarkers in Type 1 Diabetes: Challenges and Recent Advances. *Diabetes* (2019) 68:1366–79. doi: 10.2337/db19-0119
19. Chataway J, Martin K, Barrell K, Sharrack B, Stolt P, Wraith DC, et al. Effects of ATX-MS-1467 Immunotherapy Over 16 Weeks in Relapsing Multiple Sclerosis. *Neurology* (2018) 90:e955–62. doi: 10.1212/WNL.0000000000005118
20. Nel HJ, Malmström V, Wraith DC, Thomas R. Autoantigens in Rheumatoid Arthritis and the Potential for Antigen-Specific Tolerising Immunotherapy. *Lancet Rheumatol* (2020) 2:e712–23. doi: 10.1016/S2665-9913(20)30344-1
21. Kelly CP, Murray JA, Leffler DA, Getts DR, Bledsoe AC, Smithson G, et al. TAK-101 Nanoparticles Induce Gluten-Specific Tolerance in Celiac Disease: a Randomized, Double-Blind, Placebo-Controlled Study. *Gastroenterology* (2021) 161:66–80. doi: 10.1053/j.gastro.2021.03.014
22. Pathiraja V, Kuehlich JP, Campbell PD, Krishnamurthy B, Loudovaris T, Coates PT, et al. Proinsulin-Specific, HLA-DQ8, and HLA-DQ8-Transdimer-Restricted CD4+ T Cells Infiltrate Islets in Type 1 Diabetes. *Diabetes* (2015) 64:172–82. doi: 10.2337/db14-0858
23. Streeter HB, Rigden R, Martin KF, Scolding NJ, Wraith DC. Preclinical Development and First-in-Human Study of ATX-MS-1467 for Immunotherapy of MS. *Neurol Neuroimmunol Neuroinflamm* (2015) 2:e93. doi: 10.1212/NXI.0000000000000093
24. Wagar LE, Salahudeen A, Constantz CM, Wendel BS, Lyons MM, Mallajosyula V, et al. Modeling Human Adaptive Immune Responses With Tonsil Organoids. *Nat Med* (2021) 27:125–35. doi: 10.1038/s41591-020-01145-0
25. Linsley PS, Greenbaum CJ, Nepom GT. Uncovering Pathways to Personalized Therapies in Type 1 Diabetes. *Diabetes* (2021) 70:831–41. doi: 10.2337/db20-1185
26. Diggins KE, Serti E, Muir V, Rosasco M, Lu T, Balmas E, et al. Exhausted-Like CD8+ T Cell Phenotypes Linked to C-Peptide Preservation in Alefacept-Treated T1D Subjects. *JCI Insight* (2021) 6:e142680. doi: 10.1172/jci.insight.142680
27. Long SA, Thorpe J, DeBerg HA, Gersuk V, Eddy J, Harris KM, et al. Partial Exhaustion of CD8 T Cells and Clinical Response to Teplizumab in New-Onset Type 1 Diabetes. *Sci Immunol* (2016) 1:eaai7793. doi: 10.1126/sciimmunol.aai7793
28. Wiedeman AE, Muir VS, Rosasco MG, DeBerg HA, Presnell S, Haas B, et al. Autoreactive CD8+ T Cell Exhaustion Distinguishes Subjects With Slow Type 1 Diabetes Progression. *J Clin Invest* (2020) 130:480–90. doi: 10.1172/JCI126595
29. Narsale A, Lam B, Moya R, Lu T, Mandelli A, Gotuzzo I, et al. CD4+CD25+CD127hi Cell Frequency Predicts Disease Progression in Type 1 Diabetes. *JCI Insight* (2020) 6:e136114. doi: 10.1172/jci.insight.136114
30. Musthaffa Y, Hamilton-Williams EE, Nel HJ, Bergot AS, Mehdi AM, Harris M, et al. Proinsulin-Specific T-Cell Responses Correlate With Estimated c-Peptide and Predict Partial Remission Duration in Type 1 Diabetes. *Clin Trans Immunol* (2021) e1315. doi: 10.1002/cti2.1315
31. Insel RA, Dunne JL, Atkinson MA, Chiang JL, Dabelea D, Gottlieb PA, et al. Staging Presymptomatic Type 1 Diabetes: a Scientific Statement of JDRF, the Endocrine Society, and the American Diabetes Association. *Diabetes Care* (2015) 38:1964–74. doi: 10.2337/dc15-1419
32. Li Y, Tenchov R, Smoot J, Liu C, Watkins S, Zhou Q. A Comprehensive Review of the Global Efforts on COVID-19 Vaccine Development. *ACS Cent Sci* (2021) 7:512–33. doi: 10.1021/acscentsci.1c00120
33. Coppieters K, von Herrath M. The Development of Immunotherapy Strategies for the Treatment of Type 1 Diabetes. *Front Med (Lausanne)* (2018) 5:283. doi: 10.3389/fmed.2018.00283

10

Overlooked Mechanisms in Type 1 Diabetes Etiology: How Unique Costimulatory Molecules Contribute to Diabetogenesis

*David H. Wagner Jr.**

The Program in Integrated Immunology, Department of Medicine, Webb-Waring Center, University of Colorado Anschutz Medical Campus, Aurora, CO, United States

***Correspondence:**
David H. Wagner Jr.
david.wagner@ucdenver.edu

Type 1 Diabetes (T1D) develops when immune cells invade the pancreatic islets resulting in loss of insulin production in beta cells. T cells have been proven to be central players in that process. What is surprising, however, is that classic mechanisms of tolerance cannot explain diabetogenesis; alternate mechanisms must now be considered. T cell receptor (TCR) revision is the process whereby T cells in the periphery alter TCR expression, outside the safety-net of thymic selection pressures. This process results in an expanded T cell repertoire, capable of responding to a universe of pathogens, but limitations are that increased risk for autoimmune disease development occurs. Classic T cell costimulators including the CD28 family have long been thought to be the major drivers for full T cell activation. In actuality, CD28 and its family member counterparts, ICOS and CTLA-4, all drive regulatory responses. Inflammation is driven by CD40, not CD28. CD40 as a costimulus has been largely overlooked. When naïve T cells interact with antigen presenting cell CD154, the major ligand for CD40, is induced. This creates a milieu for T cell (CD40)–T cell (CD154) interaction, leading to inflammation. Finally, defined pathogenic effector cells including TH40 ($CD4^{+}CD40^{+}$) cells can express FOXP3 but are not Tregs. The cells loose FOXP3 to become pathogenic effector cells. Each of these mechanisms creates novel options to better understand diabetogenesis and create new therapeutic targets for T1D.

Keywords: autoimmunity, T cell receptor revision, costimulation, type 1 diabetes, etiology of willful acts

Medical advances in infectious diseases have been extraordinary, completely changing human history. The polio vaccine, small pox vaccine, and measles vaccine among others changed modern medicine. Success with infectious diseases has influenced and created a generalized approach to most medical problems. Unfortunately, using that approach for autoimmune disease has fared much less well. Diseases like type 1 diabetes (T1D) and multiple sclerosis (MS) have seen unpredictable and steady increases in incidence over the last half-century, with only limited treatment options and no cure options on the horizon (1). World-wide incidence of T1D has doubled over the past two decades (2). Examples of how diabetes is expanding can be described in former Soviet-Bloc countries where T1D incidence was virtually unheard of decades ago, but now has increased substantially in all age groups examined. Incidence in adults is now surprisingly high, but the highest increase was seen in children aged 0–4 years (2). Speculation as to why the incidence rate is so drastically expanding focused on the introduction of Western-Style diet, in other words high-fat, high-glucose diets (3). Other parameters, such as genetics, could not account for the increases. Like T1D, MS incidence is increasing (4), as is inflammatory bowel disease (IBD) (5), even the more rare Hashimoto's Thyroiditis is seeing steady incidence increase (6). Another alarming trend is autoimmune comorbidities. Once thought to be unlikely, different autoimmune diseases now are being diagnosed in the same patient; MS and T1D (5); MS and IBD (7); rheumatoid arthritis and T1D (8); psoriasis and T1D (9); and alopecia areata and T1D (10). This is partially due to improved diagnostic techniques, and due to longer survival of patients with autoimmune conditions.

Each autoimmune disease is disparate in symptoms and effect; nonetheless, they share immunologic mechanistic similarities. The integral components of autoimmune disease like infectious disease involve classic immune reactions. During an immunological event, foreign antigens, including viruses, bacteria, funguses, etc., are processed and presented as antigens that lead to T and other cell type activation. This process collectively creates an inflammatory microenvironment. Macrophages or dendritic cells (DCs) at the infection site take up the invading pathogen that then is processed. The pathogen is internalized by engulfment or receptor-mediated uptake, and associates with proteasomes to create antigen fragments. The order of antigenicity is protein $\gg$ DNA/RNA > carbohydrate > lipid. There are very few lipid antigens, although CD1-bearing cells are able to present lipids through the CD1 complex to activate T cells (11). Once generated, the antigen associates with MHC/HLA in the Golgi–endoplasmic reticular compartment. MHC + antigen then is exported and maintained on the cell surface. Professional antigen presenting cells (APCs) include B cells, macrophages, and DC that express the class II version of MHC. $CD4^+$ lymphocytes interact with professional APC to create localized inflammation. $CD8^+$ cells interact with MHC-class I type molecules. Under normal immune conditions, $CD8^+$ cells respond to virally infected cells. In autoimmune conditions including T1D and MS, $CD8^+$ cells can play a role in pathogenesis (12, 13). T cells that carry a specific and unique T cell receptor (TCR) recognize and respond to a specific antigen creating localized inflammation. Under septic conditions, the initial response is pro-inflammatory including activation of TH1 and/or TH17 type cells (14). Under non-septic, autoimmune conditions, the pro-inflammatory phenotype also occurs (15–18). In both scenarios, an appropriately expressed TCR is required, the problem being that in autoimmune diseases T cells arise that recognize and respond to self-antigens. The thymic microenvironment is responsible for generating mature T cells with appropriate TCRs; this means generating T cells that respond to foreign/invader antigens but do not respond to self-antigens. There are, however, medical conditions where self-antigen response is desirable. Transformed cells that result in cancers need to be targeted, and self-antigen reactive T cells perform that function. Maintaining the fine-line homeostatic balance, however, becomes the tricky part.

The interaction of TCR and MHC-Antigen is a crucial aspect of immune function, never more so than during autoimmunity. Autoaggressive T cells have been predicted to slip through the selective pressures of the thymus (19). Alternatively, it has been shown that autoaggressive TCRs can be generated in the periphery through a process termed TCR revision (20–23), thereby subverting central tolerance. It is possible that peripheral negative selection occurs and may be dysfunctional in T1D and other autoimmune diseases. TCR revision contributing to autoimmune disease development has been discussed in a previous review (24). A defining feature to peripherally generated, autoaggressive T cells is expression of CD40 (20, 21, 24–28). Relative to CD40 expression on T cells is what function(s) does it perform? A surprising outcome was the potential role as a costimulus molecule (29–31). Relative to the accepted two-signal model for T cell activation (32, 33), costimulation can play a critical, even decisive, role during autoimmunity.

THE ROLE OF COSTIMULATION AND AUTO-AGGRESSION

The necessity of costimulatory molecules for T cell activation was described in the two-signal model by Bretscher (32). Signal 1 is antigen specific, mediated by TCR interaction with an antigen/MHC complex. Signal 2 is antigen independent, mediated by receptor–ligand interactions that occur between the T cell and APC. The TCR/CD3–MHC/Ag complex with the assistance of adhesion and addressin molecules expressed on each cell type act in a velcro-like manner to adhere the cells together during antigen recognition creating what is known as the immunologic synapse (34). Signaling within the synapse is bidirectional with each cell contributing to the others full activation. Therefore, dysfunction involving either cell could result in pathogenesis. From the T cell perspective, Jenkins and Swartz suggested that TCR-mediated signals alone, without appropriate costimulus, results in a permanent non-responsive condition called anergy (35). While stimulatory signals are sent from T cell to APC within the synapse, the type of costimulation toward the T cell often dictates the immunologic outcome.

IMMUNOGLOBULIN "Ig" COSTIMULUS

One of the first described T cell costimulatory molecules was CD28, which turned out to be a member of a subfamily of proteins that includes ICOS and CTLA-4. This subfamily was categorized as "Immunoglobulin-family costimulus" due to the biochemical structure of the proteins. CD28 is expressed on most naïve, activated, and memory T cells; ICOS and CTLA-4 are expressed on activated T cells and subsets of memory cells (36). CD28 and CTLA-4 interact with CD80 (B71) and CD86 (B72) found primarily on professional APCs. ICOS interacts only with B7H expressed constitutively on naïve B cells but expression extinguishes after antigen engagement and IL-4 cytokine exposure (37). CD40 stimulation of B cells restores B7H expression (37). The fact that ICOS is limited to only B7H stimulation provides possible unique signaling outcomes. CTLA-4, unlike its counterparts, plays a role in cell regulation as opposed to cell activation (36). CTLA-4 is constitutively expressed on Tregs and is inducible on effector cells (38), including potential pathogenic effector cells (39). Study of

CTLA-4-mediated tolerance demonstrated interesting outcomes relative to endogenous and exogenous antigens. Using double transgenic mouse models, a more definitive role for CTLA-4 was determined. Mice genetically manipulated to express an ovalbumin peptide directly on islet beta cells, RIPmOVA mice on a BALB/c background, and exposed to OVA-peptide-specific T cells, DO11.TCR-transgenics, only developed diabetes if the cells originated from $RAG^{-/-}$.DO11.TCR.Tg donor mice and if OVA peptide was injected (40). If donor T cells further included a $CTLA\text{-}4^{-/-}$ background, then disease occurred independently of injected OVA. Because of CTLA-4's role as potential tolerance inducer, it was considered an ideal candidate for therapeutic development. A CTLA-4 analog was developed as a therapeutic in T1D, but has had only limited success (41, 42).

Given the potential prominence of CD28 signaling, considered crucial for T cell activation, it was assumed that CD28 would be a useful target for controlling autoimmunity. The assumption being that induced anergy, as suggested by Jenkins and Swartz, would prove therapeutic. This rationale applied to T1D and other autoimmune diseases. CD28 and B7 knockout mice were created but the results were unanticipated. $CD28^{-/-}$ and $B7^{-/-}$ mice developed extensive autoimmunity (36, 43–48). One study showed that in the experimental autoimmune encephalomyelitis model of MS, $CD28^{-/-}$ mice developed very rapid, more severe disease when challenged with disease causing MOG antigen (46). If, however, the CD40–CD154 signaling pathway was blocked, no disease development occurred (46). $CTLA\text{-}4^{-/-}$ mice likewise experience extensive, systemic autoimmunity (49, 50). Collectively these data suggested that CD28 plays a more prominent role in regulatory T cell development. In fact, CD28 is required for Treg development (43). Rather than CD28 being the "all-purpose" T cell costimulus it was originally thought to be, its part in autoaggressive T cell stimulation comes in to question.

MUCIN COSTIMULUS

Given that the Immunoglobulin family (CD28/ICOS specifically) knockouts still experienced classic T cell responses; the only viable explanation was "other" costimulatory molecules. A series of T cell potential costimulatory molecules was discovered in relation to Asthma that were defined as T-cell-immunoglobulin-domain/mucin-domain (TIM) proteins. The family is comprised of eight members, two of which occur directly on T cells (51). Only TH2 cells express TIM-1 where it plays a pro-regulatory role while TIM-3 preferentially is expressed on TH1, TC1 cells, and DC (52). TIM-3 engagement results in inhibitory signals that lead to apoptosis (52). Polymorphisms within the TIM family were examined in T1D and no positive correlations were discovered (53). The ligand for TIM-3 is galectin-9 (51). NOD mice that were treated with a plasmid encoding galectin-9 were significantly protected from diabetes (54). In another model, galectin-9 treatment induced aggregation and cell death of TH1 cells, selective loss of IFNγ producing cells and suppression of TH1 autoimmunity (55). Treating mice with anti-TIM-3 resulted in increased fatty streak formation and increased atherosclerotic plaque formation in mice (56). The problem with identifying galectin-9 as the ligand for TIM-3 is that galectins are proteins that non-specifically interact with carbohydrates. Galectin-9 for example interacts with β-galactoside sugars on proteins including CD44 (57) and CD40 (58), both of which are associated with pathogenic T cells. In addition, Galectin-9 interaction with CD40 is independent of TIM-3 (58). A study showed that activation of human T cells is not affected by the presence of galectin-9 nor to antibodies to TIM-3 (59). That result is logical given that galectin-9 can bind to any β-galactoside. Given these findings, many of the TIM-3 studies must be reconsidered in relation to autoimmunity. Galectin-9 for example can interact with any β-galoctoside and, therefore, may impact a large number of signaling pathways not just TIM-3.

TNF-RECEPTOR-SUPERFAMILY COSTIMULUS

A perhaps somewhat surprising subgroup of T cell costimulatory molecules involves members of the TNF-receptor-superfamily (TNFRSF). The initial understanding of TNFRSF costimulation was from the perspective of APCs. The early assumption was based on the determination that TNFRSF ligands or TNF-super family members largely are expressed on activated T cells and the receptors, TNF-receptors I and II, and CD40, etc., were first described on APC. TNFα is a pro-inflammatory cytokine produced by TH1 cells and macrophages (60); it occurs both as a secreted cytokine, the major form, and as a cell surface molecule (61). Both the soluble and transmembrane forms of TNFα interact with TNFR I and II (61). CD154, one of the ligands for CD40, is activation induced on T cells where its expression is temporal (18). CD154 also is expressed on APC (62), astrocytes in the CNS (63), and its major source is platelets (64). Like TNFα, CD154 occurs as both a cell surface molecule and a secreted form (65–67). Soluble CD154 is significantly increased in serum of T1D (68), and other autoimmune diseases; it may behave as a highly pro-inflammatory cytokine.

Members of the TNFRSF that act as T cell costimulatory molecules include 4-1BB and OX40. Both OX40 and 4-1BB are activation induced and promote cell survival, potential T cell memory formation, and cytokine production (69–71). In addition to expression on effector T cells, OX40 was detected on $CD25^{+}$, potential Tregs in T1D patients (72). 4-1BB performs similar function on T cells (73, 74). 4-1BB mapped to the *Idd9.3* locus in NOD mouse studies, and reportedly increases IL-2 production and improves CD3 stimulated-activation-outcomes (75–77). These data suggest that OX40 and 4-1BB are more directed toward regulatory outcomes. In that same vein, another TNFRSF member is glucocorticoid-induced-TNF-receptor-protein, GITR known as TNFRSF18. GITR is predominately associated with Tregs (38). Like OX40 and 4-1BB, GITR increases IL-2 production, and improves CD3 activation, developing the MAPK signaling cascade (38, 78). Tregs have been discriminated into innate, those that arise during thymic development (79, 80), and induced, Tregs that are created in the periphery often after exposure to IL-10, GITR expression associates with induced Tregs (38, 79–82).

CD40 (TNSFR5)

Unlike the other TNF-receptor costimulatory molecules on T cells, CD40 acts in a predominant pro-inflammatory manner (18, 27, 31, 58, 83–99). CD40 expression was first described on B cells, and when associated with IL-4, CD40 signals induce antibody class switching. While this action could be involved in autoantibody generation, such function has not been described in T1D or other autoimmune diseases. Like other TNFRSF members, CD40 signals ablate cell death and promote cell survival in B cells, performing similar function in T cells (22, 100). A major problem in understanding the scope of CD40-mediated inflammation has been a gross underestimation of CD40 expression. As studies of CD40 evolved, its expression was identified in numerous cell types. CD40 is expressed on all professional APC, B cells, but also DCs and macrophages. On DCs, it plays a central role in T cell licensing. CD40 engagement on DC switches the DC's interactions with T cells (101). DCs that are high CD40 expressers promote TH1 cell development while CD40-low or CD40-negative DCs favor Treg development (102). CD40 induces iNOS in macrophages (103), thus contributing to the innate immune arm and it induces pro-inflammatory cytokines, including TNFα, IL-1α, IL-1β, and IL-6 (17, 18, 104). CD40 expression has been described on endothelial cells (105); neural cells (106); and surprisingly on islet β cells (107–109). On each of those cell types, CD40 engagement leads to pro-inflammatory cytokine production.

While initially unexpected, CD40 expression occurs on T cells, including $CD4^+$ and $CD8^+$ cells (20–23, 26–28, 31, 39, 58, 100, 110–113). Like OX40 and 4-1BB, CD40 on $CD8^+$ cells is associated with memory cell generation (114). On $CD4^+$ cells, CD40 has been reported on naïve, effector, central, and effector memory cells (29–31), in both murine and human studies. CD40 engagement works independently of CD28 or other costimulatory molecules, inducing predominantly TH1 phenotype cytokines including TNFα and IL-6 (29), as well as GM-CSF and IL-1β (31). CD40 costimulus also induces the TH17 phenotype cytokines IL-17 and IL-21. Interestingly, the TH1 and TH17 cytokines express concomitantly in TH40 cells after CD40 engagement. Because TH40 cells produce both TH1 and TH17 cytokines, post CD40-mediated costimulus these helper cells do not fit the paradigm of either TH1 or TH17 cells, and thus have been termed TH40 cells (20–22, 27, 28, 39, 100, 112, 113).

TH40 CELLS: CD40 SERVES AS A BIOMARKER FOR AUTOAGGRESSIVE T CELLS

When isolated from diabetic or pre-diabetic NOD mice TH40 cells transfer diabetes readily and without any manipulations; thus CD40 constitutes a diabetogenic T cell biomarker (20–22, 26–28, 100). A panel of highly pathogenic, autoaggressive T cell clones, including the well described BDC2.5 and BDC6.9 clones, express CD40 (20, 21, 28). Non-diabetogenic T cell clones including BDC2.4, isolated from the same NOD spleen as BDC2.5 cells, do not express CD40 (28). Primary TH40 cells increase to significantly greater percentages and cell numbers during autoimmunity (20–22, 26, 27, 100). However, like Tregs, some CD40-expressing CD4 cells arise in the thymus (39). In NOD mice that develop spontaneous diabetes, substantial thymic increases in numbers of $CD40^+$ thymocytes were observed (111). Likewise, in a double transgenic, neo-self-antigen model, DO11.RIPmOVA mice, where TCR.Tg T cells that are specific for OVA encounter OVA on thymic medullary epithelial cells, thymic CD40 expressing $CD4^+$ cells were significantly expanded in number (39). The percentage of developing TH40 thymocytes in NOD mice was identical to that of DO11.RIPmOVA mice, suggesting that autoantigen drives the expansion of TH40 cells in the thymus. During T1D, the percentage of TH40 cells expands proportionately with increasing insulitis over time in NOD mice (29). In fact, TH40 cells proved to be diagnostic for T1D. In female NOD mice, 80% develop T1D by 18–22 weeks of age, while only 20–50% of male mice develop disease. Observations reveal that diabetic male NOD had peripheral TH40 cell numbers equivalent to that of diabetic female mice (Wagner Lab observations). Likewise, in NOD female mice that did not develop diabetes, TH40 cell numbers remain at numbers found in non-autoimmune mice. These observations suggest that breach of tolerance involves TH40 cell number expansions.

Primary TH40 cells isolated directly from the pancreatic lymph nodes or spleens of pre-diabetic and diabetic NOD mice transferred progressive insulitis and diabetes to NOD.*scid* recipients (21, 28). $CD40^-$ T cells did not transfer disease, even after removal of Tregs and additional *ex vivo* activation (20–22, 28). T cell CD40 expression is long-lived unlike classic activation molecules, i.e., CD69, CD25, or CD154. Furthermore, classic TCR-mediated activation of naïve $CD40^-$ T cells does not induce CD40 expression. Interestingly, in murine studies, TH40 cells are less susceptible to Treg suppression than non-CD40 expressing T cells (22). TH40 cells are able to express CTLA-4, one of the immunoglobulin family, pro-regulatory molecules. Using the neo-self-antigen model of T1D, TH40 (DO11 TCR^+) cells isolated from diabetic mice did not express CTLA-4, while the vast majority of $CD40^-$ T cells (also DO11 TCR^+) were $CTLA\text{-}4^+$ (39). CTLA-4 is activation induced, requiring TCR engagement (38); therefore CTLA-4 expression may be regulated by CD40-mediated signals as was demonstrated (39). Observations further show that in diabetes prone NOD mice expression of CTLA-4 is deficient (39).

BATTLE OF THE COSTIMULATORY MOLECULES

Clearly, T cells express an array of costimulatory molecules and while each can contribute to activation, the reality is that different costimulators drive the T cell in different directions. CD28, for many years, was considered the central T cell costimulatory molecule. Virtually all *in vitro* T cell stimulation/activation protocols utilized CD28 costimulation. What became a surprise was that CD28 interaction with B71 or B72 drives a more regulatory phenotype leading to production of IL-4, IL-10 and especially IL-2 (**Figure 1**). The role of IL-2 will be discussed further below. One reason that $CD28^-$ only costimulation became universally

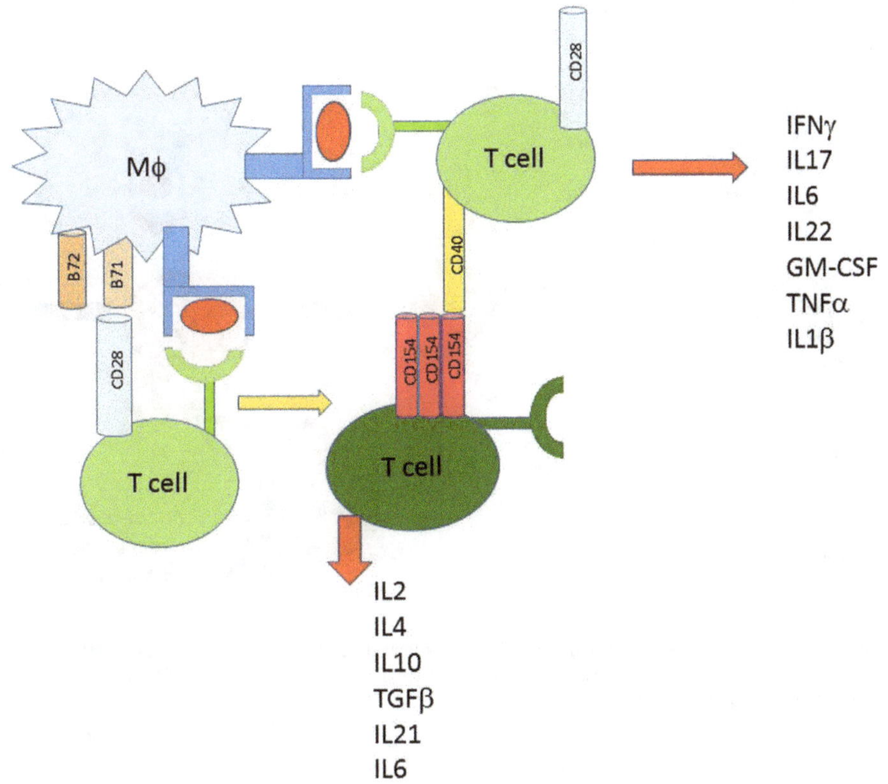

FIGURE 1 | T cell activation alternative methods. Classic 2 signal activation involves T cell interaction with antigen presenting cell. Signal one is antigen dependent and delivered to the T cell receptor by MHC/HLA and antigen. The costimulus can include CD28 interacting with B71 or B72; that outcome creates activation leading to cytokine production. When a source of CD154 is available, including from the newly activated T cells, other T cells receive a different second signal costimulus to produce inflammatory type cytokines. CD28 signals favor more regulatory type cytokines.

accepted as pro-inflammatory is that the coincident response of CD40–CD154 interaction was overlooked. When CD40 is engaged on T cells, independently of CD28 (29–31, 110) or in combination with CD28 (30, 31, 110), a TH1/TH17 pro-inflammatory phenotype results (**Figure 1**). When T cell activation occurs, signals through the synapse lead to induction of CD154 expression (115). Therefore, in the microenvironment a source for CD40–CD154 interaction in addition to CD28, costimulation is developed. In T1D compared to controls, CD40-bearing T cells, TH40 cells in particular, are over represented (20–22, 24, 27–29, 31, 39, 90, 100, 110–112, 116). The overlooked issue is T cell–T cell interactions (**Figure 1**). An activated T cell is an abundant source of CD154 and can, therefore, interact with CD40 on APC, within the immune synapse; but it also can interact with CD40 on TH40 cells. That interaction leads to inflammatory cytokine production (23, 29–31, 39, 58, 110–112), as represented in **Figure 1**. Importantly, the CD40 signal can override the CD28-mediated signal (29, 30), to drive inflammation.

THE UNINTENTIONALLY MISUNDERSTOOD ROLE OF IL-2

IL-2 discovery began from an accidental, but important happenstance involving the kidney bean extract, phytohemagglutinin (PHA). When cells in culture were treated with the extract, there was lymphocyte cellular expansion (117). The expansion was temporary, however. Over time, the substances induced by PHA that caused leukocytes to proliferate were identified as interleukins and the interleukin associated with T cell expansion specifically became known as IL-2. After this discovery, the addition of IL-2 to all T cell cultures was considered essential. To better understand T cells and IL-2 responses specifically promoting autoimmunity, IL-2 knockout mice were generated. The *a priori* hypothesis was that autoimmune disease would be completely negated, since theoretically IL-2 would be the cornerstone T cell survival cytokine. Surprisingly, IL-2$^{-/-}$ mice demonstrated that IL-2 was not the crucial cytokine for T cell development that it was thought to be (118, 119). Effector T cells develop normally in the thymus in the absence of IL-2 (120) and in fact, autoimmunity is abundant and spontaneous in those mice (121). IL-2 is, however, required for Treg development and homeostasis (120). Further study demonstrates that IL-2 promotes Treg development but does not promote pathogenic effector cell development (120). This observation creates unique problems for the vast array of T cell *in vitro* experiments where IL-2 has been added as the T cell costimulus for pathogenic effector cells. Those studies require re-visiting given that IL-2 promotes regulation.

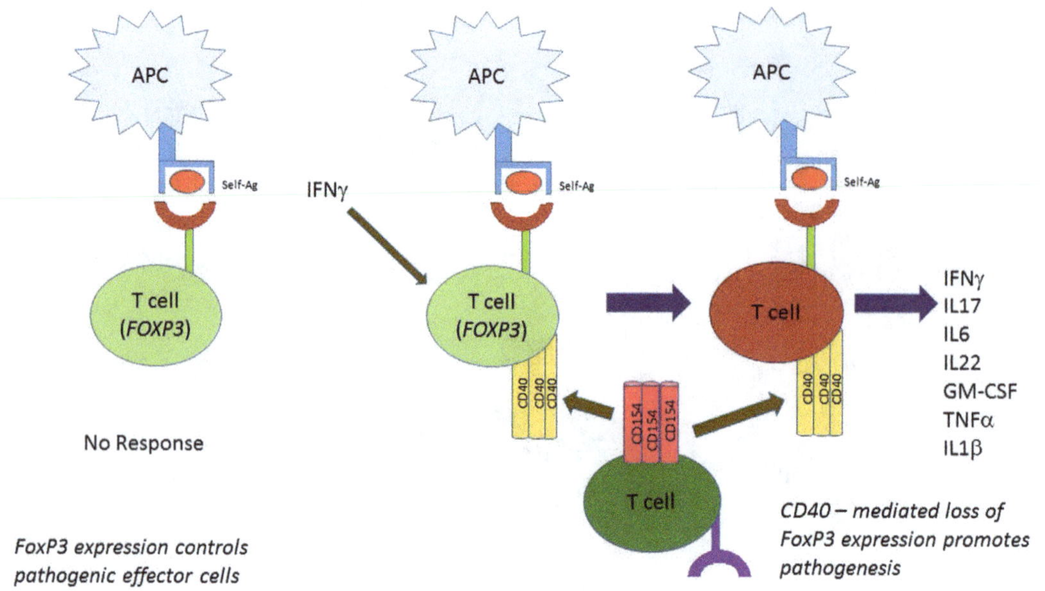

FIGURE 2 | FOXP3 as a static T cell regulator independent of Treg status. Cells other than classic Tregs express FOXP3. In the BDC2.5 T cell receptor transgenic mouse model effector, T cells express FOXP3 but in the inflammatory environment where IFNγ, etc., is produced, CD40 is induced on those cells. CD40 interaction with CD154 leads to loss of FOXP3 expression and full effector status.

ALTERNATE MECHANISMS FOR EFFECTOR T CELL REGULATION: TH40 CELLS EXPRESSING FOXP3

The BDC2.5 T cell clone rapidly and efficiently transfers diabetes to NOD.scid recipient mice (20, 28, 122). When the TCR transgenic (TCR.Tg) version of BDC2.5 was created, only about 22% of mice became diabetic in the time frame considered (123). This outcome was surprising, given the strong diabetogenicity of the BDC2.5 clone. Longitudinal studies revealed a different outcome, however. If BDC2.5.TCR transgenic mice were followed for 45 weeks, disease incidence achieved 100% (111). That finding suggests that eventual breach of tolerance occurs. TH40 cells expand rapidly in the BDC2.5.TCR.Tg mouse model, but disease kinetics are much slower than in classic NOD mice (111). The unexpected finding was that TH40 cells at younger ages contained high levels of FOXP3 (111). In this circumstance TH40 cells were not Tregs; the BDC2.5.TCR.Tg mice maintained classically defined Tregs, $CD4^{+}CD25^{hi}FOXP3^{+}$. Tregs but not TH40-$FOXP3^{+}$ cells performed regulatory functions (111). The disease defining parameter was loss of FOXP3 in TH40 cells. TH40 cells isolated from young animals had high FOXP3 levels and could not transfer diabetes; TH40 cells that rapidly and efficiently transferred diabetes were FOXP3 negative regardless of the age of the donor (111). Not only were TH40 cells disease instrumental, but CD40 itself proved to be a disease master switch. BDC2.5.TCR.Tg mice bred onto the CD40 knockout background did not develop diabetes at any age (111) and equally impressive, those mice did not exhibit insulitis (29). In addition, BDC2.5 T cells isolated from the CD40 KO mice maintained high levels of FOXP3 even after 45 weeks. These findings indicate that when CD40 levels are sufficiently controlled, effector cells are able to express FOXP3. Furthermore, that expression is independent of Treg status. If systemic CD40 levels and CD154 levels are substantially elevated, just as occurs in T1D, then effector cells loose FOXP3 to become pathogenic effector cells (**Figure 2**).

CONCLUSION

Failure of central tolerance cannot be excluded as an autoimmune mechanism. Numerous studies demonstrate that negative selection failure gives rise to peripheral pathogenic T cells. However, the overlooked mechanism of TCR revision also must be considered. This process that increases overall T cell repertoire to pathogens likewise increases risk for autoimmunity. If appropriate selective pressures are not applied in the periphery following TCR revision, then autoaggressive T cells necessarily will arise. For autoimmune disease to commence, additional criteria must be met, including perhaps HLA haplotype, CTLA-4, FOXP3 or other mechanisms of tolerance failure, etc. Within these bounds the role of costimulation is becoming evident as contributory for autoimmunity. The classic CD28 family has been thought essential for driving T cell expansions, but overlooked costimulation, CD40 in particular, is emerging as diabetogenic. TH40 cells become prominent in the NOD mouse model of T1D as well as in human T1D (20, 21, 26, 27). These cells have clearly proven to be important disease drivers. Of significance is that the CD40 molecule itself acts as a highly pro-inflammatory stimulator (29, 30). When T cell CD40 is directly engaged, T cells produce TH1 and TH2 cytokines; but when CD28 is engaged, T cells produce TH2/Treg cytokines (29, 30). Another concern is that classic tolerance mechanisms driven by Tregs or by tolerance inducing molecules, CTLA-4 and FoxP3 for example, work much less efficiently on TH40 cells derived from autoimmune backgrounds (39, 111). These findings include tolerance dysfunction in human T1D (26, 27). Full understanding of disease mechanisms leading to breach of tolerance in T1D and other autoimmune diseases is a complicated process. No one mechanism alone is causative. Nonetheless a clearer picture of those processes involving TCR development and T cell costimulation is beginning to emerge.

AUTHOR CONTRIBUTIONS

DW conceived and wrote the manuscript.

REFERENCES

1. Lerner A, Jeremias P, Matthias T. The world incidence and prevalence of autoimmune diseases is increasing. *Int J Celiac Dis* (2015) 3(4):151–5. doi:10.12691/ijcd-3-4-8
2. Battaglia M, Nigi L, Dotta F. Towards an earlier and timely diagnosis of type 1 diabetes: is it time to change criteria to define disease onset? *Curr Diab Rep* (2015) 15(12):115. doi:10.1007/s11892-015-0690-6
3. Chobot A, Polanska J, Brandt A, Deja G, Glowinska-Olszewska B, Pilecki O, et al. Updated 24-year trend of Type 1 diabetes incidence in children in Poland reveals a sinusoidal pattern and sustained increase. *Diabet Med* (2017). doi:10.1111/dme.13345
4. Marrie RA, Reider N, Cohen J, Stuve O, Trojano M, Cutter G, et al. A systematic review of the incidence and prevalence of cardiac, cerebrovascular, and peripheral vascular disease in multiple sclerosis. *Mult Scler* (2015) 21(3):318–31. doi:10.1177/1352458514564485
5. Tozzoli R, Sorrentino MC, Bizzaro N. Detecting multiple autoantibodies to diagnose autoimmune co-morbidity (multiple autoimmune syndromes and overlap syndromes): a challenge for the autoimmunologist. *Immunol Res* (2013) 56(2–3):425–31. doi:10.1007/s12026-013-8418-7
6. Pyzik A, Grywalska E, Matyjaszek-Matuszek B, Rolinski J. Immune disorders in Hashimoto's thyroiditis: what do we know so far? *J Immunol Res* (2015) 2015:979167. doi:10.1155/2015/979167
7. Kosmidou M, Katsanos AH, Katsanos KH, Kyritsis AP, Tsivgoulis G, Christodoulou D, et al. Multiple sclerosis and inflammatory bowel diseases: a systematic review and meta-analysis. *J Neurol* (2017) 264(2):254–9. doi:10.1007/s00415-016-8340-8
8. Grant WB. Epidemiology of disease risks in relation to vitamin D insufficiency. *Prog Biophys Mol Biol* (2006) 92(1):65–79. doi:10.1016/j.pbiomolbio.2006.02.013
9. Takeshita J, Grewal S, Langan SM, Mehta NN, Ogdie A, Van Voorhees AS, et al. Psoriasis and comorbid diseases: implications for management. *J Am Acad Dermatol* (2017) 76(3):393–403. doi:10.1016/j.jaad.2016.07.065
10. Huang KP, Mullangi S, Guo Y, Qureshi AA. Autoimmune, atopic, and mental health comorbid conditions associated with alopecia areata in the United States. *JAMA Dermatol* (2013) 149(7):789–94. doi:10.1001/jamadermatol.2013.3049
11. Zhang HL, Wu J, Zhu J. The immune-modulatory role of apolipoprotein E with emphasis on multiple sclerosis and experimental autoimmune encephalomyelitis. *Clin Dev Immunol* (2010) 2010:186813. doi:10.1155/2010/186813
12. Chen W, Bluestone JA, Herold KC. Achieving antigen-specific tolerance in diabetes: regulating specifically. *Int Rev Immunol* (2005) 24(5–6):287–305. doi:10.1080/08830180500379671
13. Wong FS, Dittel BN, Janeway CA Jr. Transgenes and knockout mutations in animal models of type 1 diabetes and multiple sclerosis. *Immunol Rev* (1999) 169:93–104. doi:10.1111/j.1600-065X.1999.tb01309.x
14. Lucey DR, Clerici M, Shearer GM. Type 1 and type 2 cytokine dysregulation in human infectious, neoplastic, and inflammatory diseases. *Clin Microbiol Rev* (1996) 9(4):532–62.
15. Stout RD, Watkins SK, Suttles J. Functional plasticity of macrophages: in situ reprogramming of tumor-associated macrophages. *J Leukoc Biol* (2009) 86(5):1105–9. doi:10.1189/jlb.0209073
16. Suttles J, Stout RD. Macrophage CD40 signaling: a pivotal regulator of disease protection and pathogenesis. *Semin Immunol* (2009) 21(5):257–64. doi:10.1016/j.smim.2009.05.011
17. Poe J, Wagner DH Jr, Miller RW, Stout RD, Suttles J. IL-4 and IL-10 modulation of CD40-mediated signaling of monocyte IL-1beta synthesis and rescue from apoptosis. *J Immunol* (1997) 159(2):846–52.
18. Wagner DH Jr, Stout RD, Suttles J. Role of the CD40-CD40 ligand interaction in CD4+ T cell contact-dependent activation of monocyte interleukin-1 synthesis. *Eur J Immunol* (1994) 24(12):3148–54. doi:10.1002/eji.1830241235
19. Kreuwel HT, Sherman LA. Defects in deletional tolerance of CD8+ T cells in autoimmune diabetes. *Curr Dir Autoimmun* (2001) 4:123–43. doi:10.1159/000060533
20. Vaitaitis GM, Poulin M, Sanderson RJ, Haskins K, Wagner DH Jr. Cutting edge: CD40-induced expression of recombination activating gene (RAG) 1 and RAG2: a mechanism for the generation of autoaggressive T cells in the periphery. *J Immunol* (2003) 170(7):3455–9. doi:10.4049/jimmunol.170.7.3455
21. Waid DM, Vaitaitis GM, Wagner DH Jr. Peripheral expansion of $CD4^{lo}CD40^{+}$ auto-aggressive T cells during insulin-dependent diabetes mellitus. *Eur J Immunol* (2004) 34(5):1488–97. doi:10.1002/eji.200324703
22. Waid DM, Vaitaitis GM, Pennock ND, Wagner DH Jr. Disruption of the homeostatic balance between autoaggressive (CD4+CD40+) and regulatory (CD4+CD25+FoxP3+) T cells promotes diabetes. *J Leukoc Biol* (2008) 84(2):431–9. doi:10.1189/jlb.1207857
23. Vaitaitis GM, Wagner DH Jr. CD40 interacts directly with RAG1 and RAG2 in autoaggressive T cells and Fas prevents CD40-induced RAG expression. *Cell Mol Immunol* (2013) 10(6):483–9. doi:10.1038/cmi.2013.24
24. Wagner DH. Of the multiple mechanisms leading to type 1 diabetes, T cell receptor revision may play a prominent role (is type 1 diabetes more than a single disease?). *Clin Exp Immunol* (2016) 185(3):271–80. doi:10.1111/cei.12819
25. Wagner DH Jr. Re-shaping the T cell repertoire: TCR editing and TCR revision for good and for bad. *Clin Immunol* (2007) 123(1):1–6. doi:10.1016/j.clim.2006.08.006
26. Siebert JC, Inokuma M, Waid DM, Pennock ND, Vaitaitis GM, Disis ML, et al. An analytical workflow for investigating cytokine profiles. *Cytometry A* (2008) 73(4):289–98. doi:10.1002/cyto.a.20509
27. Waid DM, Wagner RJ, Putnam A, Vaitaitis GM, Pennock ND, Calverley DC, et al. A unique T cell subset described as CD4loCD40+ T cells (TCD40) in human type 1 diabetes. *Clin Immunol* (2007) 124(2):138–48. doi:10.1016/j.clim.2007.05.003
28. Wagner DH Jr, Vaitaitis G, Sanderson R, Poulin M, Dobbs C, Haskins K. Expression of CD40 identifies a unique pathogenic T cell population in type 1 diabetes. *Proc Natl Acad Sci U S A* (2002) 99(6):3782–7. doi:10.1073/pnas.052247099
29. Vaitaitis GM, Yussman MG, Waid DM, Wagner DH. CD40-mediated signaling influences trafficking, TCR expression and T cell pathogenesis in the NOD model of type 1 diabetes. *Immunology* (2017). doi:10.1111/imm.12761
30. Vaitaitis GM, Yussman MG, Waid DM, Wagner DH. Th40 cells (CD4+CD40+ Tcells) drive a more severe form of experimental autoimmune encephalomyelitis than conventional CD4 T cells. *PLoS One* (2017) 12(2):e0172037. doi:10.1371/journal.pone.0172037

31. Waid DM, Schreiner T, Vaitaitis G, Carter JR, Corboy JR, Wagner DH Jr. Defining a new biomarker for the autoimmune component of Multiple Sclerosis: Th40 cells. *J Neuroimmunol* (2014) 270(1–2):75–85. doi:10.1016/j.jneuroim.2014.03.009
32. Bretscher P. A two-step, two-signal model for the primary activation of precursor helper T cells. *Proc Natl Acad Sci U S A* (1999) 96:185–90. doi:10.1073/pnas.96.1.185
33. Bretscher P. The two-signal model of lymphocyte activation twenty-one years later. *Immunol Today* (1992) 13:74–6. doi:10.1016/0167-5699(92)90138-W
34. Yokosuka T, Saito T. Dynamic regulation of T-cell costimulation through TCR-CD28 microclusters. *Immunol Rev* (2009) 229(1):27–40. doi:10.1111/j.1600-065X.2009.00779.x
35. Jenkins MK, Mueller D, Schwartz RH, Carding S, Bottomley K, Stadecker MJ, et al. Induction and maintenance of anergy in mature T cells. *Adv Exp Med Biol* (1991) 292:167–76. doi:10.1007/978-1-4684-5943-2_19
36. Rudd CE, Schneider H. Unifying concepts in CD28, ICOS and CTLA4 coreceptor signalling. *Nat Rev Immunol* (2003) 3(7):544–56. doi:10.1038/nri1131
37. Liang L, Porter EM, Sha WC. Constitutive expression of the B7h ligand for inducible costimulator on naive B cells is extinguished after activation by distinct B cell receptor and interleukin 4 receptor-mediated pathways and can be rescued by CD40 signaling. *J Exp Med* (2002) 196(1):97–108. doi:10.1084/jem.20020298
38. Corthay A. How do regulatory T cells work? *Scand J Immunol* (2009) 70(4):326–36. doi:10.1111/j.1365-3083.2009.02308.x
39. Carter J, Vaitaitis GM, Waid DM, Wagner DH Jr. CD40 engagement of CD4+ CD40+ T cells in a neo-self antigen disease model ablates CTLA-4 expression and indirectly impacts tolerance. *Eur J Immunol* (2012) 42(2):424–35. doi:10.1002/eji.201141880
40. Eggena MP, Walker LS, Nagabhushanam V, Barron L, Chodos A, Abbas AK. Cooperative roles of CTLA-4 and regulatory T cells in tolerance to an islet cell antigen. *J Exp Med* (2004) 199(12):1725–30. doi:10.1084/jem.20040124
41. Alegre ML, Fallarino F. Mechanisms of CTLA-4-Ig in tolerance induction. *Curr Pharm Des* (2006) 12(2):149–60. doi:10.2174/138161206775193046
42. Garyu JW, Meffre E, Cotsapas C, Herold KC. Progress and challenges for treating type 1 diabetes. *J Autoimmun* (2016) 71:1–9. doi:10.1016/j.jaut.2016.04.004
43. Bour-Jordan H, Bluestone JA. Regulating the regulators: costimulatory signals control the homeostasis and function of regulatory T cells. *Immunol Rev* (2009) 229(1):41–66. doi:10.1111/j.1600-065X.2009.00775.x
44. Chitnis T, Najafian N, Abdallah KA, Dong V, Yagita H, Sayegh MH, et al. CD28-independent induction of experimental autoimmune encephalomyelitis. *J Clin Invest* (2001) 107(5):575–83. doi:10.1172/JCI11220
45. Oliveira-dos-Santos AJ, Ho A, Tada Y, Lafaille JJ, Tonegawa S, Mak TW, et al. CD28 costimulation is crucial for the development of spontaneous autoimmune encephalomyelitis. *J Immunol* (1999) 162(8):4490–5.
46. Girvin AM, Dal Canto MC, Miller SD. CD40/CD40L interaction is essential for the induction of EAE in the absence of CD28-mediated co-stimulation. *J Autoimmun* (2002) 18(2):83–94. doi:10.1006/jaut.2001.0573
47. Girvin AM, Dal Canto MC, Rhee L, Salomon B, Sharpe A, Bluestone JA, et al. A critical role for B7/CD28 costimulation in experimental autoimmune encephalomyelitis: a comparative study using costimulatory molecule-deficient mice and monoclonal antibody blockade. *J Immunol* (2000) 164(1):136–43. doi:10.4049/jimmunol.164.1.136
48. Salomon B, Rhee L, Bour-Jordan H, Hsin H, Montag A, Soliven B, et al. Development of spontaneous autoimmune peripheral polyneuropathy in B7-2-deficient NOD mice. *J Exp Med* (2001) 194(5):677–84. doi:10.1084/jem.194.5.677
49. Chikuma S, Bluestone JA. CTLA-4 and tolerance: the biochemical point of view. *Immunol Res* (2003) 28(3):241–53. doi:10.1385/IR:28:3:241
50. van Parijs L, Perez VL, Abbas AK. Mechanisms of peripheral T cell tolerance. *Novartis Found Symp* (1998) 215:5–14.
51. Rodriguez-Manzanet R, DeKruyff R, Kuchroo VK, Umetsu DT. The costimulatory role of TIM molecules. *Immunol Rev* (2009) 229(1):259–70. doi:10.1111/j.1600-065X.2009.00772.x
52. Freeman GJ, Casasnovas JM, Umetsu DT, DeKruyff RH. TIM genes: a family of cell surface phosphatidylserine receptors that regulate innate and adaptive immunity. *Immunol Rev* (2010) 235(1):172–89. doi:10.1111/j.0105-2896.2010.00903.x
53. Bruck P, Ramos-Lopez E, Bartsch W, Bohme A, Badenhoop K. TIM-3 polymorphisms in type 1 diabetes families. *J Hum Genet* (2008) 53(6):559–64. doi:10.1007/s10038-008-0286-y
54. Chou FC, Shieh SJ, Sytwu HK. Attenuation of Th1 response through galectin-9 and T-cell Ig mucin 3 interaction inhibits autoimmune diabetes in NOD mice. *Eur J Immunol* (2009) 39(9):2403–11. doi:10.1002/eji.200839177
55. Zhu C, Anderson AC, Schubart A, Xiong H, Imitola J, Khoury SJ, et al. The Tim-3 ligand galectin-9 negatively regulates T helper type 1 immunity. *Nat Immunol* (2005) 6(12):1245–52. doi:10.1038/ni1271
56. Foks AC, Ran IA, Wasserman L, Frodermann V, Ter Borg MN, de Jager SC, et al. T-cell immunoglobulin and mucin domain 3 acts as a negative regulator of atherosclerosis. *Arterioscler Thromb Vasc Biol* (2013) 33(11):2558–65. doi:10.1161/ATVBAHA.113.301879
57. Wu C, Thalhamer T, Franca RF, Xiao S, Wang C, Hotta C, et al. Galectin-9-CD44 interaction enhances stability and function of adaptive regulatory T cells. *Immunity* (2014) 41(2):270–82. doi:10.1016/j.immuni.2014.06.011
58. Vaitaitis GM, Wagner DH Jr. Galectin-9 controls CD40 signaling through a Tim-3 independent mechanism and redirects the cytokine profile of pathogenic T cells in autoimmunity. *PLoS One* (2012) 7(6):e38708. doi:10.1371/journal.pone.0038708
59. Leitner J, Rieger A, Pickl WF, Zlabinger G, Grabmeier-Pfistershammer K, Steinberger P. TIM-3 does not act as a receptor for galectin-9. *PLoS Pathog* (2013) 9(3):e1003253. doi:10.1371/journal.ppat.1003253
60. Mountz JD, Zhou T, Su X, Cheng J, Pierson M, Bluethmann H, et al. Autoimmune disease results from multiple interactive defects in apoptosis induction molecules and signaling pathways. *Behring Inst Mitt* (1996) 97:200–19.
61. Horiuchi T, Mitoma H, Harashima S, Tsukamoto H, Shimoda T. Transmembrane TNF-alpha: structure, function and interaction with anti-TNF agents. *Rheumatology (Oxford)* (2010) 49(7):1215–28. doi:10.1093/rheumatology/keq031
62. Munroe ME. Functional roles for T cell CD40 in infection and autoimmune disease: the role of CD40 in lymphocyte homeostasis. *Semin Immunol* (2009) 21(5):283–8. doi:10.1016/j.smim.2009.05.008
63. Chen K, Huang J, Gong W, Zhang L, Yu P, Wang JM. CD40/CD40L dyad in the inflammatory and immune responses in the central nervous system. *Cell Mol Immunol* (2006) 3(3):163–9.
64. Xu H, Zhang X, Mannon RB, Kirk AD. Platelet-derived or soluble CD154 induces vascularized allograft rejection independent of cell-bound CD154. *J Clin Invest* (2006) 116(3):769–74. doi:10.1172/JCI27155
65. Prahalad S, Martins TB, Tebo AE, Whiting A, Clifford B, Zeft AS, et al. Elevated serum levels of soluble CD154 in children with juvenile idiopathic arthritis. *Pediatr Rheumatol Online J* (2008) 6:8. doi:10.1186/1546-0096-6-8
66. Russo S, Bussolati B, Deambrosis I, Mariano F, Camussi G. Platelet-activating factor mediates CD40-dependent angiogenesis and endothelial-smooth muscle cell interaction. *J Immunol* (2003) 171(10):5489–97. doi:10.4049/jimmunol.171.10.5489
67. Stumpf C, Lehner C, Eskafi S, Raaz D, Yilmaz A, Ropers S, et al. Enhanced levels of CD154 (CD40 ligand) on platelets in patients with chronic heart failure. *Eur J Heart Fail* (2003) 5(5):629–37. doi:10.1016/S1388-9842(03)00110-7
68. Jinchuan Y, Zonggui W, Jinming C, Li L, Xiantao K. Upregulation of CD40-CD40 ligand system in patients with diabetes mellitus. *Clin Chim Acta* (2004) 339(1–2):85–90. doi:10.1016/j.cccn.2003.09.007
69. Gotsman I, Sharpe AH, Lichtman AH. T-cell costimulation and coinhibition in atherosclerosis. *Circ Res* (2008) 103(11):1220–31. doi:10.1161/CIRCRESAHA.108.182428
70. Inman BA, Frigola X, Dong H, Kwon ED. Costimulation, coinhibition and cancer. *Curr Cancer Drug Targets* (2007) 7(1):15–30. doi:10.2174/156800907780006878
71. Stuart RW, Racke MK. Targeting T cell costimulation in autoimmune disease. *Expert Opin Ther Targets* (2002) 6(3):275–89. doi:10.1517/14728222.6.3.275
72. Williams CA, Murray SE, Weinberg AD, Parker DC. OX40-mediated differentiation to effector function requires IL-2 receptor signaling but not CD28, CD40, IL-12Rbeta2, or T-bet. *J Immunol* (2007) 178(12):7694–702. doi:10.4049/jimmunol.178.12.7694

73. Cannons JL, Lau P, Ghumman B, DeBenedette MA, Yagita H, Okumura K, et al. 4-1BB ligand induces cell division, sustains survival, and enhances effector function of CD4 and CD8 T cells with similar efficacy. *J Immunol* (2001) 167(3):1313–24. doi:10.4049/jimmunol.167.3.1313
74. DeBenedette MA, Wen T, Bachmann MF, Ohashi PS, Barber BH, Stocking KL, et al. Analysis of 4-1BB ligand (4-1BBL)-deficient mice and of mice lacking both 4-1BBL and CD28 reveals a role for 4-1BBL in skin allograft rejection and in the cytotoxic T cell response to influenza virus. *J Immunol* (1999) 163(9):4833–41.
75. Cannons JL, Chamberlain G, Howson J, Smink LJ, Todd JA, Peterson LB, et al. Genetic and functional association of the immune signaling molecule 4-1BB (CD137/TNFRSF9) with type 1 diabetes. *J Autoimmun* (2005) 25(1):13–20. doi:10.1016/j.jaut.2005.04.007
76. Kachapati K, Bednar KJ, Adams DE, Wu Y, Mittler RS, Jordan MB, et al. Recombinant soluble CD137 prevents type one diabetes in nonobese diabetic mice. *J Autoimmun* (2013) 47:94–103. doi:10.1016/j.jaut.2013.09.002
77. Maier LM, Smyth DJ, Vella A, Payne F, Cooper JD, Pask R, et al. Construction and analysis of tag single nucleotide polymorphism maps for six human-mouse orthologous candidate genes in type 1 diabetes. *BMC Genet* (2005) 6:9. doi:10.1186/1471-2156-6-9
78. Esparza EM, Arch RH. Signaling triggered by glucocorticoid-induced tumor necrosis factor receptor family-related gene: regulation at the interface between regulatory T cells and immune effector cells. *Front Biosci* (2006) 11:1448–65. doi:10.2741/1895
79. Peters N, Sacks D. Immune privilege in sites of chronic infection: *Leishmania* and regulatory T cells. *Immunol Rev* (2006) 213:159–79. doi:10.1111/j.1600-065X.2006.00432.x
80. Romani L. Cell mediated immunity to fungi: a reassessment. *Med Mycol* (2008) 46(6):515–29. doi:10.1080/13693780801971450
81. Meier P, Meier R, Blanc E. Influence of CD4+/CD25+ regulatory T cells on atherogenesis in patients with end-stage kidney disease. *Expert Rev Cardiovasc Ther* (2008) 6(7):987–97. doi:10.1586/14779072.6.7.987
82. Zhang GY, Hu M, Wang YM, Alexander SI. Foxp3 as a marker of tolerance induction versus rejection. *Curr Opin Organ Transplant* (2009) 14(1):40–5. doi:10.1097/MOT.0b013e32831da83c
83. Deng G, Carter J, Traystman RJ, Wagner DH, Herson PS. Pro-inflammatory T-lymphocytes rapidly infiltrate into the brain and contribute to neuronal injury following cardiac arrest and cardiopulmonary resuscitation. *J Neuroimmunol* (2014) 274(1–2):132–40. doi:10.1016/j.jneuroim.2014.07.009
84. Dole VS, Bergmeier W, Mitchell HA, Eichenberger SC, Wagner DD. Activated platelets induce Weibel-Palade-body secretion and leukocyte rolling in vivo: role of P-selectin. *Blood* (2005) 106(7):2334–9. doi:10.1182/blood-2005-04-1530
85. Gao D, Wagner AH, Fankhaenel S, Stojanovic T, Schweyer S, Panzner S, et al. CD40 antisense oligonucleotide inhibition of trinitrobenzene sulphonic acid induced rat colitis. *Gut* (2005) 54(1):70–7. doi:10.1136/gut.2003.029587
86. Huckel M, Schurigt U, Wagner AH, Stockigt R, Petrow PK, Thoss K, et al. Attenuation of murine antigen-induced arthritis by treatment with a decoy oligodeoxynucleotide inhibiting signal transducer and activator of transcription-1 (STAT-1). *Arthritis Res Ther* (2006) 8(1):R17. doi:10.1186/ar1869
87. Ju XS, Hacker C, Scherer B, Redecke V, Berger T, Schuler G, et al. Immunoglobulin-like transcripts ILT2, ILT3 and ILT7 are expressed by human dendritic cells and down-regulated following activation. *Gene* (2004) 331:159–64. doi:10.1016/j.gene.2004.02.018
88. Kang YM, Zhang X, Wagner UG, Yang H, Beckenbaugh RD, Kurtin PJ, et al. CD8 T cells are required for the formation of ectopic germinal centers in rheumatoid synovitis. *J Exp Med* (2002) 195(10):1325–36. doi:10.1084/jem.20011565
89. Kenyon NS, Chatzipetrou M, Masetti M, Ranuncoli A, Oliveira M, Wagner JL, et al. Long-term survival and function of intrahepatic islet allografts in rhesus monkeys treated with humanized anti-CD154. *Proc Natl Acad Sci U S A* (1999) 96(14):8132–7. doi:10.1073/pnas.96.14.8132
90. Kenyon NS, Fernandez LA, Lehmann R, Masetti M, Ranuncoli A, Chatzipetrou M, et al. Long-term survival and function of intrahepatic islet allografts in baboons treated with humanized anti-CD154. *Diabetes* (1999) 48(7):1473–81. doi:10.2337/diabetes.48.7.1473
91. Krzesz R, Wagner AH, Cattaruzza M, Hecker M. Cytokine-inducible CD40 gene expression in vascular smooth muscle cells is mediated by nuclear factor kappaB and signal transducer and activation of transcription-1. *FEBS Lett* (1999) 453(1–2):191–6. doi:10.1016/S0014-5793(99)00683-3
92. Luhrmann A, Tschernig T, von der Leyen H, Hecker M, Pabst R, Wagner AH. Decoy oligodeoxynucleotide against STAT transcription factors decreases allergic inflammation in a rat asthma model. *Exp Lung Res* (2010) 36(2):85–93. doi:10.3109/01902140903144138
93. Stojakovic M, Krzesz R, Wagner AH, Hecker M. CD154-stimulated GM-CSF release by vascular smooth muscle cells elicits monocyte activation – role in atherogenesis. *J Mol Med* (2007) 85(11):1229–38. doi:10.1007/s00109-007-0225-y
94. Stojanovic T, Wagner AH, Wang S, Kiss E, Rockstroh N, Bedke J, et al. STAT-1 decoy oligodeoxynucleotide inhibition of acute rejection in mouse heart transplants. *Basic Res Cardiol* (2009) 104(6):719–29. doi:10.1007/s00395-009-0028-0
95. Vabulas RM, Pircher H, Lipford GB, Hacker H, Wagner H. CpG-DNA activates in vivo T cell epitope presenting dendritic cells to trigger protective antiviral cytotoxic T cell responses. *J Immunol* (2000) 164(5):2372–8. doi:10.4049/jimmunol.164.5.2372
96. Wagner AH, Gebauer M, Guldenzoph B, Hecker M. 3-hydroxy-3-methylglutaryl coenzyme A reductase-independent inhibition of CD40 expression by atorvastatin in human endothelial cells. *Arterioscler Thromb Vasc Biol* (2002) 22(11):1784–9. doi:10.1161/01.ATV.0000037098.20829.31
97. Wagner AH, Gebauer M, Pollok-Kopp B, Hecker M. Cytokine-inducible CD40 expression in human endothelial cells is mediated by interferon regulatory factor-1. *Blood* (2002) 99(2):520–5. doi:10.1182/blood.V99.2.520
98. Wagner AH, Guldenzoph B, Lienenluke B, Hecker M. CD154/CD40-mediated expression of CD154 in endothelial cells: consequences for endothelial cell-monocyte interaction. *Arterioscler Thromb Vasc Biol* (2004) 24(4):715–20. doi:10.1161/01.ATV.0000122853.99978.b1
99. Wagner AH, Wittjen I, Stojanovic T, Middel P, Meingassner JG, Hecker M. Signal transducer and activator of transcription 1 decoy oligodeoxynucleotide suppression of contact hypersensitivity. *J Allergy Clin Immunol* (2008) 121(1):158–65.e5. doi:10.1016/j.jaci.2007.09.015
100. Vaitaitis GM, Wagner DH Jr. High distribution of CD40 and TRAF2 in Th40 T cell rafts leads to preferential survival of this auto-aggressive population in autoimmunity. *PLoS One* (2008) 3(4):e2076. doi:10.1371/journal.pone.0002076
101. Martin-Fontecha A, Baumjohann D, Guarda G, Reboldi A, Hons M, Lanzavecchia A, et al. CD40L+ CD4+ memory T cells migrate in a CD62P-dependent fashion into reactive lymph nodes and license dendritic cells for T cell priming. *J Exp Med* (2008) 205(11):2561–74. doi:10.1084/jem.20081212
102. Martin S, Agarwal R, Murugaiyan G, Saha B. CD40 expression levels modulate regulatory T cells in *Leishmania donovani* infection. *J Immunol* (2010) 185(1):551–9. doi:10.4049/jimmunol.0902206
103. Takaki H, Minoda Y, Koga K, Takaesu G, Yoshimura A, Kobayashi T. TGF-beta1 suppresses IFN-gamma-induced NO production in macrophages by suppressing STAT1 activation and accelerating iNOS protein degradation. *Genes Cells* (2006) 11(8):871–82. doi:10.1111/j.1365-2443.2006.00988.x
104. Alderson MR, Armitage RJ, Tough TW, Strockbine L, Fanslow WC, Spriggs MK. CD40 expression by human monocytes: regulation by cytokines and activation of monocytes by the ligand for CD40. *J Exp Med* (1993) 178(2):669–74. doi:10.1084/jem.178.2.669
105. Town T, Tan J, Mullan M. CD40 signaling and Alzheimer's disease pathogenesis. *Neurochem Int* (2001) 39(5–6):371–80. doi:10.1016/S0197-0186(01)00044-4
106. Suo Z, Wu M, Ameenuddin S, Anderson HE, Zoloty JE, Citron BA, et al. Participation of protease-activated receptor-1 in thrombin-induced microglial activation. *J Neurochem* (2002) 80(4):655–66. doi:10.1046/j.0022-3042.2001.00745.x
107. Haase C, Markholst H. CD40 is required for development of islet inflammation in the RIP-CD154 transgenic mouse model of type 1 diabetes. *Ann N Y Acad Sci* (2007) 1107:373–9. doi:10.1196/annals.1381.039
108. Klein D, Barbe-Tuana F, Pugliese A, Ichii H, Garza D, Gonzalez M, et al. A functional CD40 receptor is expressed in pancreatic beta cells. *Diabetologia* (2005) 48(2):268–76. doi:10.1007/s00125-004-1645-7

109. Hanninen A, Martinez NR, Davey GM, Heath WR, Harrison LC. Transient blockade of CD40 ligand dissociates pathogenic from protective mucosal immunity. *J Clin Invest* (2002) 109(2):261–7. doi:10.1172/JCI0213720
110. Vaitaitis GM, Olmstead MH, Waid DM, Carter JR, Wagner DH Jr. A CD40-targeted peptide controls and reverses type 1 diabetes in NOD mice. *Diabetologia* (2014) 57(11):2366–73. doi:10.1007/s00125-014-3342-5
111. Vaitaitis GM, Carter JR, Waid DM, Olmstead MH, Wagner DH Jr. An alternative role for Foxp3 as an effector T cell regulator controlled through CD40. *J Immunol* (2013) 191(2):717–25. doi:10.4049/jimmunol.1300625
112. Vaitaitis GM, Wagner DH Jr. CD40 glycoforms and TNF-receptors 1 and 2 in the formation of CD40 receptor(s) in autoimmunity. *Mol Immunol* (2010) 47(14):2303–13. doi:10.1016/j.molimm.2010.05.288
113. Vaitaitis G, Waid DM, Wagner D Jr. The expanding role of TNF-receptor super family member CD40 (tnfrsf5) in autoimmune disease: focus on Th40 cells. *Curr Immunol Rev* (2010) 6(2):130–7. doi:10.2174/157339510791111673
114. Bourgeois C, Rocha B, Tanchot C. A role for CD40 expression on CD8+ T cells in the generation of CD8+ T cell memory. *Science* (2002) 297(5589):2060–3. doi:10.1126/science.1072615
115. Najafian N, Khoury SJ. T cell costimulatory pathways: blockade for autoimmunity. *Expert Opin Biol Ther* (2003) 3(2):227–36. doi:10.1517/14712598.3.2.227
116. Baker RL, Wagner DH Jr, Haskins K. CD40 on NOD CD4 T cells contributes to their activation and pathogenicity. *J Autoimmun* (2008) 31(4):385–92. doi:10.1016/j.jaut.2008.09.001
117. Nowell PC. Phytohemagglutinin: an initiator of mitosis in cultures of normal human leukocytes. *Cancer Res* (1960) 20:462–6.
118. Ke Y, Ma H, Kapp JA. Antigen is required for the activation of effector activities, whereas interleukin 2 Is required for the maintenance of memory in ovalbumin-specific, CD8+ cytotoxic T lymphocytes. *J Exp Med* (1998) 187(1):49–57. doi:10.1084/jem.187.1.49
119. McDonald SA, Palmen MJ, Van Rees EP, MacDonald TT. Characterization of the mucosal cell-mediated immune response in IL-2 knockout mice before and after the onset of colitis. *Immunology* (1997) 91(1):73–80. doi:10.1046/j.1365-2567.1997.00217.x
120. Malek TR, Yu A, Zhu L, Matsutani T, Adeegbe D, Bayer AL. IL-2 family of cytokines in T regulatory cell development and homeostasis. *J Clin Immunol* (2008) 28(6):635–9. doi:10.1007/s10875-008-9235-y
121. Isakson SH, Katzman SD, Hoyer KK. Spontaneous autoimmunity in the absence of IL-2 is driven by uncontrolled dendritic cells. *J Immunol* (2012) 189(4):1585–93. doi:10.4049/jimmunol.1200342
122. Piganelli JD, Flores SC, Cruz C, Koepp J, Batinic-Haberle I, Crapo J, et al. A metalloporphyrin-based superoxide dismutase mimic inhibits adoptive transfer of autoimmune diabetes by a diabetogenic T-cell clone. *Diabetes* (2002) 51(2):347–55. doi:10.2337/diabetes.51.2.347
123. Katz JD, Wang B, Haskins K, Benoist C, Mathis D. Following a diabetogenic T cell from genesis through pathogenesis. *Cell* (1993) 74(6):1089–100. doi:10.1016/0092-8674(93)90730-E

11

Environmental Factors Contribute to β Cell Endoplasmic Reticulum Stress and Neo-Antigen Formation in Type 1 Diabetes

*Meghan L. Marré and Jon D. Piganelli**

Division of Pediatric Surgery, Department of Surgery, Children's Hospital of Pittsburgh, University of Pittsburgh, Pittsburgh, PA, United States

Correspondence:
Jon D. Piganelli
jdp51@pitt.edu

Type 1 diabetes (T1D) is an autoimmune disease in which immune-mediated targeting and destruction of insulin-producing pancreatic islet β cells leads to chronic hyperglycemia. There are many β cell proteins that are targeted by autoreactive T cells in their native state. However, recent studies have demonstrated that many β cell proteins are recognized as neo-antigens following posttranslational modification (PTM). Although modified neo-antigens are well-established targets of pathology in other autoimmune diseases, the effects of neo-antigens in T1D progression and the mechanisms by which they are generated are not well understood. We have demonstrated that PTM occurs during endoplasmic reticulum (ER) stress, a process to which β cells are uniquely susceptible due to the high rate of insulin production in response to dynamic glucose sensing. In the context of genetic susceptibility to autoimmunity, presentation of these modified neo-antigens may activate autoreactive T cells and cause pathology. However, inherent β cell ER stress and protein PTM do not cause T1D in every genetically susceptible individual, suggesting the contribution of additional factors. Indeed, many environmental factors, such as viral infection, chemicals, or inflammatory cytokines, are associated with T1D onset, but the mechanisms by which these factors lead to disease onset remain unknown. Since these environmental factors also cause ER stress, exposure to these factors may enhance production of neo-antigens, therefore boosting β cell recognition by autoreactive T cells and exacerbating T1D pathogenesis. Therefore, the combined effects of physiological ER stress and the stress that is induced by environmental factors may lead to breaks in peripheral tolerance, contribute to antigen spread, and hasten disease onset. This Hypothesis and Theory article summarizes what is currently known about ER stress and protein PTM in autoimmune diseases including T1D and proposes a role for environmental factors in breaking immune tolerance to β cell antigens through neo-antigen formation.

Keywords: type 1 diabetes, β cell, environmental factors, endoplasmic reticulum stress, posttranslation modification, neo-antigen, autoimmunity

INTRODUCTION

Type 1 diabetes (T1D) is a chronic autoimmune disease in which insulin-producing pancreatic islet β cells are targeted and destroyed by autoreactive immune cells. Autoimmune recognition of β cell antigens leads to decreased β cell mass and to the subsequent decline of insulin-mediated regulation of glucose levels in the blood. Eventually, too few β cells remain to meet the demand for insulin to maintain normal blood glucose levels. This insufficient insulin secretion leads to chronic hyperglycemia and T1D.

Type 1 diabetes is strongly associated with a genetic predisposition to autoimmunity that is conferred by single-nucleotide polymorphisms (SNPs) and gene variants found at many genetic loci. In particular, SNPs and variants in genes associated with both the innate and adaptive branches of the immune system cause failures of central and peripheral tolerance that eventually lead to autoimmune targeting of β cells. Of these loci, polymorphisms in the major histocompatibility complex (MHC) locus are most strongly associated with T1D onset (1–3). MHC proteins are crucial to central tolerance, because the antigens they present during T cell development in the thymus determine which T cells survive selection. This process directly shapes the mature adaptive immune repertoire. Strongly autoreactive T cells should be deleted upon encountering self-antigen presented by MHC during selection (4), but in individuals expressing MHC polymorphisms associated with autoimmunity, autoreactive T cells successfully mature and exit the thymus (5, 6). If peripheral tolerance mechanisms also fail, these autoreactive T cells become activated when they encounter β cell antigens in pancreatic lymph nodes. This autoimmune response destroys pancreatic β cells and ultimately causes T1D.

To better understand the processes by which the autoimmune response leads to T1D, and to identify the β cell proteins that are targeted by autoreactive T cells, researchers have studied the non-obese diabetic (NOD) mouse. These mice develop a spontaneous autoimmune diabetes that is similar in many ways to the human disease. These similarities include genetic susceptibility at the MHC locus and other immune-related loci, intra-islet infiltration of autoreactive immune cells as disease progresses, and ultimate β cell destruction (7–9). The β cell autoantigens identified using this murine model include preproinsulin (10), glutamic acid decarboxylase 65 (GAD65) (11), islet-specific glucose-6-phosphatase catalytic subunit-related protein (IGRP) (12), chromogranin A (CHgA) (13), islet amyloid polypeptide (14), zinc transporter 8 (15), and 78 kDa glucose-regulated protein (GRP78) (16) (**Table 1**). Subsequent studies confirmed the relevance of these autoantigens to human T1D (17–23) (**Table 1**). In addition, several additional autoantigens have been identified in humans but not yet confirmed in NOD mice, including tyrosine phosphatase-like insulinoma antigen 2 and IA-2β (also known as phosphatase homolog of granules from rat insulinomas) (24, 25), and islet cell autoantigen 69 (26) (**Table 1**).

The immunogenicity of these β cell autoantigens has long been attributed to failures in the mechanisms that govern immune tolerance to self-peptides. While this likely remains true, seminal studies conducted by several laboratories demonstrated that many of these β cell peptides undergo posttranslational modification (PTM). These studies propose that aberrant PTM of these β cell proteins generates so called "neo-antigens" that are then recognized as non-self by immune cells (16, 19, 23, 27–32), hastening the break in tolerance and exacerbating immune targeting and destruction of β cells. However, most of these studies did not explore the cellular processes that lead to PTM of these proteins in the context of β cell function and biology.

To address this question, our laboratory demonstrated that endoplasmic reticulum (ER) stress in the β cell leads to the activation of PTM enzymes and the modification of β cell proteins, which in turn leads to increased recognition of these β cells by diabetogenic T cells (32). ER stress in the β cell originates from various sources. For instance, the normal function of β cells (to produce and secrete insulin) causes ER stress (32–42). We demonstrated that this inherent physiological ER stress is sufficient to activate PTM enzymes and to generate β cell immunogenicity (32) (**Figure 1**). In addition, many of the environmental factors associated with T1D onset such as viral infection (43–48), chemicals (32, 49–51), reactive oxygen species (ROS) (52–55), dysglycemia (56), and inflammation (57–59) may cause β cell ER stress (**Figure 1**). Therefore, any of these environmental factors has the potential to enhance autoimmune targeting of β cells through the generation of ER stress- and PTM-dependent neo-antigens (32, 60, 61). However, the mechanisms by which these factors

TABLE 1 | β Cell autoantigens identified in murine and human T1D.

Autoantigen	Species	Reference
Preproinsulin	Mouse	(10)
	Human	(20)
Glutamic acid decarboxylase 65	Mouse	(11)
	Human	(17)
IGRP	Mouse	(12)
	Human	(22)
Chromogranin A	Mouse	(13)
	Human	(19)
Islet amyloid polypeptide	Mouse	(14)
	Human	(18)
Zinc transporter 8	Mouse	(15)
	Human	(21)
78 kDa glucose-regulated protein	Mouse	(16)
	Human	(23)
IA-2, IA-2β	Human	(24, 25)
Islet cell autoantigen 69	Human	(26)

Abbreviations: Aire, autoimmune regulator; APC, antigen-presenting cell; ATF6, activating transcription factor 6; ATP, adenosine triphosphate; Ca^{2+}, calcium; CHgA, chromogranin A; DRiP, defective ribosomal product; EAE, experimental autoimmune encephalomyelitis; ER, endoplasmic reticulum; GAD65, glutamic acid decarboxylase 65; GFP, green fluorescent protein; GRP78, 78 kDa glucose-regulated protein; IA-2, tyrosine phosphatase-like insulinoma antigen 2; IAPP, islet amyloid polypeptide; ICA69, islet cell autoantigen 69; IGF-2, insulin-like growth factor 2; IGRP, islet-specific glucose-6-phosphatase catalytic subunit-related protein; IFNγ, interferon gamma; IP_3R, inositol 1,4,5-trisphosphate receptor; IRE1, inositol-requiring protein 1; JNK, c-jun N-terminal kinase; MAP, mitogen-activated protein kinase; MHC, major histocompatibility complex; mTEC, medullary thymic epithelial cell; NET, neutrophil extracellular traps; NF-κB, nuclear factor kappa-light-chain-enhancer of activated B cells; NOD, non-obese diabetic mouse; PAD2, peptidylarginine deiminase 2; PDI, protein disulfide isomerases; PERK, protein kinase RNA (PKR)-like ER kinase; Phogrin, phosphatase homolog of granules from rat insulinomas; PTM, posttranslational modification; ROS, reactive oxygen species; RyR, ryanodine receptor; SERCA, sarco/endoplasmic reticulum Ca^{2+} ATPases; SNP, single-nucleotide polymorphisms; T1D, type 1 diabetes; Tgase2, tissue transglutaminase 2; UPR, unfolded protein response; ZnT8, zinc transporter 8.

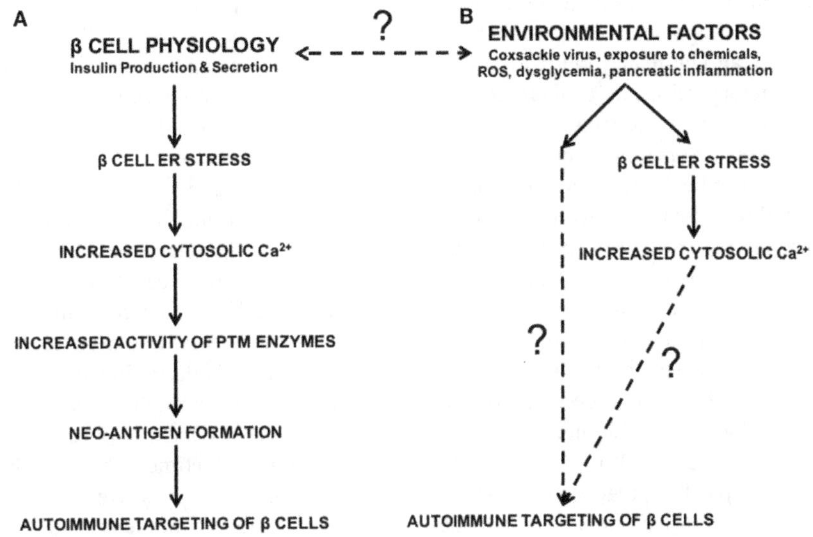

FIGURE 1 | The roles of β cell physiology and environmental favors in the autoimmune targeting of β cells in type 1 diabetes (T1D). **(A)** Normal β cell secretory physiology causes inherent endoplasmic reticulum (ER) stress, which in turn results in a release of Ca^{2+} from the ER into the cytosol. We have previously demonstrated that ER stress and its Ca^{2+} efflux lead to increased activity of Ca^{2+}-dependent posttranslational modification enzymes, formation of neo-antigens, and β cell immunogenicity (32). **(B)** In addition, many environmental factors are associated with T1D onset, such as viral infection, exposure to chemicals and reactive oxygen species, dysglycemia, and pancreatic inflammation. Although the mechanisms by which these factors lead to autoimmune targeting of β cells remain unknown, these environmental factors all cause β cell ER stress and Ca^{2+} efflux. Whether the ER stress and Ca^{2+} efflux caused by these environmental factors contributes to T1D onset, and whether this ER stress cooperates with physiological ER stress to generate neo-antigens, remain unknown.

hasten T1D onset, and whether the ER stress they cause cooperates with that caused by β cell physiology, remain unknown (**Figure 1**).

Here, we review what is known about β cell ER stress, neo-antigen formation, and the progression to pathology in T1D. We also review the role that the environmental factors associated with T1D may play in exacerbating β cell ER stress. Finally, we discuss the evidence supporting our novel hypothesis that environmental factors converge with β cell physiology to increase ER stress above a putative threshold. According to our "threshold hypothesis," ER stress must be sufficiently severe or prolonged to allow for the generation of PTM-dependent neo-antigens. We hypothesize that the convergence between β cell physiology and exposure to environmental factors increases ER stress above this threshold, leading to neo-antigen formation, β cell immunogenicity, and ultimately to the onset of T1D.

ER STRESS AND THE UNFOLDED PROTEIN RESPONSE (UPR)

The ER is primarily responsible for the proper folding and modification of proteins that are membrane bound or destined for secretion. Therefore, the ER lumen contains the molecular chaperones and the environment necessary for protein folding and PTM, including sufficient levels of adenosine triphosphate, an oxidizing environment to support disulfide bond formation, and millimolar concentrations of calcium (Ca^{2+}) (62). Proteins that are folded and modified properly exit the ER and are shuttled to their intended intra- or extracellular locations. However, proteins that become misfolded cannot exit the ER lumen. The accumulation of misfolded or aberrantly modified proteins causes ER stress.

Endoplasmic reticulum stress induces the UPR, which functions in two main modes: the adaptive UPR and the terminal UPR (63, 64). The adaptive UPR occurs early in ER stress and functions largely to alleviate ER stress and restore normal cellular homeostasis through three signaling cascades, each of which begins with the activation of protein sensors of stress in the ER membrane (65). First, protein kinase RNA (PKR)-like ER kinase (PERK) activates a signaling cascade that inhibits mRNA translation and reduces the protein burden in the lumen of the ER (66, 67). Second, activating transcription factor 6 signaling leads to increased production of new molecular chaperones to aid with the folding of accumulated misfolded proteins (68). And third, the signaling pathway initiated by inositol-requiring protein 1 increases expression of chaperones for protein folding and of proteins involved in lipid synthesis to increase ER volume (69, 70). Together, these branches of the UPR work to facilitate the proper folding of proteins that have accumulated, and also reduce the entrance of additional non-chaperone proteins into the ER lumen. In these ways, the adaptive UPR acts to allow the ER to return to normal homeostasis.

Although the adaptive UPR aims to protect the cell from the negative effects of ER stress, ER dysfunction that is excessive or extended may overcome these cytoprotective mechanisms. Under these conditions, the terminal UPR activates proapoptotic processes (71–73) leading to death of the affected cell. However, long before apoptosis pathways are activated, even temporary ER stress and the adaptive UPR may have important consequences for cellular function and physiology.

All cells undergo periods of increased protein production, which increases the ER burden, leading to misfolding or aberrant modification of nascent proteins, and ultimately to ER stress and UPR activation. However, secretory cells, due to their normal physiology, are uniquely susceptible to ER stress. These cells must produce not only the proteins necessary for normal cellular maintenance, but also the proteins to be secreted and the proteins that comprise the secretory pathway itself. Even with a larger ER volume and greater numbers of chaperones to account for this increased demand (74), the secretory function of these cells leads to significantly increased ER burden and stress.

Like other secretory cells, β cells undergo naturally high levels of ER stress due to their normal physiological role of insulin production and secretion (32–42). Indeed, increased ER stress, and its consequences for protein folding, occurs as a direct consequence of glucose sensing (37, 38). In response to increased glucose concentrations, β cells upregulate the translation of preproinsulin by 50-fold, reaching a production rate of one million molecules of preproinsulin per minute (75). These one million molecules of preproinsulin inundate the ER lumen for folding and the formation of three disulfide bonds per molecule, causing tremendous ER stress. Under these conditions, many of the insulin molecules produced by β cells become misfolded or incorrectly modified (75) (**Figure 2**). In addition to this inherent ER stress due to normal physiology, β cell ER stress may rise due to exposure to the environmental factors that are associated with T1D onset (32, 43–61) (**Figure 1**). Under these circumstances, β cell ER stress may rise above physiological levels.

Heightened β cell ER stress does not necessarily activate the terminal UPR or suggest β cell exhaustion or impending death as observed in some models (63, 76–80). Rather, β cells exhibit naturally high ER stress very early and activate the adaptive UPR long before β cell death. In a study using a reporter mouse in which green fluorescent protein is expressed with the activation of the UPR, the pancreas exhibited the highest ER stress of all tissues examined, and did so as early as day 16 of life (81). In spite of the observed ER stress and UPR activation, these mice (on the C57Bl/6 background) never succumbed to loss of β cell mass and diabetes (81). These data confirm that high levels of β cell ER stress does not necessarily activate the terminal UPR and lead to β cell failure and death. Indeed, the β cells in most individuals resolve ER stress through the proper function of the adaptive UPR and therefore maintain healthy and functional β cell mass throughout their lifetimes. Therefore, β cell death is not the only consequence of ER stress. We hypothesize that lower and more transient ER stress, and the activation of the adaptive UPR, may have consequences for β cell function and for the autoimmune targeting of β cells much earlier.

ER STRESS AFFECTS Ca^{2+}-DEPENDENT CELLULAR FUNCTIONS

In addition to its role in the folding and modification of new proteins, the ER contains the largest store of intracellular Ca^{2+} and is an important organelle for regulating Ca^{2+} concentrations,

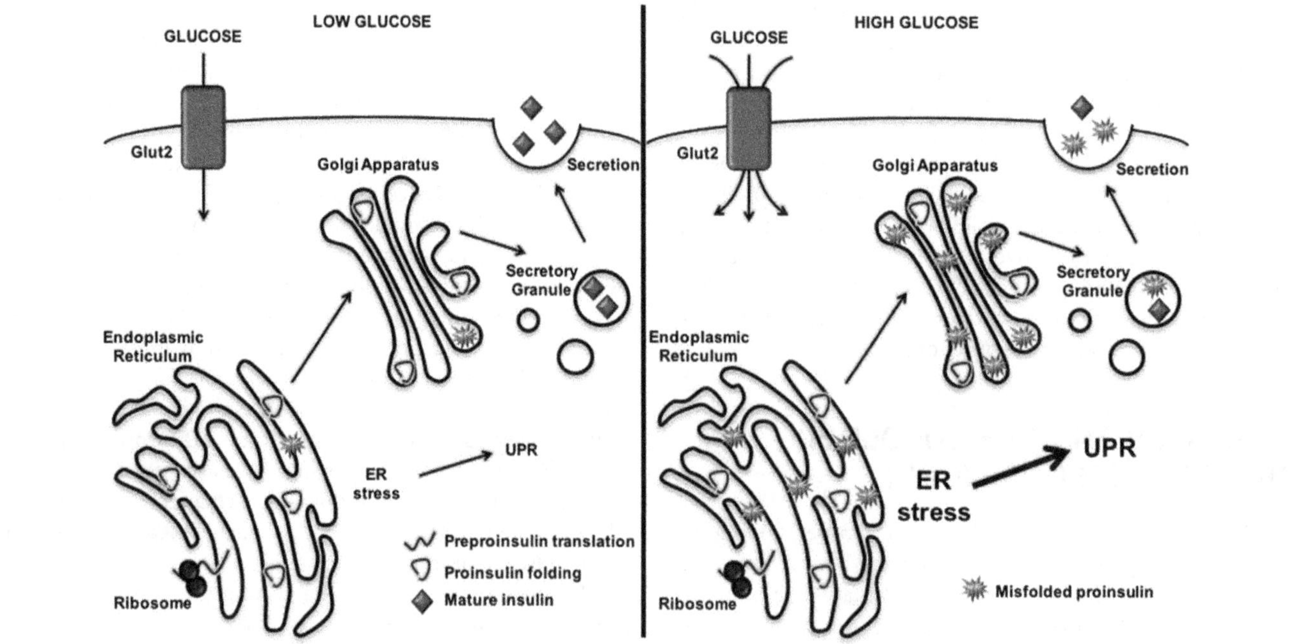

FIGURE 2 | Rising blood glucose increases misfolding of proinsulin and endoplasmic reticulum (ER) stress levels. When blood glucose levels are low, preproinsulin is translated, properly folded and modified in the ER, and secreted as mature insulin into the extracellular space. When blood glucose levels rise, β cells increase production of preproinsulin, flooding the ER lumen with one million molecules per minute that require folding and disulfide bond formation. This increased protein burden in the ER leads to misfolding of proteins and aberrant posttranslational modification, which further exacerbates ER dysfunction and activates the unfolded protein response (UPR).

and therefore Ca^{2+}-dependent processes, throughout the cell (82). One consequence of ER stress is the release of Ca^{2+} from the ER lumen into the cytosol. This Ca^{2+} efflux has important consequences for cellular physiology.

In the ER, millimolar concentrations of Ca^{2+} are necessary for proper protein folding and modification (62). Indeed, molecular chaperones that assist in protein folding and protein disulfide isomerases that facilitate the formation of disulfide bonds depend on these high Ca^{2+} concentrations (83, 84). These high concentrations of Ca^{2+} are maintained by sarco/endoplasmic reticulum Ca^{2+} ATPases (SERCA) pumps in the ER membrane that actively transport Ca^{2+} from the cytosol into the ER. When Ca^{2+} leaves the ER lumen during ER stress, the function of these proteins also decreases, further inhibiting protein folding and modification and contributing to greater ER dysfunction (85).

In the cytosol, Ca^{2+} is required for the regulation of normal cellular processes such as metabolism, vesicular trafficking, protein secretion, mRNA transcription, and apoptosis (86). To achieve the necessary cytosolic concentrations, Ca^{2+} is released from the ER by the ryanodine receptor and inositol 1,4,5-trisphosphate receptor channels. Under conditions of ER stress, the efflux of Ca^{2+} from the ER lumen increases cytosolic concentrations above normal physiological levels. This increased cytosolic Ca^{2+} can be deleterious for cellular function. For example, increased cytosolic Ca^{2+} can initiate apoptosis through activation of caspase-dependent cell death pathways (87, 88) or mitochondria-dependent pathways (89–92).

It is clear, then, that ER stress greatly affects Ca^{2+}-dependent cellular functions. While the adaptive UPR works to relieve ER stress, cytosolic Ca^{2+} still increases before ER homeostasis is regained. β cells, which are particularly susceptible to ER stress, are therefore also prone to the dysregulation of cellular processes following even a temporary efflux of Ca^{2+} from the ER. In addition, the environmental factors associated with T1D onset also lead to increased cytosolic Ca^{2+} (32, 43–61) (**Figure 1**). Therefore, we propose that the combination of physiological ER stress and that derived from environmental factors, even if transient, may have consequences for β cell health and function.

ER STRESS ACTIVATES CYTOSOLIC PTM ENZYMES

Transient ER stress and increased cytosolic Ca^{2+} concentrations can activate cytosolic Ca^{2+}-dependent enzymes, including those that mediate PTM. Activation of these PTM enzymes can have significant implications for proteins being folded in the ER. In particular, two such PTM enzymes reside in the cytosol and are activated during the ER stress Ca^{2+} flux: tissue transglutaminase 2 (Tgase2) and peptidylarginine deiminase 2 (PAD2).

Tissue transglutaminase 2 is ubiquitously expressed and resides in the cytosol (93). When activated, Tgase2 translocates to several intracellular compartments (94), including the ER (95–97) and secretory granules (98) to modify proteins through two mechanisms (99): first, Tgase2 crosslinks proteins through the formation of ε(γ-glutamyl) isopeptide bonds between glutamine and lysine residues, and second, Tgase2 mediates the deamidation of glutamine residues. Tgase2 plays important roles in the regulation of apoptosis (100, 101), gene expression (93, 102, 103), and cellular adhesion and wound healing (104–107). Of relevance to T1D, Tgase2 is expressed in and functions in β cells (32, 60).

Of the five mammalian PAD isoforms, PAD2 is the most widely expressed and is the isoform expressed in the pancreas (108). PAD2 also resides in the cytosol (109), and, similar to Tgase2, activated PAD2 is recruited to various subcellular compartments for the modification of proteins (110). PAD2 mediates the conversion of arginine to citrulline. This amino acid conversion alters the overall charge and hydrophobicity of the protein (111), causing changes in protein folding and conformation (112). PAD2 plays roles in many cellular functions, including the negative regulation of nuclear factor kappa-light-chain-enhancer of activated B cells activation (113), cytoskeleton disassembly (114), and in the formation of neutrophil extracellular traps (115).

While Ca^{2+}-dependent activation of these enzymes is necessary for normal cellular function, these enzymes also contribute to pathology in many diseases.

PTM GENERATES NEO-ANTIGENS IN AUTOIMMUNE DISEASES

Protein PTM is necessary for cellular viability and function. However, autoantigens in many different autoimmune diseases such as celiac disease (116), collagen-induced arthritis (117), multiple sclerosis/experimental autoimmune encephalomyelitis (118–121), rheumatoid arthritis (122–127), and systemic lupus erythematosus (128–131) contain PTM, suggesting that these modifications may contribute to breaks in tolerance that exacerbate disease.

Central tolerance is established during T cell development in the thymus. In the thymus, medullary thymic epithelial cells (mTECs) express peptides normally found in peripheral tissues through the function of autoimmune regulator (132–134). When these peptides are presented to developing T cells in the context of MHC molecules, T cells that respond too strongly to these self-peptides are deleted and are thus absent from the mature T cell population (4, 135–137). However, if self-proteins undergo PTM in peripheral tissues, as in the autoimmune diseases listed above, these proteins may be processed and presented differently by peripheral antigen-presenting cells (APCs) than by the mTECs (138). If such modified epitopes were not expressed and presented by mTECs, T cells that recognize these modified epitopes escape negative selection and are present in circulation as mature T cells. When these T cells encounter these neo-antigens in peripheral tissues, they become activated and lead the autoimmune targeting of peripheral tissues.

As with all peripheral tissues, peptides from β cell proteins, including insulin and insulin-like growth factor 2, are presented by mTECs to developing T cells in the thymus (5, 6, 139–142). However, the presence of T cells in the periphery that recognize islet proteins and target β cells suggests the failure of crucial tolerance mechanisms. This failure in central tolerance mechanisms may be explained by the growing body of literature that abnormal PTM increases the immunogenicity of β cell peptides in both murine and human models of T1D (**Table 2**). These studies have demonstrated that some β cell proteins undergo various modifications including oxidation (28, 143), Tgase2-mediated crosslinking by isopeptide bond (19, 29), Tgase2-mediated deamidation (30–32), PAD2-mediated citrullination (16, 23, 31), the formation of hybrid peptides (144, 145), and the formation of a defective ribosomal insulin gene product (146). Furthermore, the neo-antigens formed by these PTM elicit stronger immune responses than the native proteins (16, 19, 23, 28–31, 143, 145), suggesting an important role for these neo-antigens in precipitating disease onset. These findings have been of great importance to the understanding of T1D pathogenesis, because these studies identified novel autoantigens that are targeted in T1D. However, the mechanisms by which these neo-antigens arise in β cells was not examined.

β CELL NEO-ANTIGENS ARISE DURING ER STRESS

To begin to elucidate how PTM neo-antigens might arise in β cells, our laboratory examined the consequences of β cell ER stress for β cell immunogenicity, since β cells inherently undergo high levels of ER stress (32–42, 60, 81). To do so, we used a model system of β cell recognition by diabetogenic BDC2.5 $CD4^+$ T cells. These particular T cells were chosen because they recognize a Tgase2-modified peptide of CHgA (29) and secrete interferon gamma (IFNγ) when they encounter their PTM-dependent antigen.

Our studies demonstrated that, in primary murine islets, ER stress induced by thapsigargin [a widely accepted chemical inducer of ER stress (96, 147, 148)] contributed to heightened cytosolic Ca^{2+} concentrations, increased Tgase2 activity, and increased β cell immunogenicity (32). In fact, murine islets undergoing ER stress elicited greater IFNγ secretion from BDC2.5 T cells (32) and by all other β cell antigen-specific T cells examined (**Figure 3**), suggesting a role for Ca^{2+}-dependent PTM in immunogenicity of many other β cell antigens. This increased immunogenicity was dependent upon both Ca^{2+} and Tgase2-mediated PTM, since chelation of cytosolic Ca^{2+} or decreased expression of Tgase2 reduced this consequence of ER stress (32). These data show that β cell ER stress leads to β cell immunogenicity through Ca^{2+}-dependent PTM of endogenous proteins.

Since ER stress is inherent to β cell physiology and function (32–42, 60), we hypothesized that ER stress induced by normal physiology [e.g., dynamic glucose sensing and secretory function (33–42, 60)] may be sufficient to cause Ca^{2+}- and PTM-dependent β cell immunogenicity. Indeed, a murine insulinoma (NIT-1) that exhibited low ER stress and immunogenicity was exposed to physiological milieu by transplantation into NOD.*scid* mice. After transplant, these cells exhibited insulin secretion, ER stress, Tgase2 activity, and immunogenicity (32). These data confirm that β cell physiology and insulin secretion contributes to the autoimmune targeting of β cells (60).

Many groups have demonstrated an increase in β cell ER stress long before β cell death and T1D onset (79, 81, 149, 150). In fact, relief of ER stress has been proposed as therapeutic opportunity for preventing β cell death and maintaining euglycemia (63, 80, 151, 152). However, most researchers conclude that ER stress leads to β cell death through the terminal UPR and activation of apoptosis pathways (76, 77, 80). Ours was the first study to demonstrate that normal, physiological β cell ER stress and the adaptive UPR contribute to T1D through the formation of β cell neo-antigens. In doing so, we became the first to propose a mechanism by which β cell neo-antigens (**Table 2**) may occur (**Figure 4**).

TABLE 2 | Posttranslational modification (PTM)-mediated neo-antigen formation in type 1 diabetes.

Autoantigen	PTM	Reference
Proinsulin	Oxidation	(28, 143)
	Formation of hybrid insulin peptides	(23, 144, 145)
Chromogranin A (WE14)	Crosslinking/isopeptide bond	(19, 29)
Preproinsulin	Deamidation	(30)
Islet cell autoantigen 69	Deamidation	(30)
Zinc transporter 8	Deamidation	(30)
Phosphatase homolog of granules from rat insulinomas	Deamidation	(30)
IA-2	Deamidation	(30)
IGRP	Deamidation	(30)
Glutamic acid decarboxylase 65	Citrullination	(31)
	Deamidation	(30, 31)
78 kDa glucose-regulated protein	Citrullination	(16, 23)
Insulin	Defective ribosomal product	(146)

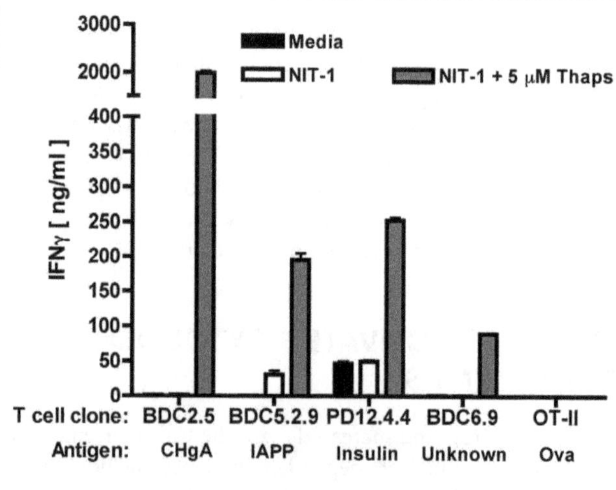

FIGURE 3 | Endoplasmic reticulum (ER) stress increases the immunogenicity of several β cell autoantigens. The immunogenicity of NIT-1 insulinoma cells treated with 5 μM thapsigargin or control for 1 h was assessed by T cell assay. Briefly, T cells (2 × 10^4), NOD.*scid* splenocytes as antigen-presenting cells (4 × 10^5), and NIT-1 cells as antigen (1 × 10^3) were combined in 200 μl in triplicate in 96-well flat-bottom tissue culture plates and incubated at 37°C for 72 h. T_H1 effector function was determined by measuring interferon gamma (IFNγ) secretion by enzyme-linked immunosorbent assay. Data are mean IFNγ secretion ± SD and are from one representative experiment of three independent experiments. For all specificities examined, NIT-1 cells undergoing ER stress elicited higher effector responses from the T cells, suggesting that ER stress contributes to the modification and greater immunogenicity of each of these proteins.

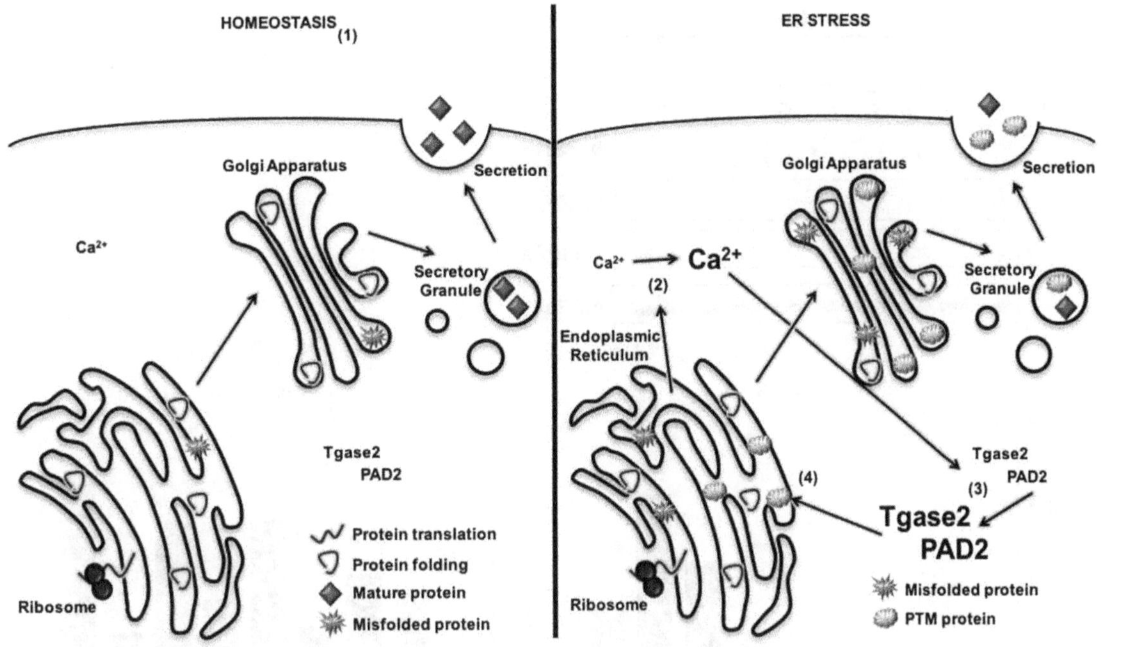

FIGURE 4 | Endoplasmic reticulum (ER) stress increases the activation of Ca^{2+}-dependent posttranslational modification (PTM) enzymes and the formation of PTM-dependent β cell neo-antigens. (1) Under homeostatic conditions, proteins are translated, folded, and packaged into secretory granules. Cytosolic Ca^{2+} and PTM enzyme activity remain low. (2) During β cell ER stress, Ca^{2+} stores are released from the ER, increasing cytosolic Ca^{2+}. (3) Increased Ca^{2+} concentrations activated Ca^{2+}-dependent enzymes tissue transglutaminase 2 (Tgase2) and peptidylarginine deiminase 2 (PAD2). (4) Active PTM enzymes modify nascent proteins. If presented to autoreactive T cells by antigen-presenting cell, modified β cell proteins break tolerance and facilitate immune recognition of β cells.

β CELL IMMUNOGENICITY REQUIRES A THRESHOLD OF ER STRESS

Endoplasmic reticulum stress occurs along a gradient. The burden of unfolded proteins in the ER lumen can vary from mild to severe, resulting in varying degrees of ER dysfunction and stress. This variance in levels of ER stress has important implications for the cellular consequences of ER stress. As discussed earlier, the strength and duration of ER stress-induced UPR signaling is a major factor in determining whether the adaptive UPR or terminal UPR is initiated (63, 64). One explanation may be that the severity and duration of ER stress affects the strength of the Ca^{2+} efflux from the ER lumen and determines whether cytosolic Ca^{2+} concentrations cross a putative threshold. Differences in cytosolic Ca^{2+} concentrations may significantly alter PTM enzyme activity, neo-antigen generation, and β cell immunogenicity.

This "threshold hypothesis" is further supported by literature that demonstrates that Tgase2 and PAD2 remain largely inactive in the cytosol, and activation requires significantly increased concentrations of cytosolic Ca^{2+}. In fact, the activation of both enzymes requires Ca^{2+} concentrations up to 100-fold higher than what is necessary for normal cellular physiology and function. Therefore, these enzymes generally become activated only under conditions of cellular distress or dysfunction, such as ER stress (96, 97, 108, 109, 147, 153, 154). Since these PTM enzymes require particular levels of cytosolic Ca^{2+} to become activated, it follows that a particular level of ER stress must be achieved before PTM-dependent neo-antigen formation can occur.

Previous work in our laboratory examined whether varying levels of ER stress lead to different degrees of β cell PTM-dependent immunogenicity. NIT-1 cells were incubated with increasing doses of thapsigargin, which increases ER stress and cytosolic Ca^{2+} by inhibiting the SERCA pumps that transport Ca^{2+} from the cytosol into the ER. As expected, thapsigargin induced ER stress and UPR activity in a dose-dependent manner (**Figure 5A**). The immunogenicity of these cells was examined by the BDC2.5 T cell clone, and T cell effector function was measured by IFNγ as previously described (32). Only the highest dose of thapsigargin elicited detectable IFNγ secretion from the T cells (**Figure 5B**). Therefore, although lower doses of thapsigargin induced ER stress, the stress (and consequences thereof) at these lower doses was not sufficient to result in β cell immunogenicity.

Tunicamycin is another chemical inducer of ER stress that blocks the initial steps of glycoprotein synthesis in the ER and thus increases the burden of unfolded proteins in the ER lumen (148). Increasing doses of tunicamycin increased ER stress in NIT-1 cells (**Figure 6A**), but to lesser degrees compared with thapsigargin (**Figure 5A**). Also, as with lower doses of thapsigargin, the lower ER stress induced by tunicamycin was not sufficient to elicit effector responses from BDC2.5 T cells (**Figure 6B**). Together, these data serve as further evidence that a particular threshold of ER stress must be reached to achieve PTM-dependent β cell immunogenicity.

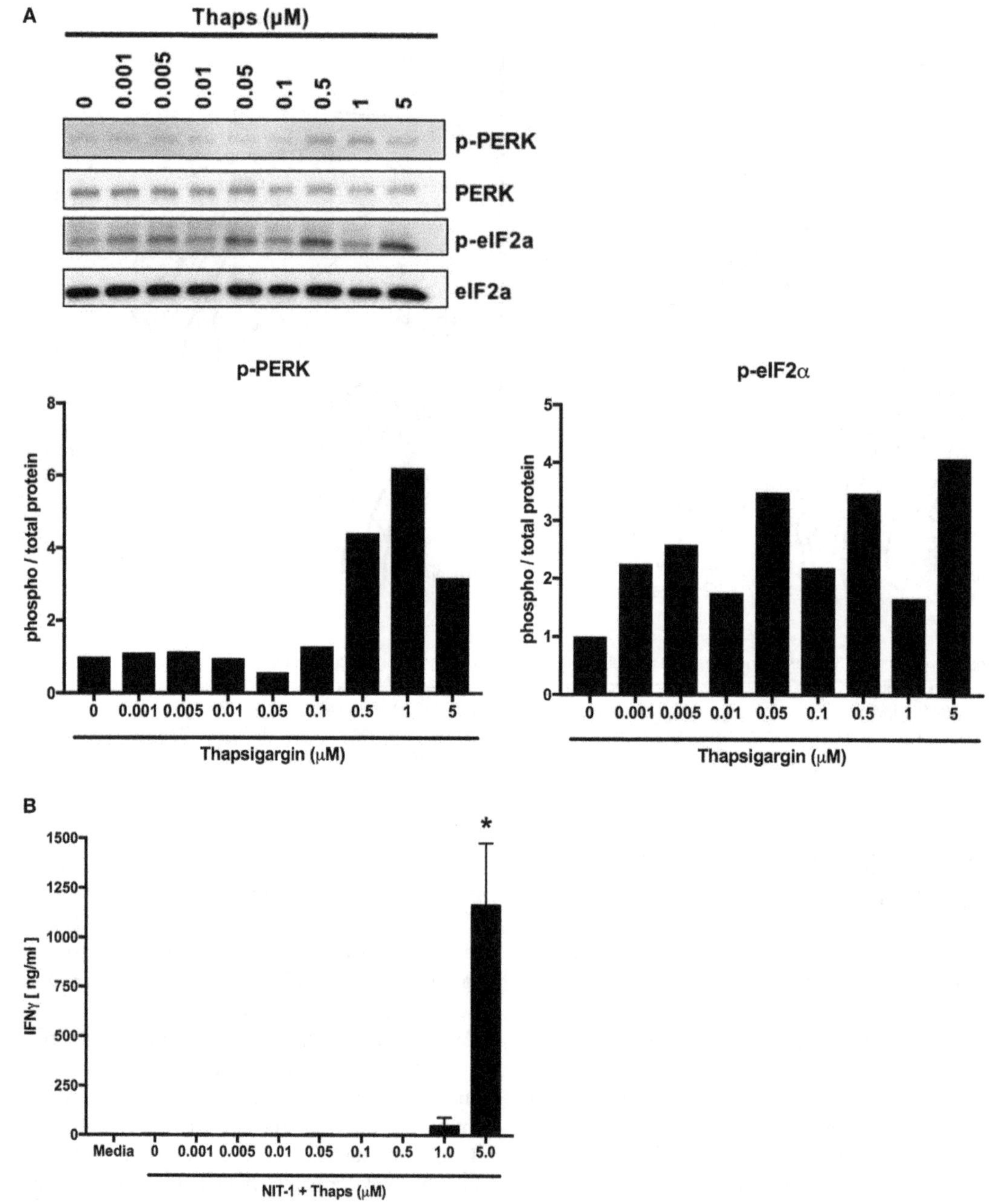

FIGURE 5 | Endoplasmic reticulum stress must increase above a threshold to induce posttranslational modification-dependent immunogenicity. **(A)** NIT-1 insulinoma cells were incubated with increasing concentrations of thapsigargin for 1 h and washed extensively. Cell lysates were analyzed for the phosphorylation of UPR proteins—protein kinase RNA (PKR)-like ER kinase (PERK) and eIF2α. Data are representative of two independent experiments. Densitometry data are phosphorylation levels normalized by total protein and relative to that in control (0 μM) treated cells. **(B)** The immunogenicity of NIT-1 cells treated with increasing concentrations of thapsigargin for 1 h was measured by BDC2.5 T cell assay. Data are mean interferon gamma (IFNγ) secretion ± SEM. $^*p < 0.05$.

ENVIRONMENTAL FACTORS ASSOCIATED WITH T1D INDUCE HEIGHTENED β CELL ER STRESS

Every pancreas undergoes ER stress (32, 81), but this stress does not lead to T1D in every individual. In fact, even in those with a genetic predisposition to autoimmunity, T1D may never occur (155) or may occur much later than expected (156, 157). These observations suggest that environmental factors may precipitate disease onset. Indeed, T1D onset is associated with several environmental factors such as viral infection (43–48), chemicals (49–51), ROS (52–55), dysglycemia (56), and inflammation (57–59). Although these environmental factors are thought to exacerbate the autoimmune targeting of β cells and hasten

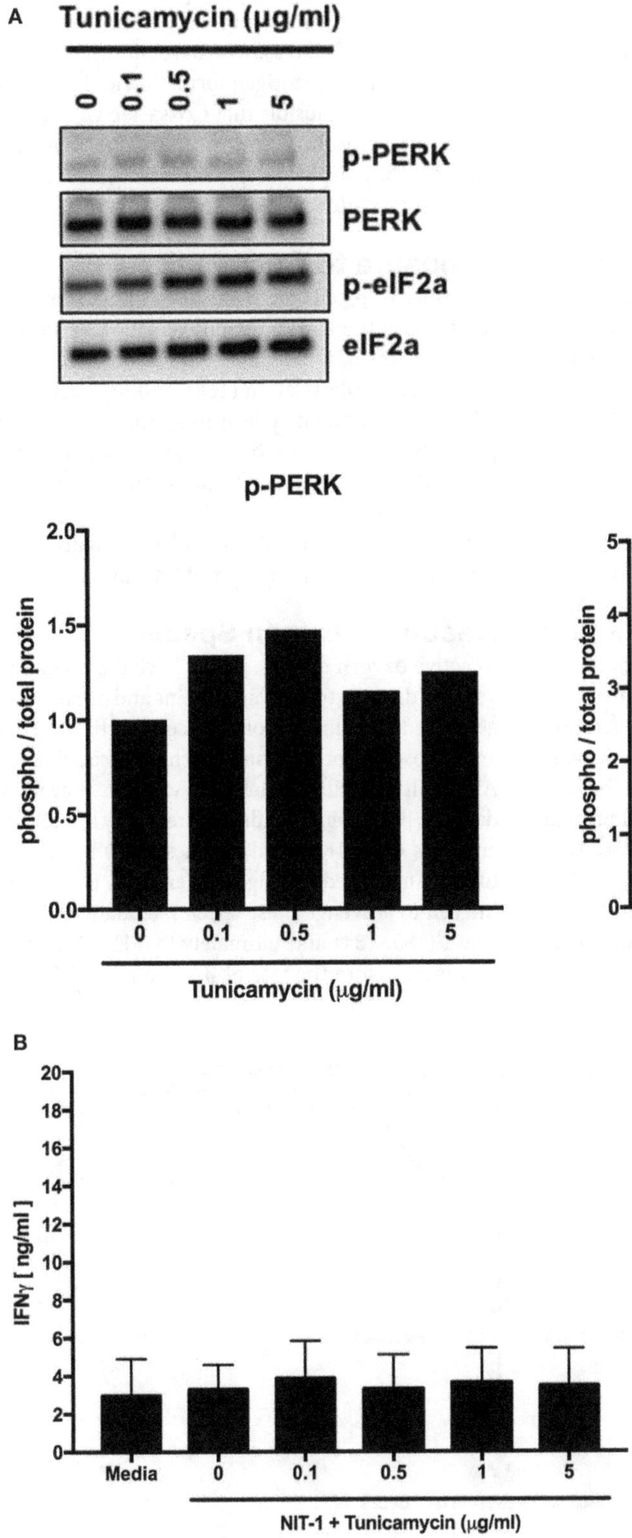

FIGURE 6 | Endoplasmic reticulum stress below a threshold does not induce posttranslational modification-dependent immunogenicity. **(A)** NIT-1 insulinoma cells were incubated with increasing concentrations of tunicamycin for 4 h and washed extensively. Cell lysates were analyzed for the phosphorylation of UPR proteins—protein kinase RNA (PKR)-like ER kinase (PERK) and eIF2α. Data are representative of two independent experiments. Densitometry data are phosphorylation levels normalized by total protein and relative to that in control (0 μg/ml) treated cells. **(B)** The immunogenicity of NIT-1 cells treated with increasing concentrations of tunicamycin for 4 h was measured by BDC2.5 T cell assay. Data are mean interferon gamma (IFNγ) secretion ± SEM.

disease onset, the mechanisms by which these environmental factors advance pathology, and whether these factors contribute to PTM-mediated neo-antigen formation, remain unknown (**Figure 1**).

As discussed earlier, β cell ER stress and Ca^{2+} flux into the cytosol must cross a threshold before Tgase2 and PAD2 can modify β cell proteins to generate neo-antigens and elicit effector responses from diabetogenic T cells. While β cell physiology causes ER stress (32–42) and this ER stress can, under some circumstances generate neo-antigens and immunogenicity (32, 60) (**Figure 1**), the discrepancy in disease onset in those genetically predisposed to autoimmunity (155–157) suggests that this physiological stress alone may not be sufficient to generate neo-antigens. Interestingly, each of the environmental factors associated with T1D also lead to an increase in β cell ER stress and cytosolic Ca^{2+}.

Coxsackie Virus

Coxsackie virus infection is associated with T1D onset. Recent onset T1D patients have viral RNA in their pancreas and higher titers of antibodies against Coxsackie virus (158, 159). Also, Coxsackie virus infection accelerates disease onset in NOD mice with established insulitis (46, 160–162), suggesting a role for Coxsackie virus in breaking immune tolerance. Studies with BDC2.5 TCR transgenic NOD mice attributed this acceleration to activation of bystander immune cells (46). These data provide a strong link between pancreatic viral infection and broken tolerance. Since BDC2.5 T cells do not recognize a viral protein (29) but rather modified CHgA, activation of BDC2.5 T cells in these mice suggests that Coxsackie virus infection may lead to PTM of endogenous β cell proteins and neo-antigen formation. Indeed, viruses cause neo-antigen generation and exacerbate pathology in other models of autoimmunity (163).

Moreover, Coxsackie virus protein 2B disrupts the ER membrane (164–166), releasing Ca^{2+} from the ER into the cytosol and causing ER stress. We have shown that β cell ER stress contributes to neo-antigen formation and immunogenicity (32). Therefore, it is plausible that Coxsackie virus may raise β cell ER stress and cytosolic Ca^{2+} concentrations above the levels attributed to normal physiology, increasing neo-antigen production through Ca^{2+}-dependent PTM.

Exposure to Chemicals

Exposure of β cells to chemicals such as alloxan and streptozotocin cause the loss of insulin secretion and β cell death (167). For each of these chemicals, β cells experience DNA damage, protein ADP ribosylation (168), and ROS generation (169–171), all of which ultimately lead to apoptosis and significant loss of β cell death. However, before apoptosis pathways are activated, ADP ribosylation and ROS cause misfolding and accumulation of nascent proteins in the ER lumen. As discussed earlier, the accumulation of misfolded and abnormally modified proteins leads to ER stress and release of Ca^{2+} into the cytosol (172, 173).

Reactive Oxygen Species

Reactive oxygen species, which have the potential to cause irreversible damage to cellular proteins and organelles (174–176), are generated both during normal β cell function (52) and when β cells are exposed to other insults such as Coxsackie virus (177–179). Although antioxidant defenses work to prevent ROS-mediated damage, β cell mitochondria express very low levels of antioxidant enzymes (180–182), making these cells particularly susceptible to ROS-mediated damage. When ROS exceeds the capacity of the cell to scavenge these species, oxidative stress leads to β cell death (183, 184) and ultimately to T1D (52, 54, 180, 185–190). However, before the loss of β cell mass, ROS leads to oxidative

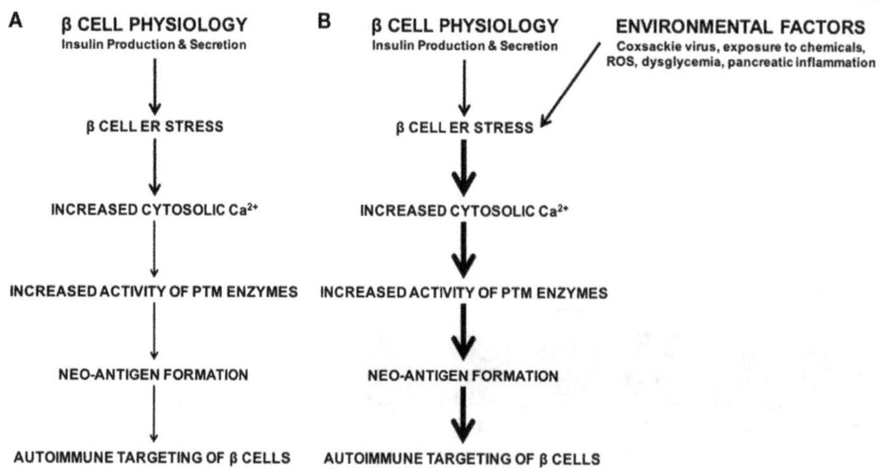

FIGURE 7 | Model. **(A)** Normal β cell secretory physiology causes inherent endoplasmic reticulum (ER) stress, which in turn results in a release of Ca^{2+} from the ER into the cytosol. This ER stress and Ca^{2+} efflux lead to increased activity of Ca^{2+}-dependent posttranslational modification (PTM) enzymes, formation of neo-antigens, and β cell immunogenicity (32). However, neo-antigen formation and immunogenicity due to inherent physiological ER stress may not be enough to cause type 1 diabetes (T1D). **(B)** The environmental factors associated with T1D onset cause β cell ER stress and Ca^{2+} efflux. The ER stress induced by these environmental factors cooperates with the physiological ER stress to raise cytosolic Ca^{2+} concentrations above a threshold to activate PTM enzymes, generate neo-antigens, cause autoimmune targeting of β cells, and precipitate T1D onset.

modification of proteins and lipids (191), and to the release of Ca^{2+} from the ER into the cytosol (192–194). Therefore, ER stress and Ca^{2+} efflux caused by ROS may lead to protein PTM and the formation for neo-antigens in β cells.

Dysglycemia

As discussed earlier, increased glucose sensing by β cells during times of dysglycemia increases insulin production and secretion (75). Normal insulin secretion raises β cell ER stress (32–42), but when blood glucose rises too high, or the hyperglycemia is too prolonged, so called "glucotoxicity" further enhances β cell ER stress. At later stages of T1D, ER stress induced by glucotoxicity is thought to be a major contributor to β cell death through the terminal UPR. However, fluctuation in blood glucose levels as β cell mass is gradually lost may also induce the adaptive UPR. In this way, glucotoxicity may, long before β cell death, contribute to Ca^{2+}- and PTM-dependent neo-antigen formation and therefore to autoimmune targeting of β cells.

Inflammation

As autoreactive immune cells infiltrate the islets to target their antigens, these activated immune cells secrete pro-inflammatory cytokines. In addition, β cells themselves release additional pro-inflammatory cytokines during viral infection (195), and cellular stress (196). These inflammatory mediators initiate signaling cascades in the β cells. For example, pro-inflammatory cytokines activate NF-kB in β cells, which inhibits the expression of other transcription factors necessary for normal β cell function (197). Also, inflammatory cytokines activate c-jun N-terminal mitogen-activated protein kinase signaling, which is associated with ER stress and Ca^{2+} release (198, 199). Finally, inflammatory cytokines reduce SERCA expression, effectively preventing the return of Ca^{2+} from the cytosol to the ER and further exacerbating ER stress (197, 200). Therefore, pancreatic inflammation may lead to β cell neo-antigen formation and exacerbate autoimmune targeting of β cells.

Therefore, we hypothesize that the ER stress generated by these environmental factors may converge with the stress caused by normal physiology to allow cytosolic Ca^{2+} to cross the necessary threshold to activate PTM enzymes and generate neo-antigens long before the terminal UPR initiates apoptosis pathways. In this way, ER stress-mediated neo-antigen formation may be a common mechanism by which these environmental factors augment autoimmune targeting of β cells and hasten T1D onset.

CONCLUSION

Type 1 diabetes is caused by the autoimmune targeting and destruction of pancreatic β cells. The autoreactive immune cells target many β cell proteins (**Table 1**) when central and peripheral tolerance fail. The mechanisms by which tolerance fails are still being elucidated, but a growing body of literature demonstrates that β cell peptides modified by Ca^{2+}-dependent PTM elicit stronger responses from autoreactive T cells than their native counterparts (16, 19, 23, 28–31, 143, 145). However, the mechanisms by which these β cell peptides become modified during β cell physiology is only beginning to be explored (32, 60).

We have previously demonstrated that β cell ER stress leads to PTM-dependent immunogenicity (32). Although this ER stress may be derived from the natural secretory physiology of the β cell (32–42), inherent, physiological ER stress alone may not sufficient to precipitate T1D onset even in those individuals harboring a genetic predisposition to autoimmunity (155–157). We therefore propose a model in which β cell ER stress leads to neo-antigen formation and immunogenicity of β cells when this ER stress reaches a critical threshold. The ER stress induced by the environmental factors associated with T1D may combine with physiological ER stress to raise cytosolic Ca^{2+} above this putative threshold, allowing for the activation of PTM enzymes and the generation of PTM-dependent neo-antigens (**Figure 7**). This convergence of with physiological stress may explain how environmental factors hasten T1D onset.

It is important to note that, although physiological and environmental factor-derived ER stress likely occurs in the β cells of all individuals, autoimmunity predominantly occurs in the context of genetic predisposition to autoimmunity. For patients who express the MHC molecules that predispose them to autoimmunity, β cell neo-antigens generated during ER stress are presented by these MHC molecules and activate the T cells that escaped negative selection during development. The activation of these T cells ultimately leads to the autoimmune destruction of the β cells and to T1D onset. However, in those without this MHC predisposition, β cell ER stress may still result in the modification of β cell proteins without leading to disease. In these patients, these neo-antigens may not be presented by APC or may not be recognized if autoreactive T cells are correctly deleted from the repertoire during negative selection in the thymus. Therefore, β cell ER stress and the subsequent neo-antigen formation likely still require genetic predisposition to autoimmunity to lead to T1D.

Our model proposes a "threshold hypothesis" according to which cytosolic Ca^{2+} must cross a particular threshold to allow for the generation of PTM-dependent β cell neo-antigens. Additional studies are necessary to confirm the cooperation between physiological ER stress and that derived from exposure to environmental factors to reach this threshold. These studies will further advance our understanding both of how neo-antigens are formed in the β cell and the mechanisms by which environmental factors hasten disease onset. Such studies may reveal novel opportunities for therapeutic intervention to prevent or delay T1D onset in at-risk patients.

MATERIALS AND METHODS

Mice

Mice were bred and housed under specific pathogen-free conditions at Rangos Research Center of Children's Hospital of Pittsburgh of University of Pittsburgh Medical Center. All experiments were approved by Institutional Animal Care and Use Committee of the University of Pittsburgh.

Cell Culture

The NIT-1 insulinoma cell line was a gift from Clayton Mathews (University of Florida) and were maintained at 37°C in a 5% CO_2

humid air incubator, in DMEM (Invitrogen) supplemented with 10% heat-inactivated fetal bovine serum (Mediatech), 10 mM HEPES buffer (Gibco), 4 mM L-glutamine (Gibco), 200 μM non-essential amino acids (Gibco), 1 mM sodium pyruvate (Gibco), 61.5 μM β-mercaptoethanol (Sigma-Aldrich), and 100 μg/ml gentamicin (Gibco).

CD4$^+$, MHC class II-restricted BDC2.5, BDC5.2.9, PD12.4.4, and BDC6.9 T cells were a gift from Kathryn Haskins (University of Colorado). T cell clones were maintained in supplemented DMEM as described previously (32, 201–203).

OT-II splenocytes were harvested and prepared in supplemented DMEM as described previously (204–208).

Induction of ER Stress

NIT-1 cells were cultured in 25 cm^2 tissue culture flasks (Greiner Bio-One) with various concentrations of thapsigargin or control for 1 h at 37°C or with various concentrations of tunicamycin or control for 4 h at 37°C. Before downstream analysis, the cells were washed extensively (50,000× original volume) to remove residual thapsigargin or tunicamycin, and removed from the flask with 0.05% trypsin–EDTA (Gibco).

T Cell Assays

T cells (2×10^4), NOD.*scid* splenocytes as APC (4×10^5), and antigen (1×10^3 dispersed NIT-1 cells) were combined in 200 μl supplemented DMEM in triplicate in 96-well flat-bottom tissue culture plates (Greiner Bio-One) and incubated at 37°C for 72 h. T_H1 effector function was determined by measuring IFNγ secretion by enzyme-linked immunosorbent assay (ELISA).

Splenocyte Assay

OT-II splenocytes (1×10^6) were combined with antigen (1×10^3 dispersed NIT-1 cells) in 200 μl supplemented DMEM in triplicate in 96-well flat-bottom tissue culture plates (Greiner Bio-One) and incubated at 37°C for 72 h as described previously (204–208). T_H1 effector function was determined by measuring IFNγ secretion by ELISA.

Enzyme-Linked Immunosorbent Assay

Interferon gamma from T cell assays was measured with murine IFNγ ELISA antibody pairs (BD Biosciences) as described previously (32, 202–204, 208). Absorbance was measured at 450 nm with a SpectraMax M2 microplate reader (Molecular Devices). Data were analyzed with SoftMax Pro (Molecular Devices).

Preparation of Cell Lysates

Cells were lysed by sonication in 50 mM Tris pH 8.0, 137 mM NaCl, 10% glycerol, 1% NP-40, 1 mM NaF, 10 μg/ml leupeptin, 10 μg/ml aprotinin, 2 mM Na_3VO_4, and 1 mM PMSF. Protein concentration was determined by bicinchoninic acid protein assay (Thermo Fisher Scientific).

Western Blotting

Lysates were separated by SDS-PAGE with 10% polyacrylamide gels and transferred to PVDF membranes. Membranes were blocked in 5% BSA in TBST for 1 h, and probed with antibodies to phosphorylated PERK (Cell Signaling Technology; 1:200), phosphorylated eIF2α (Cell Signaling Technology; 1:1,000), total PERK (Cell Signaling Technology; 1:1,000), and total eIF2α (Cell Signaling Technology; 1:1,000) overnight at 4°C. Membranes were washed and incubated with HRP-conjugated goat anti-rabbit (Cell Signaling Technology; 1:2,000) for 1 h. Chemiluminescence was detected with Luminata Crescendo Western HRP Substrate (Millipore) and analyzed with Fujifilm LAS-4000 imager and Multi Gage Software (Fujifilm Life Science).

Statistical Analysis

For ELISA, data are mean IFNγ secretion ± SD or SEM (as indicated). For Western blotting, data are representative of two experiments. Densitometry data are phosphorylation levels normalized by total and relative to that in control-treated cells. Statistical significance was determined by Student's *t*-test, and statistically significant differences are shown for $*p < 0.05$.

AUTHOR CONTRIBUTIONS

MM and JP contributed to the composition of this manuscript.

ACKNOWLEDGMENTS

The authors thank members of the Piganelli Laboratory for the review of this manuscript. In particular, the authors thank Christina P. Martins, Ethan Bassin, Dr. Gina M. Coudriet, and Dr. Dana M. Previte.

REFERENCES

1. Dorman JS, LaPorte RE, Stone RA, Trucco M. Worldwide differences in the incidence of type I diabetes are associated with amino acid variation at position 57 of the HLA-DQ beta chain. *Proc Natl Acad Sci U S A* (1990) 87(19):7370–4. doi:10.1073/pnas.87.19.7370
2. Luca D, Ringquist S, Klei L, Lee AB, Gieger C, Wichmann HE, et al. On the use of general control samples for genome-wide association studies: genetic matching highlights causal variants. *Am J Hum Genet* (2008) 82(2):453–63. doi:10.1016/j.ajhg.2007.11.003
3. Todd JA, Bell JI, McDevitt HO. HLA-DQ beta gene contributes to susceptibility and resistance to insulin-dependent diabetes mellitus. *Nature* (1987) 329(6140):599–604. doi:10.1038/329599a0
4. Hogquist KA, Jameson SC. The self-obsession of T cells: how TCR signaling thresholds affect fate 'decisions' and effector function. *Nat Immunol* (2014) 15(9):815–23. doi:10.1038/ni.2938
5. Fan Y, Rudert WA, Grupillo M, He J, Sisino G, Trucco M. Thymus-specific deletion of insulin induces autoimmune diabetes. *EMBO J* (2009) 28(18):2812–24. doi:10.1038/emboj.2009.212
6. Geenen V. Thymus and type 1 diabetes: an update. *Diabetes Res Clin Pract* (2012) 98(1):26–32. doi:10.1016/j.diabres.2012.05.023
7. Driver JP, Chen YG, Mathews CE. Comparative genetics: synergizing human and NOD mouse studies for identifying genetic causation of type 1 diabetes. *Rev Diabet Stud* (2012) 9(4):169–87. doi:10.1900/RDS.2012.9.169
8. Leiter EH. The genetics of diabetes susceptibility in mice. *FASEB J* (1989) 3(11):2231–41.
9. Tochino Y. The NOD mouse as a model of type I diabetes. *Crit Rev Immunol* (1987) 8(1):49–81.
10. Wegmann DR, Norbury-Glaser M, Daniel D. Insulin-specific T cells are a predominant component of islet infiltrates in pre-diabetic NOD mice. *Eur J Immunol* (1994) 24(8):1853–7. doi:10.1002/eji.1830240820

11. Tisch R, Yang XD, Singer SM, Liblau RS, Fugger L, McDevitt HO. Immune response to glutamic acid decarboxylase correlates with insulitis in non-obese diabetic mice. *Nature* (1993) 366(6450):72–5. doi:10.1038/366072a0
12. Lieberman SM, Evans AM, Han B, Takaki T, Vinnitskaya Y, Caldwell JA, et al. Identification of the beta cell antigen targeted by a prevalent population of pathogenic CD8+ T cells in autoimmune diabetes. *Proc Natl Acad Sci U S A* (2003) 100(14):8384–8. doi:10.1073/pnas.0932778100
13. Stadinski BD, Delong T, Reisdorph N, Reisdorph R, Powell RL, Armstrong M, et al. Chromogranin A is an autoantigen in type 1 diabetes. *Nat Immunol* (2010) 11(3):225–31. doi:10.1038/ni.1844
14. Delong T, Baker RL, Reisdorph N, Reisdorph R, Powell RL, Armstrong M, et al. Islet amyloid polypeptide is a target antigen for diabetogenic CD4+ T cells. *Diabetes* (2011) 60:2325–30. doi:10.2337/db11-0288
15. Nayak DK, Calderon B, Vomund AN, Unanue ER. ZnT8-reactive T cells are weakly pathogenic in NOD mice but can participate in diabetes under inflammatory conditions. *Diabetes* (2014) 63(10):3438–48. doi:10.2337/db13-1882
16. Rondas D, Crevecoeur I, D'Hertog W, Ferreira GB, Staes A, Garg AD, et al. Citrullinated glucose-regulated protein 78 is an autoantigen in type 1 diabetes. *Diabetes* (2015) 64(2):573–86. doi:10.2337/db14-0621
17. Baekkeskov S, Aanstoot HJ, Christgau S, Reetz A, Solimena M, Cascalho M, et al. Identification of the 64K autoantigen in insulin-dependent diabetes as the GABA-synthesizing enzyme glutamic acid decarboxylase. *Nature* (1990) 347(6289):151–6. doi:10.1038/347151a0
18. Gorus FK, Sodoyez JC, Pipeleers DG, Keymeulen B, Foriers A, Van Schravendijk CF. Detection of autoantibodies against islet amyloid polypeptide in human serum. Lack of association with type 1 (insulin-dependent) diabetes mellitus, or with conditions favouring amyloid deposition in islets. The Belgian Diabetes Registry. *Diabetologia* (1992) 35(11):1080–6. doi:10.1007/BF02221685
19. Gottlieb PA, Delong T, Baker RL, Fitzgerald-Miller L, Wagner R, Cook G, et al. Chromogranin A is a T cell antigen in human type 1 diabetes. *J Autoimmun* (2014) 50:38–41. doi:10.1016/j.jaut.2013.10.003
20. Keller RJ. Cellular immunity to human insulin in individuals at high risk for the development of type I diabetes mellitus. *J Autoimmun* (1990) 3(3):321–7. doi:10.1016/0896-8411(90)90150-Q
21. Wenzlau JM, Juhl K, Yu L, Moua O, Sarkar SA, Gottlieb P, et al. The cation efflux transporter ZnT8 (Slc30A8) is a major autoantigen in human type 1 diabetes. *Proc Natl Acad Sci U S A* (2007) 104(43):17040–5. doi:10.1073/pnas.0705894104
22. Yang J, Danke NA, Berger D, Reichstetter S, Reijonen H, Greenbaum C, et al. Islet-specific glucose-6-phosphatase catalytic subunit-related protein-reactive CD4+ T cells in human subjects. *J Immunol* (2006) 176(5):2781–9. doi:10.4049/jimmunol.176.5.2781
23. Babon JA, DeNicola ME, Blodgett DM, Crevecoeur I, Buttrick TS, Maehr R, et al. Analysis of self-antigen specificity of islet-infiltrating T cells from human donors with type 1 diabetes. *Nat Med* (2016) 22(12):1482–7. doi:10.1038/nm.4203
24. Lan MS, Wasserfall C, Maclaren NK, Notkins AL. IA-2, a transmembrane protein of the protein tyrosine phosphatase family, is a major autoantigen in insulin-dependent diabetes mellitus. *Proc Natl Acad Sci U S A* (1996) 93(13):6367–70. doi:10.1073/pnas.93.13.6367
25. Bonifacio E, Lampasona V, Genovese S, Ferrari M, Bosi E. Identification of protein tyrosine phosphatase-like IA2 (islet cell antigen 512) as the insulin-dependent diabetes-related 37/40K autoantigen and a target of islet-cell antibodies. *J Immunol* (1995) 155(11):5419–26.
26. Pietropaolo M, Castano L, Babu S, Buelow R, Kuo YL, Martin S, et al. Islet cell autoantigen 69 kD (ICA69). Molecular cloning and characterization of a novel diabetes-associated autoantigen. *J Clin Invest* (1993) 92(1):359–71. doi:10.1172/JCI116574
27. Dunne JL, Overbergh L, Purcell AW, Mathieu C. Posttranslational modifications of proteins in type 1 diabetes: the next step in finding the cure? *Diabetes* (2012) 61(8):1907–14. doi:10.2337/db11-1675
28. Mannering SI, Harrison LC, Williamson NA, Morris JS, Thearle DJ, Jensen KP, et al. The insulin A-chain epitope recognized by human T cells is post-translationally modified. *J Exp Med* (2005) 202(9):1191–7. doi:10.1084/jem.20051251
29. Delong T, Baker RL, He J, Barbour G, Bradley B, Haskins K. Diabetogenic T-Cell clones recognize an altered peptide of chromogranin A. *Diabetes* (2012) 61:3239–46. doi:10.2337/db12-0112
30. van Lummel M, Duinkerken G, van Veelen PA, de Ru A, Cordfunke R, Zaldumbide A, et al. Posttranslational modification of HLA-DQ binding islet autoantigens in type 1 diabetes. *Diabetes* (2014) 63(1):237–47. doi:10.2337/db12-1214
31. McGinty JW, Chow IT, Greenbaum C, Odegard J, Kwok WW, James EA. Recognition of posttranslationally modified GAD65 epitopes in subjects with type 1 diabetes. *Diabetes* (2014) 63(9):3033–40. doi:10.2337/db13-1952
32. Marre ML, Profozich JL, Coneybeer JT, Geng X, Bertera S, Ford MJ, et al. Inherent ER stress in pancreatic islet beta cells causes self-recognition by autoreactive T cells in type 1 diabetes. *J Autoimmun* (2016) 72:33–46. doi:10.1016/j.jaut.2016.04.009
33. Araki E, Oyadomari S, Mori M. Endoplasmic reticulum stress and diabetes mellitus. *Int Med* (2003) 42(1):7–14. doi:10.2169/internalmedicine.42.7
34. Eizirik DL, Cardozo AK, Cnop M. The role for endoplasmic reticulum stress in diabetes mellitus. *Endocr Rev* (2008) 29(1):42–61. doi:10.1210/er.2007-0015
35. Fonseca SG, Lipson KL, Urano F. Endoplasmic reticulum stress signaling in pancreatic beta-cells. *Antioxid Redox Sig* (2007) 9(12):2335–44. doi:10.1089/ars.2007.1790
36. Kim MK, Kim HS, Lee IK, Park KG. Endoplasmic reticulum stress and insulin biosynthesis: a review. *Exp Diabetes Res* (2012) 2012:509437. doi:10.1155/2012/509437
37. Lipson KL, Fonseca SG, Ishigaki S, Nguyen LX, Foss E, Bortell R, et al. Regulation of insulin biosynthesis in pancreatic beta cells by an endoplasmic reticulum-resident protein kinase IRE1. *Cell Metab* (2006) 4(3):245–54. doi:10.1016/j.cmet.2006.07.007
38. Lipson KL, Fonseca SG, Urano F. Endoplasmic reticulum stress-induced apoptosis and auto-immunity in diabetes. *Curr Mol Med* (2006) 6(1):71–7. doi:10.2174/156652406775574613
39. Ortsater H, Sjoholm A. A busy cell - endoplasmic reticulum stress in the pancreatic beta-cell. *Mol Cell Endocrinol* (2007) 277(1–2):1–5. doi:10.1016/j.mce.2007.06.006
40. Teodoro T, Odisho T, Sidorova E, Volchuk A. Pancreatic beta-cells depend on basal expression of active ATF6alpha-p50 for cell survival even under non-stress conditions. *Am J Physiol Cell Physiol* (2012) 302(7):C992–1003. doi:10.1152/ajpcell.00160.2011
41. Volchuk A, Ron D. The endoplasmic reticulum stress response in the pancreatic beta-cell. *Diabetes Obes Metab* (2010) 12(Suppl 2):48–57. doi:10.1111/j.1463-1326.2010.01271.x
42. Wu J, Kaufman RJ. From acute ER stress to physiological roles of the unfolded protein response. *Cell Death Differ* (2006) 13(3):374–84. doi:10.1038/sj.cdd.4401840
43. Atkinson MA, Bowman MA, Campbell L, Darrow BL, Kaufman DL, Maclaren NK. Cellular immunity to a determinant common to glutamate decarboxylase and Coxsackie virus in insulin-dependent diabetes. *J Clin Invest* (1994) 94(5):2125–9. doi:10.1172/JCI117567
44. Harkonen T, Lankinen H, Davydova B, Hovi T, Roivainen M. Enterovirus infection can induce immune responses that cross-react with beta-cell autoantigen tyrosine phosphatase IA-2/IAR. *J Med Virol* (2002) 66(3):340–50. doi:10.1002/jmv.2151
45. Hiemstra HS, Schloot NC, van Veelen PA, Willemen SJ, Franken KL, van Rood JJ, et al. Cytomegalovirus in autoimmunity: T cell crossreactivity to viral antigen and autoantigen glutamic acid decarboxylase. *Pro Natl Acad Sci U S A* (2001) 98(7):3988–91. doi:10.1073/pnas.071050898
46. Horwitz MS, Bradley LM, Harbertson J, Krahl T, Lee J, Sarvetnick N. Diabetes induced by Coxsackie virus: initiation by bystander damage and not molecular mimicry. *Nat Med* (1998) 4(7):781–5. doi:10.1038/nm0798-781
47. Horwitz MS, Ilic A, Fine C, Balasa B, Sarvetnick N. Coxsackieviral-mediated diabetes: induction requires antigen-presenting cells and is accompanied by phagocytosis of beta cells. *Clin Immunol* (2004) 110(2):134–44. doi:10.1016/j.clim.2003.09.014
48. Schulte BM, Kramer M, Ansems M, Lanke KH, van Doremalen N, Piganelli JD, et al. Phagocytosis of enterovirus-infected pancreatic beta-cells triggers innate immune responses in human dendritic cells. *Diabetes* (2010) 59:1182–91. doi:10.2337/db09-1071

49. Like AA, Rossini AA. Streptozotocin-induced pancreatic insulitis: new model of diabetes mellitus. *Science* (1976) 193(4251):415–7. doi:10.1126/science.180605
50. Rossini AA, Appel MC, Williams RM, Like AA. Genetic influence of the streptozotocin-induced insulitis and hyperglycemia. *Diabetes* (1977) 26(10):916–20. doi:10.2337/diab.26.10.916
51. Takasu N, Asawa T, Komiya I, Nagasawa Y, Yamada T. Alloxan-induced DNA strand breaks in pancreatic islets. Evidence for H_2O_2 as an intermediate. *J Biol Chem* (1991) 266(4):2112–4.
52. Delmastro MM, Piganelli JD. Oxidative stress and redox modulation potential in type 1 diabetes. *Clin Dev Immunol* (2011) 2011:593863. doi:10.1155/2011/593863
53. Delmastro-Greenwood MM, Tse HM, Piganelli JD. Effects of metalloporphyrins on reducing inflammation and autoimmunity. *Antioxid Redox Signal* (2014) 20(15):2465–77. doi:10.1089/ars.2013.5257
54. Piganelli JD, Flores SC, Cruz C, Koepp J, Batinic-Haberle I, Crapo J, et al. A metalloporphyrin-based superoxide dismutase mimic inhibits adoptive transfer of autoimmune diabetes by a diabetogenic T-cell clone. *Diabetes* (2002) 51:347–55. doi:10.2337/diabetes.51.2.347
55. Tse HM, Thayer TC, Steele C, Cuda CM, Morel L, Piganelli JD, et al. NADPH oxidase deficiency regulates Th lineage commitment and modulates autoimmunity. *J Immunol* (2010) 185:5247–58. doi:10.4049/jimmunol.1001472
56. Sosenko JM, Palmer JP, Rafkin-Mervis L, Krischer JP, Cuthbertson D, Mahon J, et al. Incident dysglycemia and progression to type 1 diabetes among participants in the diabetes prevention trial-type 1. *Diabetes Care* (2009) 32(9):1603–7. doi:10.2337/dc08-2140
57. Held W, MacDonald HR, Weissman IL, Hess MW, Mueller C. Genes encoding tumor necrosis factor alpha and granzyme A are expressed during development of autoimmune diabetes. *Proc Natl Acad Sci U S A* (1990) 87(6):2239–43. doi:10.1073/pnas.87.6.2239
58. Jiang Z, Woda BA. Cytokine gene expression in the islets of the diabetic biobreeding/Worcester rat. *J Immunol* (1991) 146(9):2990–4.
59. Mandrup-Poulsen T, Spinas GA, Prowse SJ, Hansen BS, Jorgensen DW, Bendtzen K, et al. Islet cytotoxicity of interleukin 1. Influence of culture conditions and islet donor characteristics. *Diabetes* (1987) 36(5):641–7. doi:10.2337/diabetes.36.5.641
60. Marre ML, James EA, Piganelli JD. Beta cell ER stress and the implications for immunogenicity in type 1 diabetes. *Front Cell Dev Biol* (2015) 3:67. doi:10.3389/fcell.2015.00067
61. McGinty JW, Marre ML, Bajzik V, Piganelli JD, James EA. T cell epitopes and post-translationally modified epitopes in type 1 diabetes. *Curr Diab Rep* (2015) 15(11):90. doi:10.1007/s11892-015-0657-7
62. Gething MJ, Sambrook J. Protein folding in the cell. *Nature* (1992) 355(6355):33–45. doi:10.1038/355033a0
63. Papa FR. Endoplasmic reticulum stress, pancreatic beta-cell degeneration, and diabetes. *Cold Spring Harb Perspect Med* (2012) 2(9):a007666. doi:10.1101/cshperspect.a007666
64. Eizirik DL, Cnop M. ER stress in pancreatic beta cells: the thin red line between adaptation and failure. *Sci Signal* (2010) 3(110):e7. doi:10.1126/scisignal.3110pe7
65. Hetz C. The unfolded protein response: controlling cell fate decisions under ER stress and beyond. *Nat Rev Mol Cell Biol* (2012) 13(2):89–102. doi:10.1038/nrm3270
66. Harding HP, Novoa I, Zhang Y, Zeng H, Wek R, Schapira M, et al. Regulated translation initiation controls stress-induced gene expression in mammalian cells. *Mol Cell* (2000) 6(5):1099–108. doi:10.1016/S1097-2765(00)00108-8
67. Harding HP, Zhang Y, Bertolotti A, Zeng H, Ron D. Perk is essential for translational regulation and cell survival during the unfolded protein response. *Mol Cell* (2000) 5(5):897–904. doi:10.1016/S1097-2765(00)80330-5
68. Haze K, Yoshida H, Yanagi H, Yura T, Mori K. Mammalian transcription factor ATF6 is synthesized as a transmembrane protein and activated by proteolysis in response to endoplasmic reticulum stress. *Mol Biol Cell* (1999) 10(11):3787–99. doi:10.1091/mbc.10.11.3787
69. Lee AH, Iwakoshi NN, Glimcher LH. XBP-1 regulates a subset of endoplasmic reticulum resident chaperone genes in the unfolded protein response. *Mol Cell Biol* (2003) 23(21):7448–59. doi:10.1128/MCB.23.21.7448-7459.2003
70. Sriburi R, Jackowski S, Mori K, Brewer JW. XBP1: a link between the unfolded protein response, lipid biosynthesis, and biogenesis of the endoplasmic reticulum. *J Cell Biol* (2004) 167(1):35–41. doi:10.1083/jcb.200406136
71. Wang XZ, Lawson B, Brewer JW, Zinszner H, Sanjay A, Mi LJ, et al. Signals from the stressed endoplasmic reticulum induce C/EBP-homologous protein (CHOP/GADD153). *Mol Cell Biol* (1996) 16(8):4273–80. doi:10.1128/MCB.16.8.4273
72. McCullough KD, Martindale JL, Klotz LO, Aw TY, Holbrook NJ. Gadd153 sensitizes cells to endoplasmic reticulum stress by down-regulating Bcl2 and perturbing the cellular redox state. *Mol Cell Biol* (2001) 21(4):1249–59. doi:10.1128/MCB.21.4.1249-1259.2001
73. Zinszner H, Kuroda M, Wang X, Batchvarova N, Lightfoot RT, Remotti H, et al. CHOP is implicated in programmed cell death in response to impaired function of the endoplasmic reticulum. *Genes Dev* (1998) 12(7):982–95. doi:10.1101/gad.12.7.982
74. Shimizu Y, Hendershot LM. Oxidative folding: cellular strategies for dealing with the resultant equimolar production of reactive oxygen species. *Antioxid Redox Signal* (2009) 11(9):2317–31. doi:10.1089/ARS.2009.2501
75. Scheuner D, Kaufman RJ. The unfolded protein response: a pathway that links insulin demand with beta-cell failure and diabetes. *Endocr Rev* (2008) 29(3):317–33. doi:10.1210/er.2007-0039
76. Araki E, Oyadomari S, Mori M. Impact of endoplasmic reticulum stress pathway on pancreatic beta-cells and diabetes mellitus. *Exp Biol Med* (2003) 228(10):1213–7. doi:10.1177/153537020322801018
77. Nozaki J, Kubota H, Yoshida H, Naitoh M, Goji J, Yoshinaga T, et al. The endoplasmic reticulum stress response is stimulated through the continuous activation of transcription factors ATF6 and XBP1 in Ins2+/Akita pancreatic beta cells. *Genes Cells* (2004) 9(3):261–70. doi:10.1111/j.1356-9597.2004.00721.x
78. Oyadomari S, Koizumi A, Takeda K, Gotoh T, Akira S, Araki E, et al. Targeted disruption of the Chop gene delays endoplasmic reticulum stress-mediated diabetes. *J Clin Invest* (2002) 109(4):525–32. doi:10.1172/JCI14550
79. Oyadomari S, Mori M. Roles of CHOP/GADD153 in endoplasmic reticulum stress. *Cell Death Differ* (2004) 11(4):381–9. doi:10.1038/sj.cdd.4401373
80. Ron D. Proteotoxicity in the endoplasmic reticulum: lessons from the Akita diabetic mouse. *J Clin Invest* (2002) 109(4):443–5. doi:10.1172/JCI15020
81. Iwawaki T, Akai R, Kohno K, Miura M. A transgenic mouse model for monitoring endoplasmic reticulum stress. *Nat Med* (2004) 10(1):98–102. doi:10.1038/nm970
82. Meldolesi J, Pozzan T. The endoplasmic reticulum Ca2+ store: a view from the lumen. *Trends Biochem Sci* (1998) 23(1):10–4. doi:10.1016/S0968-0004(97)01143-2
83. Ma Y, Hendershot LM. ER chaperone functions during normal and stress conditions. *J Chem Neuroanat* (2004) 28(1–2):51–65. doi:10.1016/j.jchemneu.2003.08.007
84. Nigam SK, Goldberg AL, Ho S, Rohde MF, Bush KT, Sherman MY. A set of endoplasmic reticulum proteins possessing properties of molecular chaperones includes Ca(2+)-binding proteins and members of the thioredoxin superfamily. *J Biol Chem* (1994) 269(3):1744–9.
85. Mekahli D, Bultynck G, Parys JB, De Smedt H, Missiaen L. Endoplasmic-reticulum calcium depletion and disease. *Cold Spring Harb Perspect Biol* (2011) 3(6):a004317. doi:10.1101/cshperspect.a004317
86. Berridge MJ, Lipp P, Bootman MD. The versatility and universality of calcium signalling. *Nat Rev Mol Cell Biol* (2000) 1(1):11–21. doi:10.1038/35036035
87. Hitomi J, Katayama T, Eguchi Y, Kudo T, Taniguchi M, Koyama Y, et al. Involvement of caspase-4 in endoplasmic reticulum stress-induced apoptosis and Abeta-induced cell death. *J Cell Biol* (2004) 165(3):347–56. doi:10.1083/jcb.200310015
88. Nakagawa T, Zhu H, Morishima N, Li E, Xu J, Yankner BA, et al. Caspase-12 mediates endoplasmic-reticulum-specific apoptosis and cytotoxicity by amyloid-beta. *Nature* (2000) 403(6765):98–103. doi:10.1038/47513
89. Gil-Parrado S, Fernandez-Montalvan A, Assfalg-Machleidt I, Popp O, Bestvater F, Holloschi A, et al. Ionomycin-activated calpain triggers apoptosis. A probable role for Bcl-2 family members. *J Biol Chem* (2002) 277(30):27217–26. doi:10.1074/jbc.M202945200
90. Hajnoczky G, Davies E, Madesh M. Calcium signaling and apoptosis. *Biochem Biophys Res Commun* (2003) 304(3):445–54. doi:10.1016/S0006-291X(03)00616-8
91. Kim MJ, Jo DG, Hong GS, Kim BJ, Lai M, Cho DH, et al. Calpain-dependent cleavage of cain/cabin1 activates calcineurin to mediate calcium-triggered

cell death. *Proc Natl Acad Sci U S A* (2002) 99(15):9870–5. doi:10.1073/pnas.152336999

92. Nakagawa T, Yuan J. Cross-talk between two cysteine protease families. Activation of caspase-12 by calpain in apoptosis. *J Cell Biol* (2000) 150(4): 887–94. doi:10.1083/jcb.150.4.887
93. Lesort M, Attanavanich K, Zhang J, Johnson GV. Distinct nuclear localization and activity of tissue transglutaminase. *J Biol Chem* (1998) 273(20): 11991–4. doi:10.1074/jbc.273.20.11991
94. Park D, Choi SS, Ha KS. Transglutaminase 2: a multi-functional protein in multiple subcellular compartments. *Amino Acids* (2010) 39(3):619–31. doi:10.1007/s00726-010-0500-z
95. Orru S, Caputo I, D'Amato A, Ruoppolo M, Esposito C. Proteomics identification of acyl-acceptor and acyl-donor substrates for transglutaminase in a human intestinal epithelial cell line. Implications for celiac disease. *J Biol Chem* (2003) 278(34):31766–73. doi:10.1074/jbc.M305080200
96. Verhaar R, Drukarch B, Bol JG, Jongenelen CA, Musters RJ, Wilhelmus MM. Increase in endoplasmic reticulum-associated tissue transglutaminase and enzymatic activation in a cellular model of Parkinson's disease. *Neurobiol Dis* (2012) 45(3):839–50. doi:10.1016/j.nbd.2011.10.012
97. Wilhelmus MM, Verhaar R, Andringa G, Bol JG, Cras P, Shan L, et al. Presence of tissue transglutaminase in granular endoplasmic reticulum is characteristic of melanized neurons in Parkinson's disease brain. *Brain Pathol* (2011) 21(2):130–9. doi:10.1111/j.1750-3639.2010.00429.x
98. Russo L, Marsella C, Nardo G, Massignan T, Alessio M, Piermarini E, et al. Transglutaminase 2 transamidation activity during first-phase insulin secretion: natural substrates in INS-1E. *Acta Diabetol* (2013) 50(1):61–72. doi:10.1007/s00592-012-0381-6
99. Facchiano F, Facchiano A, Facchiano AM. The role of transglutaminase-2 and its substrates in human diseases. *Front Biosci* (2006) 11:1758–73. doi:10.2741/1921
100. Yamaguchi H, Wang HG. Tissue transglutaminase serves as an inhibitor of apoptosis by cross-linking caspase 3 in thapsigargin-treated cells. *Mol Cell Biol* (2006) 26(2):569–79. doi:10.1128/MCB.26.2.569-579.2006
101. Fok JY, Mehta K. Tissue transglutaminase induces the release of apoptosis inducing factor and results in apoptotic death of pancreatic cancer cells. *Apoptosis* (2007) 12(8):1455–63. doi:10.1007/s10495-007-0079-3
102. Ballestar E, Abad C, Franco L. Core histones are glutaminyl substrates for tissue transglutaminase. *J Biol Chem* (1996) 271(31):18817–24. doi:10.1074/jbc.271.31.18817
103. Han JA, Park SC. Transglutaminase-dependent modulation of transcription factor Sp1 activity. *Mol Cells* (2000) 10(6):612–8. doi:10.1007/s10059-000-0612-5
104. Akimov SS, Krylov D, Fleischman LF, Belkin AM. Tissue transglutaminase is an integrin-binding adhesion coreceptor for fibronectin. *J Cell Biol* (2000) 148(4):825–38. doi:10.1083/jcb.148.4.825
105. Haroon ZA, Hettasch JM, Lai TS, Dewhirst MW, Greenberg CS. Tissue transglutaminase is expressed, active, and directly involved in rat dermal wound healing and angiogenesis. *FASEB J* (1999) 13(13): 1787–95.
106. Stephens P, Grenard P, Aeschlimann P, Langley M, Blain E, Errington R, et al. Crosslinking and G-protein functions of transglutaminase 2 contribute differentially to fibroblast wound healing responses. *J Cell Sci* (2004) 117(Pt 15):3389–403. doi:10.1242/jcs.01188
107. Verderio EA, Johnson T, Griffin M. Tissue transglutaminase in normal and abnormal wound healing: review article. *Amino Acids* (2004) 26(4):387–404. doi:10.1007/s00726-004-0094-4
108. Takahara H, Tsuchida M, Kusubata M, Akutsu K, Tagami S, Sugawara K. Peptidylarginine deiminase of the mouse. Distribution, properties, and immunocytochemical localization. *J Biol Chem* (1989) 264(22):13361–8.
109. Vossenaar ER, Zendman AJ, van Venrooij WJ, Pruijn GJ. PAD, a growing family of citrullinating enzymes: genes, features and involvement in disease. *Bioessays* (2003) 25(11):1106–18. doi:10.1002/bies.10357
110. Jang B, Shin HY, Choi JK, Nguyen du PT, Jeong BH, Ishigami A, et al. Subcellular localization of peptidylarginine deiminase 2 and citrullinated proteins in brains of scrapie-infected mice: nuclear localization of PAD2 and membrane fraction-enriched citrullinated proteins. *J Neuropathol Exp Neurol* (2011) 70(2):116–24. doi:10.1097/NEN.0b013e318207559e
111. Rogers GE, Harding HW, Llewellyn-Smith IJ. The origin of citrulline-containing proteins in the hair follicle and the chemical nature of trichohyalin, an intracellular precursor. *Biochim Biophys Acta* (1977) 495(1):159–75. doi:10.1016/0005-2795(77)90250-1
112. Tarcsa E, Marekov LN, Mei G, Melino G, Lee SC, Steinert PM. Protein unfolding by peptidylarginine deiminase. Substrate specificity and structural relationships of the natural substrates trichohyalin and filaggrin. *J Biol Chem* (1996) 271(48):30709–16. doi:10.1074/jbc.271.48.30709
113. Lee HJ, Joo M, Abdolrasulnia R, Young DG, Choi I, Ware LB, et al. Peptidylarginine deiminase 2 suppresses inhibitory {kappa}B kinase activity in lipopolysaccharide-stimulated RAW 264.7 macrophages. *J Biol Chem* (2010) 285(51):39655–62. doi:10.1074/jbc.M110.170290
114. Inagaki M, Takahara H, Nishi Y, Sugawara K, Sato C. Ca2+-dependent deimination-induced disassembly of intermediate filaments involves specific modification of the amino-terminal head domain. *J Biol Chem* (1989) 264(30):18119–27.
115. Li P, Li M, Lindberg MR, Kennett MJ, Xiong N, Wang Y. PAD4 is essential for antibacterial innate immunity mediated by neutrophil extracellular traps. *J Exp Med* (2010) 207(9):1853–62. doi:10.1084/jem.20100239
116. Molberg O, McAdam SN, Korner R, Quarsten H, Kristiansen C, Madsen L, et al. Tissue transglutaminase selectively modifies gliadin peptides that are recognized by gut-derived T cells in celiac disease. *Nat Med* (1998) 4(6): 713–7. doi:10.1038/nm0698-713
117. Corthay A, Backlund J, Broddefalk J, Michaelsson E, Goldschmidt TJ, Kihlberg J, et al. Epitope glycosylation plays a critical role for T cell recognition of type II collagen in collagen-induced arthritis. *Eur J Immunol* (1998) 28(8):2580–90. doi:10.1002/(SICI)1521-4141(199808)28:08<2580::AID-IMMU2580>3.0.CO;2-X
118. Zamvil SS, Mitchell DJ, Moore AC, Kitamura K, Steinman L, Rothbard JB. T-cell epitope of the autoantigen myelin basic protein that induces encephalomyelitis. *Nature* (1986) 324(6094):258–60. doi:10.1038/324258a0
119. Martin R, Whitaker JN, Rhame L, Goodin RR, McFarland HF. Citrulline-containing myelin basic protein is recognized by T-cell lines derived from multiple sclerosis patients and healthy individuals. *Neurology* (1994) 44(1):123–9. doi:10.1212/WNL.44.1.123
120. Wallberg M, Bergquist J, Achour A, Breij E, Harris RA. Malondialdehyde modification of myelin oligodendrocyte glycoprotein leads to increased immunogenicity and encephalitogenicity. *Eur J Immunol* (2007) 37(7):1986–95. doi:10.1002/eji.200636912
121. van Stipdonk MJ, Willems AA, Amor S, Persoon-Deen C, Travers PJ, Boog CJ, et al. T cells discriminate between differentially phosphorylated forms of alphaB-crystallin, a major central nervous system myelin antigen. *Int Immunol* (1998) 10(7):943–50. doi:10.1093/intimm/10.7.943
122. Schellekens GA, de Jong BA, van den Hoogen FH, van de Putte LB, van Venrooij WJ. Citrulline is an essential constituent of antigenic determinants recognized by rheumatoid arthritis-specific auto-antibodies. *J Clin Invest* (1998) 101(1):273–81. doi:10.1172/JCI1316
123. Masson-Bessiere C, Sebbag M, Girbal-Neuhauser E, Nogueira L, Vincent C, Senshu T, et al. The major synovial targets of the rheumatoid arthritis-specific anti-filaggrin autoantibodies are deiminated forms of the alpha- and beta-chains of fibrin. *J Immunol* (2001) 166(6):4177–84. doi:10.4049/jimmunol.166.6.4177
124. Vossenaar ER, Despres N, Lapointe E, van der Heijden A, Lora M, Senshu T, et al. Rheumatoid arthritis specific anti-Sa antibodies target citrullinated vimentin. *Arthritis Res Ther* (2004) 6(2):R142–50. doi:10.1186/ar1149
125. Vossenaar ER, Nijenhuis S, Helsen MM, van der Heijden A, Senshu T, van den Berg WB, et al. Citrullination of synovial proteins in murine models of rheumatoid arthritis. *Arthritis Rheum* (2003) 48(9):2489–500. doi:10.1002/art.11229
126. Burkhardt H, Sehnert B, Bockermann R, Engstrom A, Kalden JR, Holmdahl R. Humoral immune response to citrullinated collagen type II determinants in early rheumatoid arthritis. *Eur J Immunol* (2005) 35(5): 1643–52. doi:10.1002/eji.200526000
127. Kinloch A, Tatzer V, Wait R, Peston D, Lundberg K, Donatien P, et al. Identification of citrullinated alpha-enolase as a candidate autoantigen in rheumatoid arthritis. *Arthritis Res Ther* (2005) 7(6):R1421–9. doi:10.1186/ar1541
128. Mamula MJ, Gee RJ, Elliott JI, Sette A, Southwood S, Jones PJ, et al. Isoaspartyl post-translational modification triggers autoimmune responses to self-

proteins. *J Biol Chem* (1999) 274(32):22321–7. doi:10.1074/jbc.274.32.22321
129. Monneaux F, Lozano JM, Patarroyo ME, Briand JP, Muller S. T cell recognition and therapeutic effect of a phosphorylated synthetic peptide of the 70K snRNP protein administered in MR/lpr mice. *Eur J Immunol* (2003) 33(2):287–96. doi:10.1002/immu.200310002
130. Coudevylle N, Rokas D, Sakarellos-Daitsiotis M, Krikorian D, Panou-Pomonis E, Sakarellos C, et al. Phosphorylated and nonphosphorylated epitopes of the La/SSB autoantigen: comparison of their antigenic and conformational characteristics. *Biopolymers* (2006) 84(4):368–82. doi:10.1002/bip.20458
131. Brahms H, Raymackers J, Union A, de Keyser F, Meheus L, Luhrmann R. The C-terminal RG dipeptide repeats of the spliceosomal Sm proteins D1 and D3 contain symmetrical dimethylarginines, which form a major B-cell epitope for anti-Sm autoantibodies. *J Biol Chem* (2000) 275(22):17122–9. doi:10.1074/jbc.M000300200
132. Abramson J, Husebye ES. Autoimmune regulator and self-tolerance – molecular and clinical aspects. *Immunol Rev* (2016) 271(1):127–40. doi:10.1111/imr.12419
133. Chan AY, Anderson MS. Central tolerance to self revealed by the autoimmune regulator. *Ann N Y Acad Sci* (2015) 1356:80–9. doi:10.1111/nyas.12960
134. Ucar O, Rattay K. Promiscuous gene expression in the thymus: a matter of epigenetics, miRNA, and more? *Front Immunol* (2015) 6:93. doi:10.3389/fimmu.2015.00093
135. Starr TK, Jameson SC, Hogquist KA. Positive and negative selection of T cells. *Annu Rev Immunol* (2003) 21:139–76. doi:10.1146/annurev.immunol.21.120601.141107
136. Klein L, Kyewski B, Allen PM, Hogquist KA. Positive and negative selection of the T cell repertoire: what thymocytes see (and don't see). *Nat Rev Immunol* (2014) 14(6):377–91. doi:10.1038/nri3667
137. Palmer E. Negative selection – clearing out the bad apples from the T-cell repertoire. *Nat Rev Immunol* (2003) 3(5):383–91. doi:10.1038/nri1085
138. Doyle HA, Mamula MJ. Autoantigenesis: the evolution of protein modifications in autoimmune disease. *Curr Opin Immunol* (2012) 24(1):112–8. doi:10.1016/j.coi.2011.12.003
139. Geenen V, Lefebvre PJ. The intrathymic expression of insulin-related genes: implications for pathophysiology and prevention of type 1 diabetes. *Diabetes Metab Rev* (1998) 14(1):95–103. doi:10.1002/(SICI)1099-0895(199803)14:1<95::AID-DMR200>3.0.CO;2-W
140. Chentoufi AA, Polychronakos C. Insulin expression levels in the thymus modulate insulin-specific autoreactive T-cell tolerance: the mechanism by which the IDDM2 locus may predispose to diabetes. *Diabetes* (2002) 51(5):1383–90. doi:10.2337/diabetes.51.5.1383
141. Geenen V, Achour I, Robert F, Vandersmissen E, Sodoyez JC, Defresne MP, et al. Evidence that insulin-like growth factor 2 (IGF2) is the dominant thymic peptide of the insulin superfamily. *Thymus* (1993) 21(2):115–27.
142. Jolicoeur C, Hanahan D, Smith KM. T-cell tolerance toward a transgenic beta-cell antigen and transcription of endogenous pancreatic genes in thymus. *Proc Natl Acad Sci U S A* (1994) 91(14):6707–11. doi:10.1073/pnas.91.14.6707
143. Strollo R, Vinci C, Arshad MH, Perrett D, Tiberti C, Chiarelli F, et al. Antibodies to post-translationally modified insulin in type 1 diabetes. *Diabetologia* (2015) 58(12):2851–60. doi:10.1007/s00125-015-3746-x
144. Delong T, Wiles TA, Baker RL, Bradley B, Barbour G, Reisdorph R, et al. Pathogenic CD4 T cells in type 1 diabetes recognize epitopes formed by peptide fusion. *Science* (2016) 351(6274):711–4. doi:10.1126/science.aad2791
145. Wiles TA, Delong T, Baker RL, Bradley B, Barbour G, Powell RL, et al. An insulin-IAPP hybrid peptide is an endogenous antigen for CD4 T cells in the non-obese diabetic mouse. *J Autoimmun* (2017) 78:11–8. doi:10.1016/j.jaut.2016.10.007
146. Kracht MJ, van Lummel M, Nikolic T, Joosten AM, Laban S, van der Slik AR, et al. Autoimmunity against a defective ribosomal insulin gene product in type 1 diabetes. *Nat Med* (2017) 23(4):501–7. doi:10.1038/nm.4289
147. Ientile R, Caccamo D, Griffin M. Tissue transglutaminase and the stress response. *Amino Acids* (2007) 33:385–94. doi:10.1007/s00726-007-0517-0
148. Oslowski CM, Urano F. Measuring ER stress and the unfolded protein response using mammalian tissue culture system. *Methods Enzymol* (2011) 490:71–92. doi:10.1016/B978-0-12-385114-7.00004-0
149. Tersey SA, Nishiki Y, Templin AT, Cabrera SM, Stull ND, Colvin SC, et al. Islet beta-cell endoplasmic reticulum stress precedes the onset of type 1 diabetes in the nonobese diabetic mouse model. *Diabetes* (2012) 61(4):818–27. doi:10.2337/db11-1293
150. Zhong J, Rao X, Xu JF, Yang P, Wang CY. The role of endoplasmic reticulum stress in autoimmune-mediated beta-cell destruction in type 1 diabetes. *Exp Diabetes Res* (2012) 2012:238980. doi:10.1155/2012/238980
151. Ozcan U, Yilmaz E, Ozcan L, Furuhashi M, Vaillancourt E, Smith RO, et al. Chemical chaperones reduce ER stress and restore glucose homeostasis in a mouse model of type 2 diabetes. *Science* (2006) 313(5790):1137–40. doi:10.1126/science.1128294
152. O'Sullivan-Murphy B, Urano F. ER stress as a trigger for beta-cell dysfunction and autoimmunity in type 1 diabetes. *Diabetes* (2012) 61(4):780–1. doi:10.2337/db12-0091
153. Kojima S, Kuo TF, Tatsukawa H, Hirose S. Induction of cross-linking and silencing of Sp1 by transglutaminase during liver injury in ASH and NASH via different ER stress pathways. *Dig Dis* (2010) 28(6):715–21. doi:10.1159/000324278
154. Kuo TF, Tatsukawa H, Matsuura T, Nagatsuma K, Hirose S, Kojima S. Free fatty acids induce transglutaminase 2-dependent apoptosis in hepatocytes via ER stress-stimulated PERK pathways. *J Cell Physiol* (2012) 227(3):1130–7. doi:10.1002/jcp.22833
155. Knip M, Veijola R, Virtanen SM, Hyoty H, Vaarala O, Akerblom HK. Environmental triggers and determinants of type 1 diabetes. *Diabetes* (2005) 54(Suppl 2):S125–36. doi:10.2337/diabetes.54.suppl_2.S125
156. Barnett AH, Eff C, Leslie RD, Pyke DA. Diabetes in identical twins. A study of 200 pairs. *Diabetologia* (1981) 20(2):87–93. doi:10.1007/BF00262007
157. Verge CF, Gianani R, Yu L, Pietropaolo M, Smith T, Jackson RA, et al. Late progression to diabetes and evidence for chronic beta-cell autoimmunity in identical twins of patients with type I diabetes. *Diabetes* (1995) 44(10):1176–9. doi:10.2337/diab.44.10.1176
158. Banatvala JE, Bryant J, Schernthaner G, Borkenstein M, Schober E, Brown D, et al. Coxsackie B, mumps, rubella, and cytomegalovirus specific IgM responses in patients with juvenile-onset insulin-dependent diabetes mellitus in Britain, Austria, and Australia. *Lancet* (1985) 1(8443):1409–12. doi:10.1016/S0140-6736(85)91843-4
159. Clements GB, Galbraith DN, Taylor KW. Coxsackie B virus infection and onset of childhood diabetes. *Lancet* (1995) 346(8969):221–3. doi:10.1016/S0140-6736(95)91270-3
160. Horwitz MS, Fine C, Ilic A, Sarvetnick N. Requirements for viral-mediated autoimmune diabetes: beta-cell damage and immune infiltration. *J Autoimmun* (2001) 16(3):211–7. doi:10.1006/jaut.2000.0486
161. Drescher KM, Kono K, Bopegamage S, Carson SD, Tracy S. Coxsackievirus B3 infection and type 1 diabetes development in NOD mice: insulitis determines susceptibility of pancreatic islets to virus infection. *Virology* (2004) 329(2):381–94. doi:10.1016/j.virol.2004.06.049
162. Serreze DV, Ottendorfer EW, Ellis TM, Gauntt CJ, Atkinson MA. Acceleration of type 1 diabetes by a coxsackievirus infection requires a preexisting critical mass of autoreactive T-cells in pancreatic islets. *Diabetes* (2000) 49(5):708–11. doi:10.2337/diabetes.49.5.708
163. Doyle HA, Mamula MJ. Posttranslational modifications of self-antigens. *Ann N Y Acad Sci* (2005) 1050:1–9. doi:10.1196/annals.1313.001
164. Campanella M, de Jong AS, Lanke KW, Melchers WJ, Willems PH, Pinton P, et al. The coxsackievirus 2B protein suppresses apoptotic host cell responses by manipulating intracellular Ca2+ homeostasis. *J Biol Chem* (2004) 279(18):18440–50. doi:10.1074/jbc.M309494200
165. van Kuppeveld FJ, de Jong AS, Melchers WJ, Willems PH. Enterovirus protein 2B po(u)res out the calcium: a viral strategy to survive? *Trends Microbiol* (2005) 13(2):41–4. doi:10.1016/j.tim.2004.12.005
166. van Kuppeveld FJ, Hoenderop JG, Smeets RL, Willems PH, Dijkman HB, Galama JM, et al. Coxsackievirus protein 2B modifies endoplasmic reticulum membrane and plasma membrane permeability and facilitates virus release. *EMBO J* (1997) 16(12):3519–32. doi:10.1093/emboj/16.12.3519
167. Lenzen S. The mechanisms of alloxan- and streptozotocin-induced diabetes. *Diabetologia* (2008) 51(2):216–26. doi:10.1007/s00125-007-0886-7
168. Sandler S, Swenne I. Streptozotocin, but not alloxan, induces DNA repair synthesis in mouse pancreatic islets in vitro. *Diabetologia* (1983) 25(5):444–7. doi:10.1007/BF00282526
169. Bedoya FJ, Solano F, Lucas M. N-monomethyl-arginine and nicotinamide prevent streptozotocin-induced double strand DNA break formation in pancreatic rat islets. *Experientia* (1996) 52(4):344–7. doi:10.1007/BF01919538

170. Heikkila RE, Winston B, Cohen G. Alloxan-induced diabetes-evidence for hydroxyl radical as a cytotoxic intermediate. *Biochem Pharmacol* (1976) 25(9):1085–92. doi:10.1016/0006-2952(76)90502-5
171. Takasu N, Komiya I, Asawa T, Nagasawa Y, Yamada T. Streptozocin- and alloxan-induced H_2O_2 generation and DNA fragmentation in pancreatic islets. H_2O_2 as mediator for DNA fragmentation. *Diabetes* (1991) 40(9): 1141–5. doi:10.2337/diabetes.40.9.1141
172. Kim HR, Rho HW, Park BH, Park JW, Kim JS, Kim UH, et al. Role of Ca2+ in alloxan-induced pancreatic beta-cell damage. *Biochim Biophys Acta* (1994) 1227(1–2):87–91. doi:10.1016/0925-4439(94)90111-2
173. Park BH, Rho HW, Park JW, Cho CG, Kim JS, Chung HT, et al. Protective mechanism of glucose against alloxan-induced pancreatic beta-cell damage. *Biochem Biophys Res Commun* (1995) 210(1):1–6. doi:10.1006/bbrc.1995.1619
174. Boveris A, Oshino N, Chance B. The cellular production of hydrogen peroxide. *Biochem J* (1972) 128(3):617–30. doi:10.1042/bj1280617
175. Turrens JF. Superoxide production by the mitochondrial respiratory chain. *Biosci Rep* (1997) 17(1):3–8. doi:10.1023/A:1027374931887
176. Johnson FB, Sinclair DA, Guarente L. Molecular biology of aging. *Cell* (1999) 96(2):291–302. doi:10.1016/S0092-8674(00)80567-X
177. Yoon JW, Onodera T, Notkins AL. Virus-induced diabetes mellitus. XV. Beta cell damage and insulin-dependent hyperglycemia in mice infected with Coxsackie virus B4. *J Exp Med* (1978) 148(4):1068–80. doi:10.1084/jem.148.4.1068
178. Xie B, Zhou JF, Lu Q, Li CJ, Chen P. Oxidative stress in patients with acute Coxsackie virus myocarditis. *Biomed Environ Sci* (2002) 15(1):48–57.
179. Peterhans E, Grob M, Burge T, Zanoni R. Virus-induced formation of reactive oxygen intermediates in phagocytic cells. *Free Radic Res Commun* (1987) 3(1–5):39–46. doi:10.3109/10715768709069768
180. Lenzen S. Oxidative stress: the vulnerable beta-cell. *Biochem Soc Trans* (2008) 36(Pt 3):343–7. doi:10.1042/BST0360343
181. Lenzen S, Drinkgern J, Tiedge M. Low antioxidant enzyme gene expression in pancreatic islets compared with various other mouse tissues. *Free Radic Biol Med* (1996) 20(3):463–6. doi:10.1016/0891-5849(96)02051-5
182. Grankvist K, Marklund SL, Taljedal IB. CuZn-superoxide dismutase, Mn-superoxide dismutase, catalase and glutathione peroxidase in pancreatic islets and other tissues in the mouse. *Biochem J* (1981) 199(2):393–8. doi:10.1042/bj1990393
183. Nishikawa T, Edelstein D, Du XL, Yamagishi S, Matsumura T, Kaneda Y, et al. Normalizing mitochondrial superoxide production blocks three pathways of hyperglycaemic damage. *Nature* (2000) 404(6779):787–90. doi:10.1038/35008121
184. Welsh N, Hellerstrom C. In vitro restoration of insulin production in islets from adult rats treated neonatally with streptozotocin. *Endocrinology* (1990) 126(4):1842–8. doi:10.1210/endo-126-4-1842
185. Chen J, Gusdon AM, Thayer TC, Mathews CE. Role of increased ROS dissipation in prevention of T1D. *Ann N Y Acad Sci* (2008) 1150:157–66. doi:10.1196/annals.1447.045
186. Sivitz WI, Yorek MA. Mitochondrial dysfunction in diabetes: from molecular mechanisms to functional significance and therapeutic opportunities. *Antioxid Redox Signal* (2010) 12(4):537–77. doi:10.1089/ars.2009.2531
187. West IC. Radicals and oxidative stress in diabetes. *Diabet Med* (2000) 17(3):171–80. doi:10.1046/j.1464-5491.2000.00259.x
188. Horio F, Fukuda M, Katoh H, Petruzzelli M, Yano N, Rittershaus C, et al. Reactive oxygen intermediates in autoimmune islet cell destruction of the NOD mouse induced by peritoneal exudate cells (rich in macrophages) but not T cells. *Diabetologia* (1994) 37(1):22–31. doi:10.1007/BF00428773
189. Nerup J, Mandrup-Poulsen T, Molvig J, Helqvist S, Wogensen L, Egeberg J. Mechanisms of pancreatic beta-cell destruction in type I diabetes. *Diabetes Care* (1988) 11(Suppl 1):16–23.
190. Suarez-Pinzon WL, Szabo C, Rabinovitch A. Development of autoimmune diabetes in NOD mice is associated with the formation of peroxynitrite in pancreatic islet beta-cells. *Diabetes* (1997) 46(5):907–11. doi:10.2337/diab.46.5.907
191. Santini SA, Marra G, Giardina B, Cotroneo P, Mordente A, Martorana GE, et al. Defective plasma antioxidant defenses and enhanced susceptibility to lipid peroxidation in uncomplicated IDDM. *Diabetes* (1997) 46(11):1853–8. doi:10.2337/diab.46.11.1853
192. Favero TG, Zable AC, Abramson JJ. Hydrogen peroxide stimulates the Ca2+ release channel from skeletal muscle sarcoplasmic reticulum. *J Biol Chem* (1995) 270(43):25557–63. doi:10.1074/jbc.270.43.25557
193. Gorlach A, Klappa P, Kietzmann T. The endoplasmic reticulum: folding, calcium homeostasis, signaling, and redox control. *Antioxid Redox Signal* (2006) 8(9–10):1391–418. doi:10.1089/ars.2006.8.1391
194. Xu L, Eu JP, Meissner G, Stamler JS. Activation of the cardiac calcium release channel (ryanodine receptor) by poly-S-nitrosylation. *Science* (1998) 279(5348):234–7. doi:10.1126/science.279.5348.234
195. Schulte BM, Lanke KH, Piganelli JD, Kers-Rebel ED, Bottino R, Trucco M, et al. Cytokine and chemokine production by human pancreatic islets upon enterovirus infection. *Diabetes* (2012) 61(8):2030–6. doi:10.2337/db11-1547
196. Bottino R, Balamurugan AN, Tse H, Thirunavukkarasu C, Ge X, Profozich J, et al. Response of human islets to isolation stress and the effect of antioxidant treatment. *Diabetes* (2004) 53:2559–68. doi:10.2337/diabetes.53.10.2559
197. Cnop M, Welsh N, Jonas JC, Jorns A, Lenzen S, Eizirik DL. Mechanisms of pancreatic beta-cell death in type 1 and type 2 diabetes: many differences, few similarities. *Diabetes* (2005) 54(Suppl 2):S97–107. doi:10.2337/diabetes.54.suppl_2.S97
198. Lee H, Park MT, Choi BH, Oh ET, Song MJ, Lee J, et al. Endoplasmic reticulum stress-induced JNK activation is a critical event leading to mitochondria-mediated cell death caused by beta-lapachone treatment. *PLoS One* (2011) 6(6):e21533. doi:10.1371/journal.pone.0021533
199. Wang Q, Zhang H, Zhao B, Fei H. IL-1beta caused pancreatic beta-cells apoptosis is mediated in part by endoplasmic reticulum stress via the induction of endoplasmic reticulum Ca2+ release through the c-Jun N-terminal kinase pathway. *Mol Cell Biochem* (2009) 324(1–2):183–90. doi:10.1007/s11010-008-9997-9
200. Cardozo AK, Ortis F, Storling J, Feng YM, Rasschaert J, Tonnesen M, et al. Cytokines downregulate the sarcoendoplasmic reticulum pump Ca2+ ATPase 2b and deplete endoplasmic reticulum Ca2+, leading to induction of endoplasmic reticulum stress in pancreatic beta-cells. *Diabetes* (2005) 54(2): 452–61. doi:10.2337/diabetes.54.2.452
201. Haskins K, Portas M, Bradley B, Wegmann D, Lafferty K. T-lymphocyte clone specific for pancreatic islet antigen. *Diabetes* (1988) 37(10):1444–8. doi:10.2337/diab.37.10.1444
202. Batinic-Haberle I, Spasojevic I, Tse HM, Tovmasyan A, Rajic Z, Clair DK, et al. Erratum to: design of Mn porphyrins for treating oxidative stress injuries and their redox-based regulation of cellular transcriptional activities. *Amino Acids* (2012) 42(1):95–113. doi:10.1007/s00726-010-0603-6
203. Milton MJ, Poulin M, Mathews C, Piganelli JD. Generation, maintenance, and adoptive transfer of diabetogenic T-cell lines/clones from the nonobese diabetic mouse. *Methods Mol Med* (2004) 102:213–25. doi:10.1385/1-59259-805-6:213
204. Delmastro MM, Styche AJ, Trucco MM, Workman CJ, Vignali DA, Piganelli JD. Modulation of redox balance leaves murine diabetogenic TH1 T cells "LAG-3-ing" behind. *Diabetes* (2012) 61(7):1760–8. doi:10.2337/db11-1591
205. Previte DM, O'Connor EC, Novak EA, Martins CP, Mollen KP, Piganelli JD. Reactive oxygen species are required for driving efficient and sustained aerobic glycolysis during CD4+ T cell activation. *PLoS One* (2017) 12(4): e0175549. doi:10.1371/journal.pone.0175549
206. Sklavos MM, Coudriet GM, Delmastro M, Bertera S, Coneybeer JT, He J, et al. Administration of a negative vaccination induces hyporesponsiveness to islet allografts. *Cell Transplant* (2013) 22(7):1147–55. doi:10.3727/096368912X657233
207. Sklavos MM, Tse HM, Piganelli JD. Redox modulation inhibits CD8 T cell effector function. *Free Radic Biol Med* (2008) 45:1477–86. doi:10.1016/j.freeradbiomed.2008.08.023
208. Tse HM, Milton MJ, Schreiner S, Profozich JL, Trucco M, Piganelli JD. Disruption of innate-mediated proinflammatory cytokine and reactive oxygen species third signal leads to antigen-specific hyporesponsiveness. *J Immunol* (2007) 178:908–17. doi:10.4049/jimmunol.178.2.908

12

Endoplasmic Reticulum-Mitochondria Crosstalk and Beta-Cell Destruction in Type 1 Diabetes

Saurabh Vig[1†], Joost M. Lambooij[1,2†], Arnaud Zaldumbide[1†] and Bruno Guigas[2*†]*

[1] Department of Cell and Chemical Biology, Leiden University Medical Center, Leiden, Netherlands, [2] Department of Parasitology, Leiden University Medical Center, Leiden, Netherlands

***Correspondence:**
Bruno Guigas
b.g.a.guigas@lumc.nl
Arnaud Zaldumbide
a.zaldumbide@lumc.nl*

[†]These authors have contributed equally to this work

Beta-cell destruction in type 1 diabetes (T1D) results from the combined effect of inflammation and recurrent autoimmunity. In response to inflammatory signals, beta-cells engage adaptive mechanisms where the endoplasmic reticulum (ER) and mitochondria act in concert to restore cellular homeostasis. In the recent years it has become clear that this adaptive phase may trigger the development of autoimmunity by the generation of autoantigens recognized by autoreactive CD8 T cells. The participation of the ER stress and the unfolded protein response to the increased visibility of beta-cells to the immune system has been largely described. However, the role of the other cellular organelles, and in particular the mitochondria that are central mediator for beta-cell survival and function, remains poorly investigated. In this review we will dissect the crosstalk between the ER and mitochondria in the context of T1D, highlighting the key role played by this interaction in beta-cell dysfunctions and immune activation, especially through regulation of calcium homeostasis, oxidative stress and generation of mitochondrial-derived factors.

Keywords: endoplasmic reticulum, ER stress, mitochondria, Type 1 diabetes (T1D), beta-cell, inflammation, cytokines

INTRODUCTION

Type 1 diabetes (T1D) is an autoimmune disease that targets pancreatic beta-cells, leading to their progressive loss (1). For years, impaired thymic education or low affinity T cells were thought to be responsible of the immune attack directed against native self-proteins. However, accumulating evidence suggest that local inflammation or other forms of stress, like viral infection, toxic chemical exposure or dysglycemia, combined with genetic predisposition may lead to the generation and accumulation of aberrant or modified proteins to which central tolerance is lacking, thereby triggering autoimmunity (2–4).

The endoplasmic reticulum (ER), is the hub for protein synthesis, folding, modification and transport as well as for phospholipid and cholesterol biosynthesis (5). Alterations in ER homeostasis due to inflammatory stress, accumulation of misfolded proteins, and/or alterations in the cellular Ca^{2+} or redox balance triggers an unfolded protein response (UPR) through activation of ER transmembrane proteins [*e.g.* double-stranded RNA-activated protein kinase (PKR)-like ER kinase (PERK), inositol-requiring enzyme 1α (IRE1α) and activating transcription factor 6 (ATF6)]. These central mediators of the UPR sense the accumulation of misfolded proteins in the ER lumen and activate mechanisms to inhibit protein synthesis, restore expression of chaperones, like the 78-kDa glucose regulated protein [also known as binding immunoglobulin protein] (GRP78/BiP), and initiate ER associated degradation pathway to eliminate newly synthesized proteins through proteasome-mediated degradation (6, 7). Persistent stimulation of the UPR in response to ER stress induces apoptosis *via* activation of C/EBP homologous protein (CHOP), c-jun N-terminal kinase (JNK), death protein 5 (DP5) and other pro-apoptotic signals (8, 9). Several studies, have demonstrated that this adaptive phase disturbs (post)-transcriptional, (post)-translational and degradation processes, increasing the complexity of the beta-cell proteome and peptidome, promoting the generation of neoantigens (10, 11).

Like the ER, mitochondria are complex and dynamic cellular organelles that play a key role in beta-cell functions, notably by coupling glucose metabolism to insulin secretion, but also in regulating apoptotic cell death *via* the production of reactive oxygen species (ROS) and release of cytochrome C (12, 13). In most eukaryotic cells, including beta-cells, mitochondria form dynamic networks that are continually reshaped by fission and fusion processes, under the control of specific mitochondrial membrane anchor proteins. Induction of the mitochondria UPR (UPRmt) plays an essential role in the maintenance of the mitochondrial integrity, dynamics and function in response to various stressors (14, 15). Currently, little is known regarding the impact of pro-inflammatory stimuli on mitochondrial dynamics/bioenergetics and UPRmt in human beta-cells. Yet, the interaction between the ER and mitochondria during the adaptive mechanism to environmental stress indicates that both organelles orchestrate the communication between the beta-cells and the immune system. Therefore, further exploring the regulatory mechanisms involved in mitochondria-ER interaction and in particular those controlling Ca^{2+} homeostasis and mitochondrial homeostasis, is required for a better understanding of the pathophysiology of beta-cell failure and its immune-related consequences in T1D.

ER-MITOCHONDRIA CROSSTALK IN BETA-CELL (DYS)FUNCTIONS

The ER and mitochondria are organelles that physically interact in a highly dynamic and regulated manner, forming specific microdomains, termed mitochondria and ER contact sites (MERCs) or mitochondria-associated membranes (MAMs) when studied at the molecular level (16). It is well established that MAMs play a central role in cellular Ca^{2+} homeostasis (17–19) and, more recently, they have also been shown to regulate mitochondrial dynamics and bioenergetics (20), ROS production (21), mitochondrial-mediated apoptosis (22), and inflammation (22, 23). MAMs are composed of membrane fractions from both the ER and the outer mitochondrial membrane (OMM) containing a large range of cell-specific molecular components involved in the tethering complex (16). Alterations in the MAMs composition and abnormal ER-mitochondria interaction have been reported to be associated with different pathological conditions, especially in type 2 diabetes (T2D) where organelle miscommunication has been suggested to underlie beta-cell inflammation, cell death and impaired metabolic function (24).

ER-Mitochondria Tethering, Ca^{2+} Homeostasis and Beta-Cell Dysfunction

The regulation of Ca^{2+} homeostasis is essential for proper beta-cell functions, because of its role in driving insulin granule biogenesis, trafficking and exocytosis but also by triggering multiple intracellular signaling pathways essential for the maintenance of beta-cell identity and survival (25). Cytosolic Ca^{2+} concentration is tightly controlled and results from a balance between its cellular influx and efflux, and its intracellular uptake and release by various organelles, such as ER, Golgi and the mitochondria, through specific exchangers, pumps, and channels (**Figure 1**). It is still unclear whether the mitochondria can play a significant role in directly buffering cytosolic Ca^{2+} in a quantitative manner under physiological conditions (26). However, acute and/or long-lasting modulation of inter-organelle communication, particularly under pathological conditions, may impact Ca^{2+} homeostasis in beta-cells. As such, channeling of the cation in between subcellular compartments, notably from the ER to the mitochondria, represents another way by which large quantities of Ca^{2+} can be conveyed and exert key regulatory roles on the organelle functions. Under homeostatic conditions, a transient increase in beta-cell mitochondrial matrix Ca^{2+} levels promotes ATP production by oxidative phosphorylation (OXPHOS). This occurs principally through direct activation of several tricarboxylic acid (TCA) cycle dehydrogenases and contributes to K_{ATP} channel-mediated opening of L-type voltage-gated Ca^{2+} channels (L-VGCCs), increased cytosolic Ca^{2+} and sustained glucose-stimulated insulin secretion (GSIS) (27). However, any perturbations of this highly regulated spatio-temporal process would result in an altered mitochondrial homeostasis that may ultimately lead to bioenergetic dysfunction, enhanced oxidative stress and cell death. The ER-mitochondrial connectivity was shown to involve a set of interacting proteins located in the MAMs (**Figure 1**, insert), allowing ER and mitochondria to share their content, especially Ca^{2+}, through the 75-kDa glucose-regulated protein (GRP75)-mediated coupling of the ER inositol trisphosphate receptor (IP3R) with the mitochondrial voltage-dependent anion-selective channel 1 (VDAC1) (28). The association formed by the ER vesicle-associated membrane protein-associated protein B (VABP) with the OMM protein tyrosine phosphatase-interacting protein-51 (PTPIP51) could also contribute in the organelle interaction (29). Moreover, proteins involved in mitochondrial dynamics were also shown to be involved in this tethering, such as mitofusin 2 (MFN2) and mitochondrial fission 1 protein (FIS1). Indeed, FIS1 can directly interact with the ER B-cell receptor-associated protein 31 (Bap31), promoting Ca^{2+} transfer from ER to the mitochondria and subsequent induction of apoptosis (30).

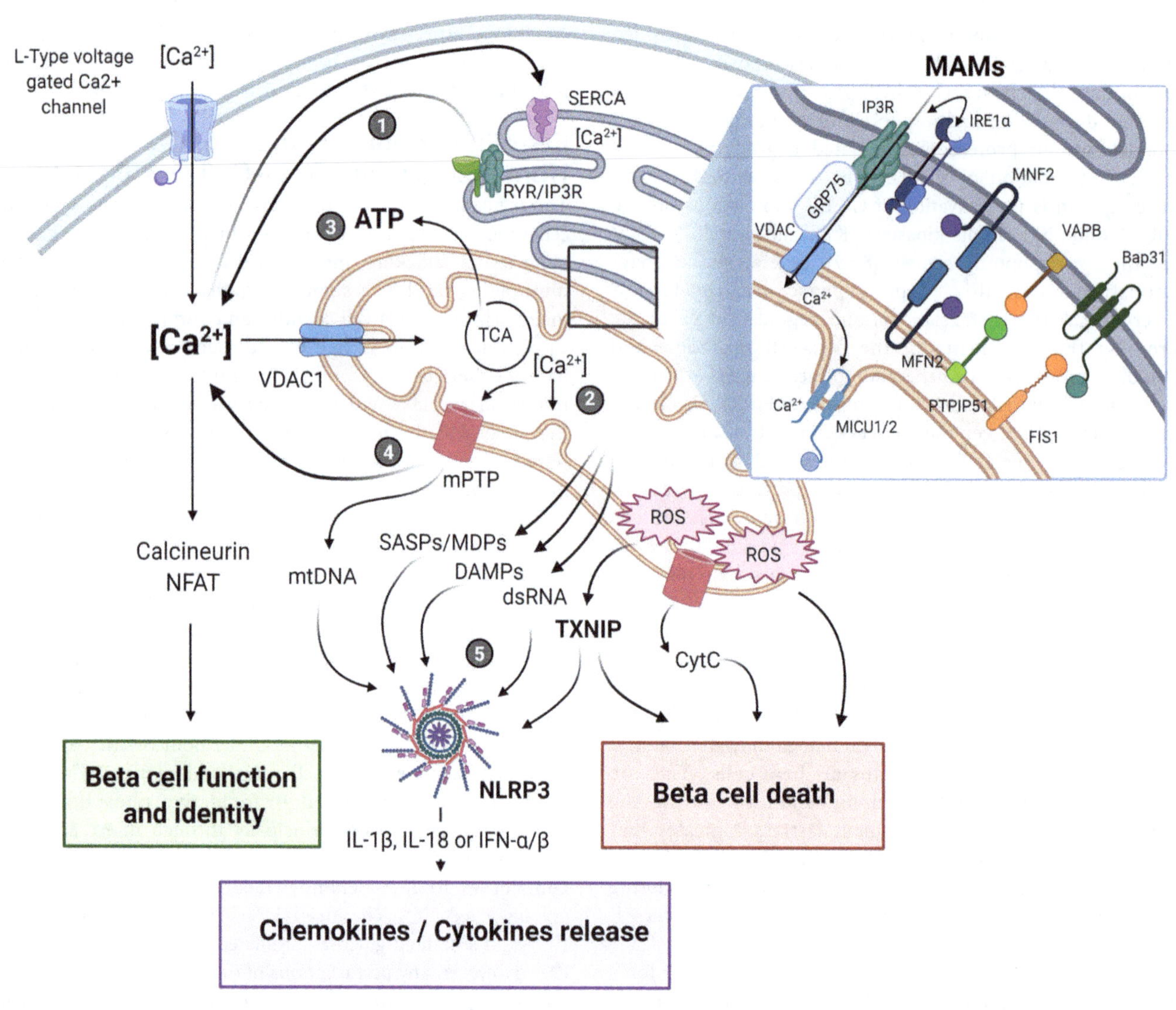

FIGURE 1 | Endoplasmic reticulum-mitochondria crosstalk in beta-cell dysfunction and immune activation in type 1 diabetes. The crosstalk between the endoplasmic reticulum (ER) and the mitochondrial network is playing a central role in cellular Ca^{2+} homeostasis and beta-cell function. The physical ER-mitochondria interaction involves a set of proteins located in the mitochondrial-associated membranes (MAMs, insert) which allows the exchange of organelle respective content. Modulation of MAM assembly has been shown to regulate mitochondrial dynamics and bioenergetics, ROS production, and release of various mitochondrial-derived factors. Alterations of these highly regulated processes in response to ER/mitochondria stress, can contribute to beta-cell dysfunction and immunogenicity by triggering apoptotic beta-cell death and NLRP3 activation, ultimately promoting pro-inflammatory cytokine/chemokine production, immune cells recruitment within the islet microenvironment, and beta-cell destruction. Upon ER stress induction, the depletion of ER Ca^{2+} store (1) induces mitochondrial Ca^{2+} accumulation (2). This increase in mitochondrial matrix Ca^{2+} concentration triggers oxidative phosphorylation and ATP production (3) in order to restore cellular and ER homeostasis. If this adaptive response fails to restore homeostasis, prolonged Ca^{2+} accumulation in the mitochondria would promote the opening of the mPTP, leading to increased mitochondrial membrane permeability and leakage of mitochondrial-derived factors, such as DAMPS, mtDNA, dsRNA (4) that ultimately activate downstream sensors/inflammasome (5). SASPs, senescence-associated secretory phenotype; DAMPs, damage-associated molecular patterns; MDPs, mitochondrial-derived peptides; ROS, reactive oxygen species; mtDNA, mitochondrial DNA; mPTP, mitochondrial permeability transition pore; CytC, cytochrome C. The figure was created with BioRender.com.

Interestingly, it has recently been reported that besides its canonical function in UPR, IRE1α also acts as a scaffold within the ER-mitochondria junction by directly interacting with IP3R, the main ER Ca^{2+} channel, ultimately affecting ER-mitochondria Ca^{2+} signaling (31). Indeed, the interaction between the respective C-terminal cytosolic domains of monomeric IRE1α and IP3R proteins within the MAMs allows for a VDAC1-mediated transfer of Ca^{2+} from the ER lumen to the mitochondrial matrix, leading to increased Ca^{2+} concentrations that trigger activation of TCA cycle and ATP production (31). Interestingly, it has been shown in pancreatic tissue sections that the number of IP3R-VDAC1 complexes assessed by *in situ* proximity ligation assay was significantly lower in beta-cells from individuals with T2D as compared to non-diabetic controls, suggesting that alterations in the ER-mitochondria interaction may contribute to beta-cell dysfunction under diabetic conditions (32). Furthermore, induction of ER stress by treatment with the long-chain fatty acid palmitate significantly reduced ER-mitochondria interactions and altered GSIS in the murine Min6-B1 beta-cell line (32). More recently, the same team has also reported that both acute or prolonged exposure to glucose may promote ER-mitochondria interactions while having opposite impact on mitochondrial Ca^{2+} homeostasis and beta-cell insulin secretion (33). Indeed, it was shown that an acute glucose challenge enhanced MAMs assembly, as evidenced by increased VDAC1-IP3R2 proximity, which was associated with higher ATP-stimulated ER-mitochondrial Ca^{2+} transfer, intramitochondrial Ca^{2+} accumulation and GSIS in rat INS-1E beta-cell line. This ER-mitochondria interaction was abolished when MAM tethering protein GRP75 was knocked down by siRNA, demonstrating that organelle coupling is crucial for beta-cell Ca^{2+} homeostasis and insulin exocytosis under homeostatic conditions (33). Counterintuitively, extending the duration of glucose exposure to mimic diabetogenic conditions also resulted in increased MAM formation in both INS-1E cells and human pancreatic islets. However, despite higher organelle interactions, chronic glucose exposure triggered ER stress and disruption of ER-mitochondrial Ca^{2+} exchange, characterized by a progressive depletion of the ER Ca^{2+} store and increased Ca^{2+} levels in fragmented mitochondria, ultimately leading to altered mitochondrial respiration and impaired GSIS (33). Remarkably, this feature also resembles the effect of pro-inflammatory cytokines in the context of T1D, with Ca^{2+} depletion in the ER being associated with enhanced protein misfolding, UPR activation, and beta-cell death (34). Of note, treatment with the ER stress inducer tunicamycin also increased VDAC1-IP3R2 interactions in INS-1E cells, suggesting that increased organelle tethering could constitute an adaptive mechanism for restoring ER-mitochondria Ca^{2+} homeostasis (33). Whether beta-cell ER stress and IRE1α-mediated UPR associated with islet inflammation in T1D would be the cause or the consequence of impaired MAM assembly that leads to altered mitochondrial Ca^{2+} homeostasis and mitochondria-mediated immune activation, remains however to be investigated.

ER-Mitochondria Crosstalk, Oxidative Stress and Beta-Cell Death

MAMs have also been identified as a critical hub in the regulation of beta-cell death, because ER stress and alterations in mitochondrial Ca^{2+} homeostasis are linked to increased local ROS production and induction of intrinsic apoptotic pathways (35, 36). IRE1α was shown to be involved in the regulation of the OMM B cell lymphoma-2 (Bcl-2) protein family. Once activated, IRE1α can bind the TNF receptor associated factor 2 (TRAF2) adaptor and activate the JNK signaling pathway, triggering apoptosis *via* upregulation of CHOP and downregulation of the anti-apoptotic protein Bcl-2 (10). Additionally, CHOP promotes Bcl-2 phosphorylation which impairs its inhibitory interaction with the pro-apoptotic proteins, Bcl-2 associated X protein (Bax) and Bcl-2 homologous antagonist killer protein (Bak). These proteins induce IP3R-mediated cytosolic release of Ca^{2+} from the ER which is next channeled into the mitochondria through VDAC1 (37, 38). This causes an increase in mitochondrial matrix Ca^{2+} concentration that triggers the opening of the mitochondrial permeability transition pore (mPTP), a non-specific channel located in the inner mitochondrial membrane (IMM), ultimately leading to cytochrome C-mediated activation of apoptotic pathway and cell death (39, 40). In addition to IRE1α, the other ER stress-driven UPR arms, involving PERK and ATF6, can also participate in MAM assembly and ER-mitochondria crosstalk. Indeed, ATF6 has been shown to promote mitochondrial biogenesis through interaction with peroxisome proliferator-activated receptor gamma coactivator 1α (PGC-1α) (41, 42), an effect that would presumably promote mitochondrial network remodeling and impact the ER-mitochondria interaction. PERK has also been reported to be located in the MAMs fraction and involved in mediating ER-mitochondria interaction during ROS-induced oxidative stress (43). Moreover, ATF4, located downstream of PERK, has been shown to regulate mitochondrial dynamics by controlling the expression of the ubiquitin ligase Parkin, that is responsible for the removal of the damaged mitochondria by mitophagy during ER stress (44). Interestingly, Parkin also mediates ER-mitochondria crosstalk during ER stress by increasing MAM microdomains assembly for maintaining intra-organelle Ca^{2+} transfer (45). In addition, ATF4 can participate to the regulation of the oxidative stress response and apoptosis in beta-cells through interaction with the transcription factor nuclear factor erythroid 2-related factor 2 (NRF2) (46–48). In fact, under inflammatory conditions, the increase in oxidative stress may lead to oxidation of cysteine residues on Kelch-like ECH associated protein 1 (KEAP1), leading to conformational changes and disruption of its interaction with NRF2. Next, NRF2 can translocate to the nucleus where it exerts a dual function. On one hand, it can form a heterodimer with ATF4 and regulate antioxidant genes (heme oxygenase-1, NAD(P)H: quinone oxidoreductase, glutathione S-transferase) and prevent cell death by activating anti-apoptotic genes (B-cell lymphoma-extra large (Bcl-xL), Bcl-2). On the other hand, it can also compete with ATF4 and inhibit its binding to the Amino Acid Responsive Element (AARE) on the CHOP promoter, ultimately limiting cytochrome C release and apoptosis (49).

Mitochondria form a very dynamic and plastic network that is continuously re-organized owing to tightly regulated processes involving fission, fusion and mitophagy-mediated clearance of dysfunctional organelles. On one hand, mitochondrial network remodeling, especially in beta-cell, is important for organelle bioenergetics and functions, including OXPHOS-driven ATP synthesis, Ca^{2+} signaling and cell survival. On the other hand, mitochondrial dynamics and their interaction with other subcellular structures are also regulated through intrinsic organelle metabolic activity and ROS production, with disrupted OXPHOS and increased oxidative stress promoting mitochondrial fission and mitophagy (50). In beta-cells, changes in the expression of mitochondrial fission/fusion proteins in response to both inflammatory and metabolic stresses have been shown to affect mitochondrial dynamic and ultrastructure, leading to impaired organelle energetics and altered beta-cell GSIS and survival (51). For instance, prolonged exposure to high glucose and/or lipotoxic environment increases the expression of the fission protein dynamin-related protein 1 (DRP1), reduces GSIS, and increases apoptotic cell death in INS-1E cells (52, 53). Similarly, DRP1 expression was found to be increased in beta-cells from dysfunctional pancreatic islets in a model of hyperglycemic T2D mice (54). In line with this, overexpression of DRP1 or FIS1 in various *in vitro* models of murine beta-cells was generally associated with increased mitochondrial fission, impaired mitochondrial bioenergetics and increased apoptosis (**Table S1**). More recently, the expression of the orphan nuclear receptor Nor1/Nr4a3, which was previously identified as a negative regulator of beta-cell mass (55), was found to be increased by proinflammatory cytokines and involved in beta-cell mitochondrial dysfunction (56). Indeed, following mitochondrial translocation, Nor1 promotes the disruption of mitochondrial network, leading to reduction in glucose oxidation and ATP production that ultimately contribute to apoptotic beta-cell death (56). By contrast, a balanced expression of the fission protein FIS1 was shown to be required for maintenance of mitochondrial network remodeling, beta-cell survival and efficient GSIS in INS-1 cells (57). Interestingly, dampening high glucose/lipid-induced beta-cell stress restores mitochondrial dynamics by increasing fusion and reducing fission, leading to decreased apoptosis in mouse islets (58).

FROM MITOCHONDRIA DYSFUNCTION TO BETA-CELL IMMUNOGENICITY?

The prokaryotic origin of mitochondria positions the organelle as a potential source of intracellular mediators that can trigger innate immunity through release of various damage-associated molecular patterns (DAMPS) and/or pathogen-associated molecular patterns (PAMPS). Among these mitochondrial-derived molecules, specific phospholipids from the OMM (59), N-formyl methionine containing peptides which are legacy from prokaryotic translation initiation phase (60), and also mitochondrial DNA (mtDNA) containing hypomethylated CpG motifs that closely resemble bacterial CpG DNA can all trigger downstream immune activation, either directly or *via* pattern recognition receptor (PRRs)-mediated activation of the inflammasome.

In response to environmental stresses that lead to altered mitochondrial homeostasis, the organelle integrity is maintained, like in the ER, by chaperones (HSP60, HSP70) and proteases (ClpXP, ATP-dependent AAA protease LON) that control protein synthesis, folding and degradation and activate antioxidant mechanisms for ROS detoxification (61). Interestingly, the humoral and T cell reactivity against both HSP60 and HSP70 reported in newly diagnosed T1D patients may illustrate the important role played by mitochondrial dysfunction and stress in triggering autoimmunity (62, 63). During ER and/or mitochondrial stress, disruption in the Ca^{2+} homeostasis opens the mPTP which may lead to cytoplasmic release of mtDNA or mitochondrial double-stranded RNA (dsRNA) from mitochondria and induction of a programmed cell death. In line with this observation, it has been shown that activation of Bax/Bak during apoptosis led to the formation of a macropores on the OMM which allows the IMM to swell out into the cytosol and release mitochondrial factors, including mtDNA and dsRNA, without caspases activation (64). Classically, the presence of cytosolic mtDNA is sensed by cyclic GMP-AMP synthase (cGAS), resulting in stimulator of interferon genes (STING) activation and downstream phosphorylation of tyrosine kinase non receptor 1 (TNK1) and interferon regulatory factor 3 (IRF3), ultimately leading to increased transcription of type 1 IFN genes (65). Alternative pathways can trigger TLR9 activation within endosomes, leading to NFκB-mediated inflammasome (NLRP1 and NLRP3) activation, increased caspase 1 activity and subsequent IL-1β and IL-18 processing (66). Although little is known on the beta-cell inflammasome, studies conducted in both INS-1E cells and human islets have shown that prototypical inflammatory cytokines of the insulitis microenvironment may differentially regulate NLRP1 and NLRP3 *via* ATF4 and NFκB pathways (67). Similarly, cytosolic accumulation of dsRNA, generated after bidirectional transcription of circular mtDNA, can be detected by several cellular sensors, including protein kinase R (PKR), retinoic acid-inducible gene I (RIG-I) and melanoma differentiation-associated protein 5 (MDA5), to inhibit protein synthesis *via* phosphorylation of the eIF2α, recruitment of TANK-binding kinase-1, inducible IκB kinase (IKKε), and activation of IFN regulatory factor 3 and 7 and NFκB, to promote type I IFN secretion (68). Altogether, these findings highlight a potential mechanism by which ER stress-induced release of mitochondrial genomic material might lead to the activation of inflammatory pathways in beta-cells, contributing to their eventual demise.

The production of IL-1β, IL-18 or IFN-α/β by islet resident innate immune cells and/or endocrine cells (69–73), among which beta-cell is probably not the major source, facilitates the recruitment of immune cells [*e.g.* monocytes/macrophages, dendritic cells (DC)] to the inflammatory microenvironment within pancreas where they might contribute to the priming and activation of adaptive immune cells (74). Type I IFNs signature has been highly associated with disease development and progression from prediabetic stage (75). Moreover, among the 50 loci linked to T1D, several are expressed in beta-cells and involved in innate immunity [*e.g.* Protein Tyrosine Phosphatase, Non-Receptor Type 2 (PTPN2), Tyrosine Kinase 2 (TYK2), Interferon Induced Helicase C Domain 1 (IFIH1) and BTB Domain and CNC Homolog 2 (BACH2)]. In addition, a recent meta-analysis comparing RNAseq data from tissues of patients with T1D (beta-cells), systemic lupus erythematosus (SLE, kidney cells), multiple sclerosis (MS, optic chiasm) and rheumatoid arthritis (RA, joint tissue), identified a type I IFN signature as a common feature, further highlighting a more global role of type I IFN signaling in the development of autoimmune disease (76).

Although it is tempting to speculate that mitochondria permeability and subsequent genetic material leakage may participate to immune activation by beta-cells, strong supportive data are currently lacking to clearly implicate these processes in T1D development. However, a recent study has reported that inhibition of VDAC1 oligomerization during mitochondrial stress reduced accumulation of cytosolic mtDNA, expression of type I IFN genes, and circulating auto antibody levels in a mouse model of SLE, highlighting the possible role of cytosolic mtDNA in triggering autoimmunity (77). Furthermore, a relation between mitochondria content and beta-cell autoimmune destruction in T1D has also been suggested by the identification of a SNP located within the mitochondrial gene for NADH dehydrogenase 2 (*mt-Nd2*) that was associated with T1D (78). In this study, the presence of the *mt-Nd2a* (resistant) allele prevented both T1D after adoptive transfer of diabetogenic CD4+ T cell clones in NOD mice and beta-cell destruction by CD8 T cells *in vitro* (78). In addition, depletion of mtDNA from βlox5 cells lowered cytokine-mediated destruction and prevented CD8 T cell-mediated cytotoxic killing (79), positioning mtDNA a potentially important trigger of beta-cell destruction.

Alterations in intracellular Ca^{2+} homeostasis by ER/mitochondria stress may also have broad consequences on the cell visibility to the immune system by generating neoantigens, through regulation of mRNA splicing and protein synthesis or proteasomal degradation (80–82). Several studies have indeed highlighted the role of Ca^{2+} as activator for post translational enzymes transglutaminase 2 (TG2) and protein arginine deiminases (PADs) involved in deamidation and citrullination, respectively. These enzymes are mainly involved in coeliac disease and RA but have also been extensively studied in the context of T1D as important component of beta-cell-directed autoimmunity (3, 83, 84). In these processes, ROS participates in the regulation of post-translation modification (PTM) enzymes, inhibiting TG2 ubiquitination in endothelial cells or controlling activity of PAD4 (85, 86). Deamidation of glutamine and asparagine residues in the insulin B chain modifies the structural properties of insulin-derived epitopes and generates perfect anchors for peptide presentation in HLA-DQ2/-DQ8 predisposing haplotype (87). Similarly, citrullination has been shown to turn the GRP78/BiP ER chaperone into an important autoantigen in T1D by an ER stress-independent mechanism involving alteration of Ca^{2+} homeostasis and activation of PADs (84). In addition, changes in cytosolic Ca^{2+} level activate nuclear factor of activated T cells (NFAT) *via* the calcineurin/calmodulin pathway which plays a critical role in beta-cell proliferation and maintenance of beta-cell mass and function. As such, immunosuppressive drugs used in islet transplantation, such as cyclosporin A or FK506, inhibit calcineurin pathway, impair beta-cell function and trigger the development of post-transplantation diabetes mellitus (New Onset Diabetes After Transplantation [NODAT]) (88). Of note, new calcineurin inhibitors, such as voclosporin, has been recently reported to have less deleterious effects on islet functions (89). Increased cytosolic Ca^{2+} also promotes phospholipase C activation and production of IP3, which stimulates Ca^{2+} mobilization and subsequent activation of protein kinase C (PKC) and downstream MAP kinases (JNK and ERK) that ultimately leads to activation of NFκB-dependent transcriptional program and increased expression of the chemokines IL8, CCL2, CXCL10 and CXCL12 (25). Although Ca^{2+} chelation had serious deleterious effect on beta-cell function and GSIS *in vitro*, it prevented DC migration to insulinoma (90) and PAD enzymes activation (4), highlighting its role as a cellular mediator in the communication with the immune compartment. This also suggests that restoration of intracellular Ca^{2+} homeostasis may inhibit immune cell trafficking to the pancreatic islets and reduce beta-cell immunogenicity. Interestingly, chemical inhibition of the NFκB pathway reduced IL-8 production by stressed human beta-cells and prevented neutrophil migration, an effect mediated by the proton exchanger GRP68 and the transcription factor RFX6 which are also involved in the regulation of Ca^{2+} homeostasis (91).

Another consequence of ER stress and mitochondria dysfunction is the induction of cell senescence (92), secondary to increased ROS production and impaired redox status (21, 93, 94). Cellular senescence is a complex cell fate response that is characterized by the release of senescence-associated secretory phenotypes (SASPs) in response to multiple types of endogenous and exogenous stressors. The SASP components are of diverse nature, including cytokines and chemokines but also a large range of soluble and insoluble factors, and can contribute to immune activation, by promoting infiltration of immune cells. Although further studies are definitely required, it has been recently reported that islets from T1D mice as well as beta-cells from T1D donors display increased markers of senescence during disease progression (95), suggesting that beta-cell senescence may be an adaptive response to prolonged cellular stress that can contribute to autoimmunity through SASPs (96). Interestingly, studies aiming at eliminating senescent beta-cells by using specific senolytic drugs show remarkable results in limiting T1D progression in mice models (95, 97). These effects were associated with reduction in insulitis and improvements of both glucose metabolism and beta-cell function (95, 97). In response to metabolic activation and stress-associated UPRmt, mitochondria can also secrete mitochondria-derived peptides (MDPs), which are small bioactive peptides encoded by mtDNA that are mainly acting as retrograde signals to regulate mitochondrial energetics (98, 99). Although supporting data are currently sparse, especially in beta-cells, one can speculate that alterations in MDPs by inflammatory microenvironment may also contribute to modulate the cell communication with the immune compartment through various signaling pathways.

CONCLUSION

Dysfunctional mitochondria has been particularly studied in the context of metabolic disorders and T2D, where it has been associated for decades to insulin resistance and beta-cell failure. Although the beta-cell failure in pancreatic islets differs in many aspect between T1D and T2D [for review (100)], the presence of an islet-specific inflammatory microenvironment characterized by elevated local concentrations of type 1 cytokines (67, 101), together with enhanced recruitment and/or activation of tissue-resident innate and adaptive immune cells (*e.g.* macrophages, B cells and T cells) (102) and accumulation of amyloid deposit (103, 104) represent common features to both pathologies. Consequently, the possibility of repurposing T2D drugs for T1D, to improve blood glucose management for relapsing metabolic and oxidative stress on beta-cells and limiting further immune destruction is worth considering. Ongoing studies using metformin, GLP-1 analogues, SGLT-2 inhibitors, or the L-VGCC inhibitor verapamil, which are either modulating mitochondrial bioenergetics/ROS/mPTP [metformin; (105–108)], ER stress [GLP-1 analogues; (109, 110)], glucose toxicity [SGLT-2 inhibitors; (111, 112)] or cellular Ca^{2+} homeostasis [verapamil; (113, 114)] are currently explored in the framework of clinical trials. These conceptually attractive novel approaches would also require further supportive mechanistic *in vitro* molecular studies in human primary beta-cells/islets and/or relevant beta-cell line models.

AUTHOR CONTRIBUTIONS

All the authors contributed equally to the review. SV and JL wrote the first draft of the manuscript. BG and AZ edited and wrote sections of the manuscript. AZ designed the figure. All authors contributed to the article and approved the submitted version.

REFERENCES

1. Ilonen J, Lempainen J, Veijola R. The heterogeneous pathogenesis of type 1 diabetes mellitus. *Nat Rev Endocrinol* (2019) 15:635–50. doi: 10.1038/s41574-019-0254-y
2. Kracht MJL, Zaldumbide A, Roep BO. Neoantigens and Microenvironment in Type 1 Diabetes: Lessons from Antitumor Immunity. *Trends Endocrinol Metab* (2016) 27:353–62. doi: 10.1016/j.tem.2016.03.013
3. Roep BO, Kracht MJ, van Lummel M, Zaldumbide A. A roadmap of the generation of neoantigens as targets of the immune system in type 1 diabetes. *Curr Opin Immunol* (2016) 43:67–73. doi: 10.1016/j.coi.2016.09.007
4. Marre ML, Piganelli JD. Environmental Factors Contribute to beta Cell Endoplasmic Reticulum Stress and Neo-Antigen Formation in Type 1 Diabetes. *Front Endocrinol (Lausanne)* (2017) 8:262. doi: 10.3389/fendo.2017.00262
5. Schwarz DS, Blower MD. The endoplasmic reticulum: structure, function and response to cellular signaling. *Cell Mol Life Sci* (2016) 73:79–94. doi: 10.1007/s00018-015-2052-6
6. Fonseca SG, Gromada J, Urano F. Endoplasmic reticulum stress and pancreatic beta-cell death. *Trends Endocrinol Metab* (2011) 22:266–74. doi: 10.1016/j.tem.2011.02.008
7. Walter P, Ron D. The unfolded protein response: from stress pathway to homeostatic regulation. *Science* (2011) 334:1081–6. doi: 10.1126/science.1209038
8. Gurzov EN, Ortis F, Cunha DA, Gosset G, Li M, Cardozo AK, et al. Signaling by IL-1beta+IFN-gamma and ER stress converge on DP5/Hrk activation: a novel mechanism for pancreatic beta-cell apoptosis. *Cell Death Differ* (2009) 16:1539–50. doi: 10.1038/cdd.2009.99
9. Nakayasu ES, Qian WJ, Evans-Molina C, Mirmira RG, Eizirik DL, Metz TO. The role of proteomics in assessing beta-cell dysfunction and death in type 1 diabetes. *Expert Rev Proteomics* (2019) 16:569–82. doi: 10.1080/14789450.2019.1634548
10. Eizirik DL, Cardozo AK, Cnop M. The role for endoplasmic reticulum stress in diabetes mellitus. *Endocr Rev* (2008) 29:42–61. doi: 10.1210/er.2007-0015
11. Thomaidou S, Zaldumbide A, Roep BO. Islet stress, degradation and autoimmunity. *Diabetes Obes Metab* (2018) 20 Suppl 2:88–94. doi: 10.1111/dom.13387
12. Chen J, Stimpson SE, Fernandez-Bueno GA, Mathews CE. Mitochondrial Reactive Oxygen Species and Type 1 Diabetes. *Antioxid Redox Signal* (2018) 29:1361–72. doi: 10.1089/ars.2017.7346
13. Las G, Oliveira MF, Shirihai OS. Emerging roles of beta-cell mitochondria in type-2-diabetes. *Mol Aspects Med* (2020) 71:100843. doi: 10.1016/j.mam.2019.100843
14. Qureshi MA, Haynes CM, Pellegrino MW. The mitochondrial unfolded protein response: Signaling from the powerhouse. *J Biol Chem* (2017) 292:13500 6. doi: 10.1074/jbc.R117.791061
15. Naresh NU, Haynes CM. Signaling and Regulation of the Mitochondrial Unfolded Protein Response. *Cold Spring Harb Perspect Biol* (2019) 11:1–17. doi: 10.1101/cshperspect.a033944
16. Herrera-Cruz MS, Simmen T. Over Six Decades of Discovery and Characterization of the Architecture at Mitochondria-Associated Membranes (MAMs). *Adv Exp Med Biol* (2017) 997:13–31. doi: 10.1007/978-981-10-4567-7_2
17. Kerkhofs M, Bittremieux M, Morciano G, Giorgi C, Pinton P, Parys JB, et al. Emerging molecular mechanisms in chemotherapy: Ca(2+) signaling at the mitochondria-associated endoplasmic reticulum membranes. *Cell Death Dis* (2018) 9:334. doi: 10.1038/s41419-017-0179-0
18. Marchi S, Bittremieux M, Missiroli S, Morganti C, Patergnani S, Sbano L, et al. Endoplasmic Reticulum-Mitochondria Communication Through Ca (2+) Signaling: The Importance of Mitochondria-Associated Membranes (MAMs). *Adv Exp Med Biol* (2017) 997:49–67. doi: 10.1007/978-981-10-4567-7_4
19. Romero-Garcia S, Prado-Garcia H. Mitochondrial calcium: Transport and modulation of cellular processes in homeostasis and cancer (Review). *Int J Oncol* (2019) 54:1155–67. doi: 10.3892/ijo.2019.4696
20. Tagaya M, Arasaki K. Regulation of Mitochondrial Dynamics and Autophagy by the Mitochondria-Associated Membrane. *Adv Exp Med Biol* (2017) 997:33–47. doi: 10.1007/978-981-10-4567-7_3
21. Janikiewicz J, Szymanski J, Malinska D, Patalas-Krawczyk P, Michalska B, Duszynski J, et al. Mitochondria-associated membranes in aging and senescence: structure, function, and dynamics. *Cell Death Dis* (2018) 9:332. doi: 10.1038/s41419-017-0105-5
22. Missiroli S, Patergnani S, Caroccia N, Pedriali G, Perrone M, Previati M, et al. Mitochondria-associated membranes (MAMs) and inflammation. *Cell Death Dis* (2018) 9:329. doi: 10.1038/s41419-017-0027-2
23. Martinvalet D. The role of the mitochondria and the endoplasmic reticulum contact sites in the development of the immune responses. *Cell Death Dis* (2018) 9:336. doi: 10.1038/s41419-017-0237-7
24. Rieusset J. The role of endoplasmic reticulum-mitochondria contact sites in the control of glucose homeostasis: an update. *Cell Death Dis* (2018) 9:388. doi: 10.1038/s41419-018-0416-1
25. Sabatini PV, Speckmann T, Lynn FC. Friend and foe: beta-cell Ca(2+) signaling and the development of diabetes. *Mol Metab* (2019) 21:1–12. doi: 10.1016/j.molmet.2018.12.007
26. Williams GS, Boyman L, Chikando AC, Khairallah RJ, Lederer WJ. Mitochondrial calcium uptake. *Proc Natl Acad Sci USA* (2013) 110:10479–86. doi: 10.1073/pnas.1300410110
27. Jung SR, Reed BJ, Sweet IR. A highly energetic process couples calcium influx through L-type calcium channels to insulin secretion in pancreatic beta-cells. *Am J Physiol Endocrinol Metab* (2009) 297:E717–27. doi: 10.1152/ajpendo.00282.2009
28. Szabadkai G, Bianchi K, Varnai P, De Stefani D, Wieckowski MR, Cavagna D, et al. Chaperone-mediated coupling of endoplasmic reticulum and mitochondrial Ca2+ channels. *J Cell Biol* (2006) 175:901–11. doi: 10.1083/jcb.200608073
29. De Vos KJ, Morotz GM, Stoica R, Tudor EL, Lau KF, Ackerley S, et al. VAPB interacts with the mitochondrial protein PTPIP51 to regulate calcium homeostasis. *Hum Mol Genet* (2012) 21:1299–311. doi: 10.1093/hmg/ddr559
30. Iwasawa R, Mahul-Mellier AL, Datler C, Pazarentzos E, Grimm S. Fis1 and Bap31 bridge the mitochondria-ER interface to establish a platform for apoptosis induction. *EMBO J* (2011) 30:556 68. doi: 10.1038/emboj.2010.346

31. Carreras-Sureda A, Jana F, Urra H, Durand S, Mortenson DE, Sagredo A, et al. Non-canonical function of IRE1 alpha determines mitochondria-associated endoplasmic reticulum composition to control calcium transfer and bioenergetics (vol 21, pg 755, 2019). *Nat Cell Biol* (2019) 21:913–3. doi: 10.1038/s41556-019-0355-9
32. Thivolet C, Vial G, Cassel R, Rieusset J, Madec AM. Reduction of endoplasmic reticulum- mitochondria interactions in beta cells from patients with type 2 diabetes. *PloS One* (2017) 12:e0182027. doi: 10.1371/journal.pone.0182027
33. Dingreville F, Panthu B, Thivolet C, Ducreux S, Gouriou Y, Pesenti S, et al. Differential Effect of Glucose on ER-Mitochondria Ca(2+) Exchange Participates in Insulin Secretion and Glucotoxicity-Mediated Dysfunction of beta-Cells. *Diabetes* (2019) 68:1778–94. doi: 10.2337/db18-1112
34. Cardozo AK, Ortis F, Storling J, Feng YM, Rasschaert J, Tonnesen M, et al. Cytokines downregulate the sarcoendoplasmic reticulum pump Ca2+ ATPase 2b and deplete endoplasmic reticulum Ca2+, leading to induction of endoplasmic reticulum stress in pancreatic beta-cells. *Diabetes* (2005) 54:452–61. doi: 10.2337/diabetes.54.2.452
35. Giorgi C, Baldassari F, Bononi A, Bonora M, De Marchi E, Marchi S, et al. Mitochondrial Ca(2+) and apoptosis. *Cell Calcium* (2012) 52:36–43. doi: 10.1016/j.ceca.2012.02.008
36. Bravo-Sagua R, Parra V, Lopez-Crisosto C, Diaz P, Quest AF, Lavandero S. Calcium Transport and Signaling in Mitochondria. *Compr Physiol* (2017) 7:623–34. doi: 10.1002/cphy.c160013
37. Bahar E, Kim H, Yoon H. ER Stress-Mediated Signaling: Action Potential and Ca (2+) as Key Players. *Int J Mol Sci* (2016) 17:1–22. doi: 10.3390/ijms17091558
38. Szegezdi E, Logue SE, Gorman AM, Samali A. Mediators of endoplasmic reticulum stress-induced apoptosis. *EMBO Rep* (2006) 7:880–5. doi: 10.1038/sj.embor.7400779
39. He J, Carroll J, Ding S, Fearnley IM, Walker JE. Permeability transition in human mitochondria persists in the absence of peripheral stalk subunits of ATP synthase. *Proc Natl Acad Sci USA* (2017) 114:9086–91. doi: 10.1073/pnas.1711201114
40. Malhotra JD, Kaufman RJ. ER stress and its functional link to mitochondria: role in cell survival and death. *Cold Spring Harb Perspect Biol* (2011) 3: a004424. doi: 10.1101/cshperspect.a004424
41. Wu J, Ruas JL, Estall JL, Rasbach KA, Choi JH, Ye L, et al. The unfolded protein response mediates adaptation to exercise in skeletal muscle through a PGC-1alpha/ATF6alpha complex. *Cell Metab* (2011) 13:160–9. doi: 10.1016/j.cmet.2011.01.003
42. Misra J, Kim DK, Choi W, Koo SH, Lee CH, Back SH, et al. Transcriptional cross talk between orphan nuclear receptor ERRgamma and transmembrane transcription factor ATF6alpha coordinates endoplasmic reticulum stress response. *Nucleic Acids Res* (2013) 41:6960–74. doi: 10.1093/nar/gkt429
43. Verfaillie T, Rubio N, Garg AD, Bultynck G, Rizzuto R, Decuypere JP, et al. PERK is required at the ER-mitochondrial contact sites to convey apoptosis after ROS-based ER stress. *Cell Death Differ* (2012) 19:1880–91. doi: 10.1038/cdd.2012.74
44. Bouman L, Schlierf A, Lutz AK, Shan J, Deinlein A, Kast J, et al. Parkin is transcriptionally regulated by ATF4: evidence for an interconnection between mitochondrial stress and ER stress. *Cell Death Differ* (2011) 18:769–82. doi: 10.1038/cdd.2010.142
45. Cali T, Ottolini D, Negro A, Brini M. Enhanced parkin levels favor ER-mitochondria crosstalk and guarantee Ca(2+) transfer to sustain cell bioenergetics. *Biochim Biophys Acta* (2013) 1832:495–508. doi: 10.1016/j.bbadis.2013.01.004
46. Chen W, Yuan C, Lu Y, Zhu Q, Ma X, Xiao W, et al. Tanshinone IIA Protects against Acute Pancreatitis in Mice by Inhibiting Oxidative Stress via the Nrf2/ROS Pathway. *Oxid Med Cell Longev* (2020) 2020:5390482. doi: 10.1155/2020/5390482
47. Sarcinelli C, Dragic H, Piecyk M, Barbet V, Duret C, Barthelaix A, et al. ATF4-Dependent NRF2 Transcriptional Regulation Promotes Antioxidant Protection during Endoplasmic Reticulum Stress. *Cancers (Basel)* (2020) 12:1–13. doi: 10.3390/cancers12030569
48. Yagishita Y, Fukutomi T, Sugawara A, Kawamura H, Takahashi T, Pi J, et al. Nrf2 protects pancreatic beta-cells from oxidative and nitrosative stress in diabetic model mice. *Diabetes* (2014) 63:605–18. doi: 10.2337/db13-0909
49. Kasai S, Yamazaki H, Tanji K, Engler MJ, Matsumiya T, Itoh K. Role of the ISR-ATF4 pathway and its cross talk with Nrf2 in mitochondrial quality control. *J Clin Biochem Nutr* (2019) 64:1–12. doi: 10.3164/jcbn.18-37
50. Frank M, Duvezin-Caubet S, Koob S, Occhipinti A, Jagasia R, Petcherski A, et al. Mitophagy is triggered by mild oxidative stress in a mitochondrial fission dependent manner. *Biochim Biophys Acta* (2012) 1823:2297–310. doi: 10.1016/j.bbamcr.2012.08.007
51. Park KS, Wiederkehr A, Kirkpatrick C, Mattenberger Y, Martinou JC, Marchetti P, et al. Selective actions of mitochondrial fission/fusion genes on metabolism-secretion coupling in insulin-releasing cells. *J Biol Chem* (2008) 283:33347–56. doi: 10.1074/jbc.M806251200
52. Men X, Wang H, Li M, Cai H, Xu S, Zhang W, et al. Dynamin-related protein 1 mediates high glucose induced pancreatic beta cell apoptosis. *Int J Biochem Cell Biol* (2009) 41:879–90. doi: 10.1016/j.biocel.2008.08.031
53. Hoppins S, Nunnari J. Cell Biology. Mitochondrial dynamics and apoptosis–the ER connection. *Science* (2012) 337:1052–4. doi: 10.1126/science.1224709
54. Reinhardt F, Schultz J, Waterstradt R, Baltrusch S. Drp1 guarding of the mitochondrial network is important for glucose-stimulated insulin secretion in pancreatic beta cells. *Biochem Biophys Res Commun* (2016) 474:646–51. doi: 10.1016/j.bbrc.2016.04.142
55. Close AF, Dadheech N, Villela BS, Rouillard C, Buteau J. The orphan nuclear receptor Nor1/Nr4a3 is a negative regulator of beta-cell mass. *J Biol Chem* (2019) 294:4889–97. doi: 10.1074/jbc.RA118.005135
56. Close AF, Dadheech N, Lemieux H, Wang Q, Buteau J. Disruption of Beta-Cell Mitochondrial Networks by the Orphan Nuclear Receptor Nor1/Nr4a3. *Cells* (2020) 9:1–15. doi: 10.3390/cells9010168
57. Schultz J, Waterstradt R, Kantowski T, Rickmann A, Reinhardt F, Sharoyko V, et al. Precise expression of Fis1 is important for glucose responsiveness of beta cells. *J Endocrinol* (2016) 230:81–91. doi: 10.1530/JOE-16-0111
58. Molina AJ, Wikstrom JD, Stiles L, Las G, Mohamed H, Elorza A, et al. Mitochondrial networking protects beta-cells from nutrient-induced apoptosis. *Diabetes* (2009) 58:2303–15. doi: 10.2337/db07-1781
59. Arnoult D, Soares F, Tattoli I, Girardin SE. Mitochondria in innate immunity. *EMBO Rep* (2011) 12:901–10. doi: 10.1038/embor.2011.157
60. Banoth B, Cassel SL. Mitochondria in innate immune signaling. *Transl Res* (2018) 202:52–68. doi: 10.1016/j.trsl.2018.07.014
61. Melber A, Haynes CM. UPR(mt) regulation and output: a stress response mediated by mitochondrial-nuclear communication. *Cell Res* (2018) 28:281–95. doi: 10.1038/cr.2018.16
62. Abulafia-Lapid R, Gillis D, Yosef O, Atlan H, Cohen IR. T cells and autoantibodies to human HSP70 in type 1 diabetes in children. *J Autoimmun* (2003) 20:313–21. doi: 10.1016/S0896-8411(03)00038-6
63. Moin ASM, Nandakumar M, Diane A, Dehbi M, Butler AE. The Role of Heat Shock Proteins in Type 1 Diabetes. *Front Immunol* (2021) 11:612584. doi: 10.3389/fimmu.2020.612584
64. McArthur K, Whitehead LW, Heddleston JM, Li L, Padman BS, Oorschot V, et al. BAK/BAX macropores facilitate mitochondrial herniation and mtDNA efflux during apoptosis. *Science* (2018) 359:1–12. doi: 10.1126/science.aao6047
65. Riley JS, Tait SW. Mitochondrial DNA in inflammation and immunity. *EMBO Rep* (2020) 21:e49799. doi: 10.15252/embr.201949799
66. Yang Y, Wang H, Kouadir M, Song H, Shi F. Recent advances in the mechanisms of NLRP3 inflammasome activation and its inhibitors. *Cell Death Dis* (2019) 10:128. doi: 10.1038/s41419-019-1413-8
67. Ghiasi SM, Dahllof MS, Osmai Y, Osmai M, Jakobsen KK, Aivazidis A, et al. Regulation of the beta-cell inflammasome and contribution to stress-induced cellular dysfunction and apoptosis. *Mol Cell Endocrinol* (2018) 478:106–14. doi: 10.1016/j.mce.2018.08.001
68. Perry AK, Chow EK, Goodnough JB, Yeh WC, Cheng G. Differential requirement for TANK-binding kinase-1 in type I interferon responses to toll-like receptor activation and viral infection. *J Exp Med* (2004) 199:1651–8. doi: 10.1084/jem.20040528
69. Anquetil F, Sabouri S, Thivolet C, Rodriguez-Calvo T, Zapardiel-Gonzalo J, Amirian N, et al. Alpha cells, the main source of IL-1beta in human pancreas. *J Autoimmun* (2017) 81:68–73. doi: 10.1016/j.jaut.2017.03.006
70. Negi S, Jetha A, Aikin R, Hasilo C, Sladek R, Paraskevas S. Analysis of beta-cell gene expression reveals inflammatory signaling and evidence of dedifferentiation following human islet isolation and culture. *PloS One* (2012) 7:e30415. doi: 10.1371/journal.pone.0030415

71. Reddy S, Krogvold L, Martin C, Holland R, Choi J, Woo H, et al. Distribution of IL-1beta immunoreactive cells in pancreatic biopsies from living volunteers with new-onset type 1 diabetes: comparison with donors without diabetes and with longer duration of disease. *Diabetologia* (2018) 61:1362–73. doi: 10.1007/s00125-018-4600-8
72. Schulte BM, Lanke KH, Piganelli JD, Kers-Rebel ED, Bottino R, Trucco M, et al. Cytokine and chemokine production by human pancreatic islets upon enterovirus infection. *Diabetes* (2012) 61:2030–6. doi: 10.2337/db11-1547
73. Westwell-Roper CY, Ehses JA, Verchere CB. Resident macrophages mediate islet amyloid polypeptide-induced islet IL-1beta production and beta-cell dysfunction. *Diabetes* (2014) 63:1698–711. doi: 10.2337/db13-0863
74. Boni-Schnetzler M, Meier DT. Islet inflammation in type 2 diabetes. *Semin Immunopathol* (2019) 41:501–13. doi: 10.1007/s00281-019-00745-4
75. Ferreira RC, Guo H, Coulson RM, Smyth DJ, Pekalski ML, Burren OS, et al. A type I interferon transcriptional signature precedes autoimmunity in children genetically at risk for type 1 diabetes. *Diabetes* (2014) 63:2538–50. doi: 10.2337/db13-1777
76. Szymczak F, Colli ML, Mamula MJ, Evans-Molina C, Eizirik DL. Gene expression signatures of target tissues in type 1 diabetes, lupus erythematosus, multiple sclerosis, and rheumatoid arthritis. *Sci Adv* (2021) 7:1–11. doi: 10.1126/sciadv.abd7600
77. Kim J, Gupta R, Blanco LP, Yang S, Shteinfer-Kuzmine A, Wang K, et al. VDAC oligomers form mitochondrial pores to release mtDNA fragments and promote lupus-like disease. *Science* (2019) 366:1531–6. doi: 10.1126/science.aav4011
78. Chen J, Gusdon AM, Piganelli J, Leiter EH, Mathews CE. mt-Nd2(a) Modifies resistance against autoimmune type 1 diabetes in NOD mice at the level of the pancreatic beta-cell. *Diabetes* (2011) 60:355–9. doi: 10.2337/db10-1241
79. Lightfoot YL, Chen J, Mathews CE. Role of the mitochondria in immune-mediated apoptotic death of the human pancreatic beta cell line betaLox5. *PloS One* (2011) 6:e20617. doi: 10.1371/journal.pone.0020617
80. Chin KV, Cade C, Brostrom CO, Galuska EM, Brostrom MA. Calcium-dependent regulation of protein synthesis at translational initiation in eukaryotic cells. *J Biol Chem* (1987) 262:16509–14. doi: 10.1016/S0021-9258(18)49285-X
81. Krebs J. The influence of calcium signaling on the regulation of alternative splicing. *Biochim Biophys Acta* (2009) 1793:979–84. doi: 10.1016/j.bbamcr.2008.12.006
82. Mukherjee R, Das A, Chakrabarti S, Chakrabarti O. Calcium dependent regulation of protein ubiquitination - Interplay between E3 ligases and calcium binding proteins. *Biochim Biophys Acta Mol Cell Res* (2017) 1864:1227–35. doi: 10.1016/j.bbamcr.2017.03.001
83. McLaughlin RJ, de Haan A, Zaldumbide A, de Koning EJ, de Ru AH, van Veelen PA, et al. Human islets and dendritic cells generate post-translationally modified islet autoantigens. *Clin Exp Immunol* (2016) 185:133–40. doi: 10.1111/cei.12775
84. Rondas D, Crevecoeur I, D'Hertog W, Ferreira GB, Staes A, Garg AD, et al. Citrullinated glucose-regulated protein 78 is an autoantigen in type 1 diabetes. *Diabetes* (2015) 64:573–86. doi: 10.2337/db14-0621
85. Luciani A, Villella VR, Vasaturo A, Giardino I, Pettoello-Mantovani M, Guido S, et al. Lysosomal accumulation of gliadin p31-43 peptide induces oxidative stress and tissue transglutaminase-mediated PPARgamma downregulation in intestinal epithelial cells and coeliac mucosa. *Gut* (2010) 59:311–9. doi: 10.1136/gut.2009.183608
86. Tatsiy O, McDonald PP. Physiological Stimuli Induce PAD4-Dependent, ROS-Independent NETosis, With Early and Late Events Controlled by Discrete Signaling Pathways. *Front Immunol* (2018) 9:2036. doi: 10.3389/fimmu.2018.02036
87. van Lummel M, Duinkerken G, van Veelen PA, de Ru A, Cordfunke R, Zaldumbide A, et al. Posttranslational modification of HLA-DQ binding islet autoantigens in type 1 diabetes. *Diabetes* (2014) 63:237–47. doi: 10.2337/db12-1214
88. Trinanes J, Ten Dijke P, Groen N, Hanegraaf M, Porrini E, Rodriguez-Rodriguez AE, et al. Tacrolimus-Induced BMP/SMAD Signaling Associates With Metabolic Stress-Activated FOXO1 to Trigger beta-Cell Failure. *Diabetes* (2020) 69:193–204. doi: 10.2337/db19-0828
89. Kolic J, Beet L, Overby P, Cen HH, Panzhinskiy E, Ure DR, et al. Differential Effects of Voclosporin and Tacrolimus on Insulin Secretion From Human Islets. *Endocrinology* (2020) 161:1–14. doi: 10.1210/endocr/bqaa162
90. Unanue ER, Ferris ST, Carrero JA. The role of islet antigen presenting cells and the presentation of insulin in the initiation of autoimmune diabetes in the NOD mouse. *Immunol Rev* (2016) 272:183–201. doi: 10.1111/imr.12430
91. Chandra V, Karamitri A, Richards P, Cormier F, Ramond C, Jockers R, et al. Extracellular acidification stimulates GPR68 mediated IL-8 production in human pancreatic beta cells. *Sci Rep* (2016) 6:25765. doi: 10.1038/srep25765
92. Wiley CD, Velarde MC, Lecot P, Liu S, Sarnoski EA, Freund A, et al. Mitochondrial Dysfunction Induces Senescence with a Distinct Secretory Phenotype. *Cell Metab* (2016) 23:303–14. doi: 10.1016/j.cmet.2015.11.011
93. Aguayo-Mazzucato C. Functional changes in beta cells during ageing and senescence. *Diabetologia* (2020) 63:2022–9. doi: 10.1007/s00125-020-05185-6
94. Moltedo O, Remondelli P, Amodio G. The Mitochondria-Endoplasmic Reticulum Contacts and Their Critical Role in Aging and Age-Associated Diseases. *Front Cell Dev Biol* (2019) 7:172. doi: 10.3389/fcell.2019.00172
95. Thompson PJ, Shah A, Ntranos V, Van Gool F, Atkinson M, Bhushan A. Targeted Elimination of Senescent Beta Cells Prevents Type 1 Diabetes. *Cell Metab* (2019) 29:1045–60.e10. doi: 10.1016/j.cmet.2019.01.021
96. Li N, Liu F, Yang P, Xiong F, Yu Q, Li J, et al. Aging and stress induced beta cell senescence and its implication in diabetes development. *Aging (Albany NY)* (2019) 11:9947–59. doi: 10.18632/aging.102432
97. Aguayo-Mazzucato C, Andle J, Lee TB Jr, Midha A, Talemal L, Chipashvili V, et al. Acceleration of beta Cell Aging Determines Diabetes and Senolysis Improves Disease Outcomes. *Cell Metab* (2019) 30:129–42 e4. doi: 10.1016/j.cmet.2019.05.006
98. Merry TL, Chan A, Woodhead JST, Reynolds JC, Kumagai H, Kim SJ, et al. Mitochondrial-derived peptides in energy metabolism. *Am J Physiol Endocrinol Metab* (2020) 319:E659–66. doi: 10.1152/ajpendo.00249.2020
99. Kim SJ, Xiao J, Wan J, Cohen P, Yen K. Mitochondrially derived peptides as novel regulators of metabolism. *J Physiol* (2017) 595:6613–21. doi: 10.1113/JP274472
100. Eizirik DL, Pasquali L, Cnop M. Pancreatic beta-cells in type 1 and type 2 diabetes mellitus: different pathways to failure. *Nat Rev Endocrinol* (2020) 16:349–62. doi: 10.1038/s41574-020-0355-7
101. Ellingsgaard H, Hauselmann I, Schuler B, Habib AM, Baggio LL, Meier DT, et al. Interleukin-6 enhances insulin secretion by increasing glucagon-like peptide-1 secretion from L cells and alpha cells. *Nat Med* (2011) 17:1481–9. doi: 10.1038/nm.2513
102. Zhou T, Hu Z, Yang S, Sun L, Yu Z, Wang G. Role of Adaptive and Innate Immunity in Type 2 Diabetes Mellitus. *J Diabetes Res* (2018) 2018:7457269. doi: 10.1155/2018/7457269
103. Beery ML, Jacobsen LM, Atkinson MA, Butler AE, Campbell-Thompson M. Islet amyloidosis in a child with type 1 diabetes. *Islets* (2019) 11:44–9. doi: 10.1080/19382014.2019.1599707
104. Westermark GT, Krogvold L, Dahl-Jorgensen K, Ludvigsson J. Islet amyloid in recent-onset type 1 diabetes-the DiViD study. *Ups J Med Sci* (2017) 122:201–3. doi: 10.1080/03009734.2017.1359219
105. Batandier C, Guigas B, Detaille D, El-Mir MY, Fontaine E, Rigoulet M, et al. The ROS production induced by a reverse-electron flux at respiratory-chain complex 1 is hampered by metformin. *J Bioenerg Biomembr* (2006) 38:33–42. doi: 10.1007/s10863-006-9003-8
106. Detaille D, Guigas B, Chauvin C, Batandier C, Fontaine E, Wiernsperger N, et al. Metformin prevents high-glucose-induced endothelial cell death through a mitochondrial permeability transition-dependent process. *Diabetes* (2005) 54:2179–87. doi: 10.2337/diabetes.54.7.2179
107. Guigas B, Detaille D, Chauvin C, Batandier C, De Oliveira F, Fontaine E, et al. Metformin inhibits mitochondrial permeability transition and cell death: a pharmacological in vitro study. *Biochem J* (2004) 382:877–84. doi: 10.1042/BJ20040885
108. Vial G, Detaille D, Guigas B. Role of Mitochondria in the Mechanism(s) of Action of Metformin. *Front Endocrinol (Lausanne)* (2019) 10:294. doi: 10.3389/fendo.2019.00294
109. Kondo M, Tanabe K, Amo-Shiinoki K, Hatanaka M, Morii T, Takahashi H, et al. Activation of GLP-1 receptor signalling alleviates cellular stresses and improves beta cell function in a mouse model of Wolfram syndrome. *Diabetologia* (2018) 61:2189–201. doi: 10.1007/s00125-018-4679-y
110. Yusta B, Baggio LL, Estall JL, Koehler JA, Holland DP, Li H, et al. GLP-1 receptor activation improves beta cell function and survival following induction of endoplasmic reticulum stress. *Cell Metab* (2006) 4:391–406. doi: 10.1016/j.cmet.2006.10.001

111. Fattah H, Vallon V. The Potential Role of SGLT2 Inhibitors in the Treatment of Type 1 Diabetes Mellitus. *Drugs* (2018) 78:717–26. doi: 10.1007/s40265-018-0901-y
112. Asahara SI, Ogawa W. SGLT2 inhibitors and protection against pancreatic beta cell failure. *Diabetol Int* (2019) 10:1–2. doi: 10.1007/s13340-018-0374-y
113. Ovalle F, Grimes T, Xu G, Patel AJ, Grayson TB, Thielen LA, et al. Verapamil and beta cell function in adults with recent-onset type 1 diabetes. *Nat Med* (2018) 24:1108–12. doi: 10.1038/s41591-018-0089-4
114. Xu G, Chen J, Jing G, Shalev A. Preventing beta-cell loss and diabetes with calcium channel blockers. *Diabetes* (2012) 61:848–56. doi: 10.2337/db11-0955

13

Isogenic Cellular Systems Model the Impact of Genetic Risk Variants in the Pathogenesis of Type 1 Diabetes

*Mark A. Wallet, Katherine E. Santostefano, Naohiro Terada and Todd M. Brusko**

Department of Pathology, Immunology, and Laboratory Medicine, University of Florida Diabetes Institute, College of Medicine, Gainesville, FL, United States

Correspondence:
Todd M. Brusko
tbrusko@ufl.edu

At least 57 independent loci within the human genome confer varying degrees of risk for the development of type 1 diabetes (T1D). The majority of these variants are thought to contribute to overall genetic risk by modulating host innate and adaptive immune responses, ultimately resulting in a loss of immunological tolerance to β cell antigens. Early efforts to link specific risk variants with functional alterations in host immune responses have employed animal models or genotype-selected individuals from clinical bioresource banks. While some notable genotype:phenotype associations have been described, there remains an urgent need to accelerate the discovery of causal variants and elucidate the molecular mechanisms by which susceptible alleles alter immune functions. One significant limitation has been the inability to study human T1D risk loci on an isogenic background. The advent of induced pluripotent stem cells (iPSCs) and genome-editing technologies have made it possible to address a number of these outstanding questions. Specifically, the ability to drive multiple cell fates from iPSC under isogenic conditions now facilitates the analysis of causal variants in multiple cellular lineages. Bioinformatic analyses have revealed that T1D risk genes cluster within a limited number of immune signaling pathways, yet the relevant immune cell subsets and cellular activation states in which candidate risk genes impact cellular activities remain largely unknown. In this review, we summarize the functional impact of several candidate risk variants on host immunity in T1D and present an isogenic disease-in-a-dish model system for interrogating risk variants, with the goal of expediting precision therapeutics in T1D.

Keywords: type 1 diabetes, autoimmunity, induced pluripotent stem cells, gene editing, genome-wide association studies, expression quantitative trait loci

INTRODUCTION

The combined genetic and environmental factors that result in type 1 diabetes (T1D) are reflected in the heterogeneous clinical presentations of the disease (1). This autoimmune process results from a complex cross-talk between cells of the innate and adaptive arms of the immune system and the target β cells within the islet microenvironment (**Figure 1**) (2). The era of genome-wide association studies (GWAS) has heralded discovery of approximately 57 independent loci conferring some component to the overall genetic risk for the development of T1D (3). This vast discovery effort has reinforced prior notions of an autoimmune basis for disease development and also has shed new light on the

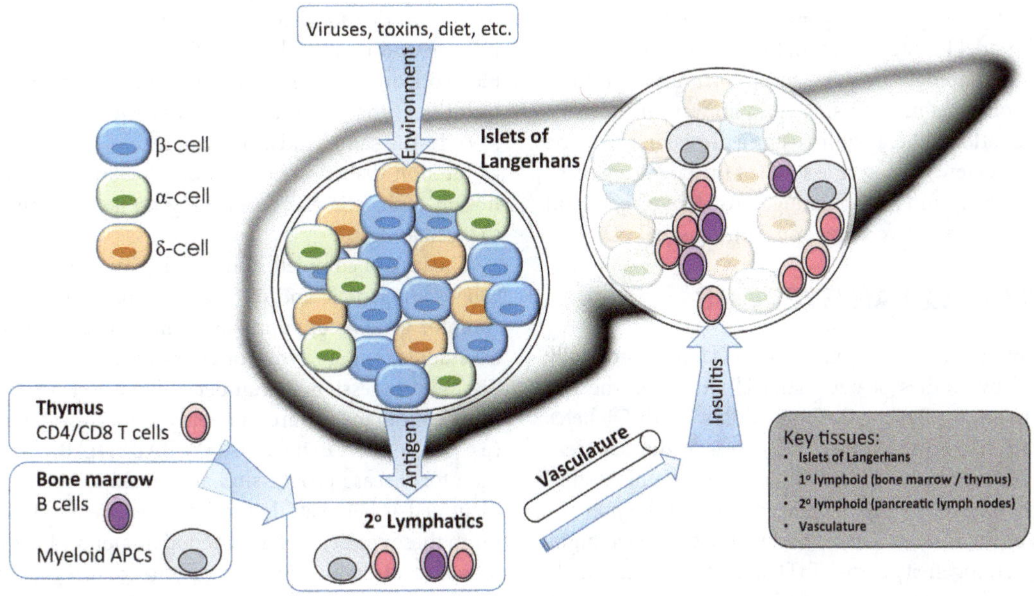

FIGURE 1 | Isogenic modeling facilitates the investigation of multiple cell types important in the pathogenesis of type 1 diabetes (T1D). A combination of environmental and genetic factors influences the overall risk for T1D. Genes conferring risk for T1D may affect the functions of β cells, immune cells, and vascular endothelium. For β cells, risk variants of some genes may alter the response to environmental triggers such as inflammatory or viral sensing, or they may alter the way that β cells cope with stress from bioenergetic demands. For immune cells, gene variants my alter the way that T and B cells are selected in primary (1°) lymphatic tissues during central tolerance, or they may alter several key events that occur during antigen-specific priming and effector differentiation in the peripheral (2°) lymphatics. Immune destruction of β cells requires homing of innate and adaptive effector populations into the pancreatic islets, so alterations to endothelial function could affect disease at this late stage. Isogenic cellular modeling can be applied to complex multifactorial diseases to facilitate a more complete understanding of which genes are expressed in any given tissue/cell type and at which developmental stage they may exert their influence on disease progression.

etiology of T1D, including support for cellular stress within β cells contributing to their demise (4). Despite these advances, there remain numerous questions regarding the mechanisms by which causal gene variants, both individually and in concert, impact immune checkpoints and β cell responses throughout the natural history of the disease. Thus, there remains a critical need in the field to address some fundamental questions regarding the single-nucleotide polymorphisms (SNPs) identified by GWAS including (1) What are the causative variants within any given tag SNP locus? (2) In what cell type(s) and developmental stage(s) are the candidate genes actively expressed? (3) What environmental stimuli modify candidate gene expression or activity? And ultimately, (4) what variants and/or pathways are amenable to therapeutic interventions?

A number of large-scale mechanistic studies to discern the impact of specific genotypes on resulting phenotypes are underway from population-based studies (5). These investigations often utilize clinical material derived from bioresource banks (i.e., genotyped clinical samples capable of recall or recovery from cryopreservation) (6). While promising results have emerged, the number of well-characterized genotype:phenotype interactions remains limited to a small fraction of the putatively identified risk loci. The paucity of functional studies validating causative SNPs can be attributed to a number of challenges including the need to acquire sufficient clinical blood volumes for functional testing, limited access to biological replicates to account for human heterogeneity (particularly with low minor allele frequency variants), and the clear potential for epistatic genetic influences. In sum, these confounding factors constitute a considerable discovery bottleneck limiting human studies by the larger research community.

Immunodeficient mouse models, so-called "humanized" mice, capable of being engrafted with primary human lymphocytes or hematopoietic stem cells (HSCs) have been proposed as a means to fill the translational gap between *in vitro* human studies and clinical trials. These rodent models display full organism level complexity yet can still be manipulated experimentally (7). Despite the powerful tool humanized mice provide when used appropriately, they still present significant constraints as a model system. Mice hold notable differences when compared to human biology, particularly when considering host immune responses in the context of TLR ligands, responses to cytokines and growth factors, and cellular trafficking (8). These factors present challenges in modeling autoimmune T1D in xenogeneic systems, where there are essential homology requirements for full effector function. These requirements include the need for lymphocyte trafficking from circulation to secondary lymphoid organs, auto-antigen priming and activation, and eventual extravasation to target β cells within islets (9). The emergence of induced pluripotent stem cell (iPSC) technologies offers an attractive alternative to humanized mice that allows the interrogation of underlying genetic defects using a vast array of relevant biological tissues and cell types avoiding both allo- and xenogeneic responses.

Isogenic cellular systems constitute a powerful experimental platform for conducting precision gene editing to create a "disease-in-a-dish" model to interrogate multifactorial diseases such as T1D. This methodology provides an opportunity to understand specific molecular mechanisms and pathways in humans to thereby derive rational therapeutics using a precision medicine approach. In this review, we describe some of the emerging technologies for generating and manipulating iPSC-derived cells and tissues to interrogate causative genes and pathways in T1D.

ISOGENIC CELLULAR SYSTEMS

Investigations into the etiopathogenesis of T1D have historically been dominated by studies of peripheral blood. Over the last decade, the Network for Pancreatic Organ donors with Diabetes (nPOD) program has provided essential access to the pancreas and lymphoid tissues from donors with T1D. Emerging studies from this program have already challenged many of the preconceived notions of the disease. Of note, nPOD tissues have highlighted disease heterogeneity across T1D donors and remarkable variability even at the level of adjacent islets within a single T1D donor (10–14). For example, early histological observations from nPOD led Dr. George Eisenbarth to refer to T1D as "vitiligo of the pancreas," in reference to intact insulin-containing islets being observed in close proximity to pseudo-atrophic islets completely devoid of insulin (15). Despite the transformative resource that nPOD provides, donor and programmatic limitations necessitate systematic prioritization of access to tissues. Hence, there is a paramount need within the field to derive cell types from renewable human cellular sources. The capacity for pluripotent and renewable cells to undergo reprogramming to generate immune subsets, endothelial cells, and neuroendocrine lineages will facilitate the modeling of cellular interactions involved in T1D disease pathogenesis (**Figure 2**).

GENETIC SUSCEPTIBILITY IN T1D

The autoimmune destruction of insulin-producing pancreatic β cells in T1D shares complex etiology with a collection of organ-specific disorders (i.e., juvenile idiopathic arthritis, alopecia areata, rheumatoid arthritis, and celiac disease, among others) (3). Though each of these diseases demonstrates unique immunopathologic mechanisms, they all share two common features: specifically, inheritance with a significant genetic contribution coming from the human leukocyte antigen (HLA) region of chromosome 6 and additional genetic risk conferred by loci dispersed throughout the genome (**Table 1**). While no single risk haplotype accurately predicts whether or not a person will develop T1D (or another autoimmune disease), there is clear genetic evidence that T1D is primarily an inherited disease with an autoimmune pathogenesis (**Figure 3**) and with additional poorly defined environmental contributions. Discordant incidence of T1D in monozygotic twins is often cited as evidence for a greater environmental role in T1D (16, 17); however, the early studies likely underestimated the concordance rates. It is now better understood that childhood-onset T1D and latent autoimmune diabetes of the adult (LADA) share overlapping genetic risk (18). Thus, long-term monitoring is essential to capture the total genetic risk for disease development. For example, one study of monozygotic twins found that by the age of 60 years, there was greater than 65% concordance for T1D—i.e., when one twin is afflicted, it is more likely that the other twin will eventually develop the disease (19). In the same study, concordance of autoantibody positivity in the non-diabetic twin was nearly 80%, again supporting the notion of genetic risk controlling the loss of immune tolerance to β cell antigens.

The lack of complete concordance may indicate an additional role for epigenetic and/or stochastic influences due to antigenic receptor gene recombination events. In addition, epidemiological studies support a role for environmental factor(s) influencing disease progression. A number of large consortium studies have been conducted or are currently underway around the world (e.g., TrialNet, TEDDY, DAISY, BABYDIAB, and Pre-Point) to monitor disease progression and potentially, intervene in those identified as being at high-risk for disease development (27–31). From these studies, environmental influences have been reported to affect disease incidence or rate of progression, including enteroviral triggers, lack of protective exposures, and the influence of various components of Westernized diets. Many of these modifying factors impact pathways with associated genetic risk variants (e.g., *Tyk2* and *IFIH1* in response to viral infections), further supporting their potential importance (32). Thus, T1D is principally a genetic disease with environmental exposures influencing progression. These combined influences support the notion of a complex multifactorial disease, yet ultimately beg the question: Why do we not better understand the etiology and pathogenesis of human T1D? Even though the human genome is complex, it is still a finite collection of variables. In principle, utilization of "big data" approaches involving GWAS, biomarker studies, and expression profiling, when paired with robust computational capabilities, should be able to reveal a clear molecular signature, and from this signature, we should be able to progress through reductionist approaches to reveal pathways of disease.

This theoretical solution to the problem of complex autoimmune diseases is hindered by a number of fundamental challenges. Foremost, heretofore there have been no experimental systems available to study individual risk variants in human subjects. For T1D, where approximately 57 different genetic regions confer some portion of genetic risk (immunobase.org, July 2017) (3, 20–26), it is not possible to study one gene at a time without incurring significant epistatic effects from other risk genes. The likelihood of finding two individuals differing at *only* one risk gene (i.e., one person with the protective allele and one person with the risk allele) while having *identical* variants at the remaining 56 risk regions is infinitesimally small. A more practical approach would be to reduce the number of genetic loci being studied to include only those with the largest odds ratios (ORs). Even here, the problem is magnified by the fact that some of the most highly associated risk genes beyond the HLA [e.g., protein tyrosine phosphatase, non-receptor type 22 (*PTPN22*)] have a low minor allele frequency, even among T1D subjects. For North American and European T1D subjects, the frequency of individuals with homozygosity for the risk variant of *PTPN22* (1858T at rs2476601) ranges from 0.6 to 3.7% (33). Moreover,

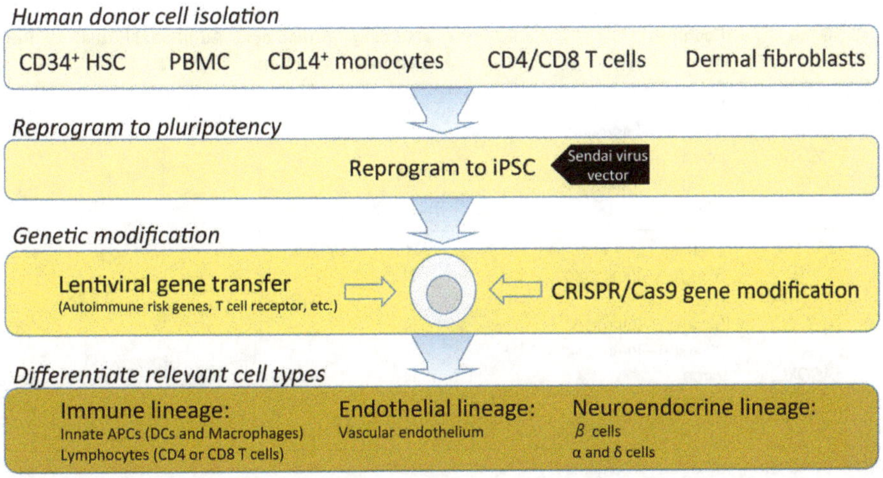

FIGURE 2 | A hypothetical outline for establishing an isogenic disease-in-a-dish workflow. Induced pluripotent stem cell (iPSC) stable cell lines can be generated from several different somatic cell types depending on specimen availability. Traditionally, dermal fibroblasts from skin biopsy were utilized; however, this is being replaced by less invasive samples such as freshly isolated or cryopreserved peripheral blood mononuclear cells (PBMCs). PBMCs can be enriched for various populations such as $CD34^+$ hematopoietic stem cells, $CD14^+$ monocytes, T cells, or reprogrammed as a bulk population. Where a pre-re-arranged T-cell receptor (TCR) is desired, antigen-specific CD4 or CD8 T cells can be used so that iPSC-derived T cells will clonally express the desired TCR with a naive T-cell phenotype. Several commercial platforms for iPSC reprogramming are currently available. Non-integrating Sendai virus vectors provide a safe and efficient means for iPSC reprogramming of human primary cells. Following reprogramming into iPSC, gene modification enables researchers to investigate disease-associated risk variants and/or over-express or knockdown genes to modulate pathways. Once gene modifications are confirmed, validated protocols for differentiation of immune, endothelial or neuroendocrine lineages are utilized to interrogate the specific effects of each gene variant in several disease-relevant cell types.

genes associated with T1D risk encode proteins that cluster within biological processes and/or pathways, posing a considerable challenge when analyzing the impact of a given risk variant.

Currently, 57 genomic regions that are defined by 104 SNPs [some SNPs identify the same linkage disequilibrium block] are significantly associated with T1D according to immunobase.org. The set of 64 T1D candidate gene variants from 57 SNP-tagged regions listed in **Table 1** was analyzed using the Protein ANalysis THrough Evolutionary Relationships gene ontology tool (pantherdb.org) (34, 35). Not surprisingly, pathway analysis revealed a significant enrichment for genes involved in immune processes ($P = 9.9E{-}11$), where 26 of the 64 candidate genes contribute to immune function. The immune system is highly dynamic and integrates signals from antigenic receptors, adhesion molecules/integrins, costimulatory molecules, and cytokine/chemokine receptors. These events in turn lead to signal transduction events that are also significantly enriched as a defined pathway. Based on our analysis, 32 of the 64 T1D candidate genes are implicated in cellular signaling ($P = 9.25E{-}03$) (Data File S1 in Supplementary Material). Considering the role of cross-talk between signaling pathways, it is evident that heterogeneous genetic risk will result in complex downstream effects on cell signaling and functions.

As a specific example of immune signaling pathway cross-talk, we consider one gene that encodes a protein with known effects on cytokine receptor signaling. *SH2B3* encodes a protein phosphatase Lnk that regulates Janus kinase/signal transducers and activators of transcription (JAK/STAT) signaling. The risk variant of *SH2B3* (T at rs3184504) encodes a modified Lnk protein where arginine at amino acid 262 is replaced by tryptophan (R262W). Lnk is a regulator of Jak2 signaling in myeloid cells (36–38), and the T1D risk SNP for *SH2B3*/Lnk is associated with altered expression of key elements of IFNγ signaling including signal transducer and activator of transcription 1 (STAT1) (39). Furthermore, the target of Lnk, Jak2, is a cytosolic protein that transduces signals from a variety of cytokine receptors including IL-6, IL-13, G-CSF, IL-12, IL-23, granulocyte-macrophage colony-stimulating factor (GM-CSF), EPO, IL-3, and IL-5 (40, 41). Thus, the specific effect(s) of Lnk^{R262W} upon immune cell function are difficult to predict. Adding to this inherent complexity, additional T1D risk genes/proteins are likely to co-regulate the same pathways as Lnk. For example, at least three T1D candidate genes, *Tyk2*, *SOCS1*, and *IL10*, encode proteins with known roles in modulating JAK/STAT signaling. The interplay of different alleles of each protein will likely modify the effect of Lnk. This example highlights the need for an experimental system that mitigates the epistatic effects of related genes/proteins so that observed phenotypes are attributed to the gene of interest alone.

In addition to the number of variants and overlapping pathways noted above, there are additional layers of complexity at the cellular level. Specifically, it is poorly characterized how a given risk variant may impact function within various innate or adaptive immune subsets. For example, a gene that regulates JAK/STAT signaling in antigen-presenting cells (APCs) such as dendritic cells (DCs) may have an entirely different biological effect in lymphocytes. Moreover, the impact of a gene variant may be combinatorial to multiple cell types that conspire to drive autoimmunity. Furthermore, some genes may affect the β cells themselves, endothelial cells, or other cells such as neurons (42).

The central pathophysiological mechanism of T1D entails at least three major tissue types—immune, endothelial, and

TABLE 1 | Genetic variants associated with type 1 diabetes and other common autoimmune diseases.

Chromosome	Marker	Gene	Feature	Coding variant	Amino acid variation	Additional notes	Region	Other associated diseases
1	rs2476601	*PTPN22*	Exon	Y	R620W		1p13.2	ATD/CRO/JIA/RA/SLE/AA/VIT
	rs6679677		3′ region—intergenic	N				
	rs6691977	*CAMSAP2*	Intron	N			1q32.1	
	rs3024505	*IL10*	3′ region—intergenic	N			1q32.1	CRO/SLE/UC/IBD
	rs3024493		Intron	N				
2	rs35667974	*IFIH1*	Exon	Y	I923V		2q24.2	PSO/SLE/UC/IBD/VIT
	rs2111485		3′ region—intergenic	N				
	rs1990760		Exon	Y	A946T			
	rs11571316	*CTLA4*	5′ region—intergenic	N			2q33.2	ATD/CEL/RA
	rs3087243		3′ region—intergenic	N				
	rs4849135	*ACOXL*	Intron	N			2q13	
	rs478222	*EFR3B*	Intron	N			2p23.3	
	rs9653442	*AFF3*	5′ region—intergenic	N			2q11.2	RA
3	rs113010081	*CCR5* and *CCRL2*	3′ region—intergenic	N			3p21.31	CEL/UC
4	rs2611215	*LINC01179*	5′ region—intergenic	N			4q32.3	
	rs75793288	*CTNNB1*	Intron	N		5′ of ADAD1 and 3′ of IL2	4q27	CEL/CRO/UC
	rs6827756		Intron	N		5′ of ADAD1 and 3′ of IL2		
	rs4505848		Intron	N		5′ of ADAD1 and 3′ of IL2		
	rs17388568	*ADAD1*	Intron	N		3′ of IL2		
	rs10517086	*No gene*	Intergenic—H3K27Ac rich	N			4p15.2	
5	rs11954020	*IL7R*	3′ region—intergenic	N			5p13.2	
6	rs9388489	*CENPW*	Intron	N			6q22.32	
	rs1538171		Intron	N				
	rs9375435		Intron	N				
	rs597325	*BACH2*	Intron	N			6q15	ATD/MS/RA
	rs11755527		Intron	N				
	rs72928038		Intron	N				
	rs924043	*No gene*	Intergenic	N			6q27	
	rs6920220	*TNFAIP3*	5′ region—intergenic	N			6q23.3	RA/SLE/UC/IBD
	rs1738074	*TAGAP*	Exon	N	SYN		6q25.3	CEL/MS
7	rs7804356	*SKAP2*	Intron	N			7p15.2	
	rs4948088	*COBL*	3′ region—intergenic	N			7p12.1	
	rs62447205	*IKZF1*	Intron	N			7p12.2	
9	rs10758593	*GLIS3*	Intron	N			9p24.2	
	rs7020673		Intron	N				
	rs6476839		Intron	N				
10	rs722988	*NRP1*	3′ region—intergenic—H3K27Ac rich	N			10p11.22	
	rs11258747	*PRKCQ*	Exon	N	SYN		10p15.1	
	rs61839660	*IL2RA*	Intron	N			10p15.1	MS/RA
	rs2104286		Intron	N				
	rs12251307	*IL2RA* and	5′ of RMB17 and 3′ of IL2RA	N				
	rs41295121	*RBM17*	5′ of RMB17 and 3′ of IL2RA	N				
	rs7090530		5′ of RMB17 and 3′ of IL2RA	N				
	rs10795791		5′ of RMB17 and 3′ of IL2RA	N				
	rs12416116	*RNLS*	Intron	N			10q23.31	
	rs10509540		3′ region—intergenic	N				
11	rs72853903	*INS*	5′ region—intergenic—H3K27Ac rich	N			11p15.5	
	rs689		Intron	N				
	rs7111341		5′ region—intergenic	N				
	rs7928968		3′ region—intergenic	N				
	rs694739	*BAD*	5′ region—intergenic	N		5′ of CCDC88B and 3′ of PRDX5	11q13.1	CRO/MS/AA

(*Continued*)

TABLE 1 | Continued

Chromosome	Marker	Gene	Feature	Coding variant	Amino acid variation	Additional notes	Region	Other associated diseases
12	rs11170466	*ITGB7*	Intron	N			12q13.13	
	rs11171739	*ERBB3*	5′ region—intergenic	N			12q13.2	AA
	rs11171710	*RAB5B*	Intron	N		5′ of IKZF4		
	rs705705	*IKZF4*	3′ region—intergenic	N				
	rs705704		3′ region—intergenic	N				
	rs2292239	*ERBB3*	Intron	N				
	rs3184504	*SH2B3*	Exon	Y	R262W		12q24.13	CEL/CRO/JIA/ PBC/RA/AA/PSC/ VIT
	rs653178	*ATXN2*	Intron	N				
	rs17696736	*NAA25*	Intron	N				
	rs10492166	*CD69*	3′ region—intergenic	N			12p13.31	
	rs4763879		Intron	N				
13	rs9585056	*GPR183*	5′ region—intergenic—H3K27Ac rich	N			13q32.3	
14	rs4900384	*LINC01550*	5′ region—intergenic	N			14q32.2	
	rs1456988		5′ region—intergenic	N				
	rs911263	*RAD51B*	Intron	N			14q24.1	PBC
	rs1465788	*ZFP36L1*	5′ region—intergenic—H3K27Ac rich	N			14q24.1	
	rs56994090	*DLK1*	3′ region—intergenic	N		Intron of MEG3	14q32.2	
	rs941576		3′ region—intergenic	N		Intron of MEG3		
15	rs12148472	*CTSH*	Intron—splice site	N			15q25.1	CEL/NAR
	rs3825932		Intron	N				
	rs34593439		Intron	N				
	rs12908309	*RASGRP1*	5′ region—intergenic	N			15q14	CRO
	rs72727394		Intron	N				
16	rs4788084	*IL27*	5′ region—intergenic	N			16p11.2	AS/CRO/IBD
	rs9924471		5′ region—intergenic	N		Intron of *SGF29*		
	rs151234	*CLN3*	Intron	N		5′ of *APOBR* and 3′ of *IL27*—K3K27Ac rich		
	rs12708716	*CLEC16A*	Intron	N			16p13.13	MS/PBC
	rs12927355		Intron	N				
	rs193778	*SOCS1*	5′ region—intergenic—H3K27Ac rich	N		3′ of *CLEC16A*, Intron of *RMI2*		
	rs8056814	*CTRB1*	5′ region—intergenic—H3K27Ac rich	N			16q23.1	
	rs7202877		5′ region—intergenic—H3K27Ac rich	N				
17	rs1052553	*MAPT*	Exon	N	SYN		17q21.31	
	rs7221109	*CCR7*	5′ region—intergenic—H3K27Ac rich	N			17q21.2	
	rs2290400	*GSDMB*	Intron	N			17q12	CRO/UC/IBD
	rs12453507		3′ region—intergenic	N				
18	rs763361	*CD226*	Exon	Y	G307S		18q22.2	MS
	rs1615504		3′ region—intergenic	N				
	rs2542151	*PTPN2*	3′ region—intergenic	N			18p11.21	CEL/CRO/UC/IBD
	rs1893217		Intron	N				
19	rs602662	*FUT2*	Exon	Y	G258S		19q13.33	CRO/IBD
	rs516246		Intron	N				
	rs402072	*PRKD2*	Intron	N			19q13.32	
	rs425105		Intron	N				
	rs12720356	*TYK2*	Exon	Y	I684S		19p13.2	CRO/JIA/MS/PBC/ PSO/RA/IBD
	rs34536443		Exon	Y	P1104A			
20	rs2281808	*SIRPG*	Intron	N			20p13	
	rs6043409		Exon	Y	V263A			
21	rs11203202	*UBASH3A*	Intron	N			21q22.3	RA/VIT
	rs11203203		Intron	N				
22	rs4820830	*HORMAD2*	Intron	N			22q12.2	
	rs5753037		3′ region—intergenic	N				
	rs229533	*C1QTNF6*	5′ region—intergenic	N		3′ of *RAC2*	22q12.3	
X	rs2664170	*GAB3*	Intron	N			Xq28	

Genes and markers were derived from immunobase.org (3, 20–26). The genes indicated in blue text were imputed from information derived from the University of California Santa Cruz genome browser (genome.ucsc.edu). Amino acid variations (red text) were identified for single nucleotide polymorphism (SNP) variants by downloading the spliced coding sequences from genome browser and translating in SnapGene software. SYN (green text) indicates synonymous variation in an exon. Genomic region and disease information displayed were derived from Immunobase. ATD, autoimmune thyroid disease; CRO, Crohn's disease; JIA, juvenile idiopathic arthritis; RA, rheumatoid arthritis; SLE, systemic lupus erythematous; AA, alopecia areata; VIT, vitiligo; UC, ulcerative colitis; IBD, inflammatory bowel disease; PSO, psoriasis; CEL, celiac disease; MS, multiple sclerosis; PBC, primary biliary cirrhosis; PSC, primary sclerosing cholangitis; NAR, non-allergic rhinitis; AS, ankylosing spondylitis.

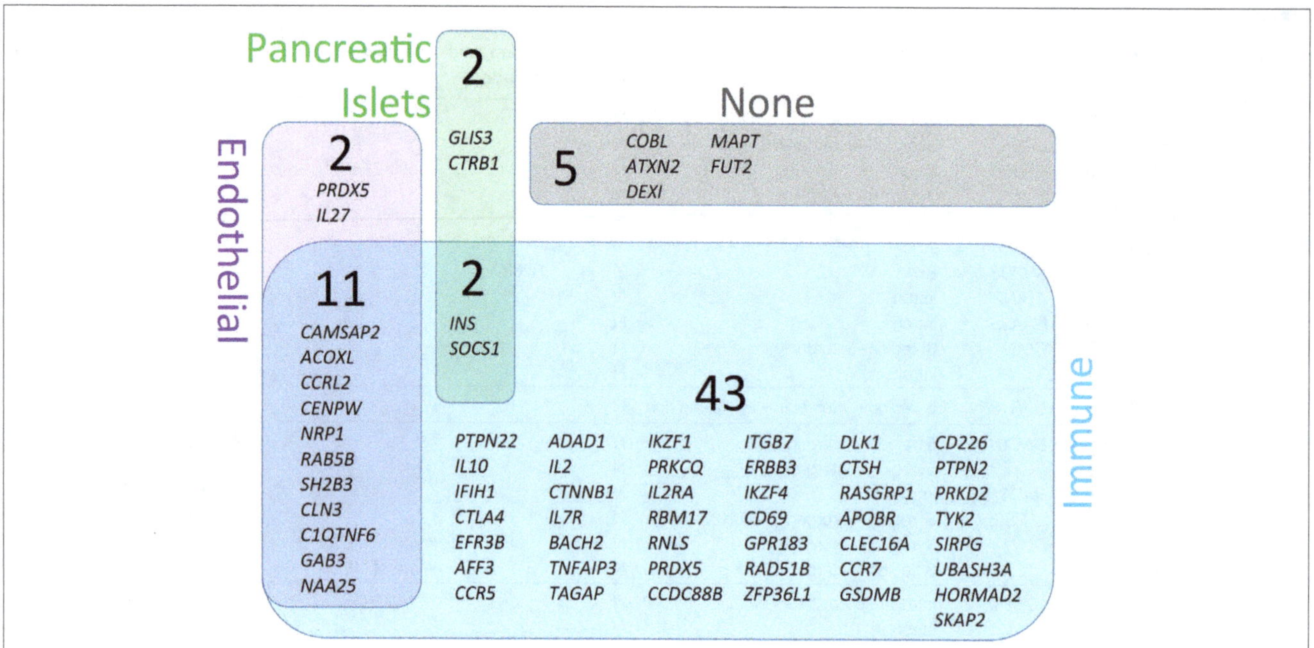

FIGURE 3 | Genetic susceptibility risk variants identified in type 1 diabetes (T1D). The current list of gene regions that have been associated with T1D through genome-wide association studies were collected from the ImmunoBase resource (www.immunobase.org). Individual single-nucleotide polymorphisms (SNPs) corresponding to candidate genes were identified from the ImmunoBase T1D data set. In addition, every SNP tag was queried on the University of California Santa Cruz Genome Browser (GRCh38; genome.ucsc.edu) to identify additional genes in each SNP-tagged region. The complete list of regions and genes are compiled in **Table 1**. Each SNP-associated gene was queried on the GeneVestigator database to identify the top 10 tissues with highest expression of each gene (genevisible.com/search). For each gene it was determined if high-expressing tissues included any one or combination of relevant tissues: immune (blue), endothelial (purple), or pancreatic islets (green). The size of regions in Venn diagram represents the relative abundance of genes expressed in each tissue type. Five genes were not highly expressed by any of the relevant tissue types (indicated as none, gray).

pancreatic (**Figure 1**). To better understand which cells are likely to be affected by each T1D candidate gene, we analyzed all genes from **Table 1** for cell/tissue expression profiles using the online GeneVisible tool (genevisible.com) (43) that queries tens of thousands of curated human gene expression experiments. As seen in **Figure 3**, the majority of T1D candidate genes are expressed most highly in immune cells, but a small number of genes are preferentially expressed in endothelial or pancreatic cell lineages. Notably, 13 genes are highly expressed in multiple lineages. Isolating the effect of candidate genes in relevant cell types should be a goal for the isogenic cellular experimental system described herein.

A number of T1D-associated SNPs encode missense mutations within gene exons, presumably altering protein stability, interactions, or function (**Table 1**); here, the path to dissect the impact of variants on biological processes is straightforward. However, the vast majority of risk loci reside in non-coding regions of the genome and careful studies must be undertaken to first dissect the causative variant(s) from each tag SNP locus and then determine whether any given SNP exerts its impact in a *cis* or *trans* manner to alter gene expression (5). One such study by Ram et al. recently applied a systems genetics approach to dissect the impact of putative risk SNPs on gene expression in purified and activated cell lines. The authors mapped *cis*-acting expression quantitative trait loci (eQTL) and found 24 non-HLA loci that significantly affected the expression of 31 transcripts in at least one cell type from Epstein–Barr virus-transformed B cells and $CD4^+$ or $CD8^+$ T cells (44). They went on to describe an additional 25 *trans*-acting loci that impacted 38 transcripts. Of note, many of the SNPs associated with risk are located within promoter or enhancer regions of their candidate gene (3). These studies provide a framework from which additional mechanistic studies can now be conducted in isogenic cellular systems.

To begin to address these challenges, the research community needs robust platforms to study the effects of individual risk alleles in various cell types under controlled conditions. With the advent of iPSC technologies and genome-editing tools, this once theoretical approach now provides an efficient method to analyze disease mechanisms and identify causal gene variants (**Figure 4**). By creating a disease-in-a-dish experimental platform, we and others have started to dissect the individual contributions of T1D risk genes in specific cell types. Harnessing this information will allow researchers to derive rational therapeutics targeting checkpoints in key pathways.

DEFECTIVE IMMUNE TOLERANCE IN T1D

Autoimmune diseases, including T1D, result from a breakdown in the pathways that maintain a state of immune homeostasis, commonly referred to as immune tolerance (1). The mechanisms controlling this process involve both central and peripheral tolerance mechanisms (e.g., thymic selection and immune checkpoints, respectively). Effective immunity requires the

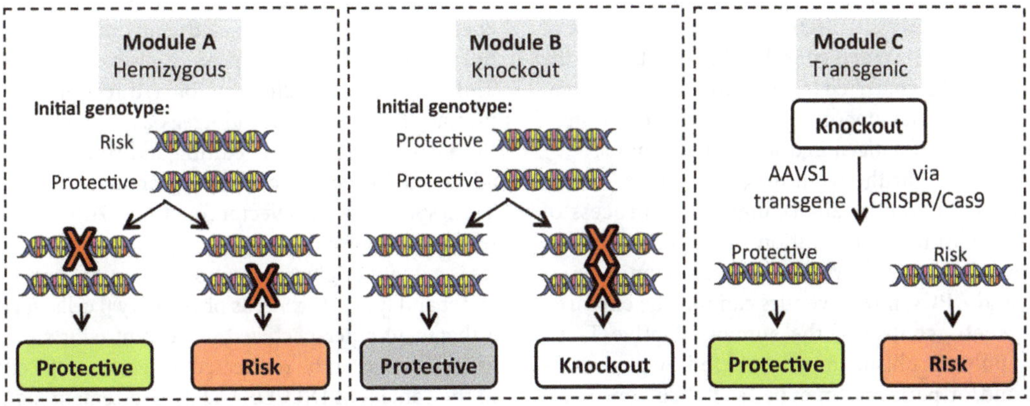

FIGURE 4 | Gene modification strategies for use in induced pluripotent stem cell (iPSC) lines. Three basic strategies can be employed for gene editing. To create single allele homozygous expression (hemizygous) lines, *Module A* targets a single allele of the gene of interest (GOI) in iPSC lines that are heterozygous for the risk variant. Targeting efficiency for hemizygous clones is approximately 20% of green fluorescent protein positive puromycin resistant clones, and allele targeting is random so that either the protective or risk allele can be modified. *Module B* generates complete knockout of the GOI on a background of homozygous protective alleles. *Module C* utilizes GOI-knockout lines to re-express either the protective or risk variant of the GOI using a CRISPR/Cas9 platform that targets integration into the adeno-associated virus integration site 1 (AAVS1) on chromosome 19.

capacity to respond to a vast array of antigens from pathogens, all while functionally limiting host responses to self-tissues and commensal microorganisms. In health, the adaptive immune system consisting of T and B lymphocytes is edited to eliminate portions of the repertoire that acquire somatically re-arranged receptors with high binding affinity for self-antigens through clonal deletion. For T cells, this process is carried out in the thymus under the control of the autoimmune regulator (AIRE) (45). Medullary thymic epithelial cells (mTECs) expressing AIRE are thought to coordinate the expression of a select number of tissue-specific self-antigens (TSAs). These TSAs, when expressed by mTEC work in concert with APCs to eliminate high-affinity autoreactive T-cell receptors (TCRs) through negative selection. The thymus is also the site for the emergence of thymic CD4$^+$ regulatory T cells (tTregs), a population of cells that express the master Treg-transcription factor FOXP3 (46). These tTregs seed the periphery, playing a key role in reinforcing immune tolerance. Rare monogenic mutations in *AIRE* and *FOXP3* result in profound autoimmune conditions, referred to as autoimmune polyglandular syndrome-1 and immunodysregulation polyendocrinopathy enteropathy X-linked syndrome (IPEX), respectively (47). T1D is a common clinical manifestation of patients presenting with these severe mutations, supporting the essential role for these transcription factors in regulating immune tolerance to β cells. To date, studies of thymic T-cell selection have largely been restricted to animal models. The development of isogenic cellular systems provides a unique opportunity to investigate molecular pathways that shape the human adaptive immune repertoire.

ISOGENIC MODELS FOR STUDYING THYMIC SELECTION

As noted earlier, the HLA region constitutes the major genetic risk locus in T1D (48). While this region has been known to confer risk for over four decades, the exact mechanisms by which variants in HLA influence disease pathogenesis remain poorly characterized. In addition to shaping the T-cell repertoire through the processes of positive and negative selection, the thymic developmental niche controls the composition and relative proportion of naive conventional T cells (Tconv) and tTregs that emerge to form the mature CD4$^+$ T cell population (49). Little is currently known about how high-risk HLA haplotypes (e.g., HLA-DR3/DR4-DQ8) shape the resulting T-cell repertoire, or for that matter, why the HLA-DRB1*15:01-DQA1*01:02-DQB1*06:02 haplotype is so dominantly protective in Caucasian populations (OR ~0.03) (50). A prevailing theory presented by Eisenbarth and colleagues suggests that the key might lie within the tri-molecular complex of HLA class II molecules presenting peptides of insulin (specifically, the insulin B-chain$_{9-23}$) for recognition by autoreactive TCRs (51). T1D DQ8 risk alleles and I-A^{g7} of the non-obese diabetic (NOD) mouse tend to share non-polar residues in place of Asp at β57 and preferentially bind peptides with acidic side chains in the P9 pocket of the MHC class II binding groove (52). Thus, these molecular interactions within distinct peptide binding pockets may either allow escape of potentially pathogenic autoreactive T-cell clones from the thymus or potentially fail to generate the proper repertoire of protective tTregs capable of maintaining tolerance.

Together with HLA, additional candidate risk genes could also have an impact on thymic T-cell development. Specifically, at least three independent variants within the *INS-IGF2* locus have been associated with risk for T1D (3). This region confers the second highest risk for disease following the HLA locus. Risk associated with the *INS* gene on chromosome 11p15.5 has been most commonly attributed to a variable number tandem repeat locus situated 596 bp 5′ of *INS* (53). Protection from the class III allele has been attributed to a markedly higher level of insulin being expressed within the thymus (54). Insulin has been proposed as a primary or triggering auto-antigen in the NOD mouse model (55) and more recently in human T1D (56). Notably, T cells reactive to both native and hybrid insulin peptides, insulin conjugated with other β cell antigens, were discovered within the islets of subjects with T1D (56–58). When considered in addition to the dominance of genetic risk conferred by the HLA, these significant observations lend additional support to the dominance of insulin epitopes as a primary auto-antigen in disease pathogenesis.

These reports highlight the need for mechanistic studies to ascertain how susceptibility alleles impact the process of thymic selection. Through the creation of isogenic systems involving human bone marrow progenitors, thymic organoids, mTECs, and APCs, novel avenues can now be explored to investigate genetic control of the human adaptive T-cell repertoire. Key polymorphisms may be altered by gene editing and genes and/or pathways may be "switched" on or off in a temporal fashion by the addition of chemical enhancers or repressors in either T-cell precursors or thymic stroma. Not only will this provide key insight into pathogenic versus regulatory receptors but could also potentially provide an opportunity for the *ex vivo* education of T cells in isogenic thymic organoids for auto- and/or allo-tolerance induction strategies following β cells regenerative or replacement therapies in T1D.

MODELING ANTIGEN-SPECIFIC T-CELL RESPONSES

Type 1 diabetes is most often described as a T-cell-mediated organ-specific autoimmune disease. This notion emanates from seminal experiments including the strong linkage to HLA, early animal model adoptive transfer experiments (59, 60), and the presence of autoreactive memory T cells within the insulitic lesion of organ donors with T1D (12, 14). Studies have been conducted to investigate and monitor autoreactive T cells in peripheral blood mononuclear cell (PBMC) of T1D subjects. To date, none of the commonly employed techniques have approached the sensitivity/specificity and level of standardization observed for autoantibody assays validated by the diabetes antibody standardization program now known as the islet autoantibody standardization program (61–66). We would speculate that the major reason(s) for this inability to identify robust T-cell biomarkers results from both technical limitations of the current assays, along with the inherent biology of T cells. Our data profiling the TCR repertoire in T1D nPOD organ donors demonstrated only modest overlap in high frequency clonotypes between the pancreatic lymph nodes and spleen (as a surrogate of PBMC) (67). This was particularly striking for $CD4^+$ T cells (mean ± SD; 9.2 ± 7.0% of clones shared), with $CD8^+$ T cells demonstrating significantly more TCR-β complementarity determining region 3 amino acid sequence overlap among different tissues (36 ± 21%).

Studies to quantify antigen-specific T cells with ELISpot or MHC-multimer reagents have demonstrated the rare nature of these cells in PBMC (in the range of 1:50,000–1:1,000,000) (68). This presents a number of challenges when trying to identify key auto-antigen targets and peptides important during the natural history of disease. To address this particular limitation, we have co-opted an approach pioneered in the cancer immunotherapy field to generate large numbers of tumor-antigen-specific T cells. Specifically, we have generated lentiviral contructs that express full TCR-α and β chains in multi-cistronic expression cassettes. This technique is effective for redirecting the specificity of primary human Tconv and Tregs as well as $CD8^+$ T cells (69). Recent advances in gene editing and receptor engineering have advanced this field to create programmable circuits for studying T-cell specificity and effector functions (70). Importantly, we have recently employed TCR gene transfer to directly test the cytotoxic activity of glucose-6-phosphatase-reactive $CD8^+$ T cells to target and lyse β-Lox5 cells or primary β cells *in vitro* (71). From a therapeutic perspective, our current efforts demonstrate that human Tregs can be redirected to recognize β cell auto-antigens in the context of DR3/DR4-DQ8 and remain highly suppressive *in vitro* to Tconv recognizing a shared peptide or in a bystander fashion (72). The application of novel single cell/clone analysis platforms, when used in concert with isogenic cellular systems, will allow researchers to quickly move from *in silico* TCR-α/β sequence information to unlimited numbers of antigen-specific T cells to expedite auto-antigen discovery and functional studies.

iPSCs can be used for yet another approach to generate a large number of antigen-specific T cells and to further study mechanisms of thymic selection. A small number of groups have successfully differentiated iPSCs into functional T cells. iPSC derived from a single $CD8^+$ T-cell clone have been re-differentiated into naive and eventually highly functional CTLs (73). This application has emerged as a particularly potent means to not only bolster the number of antigen-specific T cells but also correct the anergic and senescent phenotype common to tumor-infiltrating T cells in cancer, and while early studies were focused on generation of $CD8^+$ CTLs for targeting virus-infected cells (73) or tumors (74), the methods could be adapted to focus on auto-antigen-specific T cells. When iPSC derived from non-T cells (not bearing rearranged TCR genes) are used for T-cell differentiation, a broad diversity of TCR rearrangement events is possible (75).

Differentiation protocols for iPSC-derived T cells require culture on the murine stromal cells line OP9 expressing the Notch ligand protein DL1 (74). The quality of iPSC-derived T cells has been incrementally improved by altering culture conditions, for example activating CD4/CD8 double positive iPSC-derived thymocytes via CD3 to enhance CTL killer activity (76). Today, detailed protocols are available for the differentiation of antigen-specific $CD8^+$ T cells from iPSC (73). To date, advances in single-positive $CD4^+$ T cells have not approached the same progress as CTLs, yet efficient protocols to generate $CD4^+$ T_H-cell populations are expected. For example, advances in deriving human thymic epithelial cells from iPSCs (77) could enhance *in vitro* differentiation of $CD4^+$ and $CD8^+$ T cells by providing the full repertoire of human soluble and membrane-associated growth factors. In addition, iPSC-derived thymic epithelia will enable more precise studies of how disease-associated gene variants impact thymic selection by regulating specific processes such as auto-antigen expression during negative selection. The capacity to grow and differentiate large numbers of isogenic antigen-specific T cells (>10^9 cells), without the typical constraints of primary human T-cell clones opens up the potential for gene editing and extensive functional studies. Thus, we are nearing the point where isogenic iPSC systems can be used to study human T-cell development at a mechanistic level that was previously only attainable in animal models.

MODELING INNATE IMMUNE RESPONSES

Development of auto-antigen-specific T cells requires more than a failure of thymic negative selection. Naive T cells in the periphery must be primed by professional APCs. DCs are specialized APCs with potent abilities to initiate antigen-specific $CD4^+$ and $CD8^+$ T-cell responses. To elicit $CD4^+$ T cells priming, activation, proliferation, and effector function, DCs must first capture antigens via phagocytosis or micropinocytosis. It can be envisioned that this antigen capture in T1D manifests through DCs phagocytosing dead/dying β cells or exosomes derived from β cells.

Several genes associated with T1D risk are expressed in myeloid lineages including monocytes, macrophages, and DCs, and it is likely that at least some of the immune pathogenesis of T1D arises from the innate end of the immune system. Differences in innate immune function could emanate from dysregulated antiviral or type 1 interferon (T1-IFN) responses, altered co-stimulation, changes in antigen acquisition, or enhanced expression of pro-inflammatory cytokines. As an example, a T1-IFN response signature has been observed preceding T1D onset in high-risk populations (32). The NOD Rip-LCMV mouse model corroborates this finding, where IFN-α is critical for progression of T1D (78). Furthermore, some enteric viral infections have been associated with risk for T1D. In NOD mice, rotavirus infection can accelerate T1D in a T1-IFN-dependent manner (79). In humans, a growing number of studies have reported associations between enterovirus infection and T1D (80–84). Thus, genes that regulate the innate response to viruses including T1-IFN expression or signaling could mediate T1D risk by altering innate immune function.

T1D RISK GENES THAT MODULATE ANTIVIRAL IMMUNITY

PTPN22, commonly associated with modifying receptor signaling in T and B cells, is also reported to alter the way that DCs respond to danger signals such as bacterial lipopolysaccharide by modulating TRAF3 signaling and T1-IFN production (85). In lupus, the risk variant of *PTPN22* tagged by rs2476601, the same variant that is associated with T1D (**Table 1**), is associated with altered TLR7-induced T1-IFN production (86).

A major counter-regulator of IFN signaling is the regulatory cytokine IL-10. Indeed, IL-10 is so potent for protection of host cells from CTL-mediated killing that many DNA viruses have evolved viral homologs of IL-10 to protect them from antiviral immunity (87). The T1D risk locus defined by the SNPs rs3024504 and rs3024493 includes *IL10* (**Table 1**). A protective role for IL-10 in murine T1D has been established through transgenic NOD mice that over-express IL-10 or where exogenous administration of recombinant IL-10, plasmid DNA encoding IL-10, or cells expressing IL-10 have been used (88–90). Moreover, *in vitro*, IL-10 protects human islets from the cytotoxic effects of inflammatory cytokines (91).

From the innate arm of the immune system, variant alleles of the T1-IFN receptor downstream signaling protein Tyk2, the cytosolic viral RNA sensor IFIH1 (MDA5), the macrophage lysosomal enzyme cathepsin H, and the phosphatase *SH2B3* are also associated with risk for T1D (**Table 1**). Collectively, these genes along with *PTPN22, IL10, SOCS1* and potentially others signify a major role for innate immune responses in T1D pathogenesis. Similar to T-cell responses, isogenic systems are critical for understanding how each risk variant affects innate immune function.

ISOGENIC MODELING OF INNATE-ADAPTIVE IMMUNE INTERACTIONS

Innate APCs participate in the initiation of immune responses; however, they also play an important role in sustaining an ongoing adaptive immune response. Interaction of APCs with antigen-specific $CD4^+$ T cells provides bi-directional signals to both cell types. $CD4^+$ T helper type 1 (T_H1) cells are important enhancers of macrophage function. Secreted cytokines (e.g., IFN-γ) and membrane-associated so-stimulatory molecules [e.g., CD40 ligand (CD40L)] expressed by T_H1 cells arm macrophages to more effectively kill microbes or infected cells. In T1D pathogenesis, there are essential roles for T_H1 T cells, IFN-γ, CD40-CD40L, and intra-islet macrophages. Where IFN-γ-secreting T_H1 cells encounter macrophages in the islets of NOD mice, the macrophages become activated and produce inflammatory cytokines and reactive oxygen species that kill β cells (92).

Most human studies of macrophages and DCs rely on two sources of cells—transformed monocytic leukemia cell lines or peripheral blood monocytes isolated from venipuncture. Some studies utilize alveolar macrophages derived from broncioloaviolar lavage or other specialized macrophages that are collected and studied *ex vivo*; however, sample number and size are limiting. PBMCs, while plentiful in number, easy to differentiation into macrophages or DCs, and available from large cohorts due to the low risk of venipuncture, are not ideal for all genetotype:phenotype studies where as discussed above, isogenic systems are key. This is further complicated in monocytes, macrophages and DCs because they are non-dividing cells in culture and generally difficult to modify genetically. iPSCs offer a solution to both problems because they are relatively simple to modify by lentiviral gene delivery or CRISPR/Cas9 and they are effectively immortal in culture. Differentiation of monocytes from iPSC offers the opportunity to study individual T1D risk genes in macrophages and DCs with unprecedented clarity. Protocols for differentiation of iPSC-derived monocytes vary widely from a simple two-cytokine mix of IL-3 and macrophage colony-stimulating factor (MCSF) (93) to a complex mix of cytokines and growth factors (94). Both protocols yield monocytes that can be differentiated into macrophages or DCs using standard conditions (MCSF for macrophages; GM-CSF + IL-4 for DCs), and the differentiated cells retain functional properties of peripheral blood monocyte-derived cells. Thus, isogenic systems now allow researchers to study the effects of a gene variant in either adaptive or innate immune cells alone, but more importantly, we can now determine how T1D risk variants impact innate/adaptive immune interactions, which are more representative of *in vivo* disease etiology.

THE β CELL AND ISLET MICROENVIRONMENT

While the immune system is thought to serve as the primary pathogenic mediator of T1D, there are events leading up to that cytotoxic cell–cell interaction that must occur to facilitate autoreactive T-cell destruction of β cells. Specifically, autoreactive $CD8^+$ T cells must home from the bloodstream and tether to inflamed endothelium creating firm adhesion contacts, extravasate through the endothelial membrane into the extracellular matrix (ECM), and eventually survey the microenvironment for their cognate antigens presented by HLA class I hyperexpressing islets (95). To completely model the events driving immune destruction of β cells *in vitro*, culture systems are needed where both β cells and endothelium can be derived. Extensive research has focused on the differentiation of functional, glucose-responsive, insulin-secreting β cells from human embryonic stem cells (hES) (96–98) as well as iPSC (99–103). Established protocols rely upon multistage culture of pluripotent cells to derive definitive endoderm followed by progressive differentiation of pancreatic endoderm. Often the β cells (or β-like cells) are transplanted to immunodeficient mice where further maturation and functional development continue *in vivo* (104–106). More recently, methods have been developed to convert human fibroblasts into β-like cells by compressing the differentiation protocol so that iPSC reprogramming and differentiation of endoderm occur simultaneously (107). Many of these efforts are being carried out with the eventual goal of replacing β cell mass in T1D patients or utilizing xenotransplantation into humanized mice to model T1D pathogenesis. An alternative is to use β-like cells and immune cells from syngeneic iPSC to model immune destruction of β cells *in vitro*. This process could include endothelial layers (108–110), or ECM barriers that mimic key structures involved in immune homing *in vivo*. The advantage of this specific approach would include the ability to test novel strategies for blocking cellular adhesion, chemotaxis to inflammatory chemokines (e.g., IP-10), as well as potentially blocking degradation of the ECM needed for T-cell migration into the islet microenvironment.

ISOGENIC CELLULAR SYSTEMS: A TOOL FOR EXPEDITING TRANSLATIONAL THERAPIES

The emerging fields of iPSC and isogenic cellular systems, when coupled with genome-editing technologies, hold great potential for elucidating causative genes in complex disorders such as T1D. With at least 57 independent genetic variants contributing to overall risk, the need for experimental platforms to expedite validation of causal variants is paramount to the field of functional genomics. Before starting an iPSC project, a few considerations must be made: (1) What will be the source material for iPSC reprogramming (i.e., risk gene profile)? (2) Which of several available iPSC reprogramming methods will be utilized? and (3) What differentiation protocols are available for the cells of interest?

Each investigator must determine starting cell source and reprogramming method based on available cells and the ultimate research plan. Our group has found that $CD34^+$ HSCs isolated from peripheral blood can be efficiently reprogrammed into iPSCs using Sendai virus (**Figure 5**). This method has a few advantages over the use of PBMCs. First, $CD34^+$ progenitor cells can be isolated from fresh, non-mobilized peripheral blood and expanded *in vitro* (111). Second, the efficiency to generate iPSCs is higher with this approach versus non-sorted PBMC. We have observed that as few as 2,000 isolated $CD34^+$ HSCs yielded several iPSC colonies. Finally, the resultant iPSC will have native genetic configurations at both the TCR and immunoglobulin loci. However, $CD34^+$ cells may not always be the best source of donor material. Where a re-arranged TCR with known antigen recognition is desired, $CD4^+$ or $CD8^+$ T cells from T1D patients could be used. In addition, it is known that T-cell-derived iPSCs differentiate back into T cells more efficiently, putatively due to epigenetic memory of the lineage (73).

In addition to cell type, it is particularly important to know the T1D risk genotype(s) of donor materials. One initiative at the University of Florida Center for Cellular Reprogramming is building an iPSC resource for genomic medicine. Samples from 50 healthy donors (25 males/25 females) with genome-wide SNP typing performed using the ImmunoChip platform are being utilized to generate iPSC lines. The SNP library will include all known T1D risk variants making this cell library and others like it (e.g., the Helmsley Cellular Research Hub, cellhub.org) powerful tools for studying complex genetic traits. Such an iPSC library with SNP database will provide an extremely useful common platform for SNP validation studies in combination with conventional gene editing technologies (**Figure 4**). For example, starting from iPSC clones harboring heterozygous status for a particular SNP (**Figure 4**, Module A), an investigator can obtain SNP hemizygous clones through CRISPR/Cas9-mediated allele targeting. Using such clones, one can study the effect of SNP variations within isogenic conditions in a relatively short timeframe.

Reprogramming somatic cells into iPSC is no longer limited to the investigators who have developed various methods in their own labs. Since the initial discovery of the "Yamanaka Factors" in 2006 where four minimal genes (*Oct3/4*, *Sox2*, *c-Myc*, and *Klf4*) were identified as key iPSC reprogramming factors (112), numerous advancements in reprogramming gene delivery have been made: these include delivery of reprogramming genes as lentiviral transgenes, plasmid DNA, or messenger RNA. Each of these platforms has become commercially available in reprogramming kits so that most labs can reprogram iPSC from a variety of tissues. Our group has found most success with a Sendai virus reprogramming vector. This non-integrating and self-limiting murine parainfluenza virus delivers the four essential iPSC genes in a single polycistronic message (**Figure 5B**) (113–115). Regardless of the method used, iPSCs take on a highly pluripotent phenotype and can be used to differentiate numerous lineages.

We have highlighted earlier progress in differentiating iPSC into key immune, endocrine, and endothelial cell types.

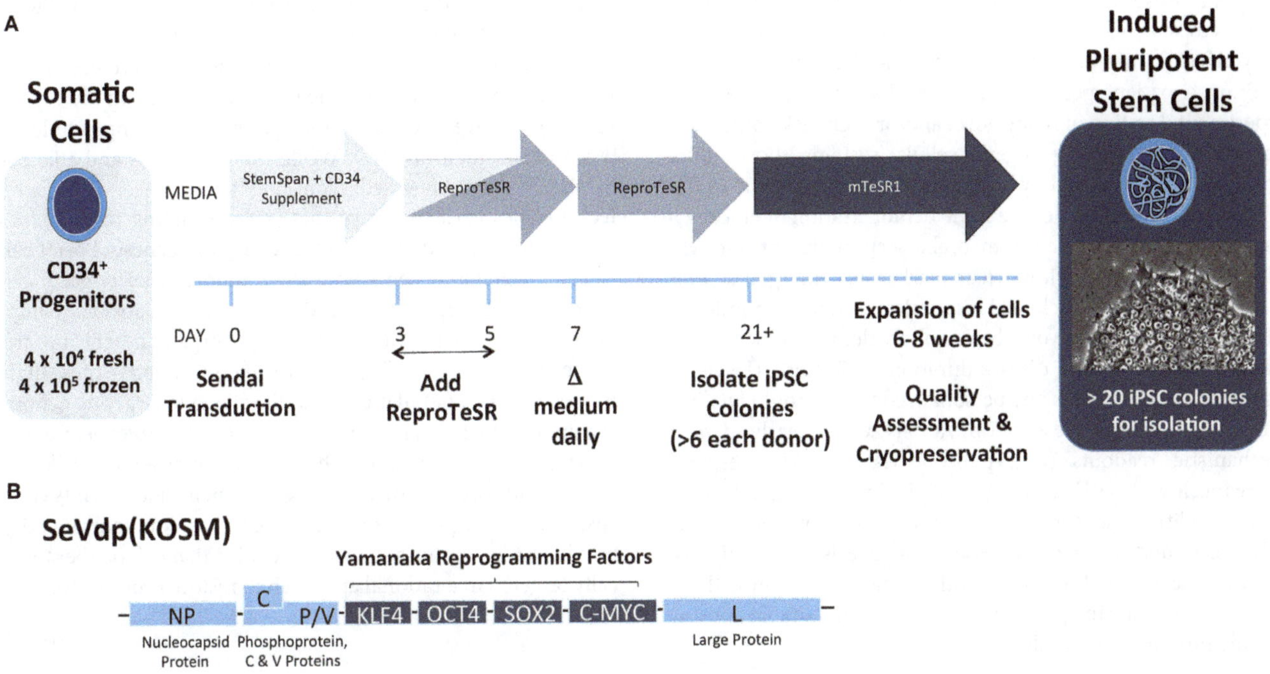

FIGURE 5 | Induced pluripotent stem cell (iPSC) reprogramming schematic from CD34+ cells using Sendai virus. **(A)** CD34+ progenitor cells are transduced with Sendai virus on day 0 and are cultured in feeder-free conditions on Matrigel-coated plates with CD34+ expansion medium (e.g., StemSpan SFEMII plus StemSpan CD34+ Expansion Supplement) for the first 3 days. Medium to support reprogramming (e.g., ReproTeSR) is added on days 3 and 5. Starting on day 7, medium is replaced daily until colonies are sufficiently large to isolate clonally, typically on day 21. After isolation, cells are cultured in PSC maintenance medium (e.g., mTeSR1) for 4–6 weeks of expansion. After expansion, iPSCs undergo assessment for pluripotency and normal karyotype and can be cryopreserved for later use. **(B)** Replication defective Sendai virus (SeVdp KOSM) contains Sendai genes NP (nucleocapsid), P (Phosphoprotein), L (large protein), C protein, V protein, and Yamanaka reprogramming genes KLF4, OCT4, SOX2, and c-MYC.

Without doubt, future applications of this approach will continue to expand as the community derives additional cell types from iPSC progenitor populations. The ability to switch between protective and susceptible variants and effectively turn genes on/off or up/down will allow the reductionist types of mechanistic studies previously only possible in gene knockout or transgenic animal models. One can certainly envision future models employing iPSC that layer increasingly complex admixtures of cells to recapitulate tissue micro-environments complete with multiple endocrine cell types, acinar tissues, microvasculature, and perhaps even innervation. We, along with others, are beginning to print living cells into liquid-like solid matrices allowing for exquisite control of cellular distribution in 3D space (116). The preliminary transcriptional profiles that have emerged from the transition from 2D culture in plastic wells to 3D cell culture have already suggested a distinct gene expression signature, more akin to that extracted from native tissues. Specific investigations using such 3D culture systems together with isogenic cellular models are needed to examine T1-IFN signaling with modulation of IFIH1 and TYK2 risk alleles as well as costimulatory pathways known to confer T1D risk (e.g., CD28/CTLA4 and CD226/TIGIT) (**Table 1**). Moreover, there will certainly be applications to reconstruct immune developmental niches to recapitulate key elements of hematopoietic development in the bone marrow, thymus, and secondary lymphoid organs. Such studies are expected to afford novel drug discovery through identification of new therapeutic targets.

The most obvious applications for stem cells in the T1D field reside in the ongoing need to replace the loss and functional inactivity of endogenous β cell mass that precipitates glucose dysregulation [reviewed in Ref. (117)]. To date, this has been accomplished through both hES- and iPSC-derived insulin-producing β cells. The capacity to model and recreate not only β cells but also functional immune populations will allow the testing of therapies to close the translational loop and prevent recurrent auto- or allo-immune rejection of transplanted β cells. Indeed, this might be accomplished by introducing genes to protect iPSC-generated β cells against apoptosis (e.g., GLIS3) (118) or to shield them from immunological attack, representing key objectives for iPSC-derived treatments in the regenerative medicine space.

Interventional trials to restore or preserve β cells in T1D have largely been driven by individual investigator sponsored trials in the context of larger consortiums (e.g., TrialNet and the Immune Tolerance Network). These efforts have largely taken the form of repurposing clinically approved drugs from other diseases or have been based on preliminary studies generated in the NOD mouse model of T1D. While these efforts are beginning to demonstrate some transient preservation of C-peptide (the serum marker co-secreted in equimolar amounts with insulin), no current therapy has yet resulted in an FDA-approved intervention capable of demonstrating long-term efficacy (119–128). We propose that additional dose finding studies using human isogenic cellular systems to screen for desired mechanistic outcomes could potentially inform clinical trial agent selection and dosing.

From a patient perspective, the notion of equipoise limits experimental testing of many novel and/or high-risk combinatorial agents. By adopting isogenic cellular systems, those limitations could be mitigated by testing and optimizing prior to trial validations. Moreover, despite some demonstration of efficacy in preliminary trials (e.g., teplizumab, abatacept, alefacept, and ATG with or without G-CSF), no clear marker has emerged *a priori* that effectively predicts clinical responders or non-responders to any particular agent beyond basic cohort demographics of age, residual C-peptide, and disease duration (127–129). The use of isogenic cellular systems and personalized testing could facilitate drug selection and dose optimizations with clearly defined mechanistic readouts (e.g., phosphorylated-STAT5 response following low-dose IL-2) (130–133). Ultimately, the advent of genomic editing and isogenic cellular systems will not only enable a deeper understanding of disease pathogenesis but should also expedite the speed of discovery and clinical translation with the hope of both restoring β cell mass and inducing durable antigen-specific immunological tolerance.

CONCLUSION

The emergence of genomic medicine has accelerated the rate of discovery with regard to the genetic basis of T1D. Multidimensional datasets now make it possible to overlay components of genetic variation, epigenetics, and transcriptional control of gene expression. Unfortunately, the vast number of associated SNPs, heterogeneity in human disease, and limits of clinical resources present a new set of challenges. There remains a paramount need to move beyond discovery of associated SNPs to a deeper understanding of causative variants to elucidate the molecular mechanisms and pathways of disease. The advent of iPSC technologies and precision gene editing now allows researchers to expedite the discovery and validation of these disease-associated variants.

Induced pluripotent stem cell technologies were initially met with great enthusiasm with the prospect of offering the capacity for regenerative medicine applications, including autologous β cell replacement in T1D. While the robustness and efficiency of these approaches will continue to advance, the current technologies exist to derive these cells, enabling researchers to build more powerful models of disease pathogenesis. Specifically, isogenic cellular systems now allow modeling of target β cells, effector T-cell populations, and the innate and stromal components that interact with both the target organ and effector arms of the immune system. The capacity to rapidly derive these highly limited and rare populations at scale, all while targeting genomic loci in a high-throughput manner is expected to expedite functional genomics in a manner heretofore not observed. A detailed understanding of the mechanisms by which gene variants confer susceptibility or protection to disease will undoubtedly identify a number of key immunological lynchpins that can be therapeutically targeted in a rational approach to restore immune tolerance to β cells in individuals with T1D.

AUTHOR CONTRIBUTIONS

MW and TB conceived the content and contributed to the writing and editing of the manuscript. KS and NT contributed to the writing and editing of the manuscript.

ACKNOWLEDGMENTS

The authors would like to thank the members of the University of Florida Diabetes Institute for insightful comments and discussions. The authors would like to thank Dr. Amanda Posgai for critical reading of the manuscript.

REFERENCES

1. Bluestone JA, Herold K, Eisenbarth G. Genetics, pathogenesis and clinical interventions in type 1 diabetes. *Nature* (2010) 464(7293):1293–300. doi:10.1038/nature08933
2. Atkinson MA, Eisenbarth GS. Type 1 diabetes: new perspectives on disease pathogenesis and treatment. *Lancet* (2001) 358(9277):221–9. doi:10.1016/S0140-6736(01)05415-0
3. Onengut-Gumuscu S, Chen WM, Burren O, Cooper NJ, Quinlan AR, Mychaleckyj JC, et al. Fine mapping of type 1 diabetes susceptibility loci and evidence for colocalization of causal variants with lymphoid gene enhancers. *Nat Genet* (2015) 47(4):381–6. doi:10.1038/ng.3245
4. Atkinson MA, Bluestone JA, Eisenbarth GS, Hebrok M, Herold KC, Accili D, et al. How does type 1 diabetes develop? The notion of homicide or beta-cell suicide revisited. *Diabetes* (2011) 60(5):1370–9. doi:10.2337/db10-1797
5. Marson A, Housley WJ, Hafler DA. Genetic basis of autoimmunity. *J Clin Invest* (2015) 125(6):2234–41. doi:10.1172/JCI78086
6. Dendrou CA, Plagnol V, Fung E, Yang JH, Downes K, Cooper JD, et al. Cell-specific protein phenotypes for the autoimmune locus IL2RA using a genotype-selectable human bioresource. *Nat Genet* (2009) 41(9):1011–5. doi:10.1038/ng.434
7. Brehm MA, Cuthbert A, Yang C, Miller DM, Diiorio P, Laning J, et al. Parameters for establishing humanized mouse models to study human immunity: analysis of human hematopoietic stem cell engraftment in three immunodeficient strains of mice bearing the IL2rγnull mutation. *Clin Immunol* (2010) 135(1):84–98. doi:10.1016/j.clim.2009.12.008
8. Zschaler J, Schlorke D, Arnhold J. Differences in innate immune response between man and mouse. *Crit Rev Immunol* (2014) 34(5):433–54. doi:10.1615/CritRevImmunol.2014011600
9. Brehm MA, Powers AC, Shultz LD, Greiner DL. Advancing animal models of human type 1 diabetes by engraftment of functional human tissues in immunodeficient mice. *Cold Spring Harb Perspect Med* (2012) 2(5):a007757. doi:10.1101/cshperspect.a007757
10. Gianani R, Campbell-Thompson M, Sarkar SA, Wasserfall C, Pugliese A, Solis JM, et al. Dimorphic histopathology of long-standing childhood-onset diabetes. *Diabetologia* (2010) 53(4):690–8. doi:10.1007/s00125-009-1642-y
11. Rowe PA, Campbell-Thompson ML, Schatz DA, Atkinson MA. The pancreas in human type 1 diabetes. *Semin Immunopathol* (2011) 33(1):29–43. doi:10.1007/s00281-010-0208-x
12. Coppieters KT, Dotta F, Amirian N, Campbell PD, Kay TW, Atkinson MA, et al. Demonstration of islet-autoreactive CD8 T cells in insulitic lesions from recent onset and long-term type 1 diabetes patients. *J Exp Med* (2012) 209(1):51–60. doi:10.1084/jem.20111187
13. Campbell-Thompson M, Fu A, Kaddis JS, Wasserfall C, Schatz DA, Pugliese A, et al. Insulitis and beta-cell mass in the natural history of type 1 diabetes. *Diabetes* (2016) 65(3):719–31. doi:10.2337/db15-0779

14. Rodriguez-Calvo T, Suwandi JS, Amirian N, Zapardiel-Gonzalo J, Anquetil F, Sabouri S, et al. Heterogeneity and lobularity of pancreatic pathology in type 1 diabetes during the prediabetic phase. *J Histochem Cytochem* (2015) 63(8):626–36. doi:10.1369/0022155415576543
15. Eisenbarth GS. Banting lecture 2009: an unfinished journey: molecular pathogenesis to prevention of type 1A diabetes. *Diabetes* (2010) 59(4):759–74. doi:10.2337/db09-1855
16. Barnett AH, Eff C, Leslie RD, Pyke DA. Diabetes in identical twins. A study of 200 pairs. *Diabetologia* (1981) 20(2):87–93. doi:10.1007/BF00262007
17. Redondo MJ, Yu L, Hawa M, Mackenzie T, Pyke DA, Eisenbarth GS, et al. Heterogeneity of type I diabetes: analysis of monozygotic twins in Great Britain and the United States. *Diabetologia* (2001) 44(3):354–62. doi:10.1007/s001250051626
18. Laugesen E, Ostergaard JA, Leslie RD; Danish Diabetes Academy Workshop and Workshop Speakers. Latent autoimmune diabetes of the adult: current knowledge and uncertainty. *Diabet Med* (2015) 32(7):843–52. doi:10.1111/dme.12700
19. Redondo MJ, Jeffrey J, Fain PR, Eisenbarth GS, Orban T. Concordance for islet autoimmunity among monozygotic twins. *N Engl J Med* (2008) 359(26):2849–50. doi:10.1056/NEJMc0805398
20. Bradfield JP, Qu HQ, Wang K, Zhang H, Sleiman PM, Kim CE, et al. A genome-wide meta-analysis of six type 1 diabetes cohorts identifies multiple associated loci. *PLoS Genet* (2011) 7(9):e1002293. doi:10.1371/journal.pgen.1002293
21. Barrett JC, Clayton DG, Concannon P, Akolkar B, Cooper JD, Erlich HA, et al. Genome-wide association study and meta-analysis find that over 40 loci affect risk of type 1 diabetes. *Nat Genet* (2009) 41(6):703–7. doi:10.1038/ng.381
22. Wellcome Trust Case Control Consortium. Genome-wide association study of 14,000 cases of seven common diseases and 3,000 shared controls. *Nature* (2007) 447(7145):661–78. doi:10.1038/nature05911
23. Cooper JD, Smyth DJ, Smiles AM, Plagnol V, Walker NM, Allen JE, et al. Meta-analysis of genome-wide association study data identifies additional type 1 diabetes risk loci. *Nat Genet* (2008) 40(12):1399–401. doi:10.1038/ng.249
24. Todd JA, Walker NM, Cooper JD, Smyth DJ, Downes K, Plagnol V, et al. Robust associations of four new chromosome regions from genome-wide analyses of type 1 diabetes. *Nat Genet* (2007) 39(7):857–64. doi:10.1038/ng2068
25. Fortune MD, Guo H, Burren O, Schofield E, Walker NM, Ban M, et al. Statistical colocalization of genetic risk variants for related autoimmune diseases in the context of common controls. *Nat Genet* (2015) 47(7):839–46. doi:10.1038/ng.3330
26. Evangelou M, Smyth DJ, Fortune MD, Burren OS, Walker NM, Guo H, et al. A method for gene-based pathway analysis using genomewide association study summary statistics reveals nine new type 1 diabetes associations. *Genet Epidemiol* (2014) 38(8):661–70. doi:10.1002/gepi.21853
27. Sosenko JM, Skyler JS, Mahon J, Krischer JP, Beam CA, Boulware DC, et al. Validation of the diabetes prevention trial-type 1 risk score in the TrialNet natural history study. *Diabetes Care* (2011) 34(8):1785–7. doi:10.2337/dc11-0641
28. Hummel S, Beyerlein A, Tamura R, Uusitalo U, Andren Aronsson C, Yang J, et al. First infant formula type and risk of islet autoimmunity in the environmental determinants of diabetes in the young (TEDDY) study. *Diabetes Care* (2017) 40(3):398–404. doi:10.2337/dc16-1624
29. Stene LC, Oikarinen S, Hyoty H, Barriga KJ, Norris JM, Klingensmith G, et al. Enterovirus infection and progression from islet autoimmunity to type 1 diabetes: the diabetes and autoimmunity study in the young (DAISY). *Diabetes* (2010) 59(12):3174–80. doi:10.2337/db10-0866
30. Ziegler AG, Meier-Stiegen F, Winkler C, Bonifacio E. Prospective evaluation of risk factors for the development of islet autoimmunity and type 1 diabetes during puberty – TEENDIAB: study design. *Pediatr Diabetes* (2012) 13(5):419–24. doi:10.1111/j.1399-5448.2011.00763.x
31. Achenbach P, Barker J, Bonifacio E. Modulating the natural history of type 1 diabetes in children at high genetic risk by mucosal insulin immunization. *Curr Diab Rep* (2008) 8(2):87–93. doi:10.1007/s11892-008-0017-y
32. Ferreira RC, Guo H, Coulson RM, Smyth DJ, Pekalski ML, Burren OS, et al. A type I interferon transcriptional signature precedes autoimmunity in children genetically at-risk of type 1 diabetes. *Diabetes* (2014) 63(7):2538–50. doi:10.2337/db13-1777
33. Bottini N, Musumeci L, Alonso A, Rahmouni S, Nika K, Rostamkhani M, et al. A functional variant of lymphoid tyrosine phosphatase is associated with type I diabetes. *Nat Genet* (2004) 36(4):337–8. doi:10.1038/ng1323
34. Mi H, Muruganujan A, Thomas PD. PANTHER in 2013: modeling the evolution of gene function, and other gene attributes, in the context of phylogenetic trees. *Nucleic Acids Res* (2013) 41(Database issue):D377–86. doi:10.1093/nar/gks1118
35. Thomas PD, Campbell MJ, Kejariwal A, Mi H, Karlak B, Daverman R, et al. PANTHER: a library of protein families and subfamilies indexed by function. *Genome Res* (2003) 13(9):2129–41. doi:10.1101/gr.772403
36. Bersenev A, Wu C, Balcerek J, Jing J, Kundu M, Blobel GA, et al. Lnk constrains myeloproliferative diseases in mice. *J Clin Invest* (2010) 120(6):2058–69. doi:10.1172/JCI42032
37. Gery S, Cao Q, Gueller S, Xing H, Tefferi A, Koeffler HP. Lnk inhibits myeloproliferative disorder-associated JAK2 mutant, JAK2V617F. *J Leukoc Biol* (2009) 85(6):957–65. doi:10.1189/jlb.0908575
38. Yoshida K, Toki T, Okuno Y, Kanezaki R, Shiraishi Y, Sato-Otsubo A, et al. The landscape of somatic mutations in Down syndrome-related myeloid disorders. *Nat Genet* (2013) 45(11):1293–9. doi:10.1038/ng.2759
39. Westra HJ, Peters MJ, Esko T, Yaghootkar H, Schurmann C, Kettunen J, et al. Systematic identification of trans eQTLs as putative drivers of known disease associations. *Nat Genet* (2013) 45(10):1238–43. doi:10.1038/ng.2756
40. Gonzales AJ, Bowman JW, Fici GJ, Zhang M, Mann DW, Mitton-Fry M. Oclacitinib (APOQUEL(®)) is a novel Janus kinase inhibitor with activity against cytokines involved in allergy. *J Vet Pharmacol Ther* (2014) 37(4):317–24. doi:10.1111/jvp.12101
41. Waters MJ, Brooks AJ. JAK2 activation by growth hormone and other cytokines. *Biochem J* (2015) 466(1):1–11. doi:10.1042/BJ20141293
42. Storling J, Pociot F. Type 1 diabetes candidate genes linked to pancreatic islet cell inflammation and beta-cell apoptosis. *Genes (Basel)* (2017) 8(2):E72. doi:10.3390/genes8020072
43. Grennan AK. Genevestigator. Facilitating web-based gene-expression analysis. *Plant Physiol* (2006) 141(4):1164–6. doi:10.1104/pp.104.900198
44. Ram R, Mehta M, Nguyen QT, Larma I, Boehm BO, Pociot F, et al. Systematic evaluation of genes and genetic variants associated with type 1 diabetes susceptibility. *J Immunol* (2016) 196(7):3043–53. doi:10.4049/jimmunol.1502056
45. Anderson MS, Venanzi ES, Chen Z, Berzins SP, Benoist C, Mathis D. The cellular mechanism of Aire control of T cell tolerance. *Immunity* (2005) 23(2):227–39. doi:10.1016/j.immuni.2005.07.005
46. Fontenot JD, Rudensky AY. Molecular aspects of regulatory T cell development. *Semin Immunol* (2004) 16(2):73–80. doi:10.1016/j.smim.2003.12.002
47. Husebye ES, Anderson MS. Autoimmune polyendocrine syndromes: clues to type 1 diabetes pathogenesis. *Immunity* (2010) 32(4):479–87. doi:10.1016/j.immuni.2010.03.016
48. Eisenbarth GS. Insulin autoimmunity: immunogenetics/immunopathogenesis of type 1A diabetes. *Ann N Y Acad Sci* (2003) 1005:109–18. doi:10.1196/annals.1288.012
49. Kieback E, Hilgenberg E, Stervbo U, Lampropoulou V, Shen P, Bunse M, et al. Thymus-derived regulatory T cells are positively selected on natural self-antigen through cognate interactions of high functional avidity. *Immunity* (2016) 44(5):1114–26. doi:10.1016/j.immuni.2016.04.018
50. Pugliese A, Boulware D, Yu L, Babu S, Steck AK, Becker D, et al. HLA-DRB1*15:01-DQA1*01:02-DQB1*06:02 haplotype protects autoantibody-positive relatives from type 1 diabetes throughout the stages of disease progression. *Diabetes* (2016) 65(4):1109–19. doi:10.2337/db15-1105
51. Sosinowski T, Eisenbarth GS. Type 1 diabetes: primary antigen/peptide/register/trimolecular complex. *Immunol Res* (2013) 55(1–3):270–6. doi:10.1007/s12026-012-8367-6
52. van Lummel M, van Veelen PA, Zaldumbide A, de Ru A, Janssen GM, Moustakas AK, et al. Type 1 diabetes-associated HLA-DQ8 transdimer accommodates a unique peptide repertoire. *J Biol Chem* (2012) 287(12):9514–24. doi:10.1074/jbc.M111.313940

53. Bennett ST, Lucassen AM, Gough SC, Powell EE, Undlien DE, Pritchard LE, et al. Susceptibility to human type 1 diabetes at IDDM2 is determined by tandem repeat variation at the insulin gene minisatellite locus. *Nat Genet* (1995) 9(3):284–92. doi:10.1038/ng0395-284
54. Pugliese A, Zeller M, Fernandez A Jr, Zalcberg LJ, Bartlett RJ, Ricordi C, et al. The insulin gene is transcribed in the human thymus and transcription levels correlated with allelic variation at the INS VNTR-IDDM2 susceptibility locus for type 1 diabetes. *Nat Genet* (1997) 15(3):293–7. doi:10.1038/ng0397-293
55. Nakayama M, Abiru N, Moriyama H, Babaya N, Liu E, Miao D, et al. Prime role for an insulin epitope in the development of type 1 diabetes in NOD mice. *Nature* (2005) 435(7039):220–3. doi:10.1038/nature03523
56. Michels AW, Landry LG, McDaniel KA, Yu L, Campbell-Thompson M, Kwok WW, et al. Islet-derived CD4 T cells targeting proinsulin in human autoimmune diabetes. *Diabetes* (2017) 66(3):722–34. doi:10.2337/db16-1025
57. Mannering SI, Harrison LC, Williamson NA, Morris JS, Thearle DJ, Jensen KP, et al. The insulin A-chain epitope recognized by human T cells is posttranslationally modified. *J Exp Med* (2005) 202(9):1191–7. doi:10.1084/jem.20051251
58. Delong T, Wiles TA, Baker RL, Bradley B, Barbour G, Reisdorph R, et al. Pathogenic CD4 T cells in type 1 diabetes recognize epitopes formed by peptide fusion. *Science* (2016) 351(6274):711–4. doi:10.1126/science.aad2791
59. Wicker LS, Todd JA, Peterson LB. Genetic control of autoimmune diabetes in the NOD mouse. *Annu Rev Immunol* (1995) 13:179–200. doi:10.1146/annurev.iy.13.040195.001143
60. Wicker LS, Miller BJ, Coker LZ, McNally SE, Scott S, Mullen Y, et al. Genetic control of diabetes and insulitis in the nonobese diabetic (NOD) mouse. *J Exp Med* (1987) 165(6):1639–54. doi:10.1084/jem.165.6.1639
61. Bingley PJ, Bonifacio E, Mueller PW. Diabetes antibody standardization program: first assay proficiency evaluation. *Diabetes* (2003) 52(5):1128–36. doi:10.2337/diabetes.52.5.1128
62. Torn C, Mueller PW, Schlosser M, Bonifacio E, Bingley PJ. Diabetes antibody standardization program: evaluation of assays for autoantibodies to glutamic acid decarboxylase and islet antigen-2. *Diabetologia* (2008) 51(5):846–52. doi:10.1007/s00125-008-0967-2
63. Schlosser M, Mueller PW, Torn C, Bonifacio E, Bingley PJ. Diabetes antibody standardization program: evaluation of assays for insulin autoantibodies. *Diabetologia* (2010) 53(12):2611–20. doi:10.1007/s00125-010-1915-5
64. Schlosser M, Mueller PW, Achenbach P, Lampasona V, Bingley PJ. Diabetes antibody standardization program: first evaluation of assays for autoantibodies to IA-2beta. *Diabetes Care* (2011) 34(11):2410–2. doi:10.2337/dc11-1161
65. Lampasona V, Schlosser M, Mueller PW, Williams AJ, Wenzlau JM, Hutton JC, et al. Diabetes antibody standardization program: first proficiency evaluation of assays for autoantibodies to zinc transporter 8. *Clin Chem* (2011) 57(12):1693–702. doi:10.1373/clinchem.2011.170662
66. Wasserfall C, Montgomery E, Yu L, Michels A, Gianani R, Pugliese A, et al. Validation of a rapid type 1 diabetes autoantibody screening assay for community based screening of organ donors to identify subjects at increased risk for the disease. *Clin Exp Immunol* (2016) 185(1):33–41. doi:10.1111/cei.12797
67. Seay HR, Yusko E, Rothweiler SJ, Zhang L, Posgai AL, Campbell-Thompson M, et al. Tissue distribution and clonal diversity of the T and B cell repertoire in type 1 diabetes. *JCI Insight* (2016) 1(20):e88242. doi:10.1172/jci.insight.88242
68. Nepom GT, Buckner JH, Novak EJ, Reichstetter S, Reijonen H, Gebe J, et al. HLA class II tetramers: tools for direct analysis of antigen-specific CD4+ T cells. *Arthritis Rheum* (2002) 46(1):5–12. doi:10.1002/1529-0131(200201)46:1<5::AID-ART10063>3.0.CO;2-S
69. Brusko TM, Koya RC, Zhu S, Lee MR, Putnam AL, McClymont SA, et al. Human antigen-specific regulatory T cells generated by T cell receptor gene transfer. *PLoS One* (2010) 5(7):e11726. doi:10.1371/journal.pone.0011726
70. Esensten JH, Bluestone JA, Lim WA. Engineering therapeutic T cells: from synthetic biology to clinical trials. *Annu Rev Pathol* (2017) 12:305–30. doi:10.1146/annurev-pathol-052016-100304
71. Newby BN, Brusko TM, Zou B, Atkinson MA, Clare-Salzler M, Mathews CE. Type 1 interferons potentiate human CD8+ T cell cytotoxicity through a STAT4 and granzyme B dependent pathway. *Diabetes* (2017):db170106. doi:10.2337/db17-0106
72. Yeh W-I, Seay HR, Newby B, Posgai AL, Moniz FB, Michels A, et al. Avidity and Bystander Suppressive Capacity of Human Regulatory T Cells Expressing De Novo Autoreactive T-Cell Receptors in Type 1 Diabetes. *Front Immunol* (2017) 8:1313. doi:10.3389/fimmu.2017.01313
73. Kaneko S. In vitro generation of antigen-specific T cells from induced pluripotent stem cells of antigen-specific T cell origin. *Methods Mol Biol* (2016) 1393:67–73. doi:10.1007/978-1-4939-3338-9_6
74. Vizcardo R, Masuda K, Yamada D, Ikawa T, Shimizu K, Fujii S, et al. Regeneration of human tumor antigen-specific T cells from iPSCs derived from mature CD8(+) T cells. *Cell Stem Cell* (2013) 12(1):31–6. doi:10.1016/j.stem.2012.12.006
75. Chang CW, Lai YS, Lamb LS Jr, Townes TM. Broad T-cell receptor repertoire in T-lymphocytes derived from human induced pluripotent stem cells. *PLoS One* (2014) 9(5):e97335. doi:10.1371/journal.pone.0097335
76. Maeda T, Nagano S, Ichise H, Kataoka K, Yamada D, Ogawa S, et al. Regeneration of CD8alphabeta T cells from T-cell-derived iPSC imparts potent tumor antigen-specific cytotoxicity. *Cancer Res* (2016) 76(23):6839–50. doi:10.1158/0008-5472.CAN-16-1149
77. Okabe M, Ito S, Nishio N, Tanaka Y, Isobe K. Thymic epithelial cells induced from pluripotent stem cells by a three-dimensional spheroid culture system regenerates functional T cells in nude mice. *Cell Reprogram* (2015) 17(5):368–75. doi:10.1089/cell.2015.0006
78. Marro BS, Ware BC, Zak J, de la Torre JC, Rosen H, Oldstone MB. Progression of type 1 diabetes from the prediabetic stage is controlled by interferon-alpha signaling. *Proc Natl Acad Sci U S A* (2017) 114(14):3708–13. doi:10.1073/pnas.1700878114
79. Pane JA, Fleming FE, Graham KL, Thomas HE, Kay TW, Coulson BS. Rotavirus acceleration of type 1 diabetes in non-obese diabetic mice depends on type I interferon signalling. *Sci Rep* (2016) 6:29697. doi:10.1038/srep29697
80. Ylipaasto P, Klingel K, Lindberg AM, Otonkoski T, Kandolf R, Hovi T, et al. Enterovirus infection in human pancreatic islet cells, islet tropism in vivo and receptor involvement in cultured islet beta cells. *Diabetologia* (2004) 47(2):225–39. doi:10.1007/s00125-003-1297-z
81. Gamble DR, Taylor KW. Seasonal incidence of diabetes mellitus. *Br Med J* (1969) 3(5671):631–3. doi:10.1136/bmj.3.5671.631
82. Schulte BM, Bakkers J, Lanke KH, Melchers WJ, Westerlaken C, Allebes W, et al. Detection of enterovirus RNA in peripheral blood mononuclear cells of type 1 diabetic patients beyond the stage of acute infection. *Viral Immunol* (2010) 23(1):99–104. doi:10.1089/vim.2009.0072
83. Gamble DR, Kinsley ML, FitzGerald MG, Bolton R, Taylor KW. Viral antibodies in diabetes mellitus. *Br Med J* (1969) 3(5671):627–30. doi:10.1136/bmj.3.5671.627
84. Laitinen OH, Honkanen H, Pakkanen O, Oikarinen S, Hankaniemi MM, Huhtala H, et al. Coxsackievirus B1 is associated with induction of beta-cell autoimmunity that portends type 1 diabetes. *Diabetes* (2014) 63(2):446–55. doi:10.2337/db13-0619
85. Wang Y, Shaked I, Stanford SM, Zhou W, Curtsinger JM, Mikulski Z, et al. The autoimmunity-associated gene PTPN22 potentiates toll-like receptor-driven, type 1 interferon-dependent immunity. *Immunity* (2013) 39(1):111–22. doi:10.1016/j.immuni.2013.06.013
86. Wang Y, Ewart D, Crabtree JN, Yamamoto A, Baechler EC, Fazeli P, et al. PTPN22 variant R620W is associated with reduced toll-like receptor 7-induced type I interferon in systemic lupus erythematosus. *Arthritis Rheumatol* (2015) 67(9):2403–14. doi:10.1002/art.39211
87. Ouyang P, Rakus K, van Beurden SJ, Westphal AH, Davison AJ, Gatherer D, et al. IL-10 encoded by viruses: a remarkable example of independent acquisition of a cellular gene by viruses and its subsequent evolution in the viral genome. *J Gen Virol* (2014) 95(Pt 2):245–62. doi:10.1099/vir.0.058966-0
88. Pennline KJ, Roque-Gaffney E, Monahan M. Recombinant human IL-10 prevents the onset of diabetes in the nonobese diabetic mouse. *Clin Immunol Immunopathol* (1994) 71(2):169–75. doi:10.1006/clin.1994.1068
89. Pop SM, Wong CP, He Q, Wang Y, Wallet MA, Goudy KS, et al. The type and frequency of immunoregulatory CD4+ T-cells govern the efficacy of antigen-specific immunotherapy in nonobese diabetic mice. *Diabetes* (2007) 56(5):1395–402. doi:10.2337/db06-0543
90. Goudy KS, Burkhardt BR, Wasserfall C, Song S, Campbell-Thompson ML, Brusko T, et al. Systemic overexpression of IL-10 induces CD4+CD25+ cell populations in vivo and ameliorates type 1 diabetes in nonobese diabetic mice in a dose-dependent fashion. *J Immunol* (2003) 171(5):2270–8. doi:10.4049/jimmunol.171.5.2270

91. Marselli L, Dotta F, Piro S, Santangelo C, Masini M, Lupi R, et al. Th2 cytokines have a partial, direct protective effect on the function and survival of isolated human islets exposed to combined proinflammatory and Th1 cytokines. *J Clin Endocrinol Metab* (2001) 86(10):4974–8. doi:10.1210/jcem.86.10.7938
92. Calderon B, Suri A, Unanue ER. In CD4+ T-cell-induced diabetes, macrophages are the final effector cells that mediate islet beta-cell killing: studies from an acute model. *Am J Pathol* (2006) 169(6):2137–47. doi:10.2353/ajpath.2006.060539
93. van Wilgenburg B, Browne C, Vowles J, Cowley SA. Efficient, long term production of monocyte-derived macrophages from human pluripotent stem cells under partly-defined and fully-defined conditions. *PLoS One* (2013) 8(8):e71098. doi:10.1371/journal.pone.0071098
94. Yanagimachi MD, Niwa A, Tanaka T, Honda-Ozaki F, Nishimoto S, Murata Y, et al. Robust and highly-efficient differentiation of functional monocytic cells from human pluripotent stem cells under serum- and feeder cell-free conditions. *PLoS One* (2013) 8(4):e59243. doi:10.1371/journal.pone.0059243
95. Richardson SJ, Rodriguez-Calvo T, Gerling IC, Mathews CE, Kaddis JS, Russell MA, et al. Islet cell hyperexpression of HLA class I antigens: a defining feature in type 1 diabetes. *Diabetologia* (2016) 59(11):2448–58. doi:10.1007/s00125-016-4067-4
96. Jiang W, Shi Y, Zhao D, Chen S, Yong J, Zhang J, et al. In vitro derivation of functional insulin-producing cells from human embryonic stem cells. *Cell Res* (2007) 17(4):333–44. doi:10.1038/cr.2007.28
97. Shi Y. Generation of functional insulin-producing cells from human embryonic stem cells in vitro. *Methods Mol Biol* (2010) 636:79–85. doi:10.1007/978-1-60761-691-7_5
98. Bose B, Shenoy SP, Konda S, Wangikar P. Human embryonic stem cell differentiation into insulin secreting beta-cells for diabetes. *Cell Biol Int* (2012) 36(11):1013–20. doi:10.1042/CBI20120210
99. Zhang D, Jiang W, Liu M, Sui X, Yin X, Chen S, et al. Highly efficient differentiation of human ES cells and iPS cells into mature pancreatic insulin-producing cells. *Cell Res* (2009) 19(4):429–38. doi:10.1038/cr.2009.28
100. Thatava T, Nelson TJ, Edukulla R, Sakuma T, Ohmine S, Tonne JM, et al. Indolactam V/GLP-1-mediated differentiation of human iPS cells into glucose-responsive insulin-secreting progeny. *Gene Ther* (2011) 18(3):283–93. doi:10.1038/gt.2010.145
101. Kunisada Y, Tsubooka-Yamazoe N, Shoji M, Hosoya M. Small molecules induce efficient differentiation into insulin-producing cells from human induced pluripotent stem cells. *Stem Cell Res* (2012) 8(2):274–84. doi:10.1016/j.scr.2011.10.002
102. Toyoda T, Mae S, Tanaka H, Kondo Y, Funato M, Hosokawa Y, et al. Cell aggregation optimizes the differentiation of human ESCs and iPSCs into pancreatic bud-like progenitor cells. *Stem Cell Res* (2015) 14(2):185–97. doi:10.1016/j.scr.2015.01.007
103. Shahjalal HM, Shiraki N, Sakano D, Kikawa K, Ogaki S, Baba H, et al. Generation of insulin-producing beta-like cells from human iPS cells in a defined and completely xeno-free culture system. *J Mol Cell Biol* (2014) 6(5):394–408. doi:10.1093/jmcb/mju029
104. Kroon E, Martinson LA, Kadoya K, Bang AG, Kelly OG, Eliazer S, et al. Pancreatic endoderm derived from human embryonic stem cells generates glucose-responsive insulin-secreting cells in vivo. *Nat Biotechnol* (2008) 26(4):443–52. doi:10.1038/nbt1393
105. Rezania A, Bruin JE, Riedel MJ, Mojibian M, Asadi A, Xu J, et al. Maturation of human embryonic stem cell-derived pancreatic progenitors into functional islets capable of treating pre-existing diabetes in mice. *Diabetes* (2012) 61(8):2016–29. doi:10.2337/db11-1711
106. Szot GL, Yadav M, Lang J, Kroon E, Kerr J, Kadoya K, et al. Tolerance induction and reversal of diabetes in mice transplanted with human embryonic stem cell-derived pancreatic endoderm. *Cell Stem Cell* (2015) 16(2):148–57. doi:10.1016/j.stem.2014.12.001
107. Zhu S, Russ HA, Wang X, Zhang M, Ma T, Xu T, et al. Human pancreatic beta-like cells converted from fibroblasts. *Nat Commun* (2016) 7:10080. doi:10.1038/ncomms10080
108. Peters EB. Endothelial progenitor cells for the vascularization of engineered tissues. *Tissue Eng B Rev* (2017). doi:10.1089/ten.teb.2017.0127
109. Kurokawa YK, Yin RT, Shang MR, Shirure VS, Moya ML, George SC. Human iPS-derived endothelial cells for 3D microphysiological systems. *Tissue Eng C Methods* (2017) 23(8):474–84. doi:10.1089/ten.tec.2017.0133
110. Wong WT, Huang NF, Botham CM, Sayed N, Cooke JP. Endothelial cells derived from nuclear reprogramming. *Circ Res* (2012) 111(10):1363–75. doi:10.1161/CIRCRESAHA.111.247213
111. Koizumi K, Sawada K, Yamaguchi M, Notoya A, Tarumi T, Takano H, et al. In vitro expansion of CD34+/CD41+ cells from human peripheral blood CD34+/CD41- cells: role of cytokines for in vitro proliferation and differentiation of megakaryocytic progenitors. *Exp Hematol* (1998) 26(12):1140–7.
112. Takahashi K, Yamanaka S. Induction of pluripotent stem cells from mouse embryonic and adult fibroblast cultures by defined factors. *Cell* (2006) 126(4):663–76. doi:10.1016/j.cell.2006.07.024
113. Nakanishi M, Otsu M. Development of Sendai virus vectors and their potential applications in gene therapy and regenerative medicine. *Curr Gene Ther* (2012) 12(5):410–6. doi:10.2174/156652312802762518
114. Nishimura K, Segawa H, Goto T, Morishita M, Masago A, Takahashi H, et al. Persistent and stable gene expression by a cytoplasmic RNA replicon based on a noncytopathic variant Sendai virus. *J Biol Chem* (2007) 282(37):27383–91. doi:10.1074/jbc.M702028200
115. Nishimura K, Sano M, Ohtaka M, Furuta B, Umemura Y, Nakajima Y, et al. Development of defective and persistent Sendai virus vector: a unique gene delivery/expression system ideal for cell reprogramming. *J Biol Chem* (2011) 286(6):4760–71. doi:10.1074/jbc.M110.183780
116. Bhattacharjee T, Zehnder SM, Rowe KG, Jain S, Nixon RM, Sawyer WG, et al. Writing in the granular gel medium. *Sci Adv* (2015) 1(8):e1500655. doi:10.1126/sciadv.1500655
117. Pipeleers D, Robert T, De Mesmaeker I, Ling Z. Concise review: markers for assessing human stem cell-derived implants as beta-cell replacement in type 1 diabetes. *Stem Cells Transl Med* (2016) 5(10):1338–44. doi:10.5966/sctm.2015-0187
118. Nogueira TC, Paula FM, Villate O, Colli ML, Moura RF, Cunha DA, et al. GLIS3, a susceptibility gene for type 1 and type 2 diabetes, modulates pancreatic beta cell apoptosis via regulation of a splice variant of the BH3-only protein Bim. *PLoS Genet* (2013) 9(5):e1003532. doi:10.1371/journal.pgen.1003532
119. Daifotis AG, Koenig S, Chatenoud L, Herold KC. Anti-CD3 clinical trials in type 1 diabetes mellitus. *Clin Immunol* (2013) 149(3):268–78. doi:10.1016/j.clim.2013.05.001
120. Hagopian W, Ferry RJ Jr, Sherry N, Carlin D, Bonvini E, Johnson S, et al. Teplizumab preserves C-peptide in recent-onset type 1 diabetes: two-year results from the randomized, placebo-controlled Protege trial. *Diabetes* (2013) 62(11):3901–8. doi:10.2337/db13-0236
121. Herold KC, Gitelman SE, Ehlers MR, Gottlieb PA, Greenbaum CJ, Hagopian W, et al. Teplizumab (anti CD3 mAb) treatment preserves C-peptide responses in patients with new-onset type 1 diabetes in a randomized controlled trial: metabolic and immunologic features at baseline identify a subgroup of responders. *Diabetes* (2013) 62(11):3766–74. doi:10.2337/db13-0345
122. Vudattu NK, Herold KC. Treatment of new onset type 1 diabetes with teplizumab: successes and pitfalls in development. *Expert Opin Biol Ther* (2014) 14(3):377–85. doi:10.1517/14712598.2014.881797
123. Orban T, Bundy B, Becker DJ, Dimeglio LA, Gitelman SE, Goland R, et al. Costimulation modulation with abatacept in patients with recent-onset type 1 diabetes: follow-up 1 year after cessation of treatment. *Diabetes Care* (2014) 37(4):1069–75. doi:10.2337/dc13-0604
124. Pescovitz MD, Greenbaum CJ, Bundy B, Becker DJ, Gitelman SE, Goland R, et al. B-lymphocyte depletion with rituximab and beta-cell function: two-year results. *Diabetes Care* (2014) 37(2):453–9. doi:10.2337/dc13-0626
125. Rigby MR, Harris KM, Pinckney A, DiMeglio LA, Rendell MS, Felner EI, et al. Alefacept provides sustained clinical and immunological effects in new-onset type 1 diabetes patients. *J Clin Invest* (2015) 125(8):3285–96. doi:10.1172/JCI81722
126. Haller MJ, Gitelman SE, Gottlieb PA, Michels AW, Rosenthal SM, Shuster JJ, et al. Anti-thymocyte globulin/G-CSF treatment preserves β cell function in patients with established type 1 diabetes. *J Clin Invest* (2015) 125(1):448–55. doi:10.1172/JCI78492
127. Haller MJ, Gitelman SE, Gottlieb PA, Michels AW, Perry DJ, Schultz AR, et al. Antithymocyte globulin plus G-CSF combination therapy leads to sustained immunomodulatory and metabolic effects in a subset of responders with

established type 1 diabetes. *Diabetes* (2016) 65(12):3765–75. doi:10.2337/db16-0823

128. Gitelman SE, Gottlieb PA, Felner EI, Willi SM, Fisher LK, Moran A, et al. Antithymocyte globulin therapy for patients with recent-onset type 1 diabetes: 2 year results of a randomised trial. *Diabetologia* (2016) 59(6):1153–61. doi:10.1007/s00125-016-3917-4
129. Tooley J, Vudattu N, Choi J, Cotsapas C, Devine L, Raddassi K, et al. Changes in T-cell subsets identify responders to FcR-nonbinding anti-CD3 mAb (teplizumab) in patients with type 1 diabetes. *Eur J Immunol* (2016) 46(1):230–41. doi:10.1002/eji.201545708
130. Bell CJ, Sun Y, Nowak UM, Clark J, Howlett S, Pekalski ML, et al. Sustained in vivo signaling by long-lived IL-2 induces prolonged increases of regulatory T cells. *J Autoimmun* (2015) 56:66–80. doi:10.1016/j.jaut.2014.10.002
131. Klatzmann D, Abbas AK. The promise of low-dose interleukin-2 therapy for autoimmune and inflammatory diseases. *Nat Rev Immunol* (2015) 15(5):283–94. doi:10.1038/nri3823
132. Hulme MA, Wasserfall CH, Atkinson MA, Brusko TM. Central role for interleukin-2 in type 1 diabetes. *Diabetes* (2012) 61(1):14–22. doi:10.2337/db11-1213
133. Long SA, Rieck M, Sanda S, Bollyky JB, Samuels PL, Goland R, et al. Rapamycin/IL-2 combination therapy in patients with type 1 diabetes augments Tregs yet transiently impairs beta-cell function. *Diabetes* (2012) 61(9):2340–8. doi:10.2337/db12-0049

14

Impact of Diabetes in Patients Diagnosed with COVID-19

Mohamed Abu-Farha[1†], Fahd Al-Mulla[2†], Thangavel Alphonse Thanaraj[2†], Sina Kavalakatt[1], Hamad Ali[2,3], Mohammed Abdul Ghani[4] and Jehad Abubaker[1*]*

[1] Department of Biochemistry and Molecular Biology, Dasman Diabetes Institute, Dasman, Kuwait, [2] Department of Genetics and Bioinformatics, Dasman Diabetes Institute, Dasman, Kuwait, [3] Department of Medical Laboratory Sciences, Faculty of Allied Health Sciences, Health Sciences Center, Kuwait University, Jabriya, Kuwait, [4] Diabetes Division, University of Texas Health Science Center at San Antonio, San Antonio, TX, United States

***Correspondence:**
Fahd Al-Mulla
fahd.almulla@dasmaninstitute.org
Jehad Abubaker
jehad.abubakr@dasmaninstitute.org

[†]These authors have contributed equally to this work

COVID-19 is a disease caused by the coronavirus SARS-CoV-2 (Severe Acute Respiratory Syndrome Coronavirus-2), known as a highly contagious disease, currently affecting more than 200 countries worldwide. The main feature of SARS-CoV-2 that distinguishes it from other viruses is the speed of transmission combined with higher risk of mortality from acute respiratory distress syndrome (ARDS). People with diabetes mellitus (DM), severe obesity, cardiovascular disease, and hypertension are more likely to get infected and are at a higher risk of mortality from COVID-19. Among elderly patients who are at higher risk of death from COVID-19, 26.8% have DM. Although the reasons for this increased risk are yet to be determined, several factors may contribute to type-2 DM patients' increased susceptibility to infections. A possible factor that may play a role in increasing the risk in people affected by diabetes and/or obesity is the impaired innate and adaptive immune response, characterized by a state of chronic and low-grade inflammation that can lead to abrupt systemic metabolic alteration. SARS patients previously diagnosed with diabetes or hyperglycemia had higher mortality and morbidity rates when compared with patients who were under metabolic control. Similarly, obese individuals are at higher risk of developing complications from SARS-CoV-2. In this review, we will explore the current and evolving insights pertinent to the metabolic impact of coronavirus infections with special attention to the main pathways and mechanisms that are linked to the pathophysiology and treatment of diabetes.

Keywords: coronavirus disease (COVID-19), type 2 diabetes, angiotensin converting enzyme2 (ACE2), Furin, transmembrane protease, serine 2 (TMPRSS2), metformin, interferon induced membrane (IFITM3)

Abbreviations: SARS-CoV-2, severe acute respiratory syndrome coronavirus-2; ARDS, acute respiratory distress syndrome; DM, diabetes mellitus; MERS-CoV, middle east respiratory syndrome coronavirus; COPD, chronic obstructive pulmonary disease; CVD, cardiovascular disease; CKD, chronic kidney disease; ACE2, angiotensin-converting enzyme 2; T2DM, type-2 dm; TNF-α, tumor necrosis factor alpha; MCP-1, monocyte chemoattractant protein-1; IL-6, interleukin-6; rhACE2, recombinant angiotensin-converting enzyme 2; TCZ, tocilizumab; IFITM, interferon-induced transmembrane; ADAM17, a disintegrin and metallopeptidase domain 17; GRP78, glucose regulated protein 78; SBDβ, GRP78 substrate binding domain; βDKA, Diabetic Ketoacidosis; DPP-4i, Dipeptidyl peptidase 4 inhibitor; AICAR, 5-Aminoimidazole-4-carboxamide ribonucleotide.

WORSE OUTCOMES IN COVID-19 PATIENTS AFFECTED BY OBESITY AND DIABETES

COVID-19 is caused by the coronavirus SARS-CoV-2 and has emerged as a fast-spreading contagious disease affecting most countries across the globe (1). SARS-CoV-2 is the third coronavirus appearance in human history following severe acute respiratory syndrome coronavirus (SARS-CoV) and the Middle East respiratory syndrome coronavirus (MERS-CoV) (2, 3). Coronaviruses are a family of enveloped viruses encoded by a single-stranded positive-sense RNA genome and named for the crown-like appearance of their virions under the electron microscope. The key feature of SARS-CoV-2 that differentiates it from other viruses is its transmissibility combined with a greater risk of mortality due to the acute respiratory distress syndrome (ARDS). Signs and symptoms of SARS-CoV-2 infections range from mild/asymptomatic infections (20-86% of all infections), restricted to the upper respiratory tract (20–86% of all infections), to severe respiratory distress characterized by the spread of infection to the lower airways leading to regional inflammation and pneumonia. This is manifested particularly in patients with comorbidities such as chronic obstructive pulmonary disease (COPD), asthma, diabetes, hypertension, and cardiovascular disease (CVD) (4, 5). Significantly, Maddaloni et al. suggested an increased prevalence of COPD and of chronic kidney disease (CKD) in Covid-19 patients with diabetes (6).

People with diabetes mellitus (DM), severe obesity, CVD, and hypertension are at a higher risk of poor outcome from COVID-19 (4, 7–10). The reasons underlying this increased risk have not been determined. However, a panoply of factors may contribute to type-2 DM (T2DM) patient increased risk of poor outcomes of COVID-19 disease (**Figure 1**). Individuals affected by diabetes and/or obesity generally have an impaired innate and adaptive immune response, characterized by a state of chronic low-grade inflammation (11), which can lead to abrupt systemic metabolic alteration, characterized by higher levels of leptin (a proinflammatory adipokine) and lower adiponectin (an anti-inflammatory adipokine) (12–16). An unfavorable hormone environment also contributes to dysregulation of the immune response (17). Typically, obese people have defective innate immunity manifested by enhanced production of several proinflammatory cytokines, such as tumor necrosis factor alpha (TNF-α), monocyte chemoattractant protein-1 (MCP-1), and interleukin-6 (IL-6) (18). Upon antigen exposure, obesity-related chronic inflammation reduces the activation of macrophages and dampens proinflammatory cytokine production (19). This exceptional obesogenic state may partly

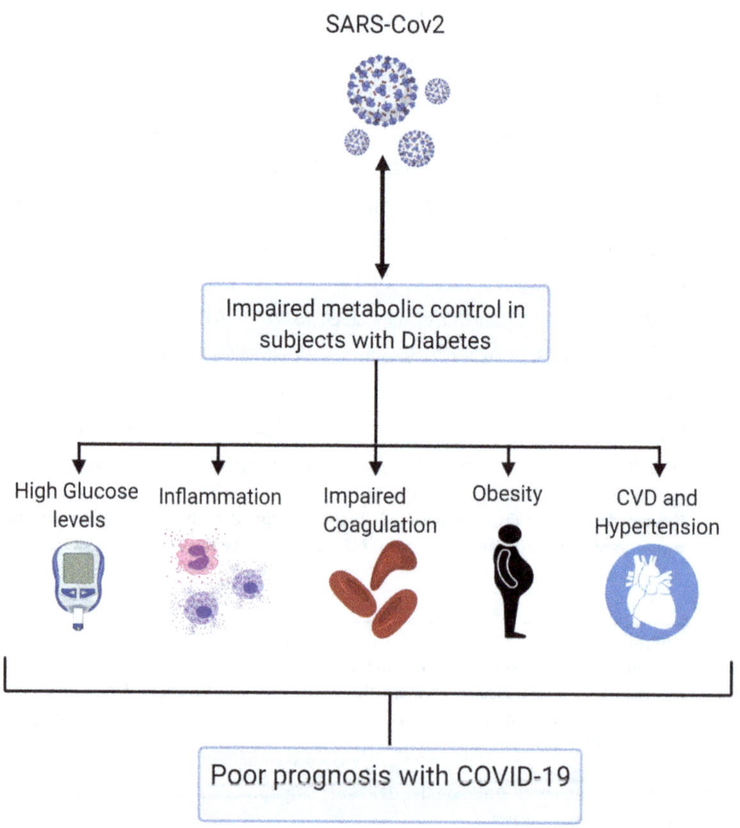

FIGURE 1 | A schematic model summarizing the various mechanisms by which diabetes can impact on COVID-19 poor outcome.

explain the presence of antiviral-resistance and vaccine-escape deviations in the obese population (19, 20). Moreover, B- and T-cell responses are weakened in obese patients and even more so in obese patients with diabetes (21). After analyzing a case cohort of 70,000 individuals infected with COVID-19, the Chinese Centre for Disease Control and Prevention reported augmented mortality in individuals with diabetes, increasing from 2.3% in the general population to 7.3% in people with diabetes (22). Interestingly, earlier studies demonstrated that individuals with diabetes exhibit a similar high risk for SARS and MERS (23, 24). Among patients infected with the SARS virus, it has been shown that histories of diabetes and hyperglycemia are independent predictors of mortality and morbidity and that metabolic control might improve their prognosis (24). Moreover, hyperglycemia is a strong prognostic predictor of outcome in hospitalized patients with COVID-19. Earlier studies showed that hyperglycemic patients with COVID-19 displayed higher cumulative incidence of severe disease than normoglycemic controls (25, 26). Possible mechanisms for this increased mortality include hyperglycemia-induced changes in the immune system and increases in inflammatory cytokines (27). Furthermore, among elderly individuals who were at higher risk of death from COVID-19, 26.8% had diabetes (4). In the United States, 10.5% of the total population has diabetes (4). Similarly, obese individuals are at higher risk of developing complications from SARS-CoV-2 (28, 29).

In this review, we will discuss current and growing perceptions pertinent to the metabolic impact of coronavirus infections while paying special attention to the main pathways and mechanisms that are connected to the pathophysiology and treatment of diabetes.

Hypertension is another predictor of poor outcomes in COVID-19 patients. This may be due to the SARS-CoV-2 binding to the angiotensin-converting enzyme 2 (ACE2) in human epithelial lung cells, potentially involved in ARDS. Ace2 KO mice display severe pathology of ARDS (30). An earlier report has shown that recombinant angiotensin-converting enzyme 2 (rhACE2) can attenuate arterial hypoxemia and pulmonary blood flow in a piglet model of lipopolysaccharide-induced ARDS (31). ACE2 exerts its functions through cleaving either Angiotensin I or Angiotensin II into inactive Angiotensin (1–9) and Angiotensin (1–7) respectively. Angiotensin (1–9) gets further metabolized into Angiotensin (1–7). Angiotensin (1–7) is a vasodilator. Hence, ACE2 counteracts the vasoconstrictor effects of the ACE-Angiotensin II axis. Angiotensin-converting enzyme inhibitors (ACEi) and/or angiotensin receptor blockers (ARBs) may interfere with angiotensin-converting enzyme 2 expression and/or activity. Thus, as recommended by several medical associations, and in light of more scientific evidence supporting their beneficial/non-harmful impact, ACEis/ARBs should be continued in COVID-19 patients (32–34). Moreover, the impact of metabolic syndrome (MS) and its comorbidities on COVID-19 prognosis must be considered. Yet, MS by definition is a set of metabolic disorders that include insulin resistance, dyslipidemia, central obesity and hypertension. All are risk factors for the development of type-2 diabetes and cardiovascular diseases (35). In 2017, it was estimated that MS affected 20% of North American population, 25% of European population and approximately 15% of Chinese population (36). Considering the presence of MS across different ethnicities and continents, more future studies focusing on the effect of MS on COVID-19 outcomes are needed.

Studies from different countries have demonstrated a varying prevalence of diabetes, other comorbidities, and mortality among patients infected with COVID-19. **Table 1** summarizes the

TABLE 1 | Prevalence (%) of comorbidities in COVID-19 infected patients.

Study	Sample size (n)	Diabetes (%)	CVD (%)	HTN (%)	CKD (%)	Ref
Li B et al.	1,527	9.7	16.4	17.1	NR	(5)
Covid-19 group, Italy	481	33.9	30.1	73.8	20.2	(37)
Onder et al.	355	35.5	42.5	NR	NR	(7)
Zhou et al.	191	19	8	30	1	(8)
Wu C et al.	201	10.9	4	19.4	1	(9)
Guan et al.	1,099	7.4	3.8	15	0.7	(10)
Bhatraju et al.	24	58	NR	NR	21	(38)
CDC, USA	7,162	10.9	9	NR	3	(39)
Zhang et al.	140	12.1	8.6	30	1.4	(40)
Liu J et al.	61	8.2	1.6	19.7	NR	(41)
Guo et al.	187	15	11.2	32.6	3.2	(42)
Huang et al.	41	19.5	15	14.6	NR	(43)
Chen N et al.	99	12.1	40	NR	NR	(44)
Wang et al.	138	10.1	19.6	31.2	2.9	(45)
Yang J et al.	Meta-analysis of eight studies n = 46,248	0.08	0.05	0.17	NR	(46)
Yang X et al.	52	17	23	NR	NR	(47)
Liu K et al.	137	10.2	7.3	9.5	NR	(41)
Chen T et al.	274	17	8	34	1	(48)
CDC China	20,982	5.3	4.2	12.8	NR	(49)
Singh et al.	Meta-analysis of 10 studies = 2,209	0.11	0.07	0.21	NR	(50)
Hu Y et al.	Meta-analysis of 21 studies n = 47,344	7.7	4.7	15.6	2.1	(37)

CVD, cardiovascular disease; HTN, hypertension; CKD, chronic kidney disease; NR, not reported; CDC, Centers for Disease Control and Prevention.

TABLE 2 | Prevalence of diabetes amongst non-severe and severe COVID-19 infected patients.

Study	Sample size(n)	DM (%)	ICU admission (Severe/ Critical) (%)*	Significance p value of non-severe *vs* severe COVID	Ref.
Wu et al.	201	10.90%	19.00%	0.002	(9)
Guan et al.	1,099	7.40%	16.20%	NR	(10)
CDC, USA	7,162	10.90%	32.00%	NR	(39)
Zhang et al.	140	12.10%	13.80%	0.615	(40)
Huang et al.	41	15%	25.00%	0.160	(43)
Wang et al.	138	10.10%	22.20%	0.009	(45)
Liu J et al.	61	8.20%	17.60%	0.094	(41)
Hu Y et al.	Meta-analysis of 21 studies n = 47,344	7.70%	44.50%	NR	(37)

DM, diabetes mellitus; Ref., references; CDC, Centers for Disease Control and Prevention.
**% is calculated from total population with COVID-19.*

prevalence of comorbidities among patients with COVID-19, and **Tables 2** and **3** summarize the prevalence of diabetes and other comorbidities among patients with severe *versus* mild COVID-19 symptoms and among survivors *versus* non-survivors of COVID-19. Overall, it was reported that the proportion of people affected by diabetes among COVID-19 patients was from 5.3% to 20%. Although the COVID-19 surveillance group in Italy showed a higher prevalence of comorbidities such as hypertension and diabetes (73% and 34%, respectively), other studies from China showed a 9 to 15% prevalence rate. Bhatraju et al. (38). reported that US patients had morbidity rates similar to patients in Italy. However, it is important to note that Bhatraju et al. included only critically ill patients from the Seattle area. Differences in the characteristics of patients included in the studies could explain the difference in the prevalence of comorbidities among various cohorts. Data also show that the presence of diabetes is associated with a high risk of severe to critical illness in 14 to 32% of patients with COVID-19 (39, 40). Other studies showed higher rate of admission into the intensive care unit (ICU) among people who were diagnosed with diabetes or other comorbidities when compared with non-ICU patients (22.2 *vs* 5.9%) (45). Furthermore, mortality rates among COVID-19 patients with various comorbidities when compared to those without any comorbidities were 15 *vs* 2.3%, respectively (43–45). Notably, several studies showed that diabetes is strongly associated with increased risk of mortality due to COVID-19 as compared with COVID-19 patients without diabetes and other comorbidities (22–31 *vs* 2–4%) (8, 10, 47). Zhou et al. also showed that the mortality rate among COVID-19 patients with diabetes was higher than the overall mortality rate with the viral infection (8). Wu et al. showed that diabetes was associated with a hazard ratio of 2.3 for ARDS (9). Other studies associated diabetes to the severity of COVID-19 (51). Hence, it was proposed that the course of treatment and prognosis should be stratified based on occurrence or absence of comorbidities (52).

In Italy, patients with diabetes showed high prevalence, severity of disease and mortality during SARS-COV-2 infection as well as higher rates of ICU admission. They frequently reported respiratory symptoms and were at increased risk of numerous pulmonary diseases, such as COPD, bronchial severe asthma and idiopathic pulmonary fibrosis (53, 54). Thus, we speculate that the complicated alveolar-capillary network of lungs could be targeted by diabetes micro-vascular injury. Recently, continuous experimental therapy with monoclonal antibody against the IL-6 receptor (tocilizumab, TCZ) in Italy seems to have positive effects on severe lung disease and prognosis in patients with COVID-19. Hence, TCZ could be administered to patients with diabetes during the SARS-COV-2 infection (55). However, an earlier study showed that at admission, hyperglycemic (n = 31) *vs.* normoglycemic (n = 47) patients had fivefold higher IL-6 levels, which persisted even after TCZ administration ($P < 0.05$) (56). Interestingly, in a risk-adjusted Cox regression analysis, TCZ in hyperglycemic patients failed to reduce risk of severe outcomes as it did in normoglycemic patients ($P < 0.009$). Thus, hyperglycemia could result in an unfavorable effect on hospital admission, clinical outcomes and drug therapy (25, 26, 56). It is possible that comorbidities associated with diabetes (*e.g.*, obesity, hypertension, and CVD) contribute to increased morbidity and mortality due to COVID-19. Diabetes was associated with COVID-19 poor outcomes (51) and with increased time required for viral clearance (4). Increased expression of ACE2, furin, and IL-6 and impaired T-cell function are several factors that were associated with the risk and severity of SARS-CoV2 infection in individuals with diabetes (57).

COVID-19 could cause endothelial dysfunction and a hyper-coagulation state. This condition is intensified by hypoxia, which augments thrombosis by both increasing blood viscosity and hypoxia-inducible transcription factors (HIF) (58, 59). Consequently, these could lead to pulmonary embolism with occlusion and micro-thrombosis in pulmonary vessels, as detected in critically ill COVID-19 patients (59). It is also

TABLE 3 | Prevalence of diabetes among non-survivor and survivor COVID-19 infected patients.

Study	Sample size (n)	DM in entire cohort (%)	DM (%) in non-survivors	DM (%) in survivors	Mortality rate	Ref.
Zhou et al.	191	19%	31.00%	14.00%	OR 2.8(1.35 to 6.05) p < 0.001	(8)
Wu et al.	88	18.2%	25.00%	12.50%	HR 1.58(0.80 to 3.13), p = 0.19	(22)
Guan et al.	1,099	7.4%	26.90%	6.10%	NR	(10)
Yang X et al.	52	17%	22%	10%	NR	(47)
Chen N et al.	274	17%	21.00%	14.00%	NR	(44)

reported that COVID-19 is associated with increased incidence of coagulation as well as thrombotic and inflammatory events (60), which was responsible, at least in part, for the severe morbidity and mortality. This suggests that COVID-19 activates yet another unidentified mechanism, which is involved in the coagulation process. Interestingly, it is well established that diabetes is a state of increased coagulability; where increased plasminogen activator inhibitor-1 is a consistent finding in patients with diabetes. Thus, increased coagulability in diabetes may be a possible mechanism that links diabetes to severity of COVID-19.

POSSIBLE MECHANISMS THAT PREDISPOSE COVID-19 PATIENTS WITH DIABETES AND/OR OBESITY TO POOR OUTCOMES

Considering the high incidence of obesity, hypertension, and CVD in patients with diabetes, it remains unclear whether diabetes is an independent contributor to the higher morbidity and mortality associated with COVID-19 (7–10). Maddaloni et al. have shown that patients with cardiometabolic multimorbidity, and not diabetes or CVD alone, experience worse COVID-19 outcomes (61). Nevertheless, plasma glucose levels and diabetes are independent predictors of mortality and morbidity in patients with SARS (24, 62). Mechanisms that likely increase the vulnerability for COVID-19 in DM patients comprise increased binding affinity and efficient virus entry, reduced viral clearance, weakened T-cell role, increased susceptibility to cytokine storm disorder, and the existence of CVD. Lung cells, including pneumocytes, are the main cellular sites for coronavirus entrance and inflammation (63). They express key proteins that enable coronavirus entry into cells, such as ACE2, transmembrane protease serine 2 (TMPRSS2), furin, and dipeptidyl peptidase-4 (DPP4). ACE2 and DPP4 also have established multiple metabolic activities linked to the pharmacologic and physiologic control of cardiovascular and glucose homeostasis and DPP4 inhibitors are used extensively in diabetes therapy (28).

Increased ACE2 expression in pulmonary cells, kidney, myocardium, and pancreas may mediate increased cellular binding of SARS-CoV-2 (64–66). The increased expression of ACE2 in these tissues is well documented in animal models of diabetes (67, 68). Although insulin administration downregulates ACE2 expression (46, 68), other hypoglycemic agents such as glucagon-like peptide-1 (GLP-1) agonists and thiazolidinediones (pioglitazone), anti-hypertensive drugs such as statins, and ACE inhibitors increase ACE2 expression (69–73). Recently, Rao et al. investigated illnesses or traits that may be connected to increased ACE2 expression in the lung. Using a phenome-wide Mendelian randomization analyses, they identified the association between diabetes and higher lung ACE2 expression (74). Moreover, circulating levels of furin (cellular protease) were found to be higher in patients with type-2 diabetes (75). The findings of these studies support the hypothesis that COVID-19 patients with diabetes are predisposed to poor outcomes. Furthermore, a recent study stated that clearance of SARS-CoV-2 was delayed in patients with diabetes (76). However, more extensive studies are needed to confirm this finding.

HOW ARE THE DIFFERENT HOST-CELLULAR PROTEINS INVOLVED IN SARS-COV-2 INFECTION ASSOCIATED WITH DIABETES?

Apart from ACE2, a number of other host-cellular protein components are thought to have the ability to regulate the entry of SARS-COV-2; such components are known to be involved in the pathogenesis of diabetes, as illustrated in **Figure 2** and as described below.

ACE2

ACE2 acts as the receptor for the binding of SARS-CoV-2 with the host cell. It is already known that the binding of the SARS coronavirus to its receptor damages islets and causes acute diabetes (77). Clinical data, which includes patients with mild and severe COVID-19, established the existence of mild pancreatitis (78). Diabetes and hypertension (common comorbidities associated with COVID-19) are often treated with ACE inhibitors and angiotensin II type-I receptor blockers. Studies have reported that the expression of ACE2 is elevated in people with diabetes treated with these medications (79, 80). The higher levels of ACE2 can thus facilitate critical illness in COVID-19 patients (81).

Furin

Furin cleaves cell surface proteins. The SARS-CoV-2 S-protein S1/S2 cleavage site is the target for furin during infection. This cleavage is critical, as it allows the fusion sequences on the COVID-19 spike protein to be exposed for the fusion of the virus with the host cell membranes (1, 65, 82). Thus, high levels of furin enhance the ability of the virus to enter the host cell. It is known that individuals with high plasma furin concentrations have a pronounced dysmetabolic phenotype and elevated risk of diabetes and premature mortality (75, 83). A point mutation at the furin cleavage site in the insulin pro-receptor was seen in an individual with extreme insulin-resistant diabetes (84). Furthermore, variations in the furin gene have been associated with decreased triglyceride and increased high-density lipoprotein cholesterol levels (85). Furin has an impact on the pancreas, as verified by previous studies, which demonstrated that furin controls the growth of pancreatic β-cells (86). It also plays a role in granular acidification in the endocrine pancreas *via* impaired processing of Ac45 (87). We have previously identified a higher proportion of damaging variations in the furin gene in the Arab population as compared with Europeans (88), which is a population with high rates of diabetes that requires special attention during this pandemic (89).

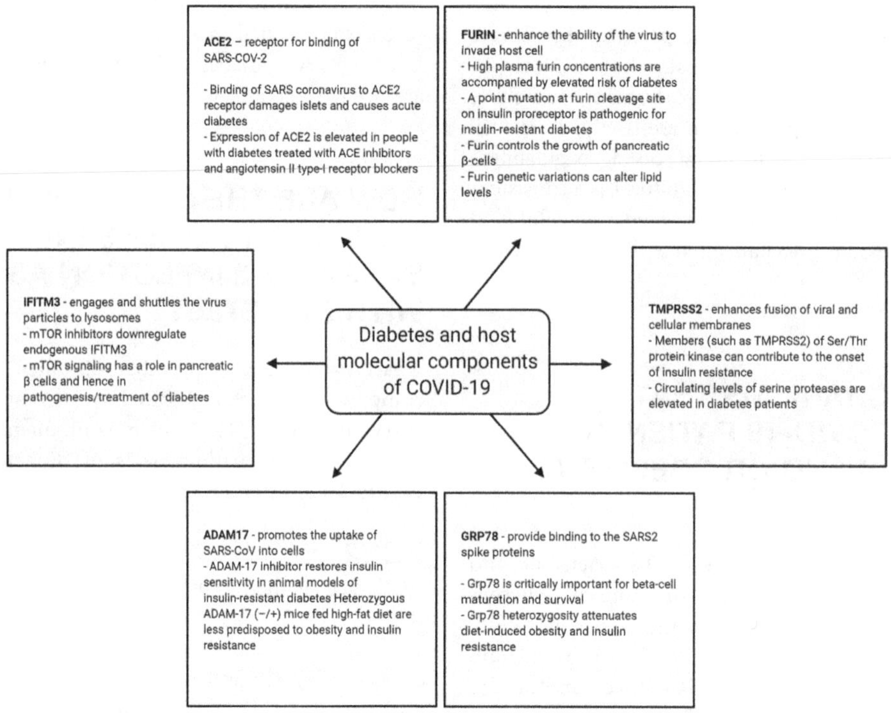

FIGURE 2 | Illustration of association of the different host-cellular proteins involved in SARS-COV-2 infection with diabetes.

TMPRSS2

SARS-CoV-2 uses the SARS-CoV receptor ACE2 for entry, and the serine protease TMPRSS2 is required for S-protein priming, which entails S-protein cleavage at the S1/S2 and the S2′ site and allows fusion of viral and cellular membranes. TMPRSS2 belongs to the family of serine proteases. It is now known that ser/thr protein kinases contribute to the onset of insulin resistance *via* the introduction of phosphorylation-based negative feedback control mechanisms, which disengage the insulin receptor from its downstream effectors (90). Circulating levels of serine proteases, such as granzyme B, are elevated in diabetes patients (91). Hence, it can be assumed that the increased activity of TMPRSS2 can increase the viral entry in the host.

IFITM3

Interferon-induced transmembrane (IFITM) proteins are important effectors that inhibit viral infections. IFITM3 directly engages and shuttles the incoming virus particles to lysosomes. It is known that the MERS-CoV entry into host cells is sensitive to inhibition by IFITM proteins (particularly IFITM3) and that the cellular context and/or IFITM expression levels can affect the efficiency of inhibition (92, 93). IFITM3 is now indicated as a novel entry site in the SARS-CoV-2 domain as well (94, 95). Inhibitors of the mammalian target of rapamycin (mTOR), such as rapamycin, downregulate endogenous IFITM3 through a lysosomal degradation pathway in hematopoietic and non-hematopoietic cells (96). Interestingly, mTOR signaling has a role in pancreatic β cells and immune cells, and hence it is also involved in the pathogenesis and treatment of diabetes (97).

Adam17

In the context of SARS-CoV infection, it has been proposed that SARS-S binding to ACE2 triggers shedding of ACE2 *via* the disintegrin and metallopeptidase domain 17 (ADAM17) protein to release the extracellular domain of ACE2 into the extracellular space. This process promotes the uptake of SARS-CoV into cells (98, 99). It is now further proposed that the inhibition of ADAM17 may exert a protective effect on COVID-19 (100). ADAM17 is a metalloprotease and disintegrin that lodges in the plasma membrane in several cell types and can cleave a wide variety of cell surface proteins. In this way, ADAM17 can influence several physiological and pathological processes (101). In animal models of insulin-resistant diabetes, the intraperitoneal injection of ADAM-17 inhibitor, restored insulin sensitivity through the inhibition of TNF-α (102). Consistent with these findings, Serino et al. demonstrated that heterozygous ADAM-17 (−/+) mice fed a high-fat diet were less predisposed to obesity and insulin resistance than their wild-type littermates (103).

Other Players: GRP78 and CD147

It appears that apart from the ACE2 receptor entry mode, SARS-CoV-2 may use the protease called TMPRSS2 to enter the cells; some researchers speculate that there can be at least 8 other different proteases. It is also proposed that other receptors such as glucose regulated protein 78 (GRP78 receptors) may provide binding to the SARS-CoV-2 spike proteins. Protein–protein docking studies revealed that four regions of the spike protein can fit tightly in the GRP78 substrate binding domain β (SBDβ) (104). Grp78 is critically important for β-cell maturation and survival; it is demonstrated that Grp78 heterozygosity attenuates diet-induced obesity and insulin resistance (105). It is also possible that other receptors mediate the entry of SARS-CoV-2, such as CD147 into T cells. Also called Basigin or EMMPRIN, CD147 is a transmembrane glycoprotein that belongs to the immunoglobulin superfamily on the surface of T lymphocytes (106). A recent study reported that it is a novel invasive route for SARS-CoV-2 entry (106, 107). CD147 is essential for diabetes-associated recombinant tissue-plasminogen activator (rt-PA)-induced hemorrhagic transformation, and reduced CD147 glycosylation is an encouraging therapy for neurovascular-unit repair following rt-PA treatment of diabetes patients (108).

USE OF GLUCOSE-LOWERING THERAPIES IN COVID-19 PATIENTS WITH DIABETES

Lack of specific and effective therapeutics is the major challenge in dealing with COVID-19 patients that are suffering from severe comorbidities such as diabetes. In the absence of specific medication for COVID-19 patients, it is essential to evaluate the applicability of drugs in practice for various comorbidities. Diabetes is one of the major comorbidities of COVID-19 patients who developed ARDS (43). It was originally thought that some anti-diabetes treatment (such as metformin, PPARs, DPP4 inhibitors, GLP-1R agonists, SGLT2 inhibitors and insulin therapy) could influence the course of COVID-19; however, no convincing evidence has emerged to support this view.

GLP-1R Agonists

GLP-1R agonists target many anti-inflammatory pathways in animals and lessen systemic inflammation in individuals affected by diabetes and obesity (109). These drugs decrease pulmonary type-2 immune cytokine reactions and the degree of lung injury in mice after respiratory viral infection (110). Thus, GLP-1-based drugs possess strong anti-inflammatory effects in lungs and could become possible repurposed drugs, useful to treat COVID-19 patients with ARDS (111). However, the beneficial effects of these drugs remain to be convincingly established in COVID-19.

SGLT2 Inhibitors

Based on the findings that showed the organ-protective effects of SGLT-2 inhibitors (112), in addition to their glycemic benefits, these drugs were proposed to provide benefits in COVID-19 settings. However, these inhibitors were also known to lead to risk of dehydration and euglycemic Diabetic Ketoacidosis (DKA) (112). Though SGLT2 inhibitors may be potentially beneficial as organ protective agents in COVID-19, there is no completed clinical trial to assess the risk/benefit balance of using these inhibitors in COVID-19 patients. Thus, caution needs to be exercised when these inhibitors are used (113). It is advisable to re-evaluate or discontinue SGLT2 inhibitors upon hospital admission of unstable patients with severe SARS-CoV-2 infection.

Insulin Therapy

Given that insulin therapy has an optimal glucose-lowering effect in patients affected by diabetes, it is suggested that insulin is the treatment of choice in hospitalized COVID-19 patients with diabetes (114, 115). As stated in the American Diabetes Association guidelines, basal insulin or a basal plus bolus correction insulin regimen is the favorite treatment for noncritically ill hospitalized patients. Continuous intravenous insulin infusion is preferred in critically ill patients. A target glucose range of 7.8–10.0 mmol/L is recommended for both critically and noncritically ill patients (114). Moreover, a recent study examined the effects of optimal glycemic control using insulin therapy in patients with hyperglycemia affected by COVID-19 (25). Fifty-nine patients with COVID-19 hospitalized with moderate disease were stratified into hyperglycemic and normoglycemic groups based on glycemia measure of >7.77 mmol/L at the time of hospital admission. Their data showed that patients with hyperglycemia treated with insulin infusion had a lower risk of severe disease outcome than patients without insulin infusion. Accordingly, insulin infusion may be an effective method for reaching glycemic control and improving outcomes in patients with COVID-19 (25). Consistently, Bornstein et al. recommended insulin treatment for diabetic patients with severe COVID-19 (116). However, a recent study examining the effects of insulin therapy in hospitalized diabetic patients with COVID-19 reported a greater than threefold risk of mortality and severe outcome in treated patients (117). Thus, it remains unclear whether insulin therapy worsens COVID-19 outcomes or if these results were caused by a patient selection bias (note. patients with diabetes receiving insulin tend to have longer duration of disease with a higher rate of comorbidities).

ACE2 and DPP4

DPP4 (CD26), a transmembrane ectopeptidase, acts as a co-receptor for a subset of coronaviruses including MERS-CoV. Its activity can potentially modulate the levels and activity of many immunomodulatory cytokines and chemokines (118). Although ACE2 and DPP4 are crucial modulators of glucose homeostasis, there is no convincing evidence to propose that medications regulating the ACE2- or DPP4-linked pathways yield obvious benefit or harm during coronavirus infections. Several studies have evaluated whether DPP4i are associated to improved Covid-19 outcomes, with apparently opposing results. Some groups have shown that patients with COVID-19 who were on Dipeptidyl peptidase 4 inhibitor (DPP-4is) had a similar disease outcome as those who were not (119–121). Instead, Solerte et al. have found that sitagliptin (DPP-4i) treatment at the time of admission was associated with improved clinical outcomes and reduced mortality, compared to standard-of-care treatment (122). ACE2 decoy receptors or antibodies targeting ACE2 can be promising tools to block the viral cell-entry. However, the impact of these drugs on metabolic parameters has not been sensibly investigated and requires further investigation (123).

CONCLUSION

Evidence implies that obesity and diabetes are leading risk factors that affect the severity of disease caused by coronaviruses infections, such as COVID-19. Among patients infected with the SARS-CoV-2, history has shown that diabetes and hyperglycemia are independent predictors for mortality and morbidity, and that glycemic control might improve patient prognosis. The risk seen among people with diabetes may be due to insulin resistance, inflammation, or hypercoagulation, or owed to underlying obesity, which may lead to adverse outcome.

Several classes of anti-obesity and anti-diabetes medications (such as metformin, 5-Aminoimidazole-4-carboxamide ribonucleotide (AICAR), and PPARγ agonists) are known to modulate the immune system and result in improved insulin sensitivity. Hence, further investigations are warranted to address their use alone or in combination with other antiviral/ immunomodulatory drugs in the treatment of COVID-19. Moreover, GLP-1R agonists and DPP4 inhibitors are known to mediate anti-inflammatory effects in human patients, while controlling glucose levels in hospitalized patients (124) Nevertheless, there is no convincing evidence advocating the use of these drugs as replacements for insulin in severely ill COVID-19 patients. The fast-growing medical information pertaining to the COVID-19 pandemic entails continuing scrutiny to assess the practical use, risks, and advantages of these anti-hyperglycemic drugs and any other associated medications generally used to treat diabetic people, who are at higher risk of coronavirus infections.

AUTHOR CONTRIBUTIONS

MA-F, FA-M, TT, SK, HA, MA, and JA contributed to the design, writing, and planning of the manuscript. All authors contributed to the article and approved the submitted version.

REFERENCES

1. Walls AC, Park YJ, Tortorici MA, Wall A, Mcguire AT, Veesler D. Structure, Function, and Antigenicity of the SARS-CoV-2 Spike Glycoprotein. *Cell* (2020) 181(2):281–292.e6. doi: 10.1016/j.cell.2020.02.058
2. Zhou J, Chu H, Chan JF, Yuen KY. Middle East respiratory syndrome coronavirus infection: virus-host cell interactions and implications on pathogenesis. *Virol J* (2015) 12:218. doi: 10.1186/s12985-015-0446-6
3. Chan JF, Lau SK, To KK, Cheng VC, Woo PC, Yuen KY. Middle East respiratory syndrome coronavirus: another zoonotic betacoronavirus causing SARS-like disease. *Clin Microbiol Rev* (2015) 28(2):465–522. doi: 10.1128/CMR.00102-14
4. Muniyappa R, Gubbi S. COVID-19 pandemic, coronaviruses, and diabetes mellitus. *Am J Physiol Endocrinol Metab* (2020) 318(5):E736–e741. doi: 10.1152/ajpendo.00124.2020
5. Li B, Yang J, Zhao F, Zhi L, Wang X, Liu L, et al. Prevalence and impact of cardiovascular metabolic diseases on COVID-19 in China. *Clin Res Cardiol* (2020) 109(5):531–8. doi: 10.1007/s00392-020-01626-9
6. Maddaloni E, D'onofrio L, Alessandri F, Mignogna C, Leto G, Pascarella, et al. Clinical features of patients with type 2 diabetes with and without Covid-19: a case control study (CoViDiab I). *Diabetes Res Clin Pract* (2020) p:108454. doi: 10.1016/j.diabres.2020.108454
7. Onder G, Rezza G, Brusaferro S. Case-Fatality Rate and Characteristics of Patients Dying in Relation to COVID-19 in Italy. *JAMA* (2020) 323 (18):1775–6. doi: 10.1001/jama.2020.4683
8. Zhou F, Yu T, Du R, Fan G, Liu Y, Liu Z, et al. Clinical course and risk factors for mortality of adult inpatients with COVID-19 in Wuhan, China: a retrospective cohort study. *Lancet* (2020) 395(10229):1054–62. doi: 10.1016/ S0140-6736(20)30566-3
9. Wu C, Chen X, Cai Y, Xia J, Zhou X, Xu S, et al. Risk Factors Associated With Acute Respiratory Distress Syndrome and Death in Patients With Coronavirus Disease 2019 Pneumonia in Wuhan, China. *JAMA Intern Med* (2020) 180(7):934–43. doi: 10.1001/jamainternmed.2020.0994
10. Guan WJ, Ni ZY, Hu Y, Liang WH, Ou. Clinical Characteristics of Coronavirus Disease 2019 in China. *N Engl J Med* (2020) 382(18):1708–20. doi: 10.1056/NEJMoa2002032
11. Andersen CJ, Murphy KE, Fernandez ML. Impact of Obesity and Metabolic Syndrome on Immunity. *Adv Nutr* (2016) 7(1):66–75. doi: 10.3945/ an.115.010207
12. Francisco V, Ruiz-Fernández C, Pino J, Mera A, González-Gay MA, Gómez, et al. Adipokines: Linking metabolic syndrome, the immune system, and arthritic diseases. *Biochem Pharmacol* (2019) 165:196–206. doi: 10.1016/ j.bcp.2019.03.030
13. Francisco V, Pino J, Campos-Cabaleiro V, Ruiz-Fernández C, Mera A, Gonzalez-Gay MA, et al. Obesity, Fat Mass and Immune System: Role for Leptin. *Front Physiol* (2018) 9:640. doi: 10.3389/fphys.2018.00640
14. Andrade-Oliveira V, Câmara NO. Adipokines as drug targets in diabetes and underlying disturbances. *J Diabetes Res* (2015) 2015:681612. doi: 10.1155/ 2015/681612
15. Bremer AA, Jialal I. Adipose tissue dysfunction in nascent metabolic syndrome. *J Obes* (2013) 2013:393192. doi: 10.1155/2013/393192
16. Faber DR, de Groot PG, Visseren FL. Role of adipose tissue in haemostasis, coagulation and fibrinolysis. *Obes Rev* (2009) 10(5):554–63. doi: 10.1111/ j.1467-789X.2009.00593.x
17. Ouchi N, Parker JL, Lugus JJ, Walsh K. Adipokines in inflammation and metabolic disease. *Nat Rev Immunol* (2011) 11(2):85–97. doi: 10.1038/ nri2921
18. Richard C, Wadowski M, Goruk S, Cameron L, Sharma AM, Field CJ. Individuals with obesity and type 2 diabetes have additional immune dysfunction compared with obese individuals who are metabolically healthy. *BMJ Open Diabetes Res Care* (2017) 5(1):e000379. doi: 10.1136/ bmjdrc-2016-000379
19. Luzi L, Radaelli MG. Influenza and obesity: its odd relationship and the lessons for COVID-19 pandemic. *Acta Diabetol* (2020) 57(6):759–64. doi: 10.1007/s00592-020-01522-8
20. Karlsson EA, Hertz T, Johnson C, Mehle A, Krammer F, Schultz-Cherry S, et al. Obesity Outweighs Protection Conferred by Adjuvanted Influenza Vaccination. *mBio* (2016) 7(4):e01144-16. doi: 10.1128/ mBio.01144-16
21. Magdy Beshbishy A, Hetta HF. Factors Associated with Increased Morbidity and Mortality of Obese and Overweight COVID-19 Patients. *Biol (Basel)* (2020) 9(9):280. doi: 10.3390/biology9090280
22. Wu Z, McGoogan JM. Characteristics of and Important Lessons From the Coronavirus Disease 2019 (COVID-19) Outbreak in China: Summary of a Report of 72 314 Cases From the Chinese Center for Disease Control and Prevention. *Jama* (2020) 323(13):1239–42. doi: 10.1001/jama.2020.2648
23. Kulcsar KA, Coleman CM, Beck SE, Frieman MB. Comorbid diabetes results in immune dysregulation and enhanced disease severity following MERS-CoV infection. *JCI Insight* (2019) 4(20):e131774. doi: 10.1172/ jci.insight.131774
24. Yang JK, Zheng Y, Gou X, Pu K, Chen Z, Guo Q, et al. Plasma glucose levels and diabetes are independent predictors for mortality and morbidity in

patients with SARS. *Diabetes Med* (2006) 23(6):623–8. doi: 10.1111/j.1464-5491.2006.01861.x

25. Sardu C, D'onofrio N, Balestrieri ML, Barbieri M, Rizzo MR, Messina V, et al. Outcomes in Patients With Hyperglycemia Affected by COVID-19: Can We Do More on Glycemic Control? *Diabetes Care* (2020) 43(7):1408–15. doi: 10.2337/dc20-0723
26. Sardu C, D'onofrio N, Balestrieri ML, Barbieri M, Rizzo MR, Messina V, et al. Hyperglycaemia on admission to hospital and COVID-19. *Diabetologia* (2020) 63(11):2486–7. doi: 10.1007/s00125-020-05216-2
27. Schuetz P, Castro P, Shapiro NI. Diabetes and sepsis: preclinical findings and clinical relevance. *Diabetes Care* (2011) 34(3):771–8. doi: 10.2337/dc10-1185
28. Drucker DJ. Coronavirus Infections and Type 2 Diabetes-Shared Pathways with Therapeutic Implications. *Endocr Rev* (2020) 41(3):bnaa011. doi: 10.1210/endrev/bnaa011
29. Ryan DH, Ravussin E. COVID 19 and the Patient with Obesity - The Editors Speak Out. *Obesity* (2020) 28(5):847. doi: 10.1002/oby.22808
30. Imai Y, Kuba K, Rao S, Huan Y, Guo F, Guan B, et al. Angiotensin-converting enzyme 2 protects from severe acute lung failure. *Nature* (2005) 436(7047):112–6. doi: 10.1038/nature03712
31. Treml B, Neu N, Kleinsasser A, Gritsch C, Finsterwalder T, Geiger R, et al. Recombinant angiotensin-converting enzyme 2 improves pulmonary blood flow and oxygenation in lipopolysaccharide-induced lung injury in piglets. *Crit Care Med* (2010) 38(2):596–601. doi: 10.1097/CCM.0b013e3181c03009
32. Bosso M, Thanaraj TA, Abu-Farha M, Alanbaei M, Abubaker J, Al-Mulla F. The Two Faces of ACE2: The Role of ACE2 Receptor and Its Polymorphisms in Hypertension and COVID-19. *Mol Ther Methods Clin Dev* (2020) 18:321–7. doi: 10.1016/j.omtm.2020.06.017
33. Vaduganathan M, Vardeny O, Michel T, Mcmurray JJV. Renin-Angiotensin-Aldosterone System Inhibitors in Patients with Covid-19. *N Engl J Med* (2020) 382(17):1653–9. doi: 10.1056/NEJMsr2005760
34. Sardu C, Maggi P, Messina V, Iuliano P, Sardu A, Iovinella V, et al. Could Anti-Hypertensive Drug Therapy Affect the Clinical Prognosis of Hypertensive Patients With COVID-19 Infection? Data From Centers of Southern Italy. *J Am Heart Assoc* (2020) 9(17):e016948. doi: 10.1161/JAHA.120.016948
35. Grundy SM, Cleeman JI, Daniels SR, Donato KA, Eckel RH, Franklin BA, et al. Diagnosis and management of the metabolic syndrome: an American Heart Association/National Heart, Lung, and Blood Institute Scientific Statement. *Circulation* (2005) 112(17):2735–52. doi: 10.1161/CIRCULATIONAHA.105.169404
36. Costa FF, Rosário WR, Ribeiro Farias AC, De Souza RG, Duarte GondimRS, Barroso WA. Metabolic syndrome and COVID-19: An update on the associated comorbidities and proposed therapies. *Diabetes Metab Syndr* (2020) 14(5):809–14. doi: 10.1016/j.dsx.2020.06.016
37. Hu Y, Sun J, Dai Z, Deng H, Li X, Huang Q, et al. Prevalence and severity of corona virus disease 2019 (COVID-19): A systematic review and meta-analysis. *J Clin Virol* (2020) 127:104371. doi: 10.1016/j.jcv.2020.104371
38. Bhatraju PK, Ghassemieh BJ, Nichols M, Kim R, Jerome, KR, Nalla, et al. Covid-19 in Critically Ill Patients in the Seattle Region - Case Series. *N Engl J Med* (2020) 382(21):2012–22. doi: 10.1056/NEJMoa2004500
39. CDC Covid-19 response team. Preliminary Estimates of the Prevalence of Selected Underlying Health Conditions Among Patients with Coronavirus Disease 2019 - United States, February 12-March 28, 2020. *MMWR Morb Mortal Wkly Rep* (2020) 69(13):382–6. doi: 10.15585/mmwr.mm6913e2
40. Zhang JJ, Dong X, Cao YY, Yuan YD, Yang YB, Yan YQ, et al. Clinical characteristics of 140 patients infected with SARS-CoV-2 in Wuhan, China. *Allergy* (2020) 75(7):1730–41. doi: 10.1111/all.14238
41. Liu K, Fang YY, Deng Y, Liu W, Wang MF, Ma JP, et al. Clinical characteristics of novel coronavirus cases in tertiary hospitals in Hubei Province. *Chin Med J (Engl)* (2020) 133(9):1025–31. doi: 10.1097/CM9.0000000000000744
42. Guo T, Fan Y, Chen M, Wu X, Zhang L, He T, et al. Cardiovascular Implications of Fatal Outcomes of Patients With Coronavirus Disease 2019 (COVID-19). *JAMA Cardiol* (2020) 5(7):811–8. doi: 10.1001/jamacardio.2020.1017
43. Huang C, Wang Y, Li X, Ren L, Zhao J, Hu Y, et al. Clinical features of patients infected with 2019 novel coronavirus in Wuhan, China. *Lancet* (2020) 395(10223):497–506. doi: 10.1016/S0140-6736(20)30183-5
44. Chen N, Zhou M, Dong X, Qu J, Gong F, Han Y, et al. Epidemiological and clinical characteristics of 99 cases of 2019 novel coronavirus pneumonia in Wuhan, China: a descriptive study. *Lancet* (2020) 395(10223):507–13. doi: 10.1016/S0140-6736(20)30211-7
45. Wang D, Hu B, Hu C, Zhu F, Liu X, Zhang J, et al. Clinical Characteristics of 138 Hospitalized Patients With 2019 Novel Coronavirus-Infected Pneumonia in Wuhan, China. *Jama* (2020) 323(11):1061–9. doi: 10.1001/jama.2020.1585
46. Yang J, Zheng Y, Gou X, Pu K, Chen Z, Guo Q, et al. Prevalence of comorbidities and its effects in patients infected with SARS-CoV-2: a systematic review and meta-analysis. *Int J Infect Dis* (2020) 94:91–5. doi: 10.1016/j.ijid.2020.03.017
47. Yang X, Yu Y, Xu J, Shu H, Xia J, Liu H, et al. Clinical course and outcomes of critically ill patients with SARS-CoV-2 pneumonia in Wuhan, China: a single-centered, retrospective, observational study. *Lancet Respir Med* (2020) 8(5):475–81. doi: 10.1016/S2213-2600(20)30079-5
48. Chen T, Wu D, Chen H, Yan W, Yang D, Chen G, et al. Clinical characteristics of 113 deceased patients with coronavirus disease 2019: retrospective study. *BMJ* (2020) 368:m1091. doi: 10.1136/bmj.m1091
49. Disease control and prevention. The epidemiological characteristics of an outbreak of 2019 novel coronavirus diseases (COVID-19) in China. *Zhonghua Liu Xing Bing Xue Za Zhi* (2020) 41(2):145–51. doi: 10.3760/cma.j.issn.0254-6450.2020.02.003
50. Singh AK, Gupta R, Ghosh A, Misra A. Diabetes in COVID-19: Prevalence, pathophysiology, prognosis and practical considerations. *Diabetes Metab Syndr* (2020) 14(4):303–10. doi: 10.1016/j.dsx.2020.04.004
51. Ali H, Alshukry A, Bu Abbas M, Ali Y, Alahmad B, Al-Shammari AA, et al. Clinical Characteristics and Outcomes of Diabetic COVID-19 patients in Kuwait. *medRxiv* (2020) p:2020.08.20.20178525.
52. Wang T, Du Z, Zhu F, Cao Z, An Y, Gao Y, et al. Comorbidities and multi-organ injuries in the treatment of COVID-19. *Lancet* (2020) 395(10228):e52. doi: 10.1016/S0140-6736(20)30558-4
53. Carsana L, Sonzogni A, Nasr A, Rossi RS, Pellegrinelli A, Zerbi P, et al. Pulmonary post-mortem findings in a series of COVID-19 cases from northern Italy: a two-centre descriptive study. *Lancet Infect Dis* (2020) 20 (10):1135–40. doi: 10.1016/S1473-3099(20)30434-5
54. Poletti V, Capozzolo A. Respiratory Rehabilitation in the COVID-19 Era. *Respiration* (2020) 99(6):461–2. doi: 10.1159/000509558
55. Sardu C, Gargiulo G, Esposito G, Paolisso G, Marfella R. Impact of diabetes mellitus on clinical outcomes in patients affected by Covid-19. *Cardiovasc Diabetol* (2020) 19(1):76. doi: 10.1186/s12933-020-01047-y
56. Marfella R, Paolisso P, Sardu C, Bergamaschi L, D'angelo EC, Barbieri, et al. Negative impact of hyperglycaemia on tocilizumab therapy in Covid-19 patients. *Diabetes Metab* (2020). 46(5):403–405. doi: 10.1016/j.diabet.2020.05.005
57. Feng SQ, Chen XD, Xia T, Gan L, Qiu H, Dai MH, et al. Cloning, chromosome mapping and expression characteristics of porcine ANGPTL3 and -4. *Cytogenet Genome Res* (2006) 114(1):44–9. doi: 10.1159/000091927
58. Gupta N, Zhao YY, Evans CE. The stimulation of thrombosis by hypoxia. *Thromb Res* (2019) 181:77–83. doi: 10.1016/j.thromres.2019.07.013
59. Sardu C, Gambardella J, Morelli MB, Wang, X, Marfella R, Santulli G. Hypertension, Thrombosis, Kidney Failure, and Diabetes: Is COVID-19 an Endothelial Disease? A Comprehensive Evaluation of Clinical and Basic Evidence. *J Clin Med* (2020) 9(5):1417. doi: 10.3390/jcm9051417
60. Alshukry A, Ali H, Ali Y, Al-Taweel T, Abu-Farha M, Abubaker J, et al. Clinical characteristics of Coronavirus Disease 2019 (COVID-19) patients in Kuwait. *medRxiv* (2020) p:2020.06.14.20131045. doi: 10.1101/2020.10.11.20210740
61. Maddaloni E, D'onofrio L, Alessandri F, Mignogna C, Leto G, Pascarella G, et al. Cardiometabolic multimorbidity is associated with a worse Covid-19 prognosis than individual cardiometabolic risk factors: a multicentre retrospective study (CoViDiab II). *Cardiovasc Diabetol* (2020) 19(1):164. doi: 10.1186/s12933-020-01140-2
62. Alahmad B, Al-Shammari AA, Bennakhi A, Al-Mulla F, Ali H. Fasting Blood Glucose and COVID-19 Severity: Nonlinearity Matters. *Diabetes Care* (2020) dc201941. doi: 10.2337/dc20-1941
63. Hamming I, Timens W, Bulthuis ML, Lely AT, Navis G, Van Goor H. Tissue distribution of ACE2 protein, the functional receptor for SARS coronavirus.

A first step in understanding SARS pathogenesis. *J Pathol* (2004) 203 (2):631–7. doi: 10.1002/path.1570
64. Verdecchia P, Cavallini C, Spanevello A, Angeli F. The pivotal link between ACE2 deficiency and SARS-CoV-2 infection. *Eur J Intern Med* (2020) 76:14–20. doi: 10.1016/j.ejim.2020.04.037
65. Lukassen S, Chua RL, Trefzer T, Kahn NC, Schneider MA, Muley T, et al. SARS-CoV-2 receptor ACE2 and TMPRSS2 are primarily expressed in bronchial transient secretory cells. *EMBO J* (2020) 39(10):e105114. doi: 10.15252/embj.20105114
66. Zou X, Chen K, Zou J, Han P, Hao J, Han Z. Single-cell RNA-seq data analysis on the receptor ACE2 expression reveals the potential risk of different human organs vulnerable to 2019-nCoV infection. *Front Med* (2020) 14(2):185–92. doi: 10.1007/s11684-020-0754-0
67. Roca-Ho H, Riera M, Palau V, Pascual J, Soler MJ. Characterization of ACE and ACE2 Expression within Different Organs of the NOD Mouse. *Int J Mol Sci* (2017) 18(3):563. doi: 10.3390/ijms18030563
68. Wysocki J, Ye M, Soler MJ, Gurley SB, Xiao HD, BernsteinKE, et al. ACE and ACE2 activity in diabetic mice. *Diabetes* (2006) 55(7):2132–9. doi: 10.2337/db06-0033
69. Romaní-Pérez M, Outeiriño-Iglesias V, Moya CM, Santisteban P, González-Matípas LC, Vigo E, et al. Activation of the GLP-1 Receptor by Liraglutide Increases ACE2 Expression, Reversing Right Ventricle Hypertrophy, and Improving the Production of SP-A and SP-B in the Lungs of Type 1 Diabetes Rats. *Endocrinology* (2015) 156(10):3559–69. doi: 10.1210/en.2014-1685
70. Tikoo K, Patel G, Kumar S, Karpe PA, Sanghavi M, Malek V, et al. Tissue specific up regulation of ACE2 in rabbit model of atherosclerosis by atorvastatin: role of epigenetic histone modifications. *Biochem Pharmacol* (2015) 93(3):343–51. doi: 10.1016/j.bcp.2014.11.013
71. Zhang W, Xu YZ, Liu B, Wu R, Yang YY, Xiao XQ, et al. Pioglitazone upregulates angiotensin converting enzyme 2 expression in insulin-sensitive tissues in rats with high-fat diet-induced nonalcoholic steatohepatitis. *ScientificWorldJournal* (2014) 2014:603409. doi: 10.1155/2014/603409
72. Wösten-van Asperen RM, Lutter R, Specht PA, Moll GN, Van Woensel JB, Van Der Loos, et al. Acute respiratory distress syndrome leads to reduced ratio of ACE/ACE2 activities and is prevented by angiotensin-(1-7) or an angiotensin II receptor antagonist. *J Pathol* (2011) 225(4):618–27. doi: 10.1002/path.2987
73. Ferrario CM, Jessup J, Chappell MC, Averill DB, Brosnihan KB, Tallant EA, et al. Effect of angiotensin-converting enzyme inhibition and angiotensin II receptor blockers on cardiac angiotensin-converting enzyme 2. *Circulation* (2005) 111(20):2605–10. doi: 10.1161/CIRCULATIONAHA.104.510461
74. Rao S, Lau A, So HC. Exploring Diseases/Traits and Blood Proteins Causally Related to Expression of ACE2, the Putative Receptor of SARS-CoV-2: A Mendelian Randomization Analysis Highlights Tentative Relevance of Diabetes-Related Traits. *Diabetes Care* (2020) 43(7):1416–26. doi: 10.2337/dc20-0643
75. Fernandez C, Ryså J, Almgren P, Nilsson J. Plasma levels of the proprotein convertase furin and incidence of diabetes and mortality. *J Intern Med* (2018) 284(4):377–87. doi: 10.1111/joim.12783
76. Chen X, Hu W, Ling J, Mo P, Zhang Y, Jiang Q, et al. Hypertension and Diabetes Delay the Viral Clearance in COVID-19 Patients. *medRxiv* (2020) p:2020.03.22.20040774. doi: 10.1101/2020.03.22.20040774
77. Yang JK, Lin SS, Ji XJ, Guo LM. Binding of SARS coronavirus to its receptor damages islets and causes acute diabetes. *Acta Diabetol* (2010) 47(3):193–9. doi: 10.1007/s00592-009-0109-4
78. Liu F, Long X, Zou W, Fang M, Wu W, Li W, et al. Highly ACE2 Expression in Pancreas May Cause Pancreas Damage After SARS-CoV-2 Infection. *medRxiv* (2020) p:2020.02.28.20029181. doi: 10.1101/2020.02.28.20029181
79. Wan Y, Shang J, Graham R, Baric RS, Li F. Receptor Recognition by the Novel Coronavirus from Wuhan: an Analysis Based on Decade-Long Structural Studies of SARS Coronavirus. *J Virol* (2020) 94(7):e00127-20. doi: 10.1128/JVI.00127-20
80. Li XC, Zhang J, Zhuo JL. The vasoprotective axes of the renin-angiotensin system: Physiological relevance and therapeutic implications in cardiovascular, hypertensive and kidney diseases. *Pharmacol Res* (2017) 125(Pt A):21–38. doi: 10.1016/j.phrs.2017.06.005
81. Fang L, Karakiulakis G, Roth M. Are patients with hypertension and diabetes mellitus at increased risk for COVID-19 infection? *Lancet Respir Med* (2020) 8(4):e21. doi: 10.1016/S2213-2600(20)30116-8
82. Braun E, Sauter D. Furin-mediated protein processing in infectious diseases and cancer. *Clin Transl Immunol* (2019) 8(8):e1073. doi: 10.1002/cti2.1073
83. Harlid S, Myte R, Van Guelpen B. The Metabolic Syndrome, Inflammation, and Colorectal Cancer Risk: An Evaluation of Large Panels of Plasma Protein Markers Using Repeated, Prediagnostic Samples. *Mediators Inflammation* (2017) 2017:4803156. doi: 10.1155/2017/4803156
84. Bravo DA, Gleason JB, Sanchez RI, Roth RA, Fuller RS. Accurate and efficient cleavage of the human insulin proreceptor by the human proprotein-processing protease furin. Characterization and kinetic parameters using the purified, secreted soluble protease expressed by a recombinant baculovirus. *J Biol Chem* (1994) 269(41):25830–7.
85. Ueyama C, Horibe H, Yamase Y, Fujimaki T, Oguri M, Kato K, et al. Association of FURIN and ZPR1 polymorphisms with metabolic syndrome. *BioMed Rep* (2015) 3(5):641–7. doi: 10.3892/br.2015.484
86. Kayo T, Sawada Y, Suda M, Konda Y, Izumi T, Tanaka S, et al. Proprotein-processing endoprotease furin controls growth of pancreatic beta-cells. *Diabetes* (1997) 46(8):1296–304. doi: 10.2337/diabetes.46.8.1296
87. Louagie E, Taylor NA, Flamez D, Roebroek AJ, Bright NA, Meulemans S, et al. Role of furin in granular acidification in the endocrine pancreas: identification of the V-ATPase subunit Ac45 as a candidate substrate. *Proc Natl Acad Sci U S A* (2008) 105(34):12319–24. doi: 10.1073/pnas.0800340105
88. Al-Mulla F, Mohammad A, Al Madhoun A, Haddad D, Ali H, Eaaswarkhanth M, et al. A comprehensive germline variant and expression analyses of ACE2, TMPRSS2 and SARS-CoV-2 activator FURIN genes from the Middle East: Combating SARS-CoV-2 with precision medicine. *bioRxiv* (2020) p:2020.05.16.099176. doi: 10.1101/2020.05.16.099176
89. Flint SW, Tahrani AA. COVID-19 and obesity-lack of clarity, guidance, and implications for care. *Lancet Diabetes Endocrinol* (2020) 8(6):474–5. doi: 10.1016/S2213-8587(20)30156-X
90. Zick Y. Role of Ser/Thr kinases in the uncoupling of insulin signaling. *Int J Obes Relat Metab Disord* (2003) 27 Suppl 3:S56–60. doi: 10.1038/sj.ijo.0802503
91. El Mesallamy HO, Hamdy NM, Mostafa DM, Amin AI. The serine protease granzyme B as an inflammatory marker, in relation to the insulin receptor cleavage in human obesity and type 2 diabetes mellitus. *J Interferon Cytokine Res* (2014) 34(3):179–86. doi: 10.1089/jir.2013.0059
92. Spence JS, He R, Hoffmann HH, Das T, Thinon E, Rice CM, et al. IFITM3 directly engages and shuttles incoming virus particles to lysosomes. *Nat Chem Biol* (2019) 15(3):259–68. doi: 10.1038/s41589-018-0213-2
93. Wrensch F, Winkler M, Pöhlmann S. IFITM proteins inhibit entry driven by the MERS-coronavirus spike protein: evidence for cholesterol-independent mechanisms. *Viruses* (2014) 6(9):3683–98. doi: 10.3390/v6093683
94. Thevarajan I, Nguyen THO, Koutsakos M, Druce J, Caly L, Van De Sandt CE, et al. Breadth of concomitant immune responses prior to patient recovery: a case report of non-severe COVID-19. *Nat Med* (2020) 26:(4):453–5. doi: 10.1038/s41591-020-0819-2
95. Hoffmann M, Kleine-Weber H, Schroeder S, Krüger N, Herrler T, Erichsen S, et al. SARS-CoV-2 Cell Entry Depends on ACE2 and TMPRSS2 and Is Blocked by a Clinically Proven Protease Inhibitor. *Cell* (2020) 181(2):271–280.e8. doi: 10.1016/j.cell.2020.02.052
96. Shi G, Ozog S, Torbett BE, Compton AA. mTOR inhibitors lower an intrinsic barrier to virus infection mediated by IFITM3. *Proc Natl Acad Sci U S A* (2018) 115: (43):E10069–e10078. doi: 10.1073/pnas.1811892115
97. Tuo Y, Xiang M. mTOR: A double-edged sword for diabetes. *J Leukoc Biol* (2018) 106(2):385–95. doi: 10.1002/JLB.3MR0317-095RR
98. Haga S, Nagata N, Okamura T, Yamamoto N, Sata T, Yamamoto N, et al. TACE antagonists blocking ACE2 shedding caused by the spike protein of SARS-CoV are candidate antiviral compounds. *Antiviral Res* (2010) 85 (3):551–5. doi: 10.1016/j.antiviral.2009.12.001
99. Haga S, Yamamoto N, Nakai-Murakami C, Osawa Y, Tokunaga K, Sata T, et al. Modulation of TNF-alpha-converting enzyme by the spike protein of SARS-CoV and ACE2 induces TNF-alpha production and facilitates viral entry. *Proc Natl Acad Sci U S A* (2008) 105(22):7809–14. doi: 10.1073/pnas.0711241105

100. Palau V, Riera M, Soler MJ. ADAM17 inhibition may exert a protective effect on COVID-19. *Nephrol Dial Transplant* (2020) 35(6):1071–2. doi: 10.1093/ndt/gfaa093
101. Xu J, Mukerjee S, Silva-Alves CR, Carvalho-Galvão A, Cruz JC, Balarini, et al. A Disintegrin and Metalloprotease 17 in the Cardiovascular and Central Nervous Systems. *Front Physiol* (2016) 7:469. doi: 10.3389/fphys.2016.00469
102. Togashi N, Ura N, Higashiura K, Murakami H, Shimamoto K. Effect of TNF-alpha–converting enzyme inhibitor on insulin resistance in fructose-fed rats. *Hypertension* (2002) 39(2 Pt 2):578–80. doi: 10.1161/hy0202.103290
103. Serino M, Menghini R, Fiorentino L, Amoruso R, Mauriello A, Lauro D, et al. Mice heterozygous for tumor necrosis factor-alpha converting enzyme are protected from obesity-induced insulin resistance and diabetes. *Diabetes* (2007) 56(10):2541–6. doi: 10.2337/db07-0360
104. Ibrahim IM, Abdelmalek DH, Elshahat ME, Elfiky AA. COVID-19 spike-host cell receptor GRP78 binding site prediction. *J Infect* (2020) 80(5):554–62. doi: 10.1016/j.jinf.2020.02.026
105. Ye R, Jung DY, Jun JY, Li J, Luo S, Ko HJ, et al. Grp78 heterozygosity promotes adaptive unfolded protein response and attenuates diet-induced obesity and insulin resistance. *Diabetes* (2010) 59(1):6–16. doi: 10.2337/db09-0755
106. Koch C, Staffler G, Hüttinger R, Hilgert I, Prager E, Cerný J, et al. T cell activation-associated epitopes of CD147 in regulation of the T cell response, and their definition by antibody affinity and antigen density. *Int Immunol* (1999) 11(5):777–86. doi: 10.1093/intimm/11.5.777
107. Ulrich H, Pillat MM. CD147 as a Target for COVID-19 Treatment: Suggested Effects of Azithromycin and Stem Cell Engagement. *Stem Cell Rev Rep* (2020) 16(3):434–40. doi: 10.1007/s12015-020-09976-7
108. Xie Y, Wang Y, Ding H, Guo M, Wang X, Dong Q, et al. Highly glycosylated CD147 promotes hemorrhagic transformation after rt-PA treatment in diabetes: a novel therapeutic target? *J Neuroinflammation* (2019) 16(1):72. doi: 10.1186/s12974-019-1460-1
109. Drucker DJ. Mechanisms of Action and Therapeutic Application of Glucagon-like Peptide-1. *Cell Metab* (2018) 27(4):740–56. doi: 10.1016/j.cmet.2018.03.001
110. Bloodworth MH, Rusznak M, Pfister CC, Zhang J, Bastarache L, Calvillo SA, et al. Glucagon-like peptide 1 receptor signaling attenuates respiratory syncytial virus-induced type 2 responses and immunopathology. *J Allergy Clin Immunol* (2018) 142(2):683–7.e12. doi: 10.1016/j.jaci.2018.01.053
111. Jin T, Liu M. Letter to the editor: Comment on GLP-1-based drugs and COVID-19 treatment. *Acta Pharm Sin B* (2020) 10(7):1249–50. doi: 10.1016/j.apsb.2020.05.006
112. Chatterjee S. SGLT-2 inhibitors for COVID-19 - A miracle waiting to happen or just another beat around the bush? *Prim Care Diabetes* (2020) 14(5):564–5. doi: 10.1016/j.pcd.2020.05.013
113. Fernandez-Fernandez B, D'Marco L. Exploring Sodium Glucose Co-Transporter-2 (SGLT2) Inhibitors for Organ Protection in COVID-19. *J Clin Med* (2020) 9(7):2030. doi: 10.3390/jcm9072030
114. American diabetes association15. Diabetes Care in the Hospital: Standards of Medical Care in Diabetes-2020. *Diabetes Care* (2020) 43(Suppl 1):S193–s202. doi: 10.2337/dc20-S015
115. Papadokostaki E, Tentolouris N, Liberopoulos E. COVID-19 and diabetes: What does the clinician need to know? *Prim Care Diabetes* (2020) 14(5):558–63. doi: 10.1016/j.pcd.2020.06.010
116. Bornstein SR, Rubino F, Khunti K, Mingrone G, Hopkins D, Birkenfeld AL, et al. Practical recommendations for the management of diabetes in patients with COVID-19. *Lancet Diabetes Endocrinol* (2020) 8(6):546–50. doi: 10.1016/S2213-8587(20)30223-0
117. Chen Y, Yang D, Cheng B, Chen J, Peng A, Yang C, et al. Clinical Characteristics and Outcomes of Patients With Diabetes and COVID-19 in Association With Glucose-Lowering Medication. *Diabetes Care* (2020) 43 (7):1399–407. doi: 10.2337/dc20-0660
118. Mulvihill EE, Drucker DJ. Pharmacology, physiology, and mechanisms of action of dipeptidyl peptidase-4 inhibitors. *Endocr Rev* (2014) 35(6):992–1019. doi: 10.1210/er.2014-1035
119. Fadini GP, Morieri ML, Longato E, Bonora BM, Pinelli S, Selmin E, et al. Exposure to dipeptidyl-peptidase-4 inhibitors and COVID-19 among people with type 2 diabetes: A case-control study. *Diabetes Obes Metab* (2020). doi: 10.1111/dom.14097
120. Strollo R, Maddaloni E, Dauriz M, Pedone C, Buzzetti R, Pozzilli P, et al. Use of DPP4 inhibitors in Italy does not correlate with diabetes prevalence among COVID-19 deaths. *Diabetes Res Clin Pract* (2020), 108444. doi: 10.1016/j.diabres.2020.108444
121. Cariou B, Hadjadj S. Phenotypic characteristics and prognosis of inpatients with COVID-19 and diabetes: the CORONADO study. *Diabetologia* (2020) 63(8):1500–15. doi: 10.1007/s00125-020-05180-x
122. Solerte SB, D'addio F, Trevisan R, Lovati E, Rossi A, Pastore I, et al. Sitagliptin Treatment at the Time of Hospitalization Was Associated With Reduced Mortality in Patients With Type 2 Diabetes and COVID-19: A Multicenter, Case-Control, Retrospective, Observational Study. *Diabetes Care* (2020) dc201521. doi: 10.2337/dc20-1521
123. Monteil V, Kwon H, Prado P, Hagelkrüys A, Wimmer RA, Stahl M, et al. Inhibition of SARS-CoV-2 Infections in Engineered Human Tissues Using Clinical-Grade Soluble Human ACE2. *Cell* (2020) 181(4):905–913.e7. doi: 10.1016/j.cell.2020.04.004
124. Mozafari N, Azadi S, Mehdi-Alamdarlou S, Ashrafi H, et al. Inflammation: A bridge between diabetes and COVID-19, and possible management with sitagliptin. *Med Hypotheses* (2020) 143:110111. doi: 10.1016/j.mehy.2020.110111

15

Identification of Sorafenib as a Treatment for Type 1 Diabetes

Qin Zeng[1,2†], Jianfeng Song[1,2†], Dandan Wang[1,2], Xiaoxiao Sun[1,2], Yalun Xiao[1,2], Haowei Zhang[1,2], Yang Xiao[1,2], Zhiguang Zhou[1,2] and Tuo Deng[1,2,3*]*

[1] National Clinical Research Center for Metabolic Diseases, and Department of Metabolism and Endocrinology, The Second Xiangya Hospital of Central South University, Changsha, China, [2] Key Laboratory of Diabetes Immunology, Ministry of Education, and Metabolic Syndrome Research Center, The Second Xiangya Hospital of Central South University, Changsha, China, [3] Clinical Immunology Center, The Second Xiangya Hospital of Central South University, Changsha, China

***Correspondence:**
Tuo Deng
dengtuo@csu.edu.cn
Zhiguang Zhou
zhouzhiguang@csu.edu.cn

[†]These authors have contributed equally to this work

Th1 cell activation is considered a key mediator of the pathogenesis of type 1 diabetes. Targeting IL-12-induced Th1 cell differentiation seems to be an effective way to block the development of type 1 diabetes. However, given the critical function of Th1 in the immune system, the potential side effects hinder the application of anti-Th1 therapy in the treatment of type 1 diabetes. To identify safe anti-Th1 treatment(s), we screened the FDA-approved tyrosine kinase inhibitor (TKI) drug library using an IL-12-induced Th1 differentiation cell model. We found that among the TKIs with little effect on T cell viability, sorafenib is the top contender for the inhibition of Th1 differentiation. Treatment of NOD mice with sorafenib significantly impeded the development of type 1 diabetes and ameliorated insulitis, which coincided with a specifically decreased accumulation of Th1 cell population in the pancreas but not in peripheral immune organs. Mechanistically, sorafenib indirectly inhibited janus kinase 2 (JAK2) activity and blocked IL-12-induced phosphorylations of JAK2 and signal transducer and activator of transcription 4 (STAT4). Since sorafenib is classified as an FDA-approved drug, it serves as a preliminary lead point for additional experimentation and may be a promising therapy for type 1 diabetes in humans.

Keywords: type 1 diabetes, Th1, sorafenib, IL-12, NOD mice

INTRODUCTION

Type 1 diabetes is an immune-mediated disease characterized by the impairment of insulin-producing pancreatic beta cells. Since the destruction of beta cells in type 1 diabetes is mainly mediated by pathogenic autoreactive T cells, targeting autoreactive T cells shows promise in treating type 1 diabetes. T cell-based immunotherapies, such as an anti-CD3 monoclonal antibody, CTLA4-Ig fusion protein and low-dose anti-thymocyte globulin, have emerged for the treatment of type 1 diabetes (1). These immunotherapies indeed have shown some benefits in human clinical trials, but

Abbreviations: APCs, antigen-presenting cells; Cy, Cyclophosphamide; I-A2, insulinoma-associated antigen 2; JAK2, janus kinase 2; LADA, latent autoimmune diabetes in adults; MLN, mesenteric lymph node; PBMCs, Peripheral blood mononuclear cells; PDGFR, platelet derived growth factor receptor; PLNs, pancreatic lymph nodes; PPI, preproinsulin; STAT4, signal transducer and activator of transcription 4; TKI, tyrosine kinase inhibitor; Tregs, regulatory T cells; TYK2, tyrosine kinase 2; VEGFR, vascular endothelial growth factor receptor; ZnT8, zinc transporter 8; Cy, cyclophosphamide; MLN, mesenteric lymph node; PMBC, peripheral blood mononuclear cells.

their systemic immunosuppressive effects and transient efficiency limit the success of application. In the face of an increasing type 1 diabetes population, it is urgent to development more effective and safer T cell-based immunotherapies.

In the early stage of type 1 diabetes, antigen-presenting cells (APCs) present autoantigens such as preproinsulin (PPI), insulinoma-associated antigen 2 (I-A2), GAD, and zinc transporter (ZnT8) to $CD4^+$ T cells (2). Meanwhile, APCs secrete IL-12 to trigger the differentiation of naïve $CD4^+$ T cells into Th1 cells. The Th1 cells produce inflammatory cytokines including IFN-γ and IL-2 to activate $CD8^+$ cytotoxic T lymphocytes and macrophages (3), and cooperate with them to attack pancreatic beta cells. Transfer of pathogenic Th1 cells into neonatal NOD mice initiated the onset of type 1 diabetes (4), while the depletion of Th1 cells by disrupting Tbet, a key transcription factor for Th1 cell polarization, effectively blocked insulitis and type 1 diabetes in NOD mice (5). Therefore, Th1 cell population is a critical mediator of type 1 diabetes pathogenesis. IL-12 is a key cytokine for the induction of Th1 cell differentiation, and IL-12-induced signal transducer and activator of transcription 4 (STAT4) activation is a paramount signaling pathway for Th1 cell differentiation (6). In NOD mice, daily administration of IL-12 increased type 1 diabetes incidence (7), while addition of an IL-12 antagonist decreased type 1 diabetes incidence (8, 9). In addition, disruption of STAT4 activation prevented the development of type 1 diabetes in NOD mice completely (10). In humans, *IL-12b* was identified as a susceptible type 1 diabetes gene (11). These studies suggest that IL-12 played an essential role, inducing Th1 cell differentiation in pathogenesis of type 1 diabetes. Therefore, targeting the IL-12/STAT4 axis to suppress Th1 cell may be an effective strategy for the treatment of type 1 diabetes.

Tyrosine kinases possess a catalytic subunit that transfers a phosphate group from ATP to one or more tyrosine residues in a protein, leading to conformational changes, affecting protein function. They are important mediators of the signaling transduction, regulating cellular activity such as cell division, differentiation, apoptosis, and metabolism, in response to external and internal stimuli (12, 13). Due to multiple functions of tyrosine kinases in a variety of biological processes, tyrosine kinase inhibitors (TKIs) have been developed for the treatment of many diseases, including cancer, autoimmune and inflammatory diseases, degenerative disease and infectious disease (14, 15). Up until now, 39 TKIs have been approved by FDA, and more are being tested in clinical trials (16). IL-12/STAT4 pathway is directly mediated by a tyrosine kinase, janus kinase 2 (JAK2) (17, 18), and may be indirectly regulated by tyrosine kinase 2 (TYK2) or other tyrosine kinases (19, 20). To identify new and safe Th1 cell differentiation inhibitors that can be used to treat type 1 diabetes, we screened the FDA-approved TKI drug sub-library in an *in-vitro* cell culture model of IL-12-induced Th1 cell differentiation. We found that sorafenib, a TKI mainly targeting Raf for the treatment of renal and liver cancers, strongly blocked IL-12-induced Th1 cell differentiation by inhibiting the phosphorylations of JAK2 and STAT4. Treatment with sorafenib in NOD mice inhibited Th1 cell accumulation in the pancreas, and prevented insulitis and diabetes. These results suggest that sorafenib may be a potential treatment for type 1 diabetes.

MATERIAL AND METHODS

Experimental Animals

Female NOD mice were purchased from the Model Animal Research Center of Nanjing University (Nanjing, China), 017581-B6.129S4-*Ifng*$^{tm3.1Lky}$/J (GREAT) mice were purchased from the Jackson Laboratory (Bar Harbor, ME, USA), C57BL/6J mice were purchased from Slac Laboratory Animal Inc (Shanghai, China). All mice were housed in a specific-pathogen-free animal facility at Central South University (Changsha, China). 12-week-old female NOD mice were monitored for blood glucose twice per week and considered diabetic after two consecutive blood glucose readings were >250 mg/dl. All animal experiments were performed in accordance with the guidelines from the Department of Laboratory Animal Science, Central South University.

Drugs and Treatments

Sorafenib tosylate (Nexavar) tablets were purchased from Byer (Leverkusen, Germany) and suspended in 1% sodium carboxymethyl cellulose for *in vivo* use. Eight-week-old female NOD mice were treated with 10 mg/kg body weight of sorafenib or vehicle once daily by oral gavage. Administration time varies by experiment. Cyclophosphamide (Cy, Sigma-Aldrich, St. Louis, MO) was diluted to 35 mg/ml with 0.9% sodium chloride solution before i.p. for the treatment of 12-week-old mice (300 mg/kg) to induce the onset of diabetes in female NOD mice. For the therapeutic treatment, diabetic female NOD mice were treated with 10 or 50 mg/kg body weight of sorafenib or vehicle once daily by oral gavage for three weeks.

Histological Analysis of Insulitis

Pancreatic tissues from vehicle-treated or sorafenib-treated mice were fixed with 4% paraformaldehyde, embedded in paraffin, and 5-μm-thick sections were stained with hematoxylin and eosin. Insulitis scores were calculated by using the following scale: 0 = no infiltrate, 1 = peri-insulitis, 2 = moderate insulitis (<50%), 3 = severe insulitis (>50%).

Isolation of Lymphocytes From Tissues and Intracellular Staining

The pancreas was dissected from vehicle and sorafenib-treated mice, and digested in 1.5 mg/ml collagenase IV (Worthington Biochemical, Lakewood, NJ) for 45 min at 37°C. Pancreatic lymph nodes (PLNs) and spleens were mechanically disrupted. Cells were filtered through a 70 μm filter to get single cell suspension. Lymphocytes from tissues were stimulated for 6 h with phorbol myristate acetate (50 ng/ml) and ionomycin (5 μM) in the presence of brefeldin A and monensin (Biolegend, San Diego, CA, USA). Cells were collected to stain with antibodies, and then fixed and permeabilized in cytofix/cytoperm buffer (BD Biosciences, San Jose, CA).

Mouse T Cell Isolation and Th1 Differentiation

Naive $CD4^+$ T cells from the spleens of 6-8 weeks old male GREAT mice were prepared using magnetic bead cell sorting (Miltenyi Biotec, Bergisch-Gladbach, Germany). The purity of $CD4^+CD44^{low}CD62L^{high}$ T cell subset was validated by flow cytometry. These naïve $CD4^+$ T cells were stimulated with 5 µg/ml pre-coated anti-CD3ϵ antibody (Biolegend) and 1 µg/ml soluble anti-CD28 antibody (Biolegend) in culture medium containing 10 ng/ml IL-12 (Peprotech, Cranbury, NJ, USA), 10 ng/ml IL-2 (Peprotech) and 10 µg/ml anti–IL-4 antibody (BD Biosciences) for 3 days. The culture medium was RPMI 1640 medium (plus 50 µM β-mercaptoethanol) supplemented with 10% FBS, 1% GlutaMax, and 1% Pen/Strep (Gibco, Shanghai, China). 1×10^5 naive $CD4^+$ T cells were cultured in 96-well plates with 100 µl culture medium per well.

Human T Cell Isolation and Th1 Differentiation

Healthy volunteers were recruited from the medical students at the Second Xiangya Hospital and written informed consent was obtained. Human study was approved by the Ethics Committee of the Second Xiangya Hospital of Central South University. Peripheral blood mononuclear cells (PBMCs) from the peripheral blood of healthy volunteers were separated by Histopaque (Sigma-Aldrich, St. Louis, MO). Naive $CD4^+$ T cells from PBMC were isolated by negative selection using Miltenyi beads according to the manufacturer's instructions. The purity of $CD4^+CD45RA^+CD45RO^-$ T cell subset was validated by flow cytometry. The purified naïve $CD4^+$ T cells were stimulated with 5 µg/ml pre-coated anti-CD3ϵ antibody (Biolegend) and 2 µg/ml soluble anti-CD28 antibody (Biolegend) in culture medium containing 10 ng/ml IL-12 (Peprotech, Cranbury, NJ, USA), 10 ng/ml IL-2 (Peprotech) and 10 µg/ml anti–IL-4 antibody (eBioscience) for 5 days. The culture medium was RPMI 1640 medium supplemented with 10% FBS, 1% GlutaMax, and 1% Pen/Strep (Gibco, Shanghai, China). 1×10^5 naive $CD4^+$ T cells were cultured in 96-well plates with 100 µl culture medium per well. The culture medium was refreshed on day 3.

Drug Screen

The FDA-approved TKI drug library was purchased from Selleck Chemicals (Houston, TX, USA), and was dissolved in DMSO or water to get a 10 mM concentration for screening. Naive $CD4^+$ T cells were prepared from the spleens of 8-week-old male GREAT mice, 1×10^5 Th0 cells/well were plated into 96-well plates and cultured for 72 h. Th0 cells were cultured with Th1 differentiation medium containing 10 µM of individual FDA-approved TKI drug, and the IFN-γ–expressing Th1 cells were defined by detection of YFP expression.

Cell Viability Assay

Cell viability of Th0 cells was performed using standard trypan blue exclusion method and ATP chemiluminescence assay. After isolation of naïve $CD4^+$ T cells (Th0) cells, 5×10^4 Th0 cells/well were plated into 96-well plates and cultured for 48 h. Viable cells were assessed by trypan blue staining. Similarly, 1×10^3 Th0 cells/well were plated into opaque 96-well plates and cultured for 48 h, and then detected by using the CellTiter-Lumi™ luminescent cell viability assay kit (Beyotime, Beijing, China), the absorbance of 570 nm was measured using a microplate reader (Enspire Multimode Plate Reader, Perkin Elmer).

E. coli-Infection Mouse Model

Eight weeks old male C57BL/6J mice were treated with 10 mg/kg body weight of sorafenib or vehicle once daily by oral gavage. Two days after sorafenib treatment, C57BL/6J mice were injected intraperitoneally with 0.2 ml of suspensions of *E. coli* (ATCC 8739) at 10^7 CFU. Bacteria were harvested by centrifugation at 4000 rpm for 15 min and washed twice in PBS, and then diluted in PBS to obtain the desired concentration for infection experiments. To determine injection success, bacteria in peritoneal lavage fluid from the infected mice were collected at 24 hours after infection, and cultured overnight at 37°C on Luria-Bertani Agar plates.

In-Vitro Kinase Assay

Enzyme activity was measured using mobility shift assay in duplicate in 384-well plates. Dilution series of ten different concentrations were diluted in DMSO. Sorafenib was diluted to 50X of the final desired highest inhibitor concentration in DMSO, 10 µl of the compound was mixed with 90 µl of 1x kinase buffer to each well of the 96-well plate for shaking 10 min, then the mixture was transferred to a 384-well plate in duplicates. After assay plate preparation, enzyme solution and carboxyfluorescein-labeled peptide and ATP were added into the assay plate in turn. Luminescence signal was measured on Caliper (Perkin Elmer).

Real-Time Quantitative PCR

Total RNA was extracted from the pancreas using the Trizol reagent (Invitrogen, Life Technologies, NY) following manufacturer's instructions. cDNA was synthesized using the cDNA Synthesis Kit (Thermo-Fisher Scientific, MA) and primers (Sangon Biotech Shanghai, China). RT-qPCR was performed using the FastStart Universal Master mix (Roche, Germany) in an ABI ViiA 7 Real-Time Polymerase Chain Reaction System. Relative gene expression levels were normalized to housing-keeping gene beta-actin. The following primers were used: mouse Tbet (Tbx21; forward: 5'-TTCAACCAGCACCAGACAG-3', reverse: 5'-AGACCACATCCACAAACATCC-3'), mouse IFN-γ (Ifng; forward: 5'-CTTTGGACCCTCTGACTTGAG-3', reverse: 5'-TCTTCCACATCTATGCCACTTG-3'), mouse IL-1β (forward: 5'-TGAAATGCCACCTTTTGACAG-3', reverse: 5'-CACGGGAAAGACACAGGTAG-3'), mouse IL-6 (forward: 5'-TGGAAATGAGAAAAGAGTTGTGC-3', reverse: 5'-CTCTGAAGGACTC

TGGCTTTG-3'), mouse TNF-α (forward: 5'-CTTCTG TCTACTGAACTTCGGG-3', reverse: 5'-TGTCTTTGAGA TCCATGCCG-3'), mouse Bcl6 (forward: 5'-CCATACAAAT GTGATCGCTGC-3', reverse: 5'- GTAGGGCTTTTCT CCAGAGTG-3'), mouse Rorc (forward: 5'-GCACCAACCT CTTTTCACG-3', reverse: 5'-ACGACTTCCATTGCTCCTG-3'), mouse Foxp3 (forward: 5'-ACCCAGGAAAGACAGCAAC-3', reverse: 5'-CTTCTCCTTTTCCAGCTCCAG-3'), mouse Gata3 (forward: 5'-CTTATCAAGCCCAAGCGAAG-3', reverse: 5'-TCGATTTGCTAGACATCTTCCG-3'), mouse IL-21 (forward: 5'-ATCATTGACCTCGTGGCC-3', reverse: 5'-CTTCGG GTCCTATGTGTTCTAG-3'), mouse Stat4 (forward: 5'-CTGGGAGTAAAGGAAACGAGG-3', reverse: 5'-GCTG GTCTCTAGGTTAATGGTG-3'), mouse Jak2 (forward: 5'-TGAGGCCACCAGTAAAAGACA-3', reverse: 5'-TTTTG CCAGACAAGAGTGATG-3'), mouse beta-actin (forward: 5'-ACCGTGAAAAGATGACCCAG-3', reverse: 5'-GAGCA TAGCCCTCGTAGATG-3').

In-Vitro Phosphorylation Assay

The purified naive CD4$^+$ T cells were cultured in RPMI 1640 with 10% FBS and 1% Pen/Strep. 2×10^6 Th0 cells/well were pre-treated with gradient concentrations of sorafenib for 3 h and then stimulated with 10 ng/ml IL-12 for 5 min to induce the phosphorylations of JAK2 and STAT4. Finally, cell extracts were collected for western blots analysis.

Western Blots Analysis

Total protein was extracted using RIPA buffer containing a cocktail of proteinase and phosphatase inhibitors (Sigma-Aldrich). Protein concentration was measured using BCA kit (Thermo Scientific, Pierce) and 30 μg/lane of total protein was loaded onto 10% polyacrylamide gels. The membranes were first incubated with following anti-phosphotyrosine antibodies at 4°C overnight: anti-pJAK2 (Cell Signaling Technology, Cat#3771, dilute 1:1000) and anti-pSTAT4 (Santa Cruz, Cat#sc-28296, dilute 1:100). The membranes were subsequently stripped using a solution containing 100 mM β-mercaptoethanol, 2% SDS, and 62.5 mM Tris-HCl (pH 7.6) at 50°C for 30 min, and re-incubated with anti-JAK2 (Cell Signaling Technology, Cat#3230, dilute 1:1000) or anti-STAT4 (Cell Signaling Technology, Cat#2653, dilute 1:1000) antibodies at 4°C overnight.

Flow Cytometry

Cells were stained with fluorochrome-conjugated mAbs and analyzed on CYTEK northern lights NL-3000 or BD FACS Canto II. For surface markers detection, cells were incubated with FcR blocking antibody (Biolegend, Cat#101302 and 422302) for 15 min at room temperature, and stained with antibodies against surface markers for 30 min at 4°C in the dark. Stained cells were washed in PBS and then incubated with 7-AAD viability staining solution (Biolegend, Cat#420404) for 5 min at room temperature. For intracellular staining, cells were incubated with Zombie NIR (Biolegend, Cat#423106) for 15 min at room temperature, and then blocked with CD16/32 antibody and stained with fluorochrome-labeled mAbs against cell-surface antigens for 30 min at 4°C. Cells subsequently were fixed and permeabilized with foxp3/transcription factor staining buffer set (eBioscience, 00-5523-00) or cytofix/cytoperm buffer, and stained with fluorochrome-conjugated antibodies for an additional 30 minutes at 4°C in the dark. The following mAbs were used: CD45 (Biolegend, Cat#103108, 103132 and BD, Cat#562420), CD3e (Biolegend, Cat#100330, 100306, 100216), CD4 (Biolegend, Cat#100406, 100408, 100414, 980804 and eBioscience, Cat#11-0049-41), CD8a (Biolegend, Cat#100721), IFN-γ (Biolegend, Cat#505810, 505832 and 502512), IL-4 (Biolegend, Cat# 504123), IL-17A (Biolegend, Cat#506903), CD25 (Biolegend, Cat#102012 and eBioscience, Cat#56-0251-80), Foxp3 (Biolegend, Cat#126403 and eBioscience, Cat#17-57773-82), CD62L (Biolegend, Cat#104427), CD44 (Biolegend, Cat#103012), CD45RA (Biolegend, Cat#983002) and CD45RO (Biolegend, Cat#304230). Data were analyzed using FlowJo software.

Statistical Analysis

Data are presented as means ± SEM. Statistical analysis was performed using SPSS Version 19.0 software (Chicago, IL, USA). Diabetes incidence was compared using log-rank test. Insulitis was analyzed with χ^2 test. The other group differences were analyzed with 2-tailed Student's t test.

RESULTS

Sorafenib Inhibits IL-12-Induced Th1 Cell Differentiation

To identify new inhibitors of Th1 cell differentiation, we utilized the 'GREAT' (IFN-γ reporter with endogenous polyA transcript) mice model (21), which allows analysis of IFN-γ–expressing cells through the detection of YFP expression. We screened a mini compound library including all TKI drugs approved by FDA between 2001 and 2019 (**Supplementary Figures 1A–C**). To exclude the TKIs with significant cytotoxicity to T cells, we assessed the toxic effects of TKIs on T cells first. We found that 10 TKIs have minimal cytotoxic effects on T cells at a concentration of 10 μM. Among them, sorafenib, an oral multikinase inhibitor with antitumor properties, was identified as the most potent inhibitor of IL-12-induced Th1 cell differentiation. As shown in **Figures 1A, B**, sorafenib inhibited IL-12-induced Th1 cell differentiation in a dose-dependent manner. The gating strategy and purity of sorted mouse naïve CD4$^+$ T cells were shown in **Supplementary Figures 2A, B**. To confirm that the inhibitory effect of sorafenib on Th1 cell differentiation was not due to cytotoxicity, we treated naïve CD4$^+$ T (Th0) cells with different doses of sorafenib for 2 days and examined the viability of naïve CD4$^+$ T cells by performing an ATP chemiluminescence assay. We found that the number of viable cells did not differ by the treatment of 10 μM of sorafenib (**Figure 1C**), which strongly inhibited IL-12-induced Th1 cell differentiation. However, sorafenib was not able to inhibit IFN-γ production in Th1 cells at non-toxic doses (**Supplementary**

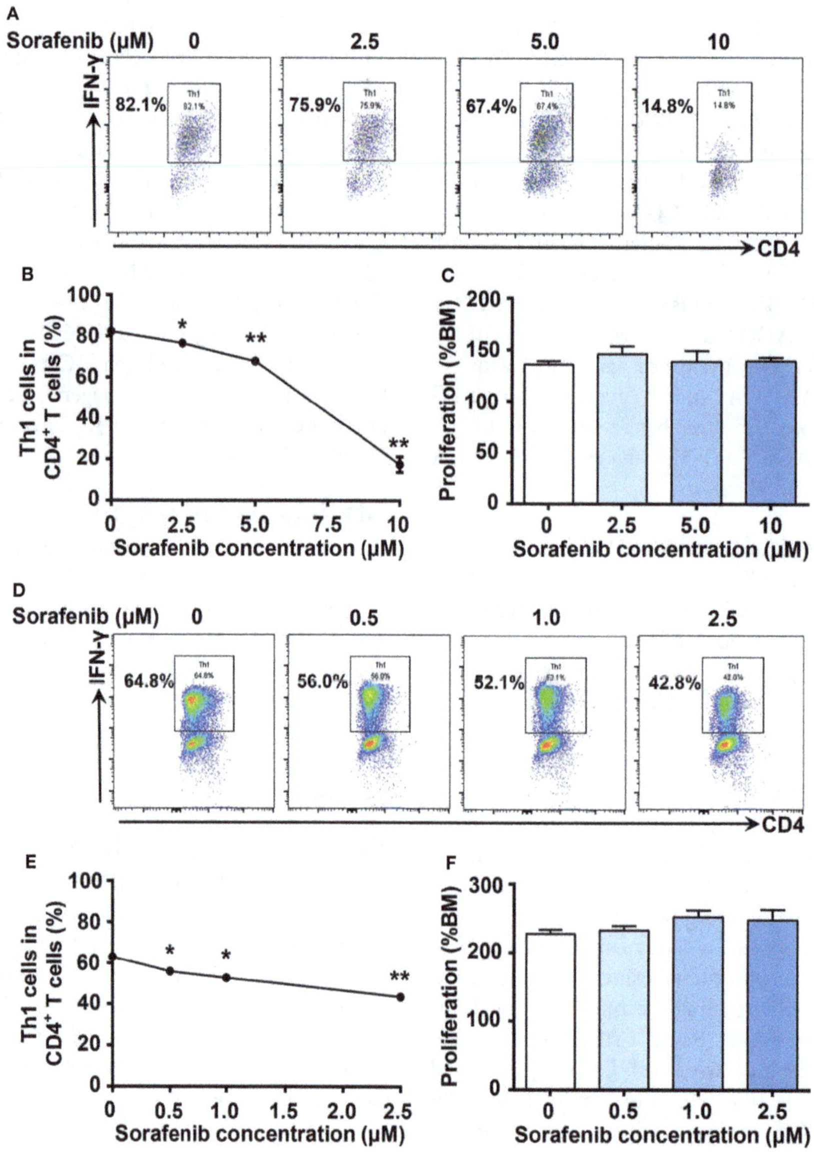

FIGURE 1 | Sorafenib inhibits IL-12-induced Th1 cell differentiation in a dose-dependent manner in both mice and humans. **(A, B)** Flow cytometry analysis of Th1 cells in mouse naïve splenic CD4$^+$ T cells stimulated with IL-12 in medium containing different concentrations of sorafenib as indicated. **(C)** CellTiter-Lumi assay to assess viable cells in the naïve splenic Th0 cells cultured in medium containing different concentrations of sorafenib as indicated. **(D, E)** Flow cytometry analysis of Th1 cells in human naïve PBMC CD4$^+$ T cells stimulated with IL-12 in medium containing different concentrations of sorafenib as indicated. **(F)** CellTiter-Lumi assay to assess viable cells in the naïve PBMC Th0 cells cultured in medium containing different concentrations of sorafenib as indicated. BM, blank medium. Data are representative of 3 independent experiments. Data represent means ± s.e.m; $^*P < 0.05$ or $^{**}P < 0.01$ versus 0 μM by t-test.

Figures 3A, B). To determine whether sorafenib inhibits Th1 cell differentiation in humans, naïve CD4$^+$ T cells were isolated from PBMC of healthy donors by cell sorting and subsequently were differentiated into Th1 cells by IL-12 stimulation. The gating strategy and purity of sorted naïve CD4$^+$ T cells were shown in **Supplementary Figures 2C, D**. As shown in **Figures 1D–F**, sorafenib effectively inhibited IL-12-induced Th1 cell differentiation in human T cells without altering their viability. Collectively, our results indicate that sorafenib is a strong inhibitor of Th1 differentiation.

Sorafenib Administration Prevents Development of Type 1 Diabetes

Type 1 diabetes is characterized by the activation of pathogenic autoreactive Th1 cells in the pancreas (3). To investigate whether sorafenib inhibits the development of type 1 diabetes, sorafenib was administered to NOD mice, a widely used type 1 diabetes mice model, once daily by oral gavage at a dose of 10 mg/kg body weight. Oral administration was initiated at 8 weeks of age and continued to 20 weeks of age. During the development of natural diabetes, vehicle-treated mice had a higher incidence (32%) than sorafenib-treated mice (19%) at 17 weeks of age, and the gap between two groups grew over time. By 32 weeks of age, the endpoint of this experiment, 43% of the mice treated with sorafenib were diabetic, as opposed to 74% of the vehicle-treated mice (**Figure 2A**). Next, we assessed the effects of sorafenib on cyclophosphamide (Cy)-induced type 1 diabetes. Cy treatment leads to a rapid onset of type 1 diabetes both in human and NOD mice through suppression of regulatory T cells (Tregs) (22–25). Our data showed that more than half of the vehicle-treated mice developed diabetes within 6 weeks after Cy injection, in contrast, only 24% of the sorafenib-treated mice developed diabetes during the same period (**Figure 2B**). Notably, the protective effects of sorafenib persisted and lasted for at least 5 weeks after cessation of oral administration (**Figure 2B**), suggesting that the short-term treatment had prolonged beneficial effects on the development of diabetes in this setting. Pancreatic islets were examined in vehicle-treated and sorafenib-treated prediabetic mice. After 2 weeks of Cy treatment, the mononuclear cell accumulation was less evident in the sorafenib-treated group when compared with the vehicle-treated group (**Figure 2C**), and mice treated with sorafenib showed a significantly lower insulitis score compared with the control mice (**Figure 2D**). Collectively, these results show that sorafenib impedes the development of type 1 diabetes and alleviates insulitis in NOD mice.

Sorafenib Administration Diminishes Th1 Cells Accumulation in Pancreas but Not in Peripheral Immune Organs in NOD Mice

T cells play an important role in the development of type 1 diabetes (2). Our data (**Figure 1**) has shown sorafenib inhibits Th1 cell differentiation *in vitro*. To examine the effects of sorafenib on T cells *in vivo*, 8-week-old prediabetic NOD mice were treated with a therapeutic dose of sorafenib (10 mg/kg/day) for 6 weeks. These mice were injected with Cy 4 weeks after the beginning of the sorafenib treatment to promote accumulation of Th1 cells in pancreas. At the end of the sorafenib treatment, the T cells in the spleen, PLN and pancreas from the vehicle-treated or sorafenib-treated mice were analyzed with flow cytometry. Preventative treatment of sorafenib did not alter the $CD4^+$ and $CD8^+$ T cell ratio (data not shown) in spleen or PLNs, nor the $CD4^+$ T cell subsets such as Th1, Th2, Th17 cell and Tregs populations (**Supplementary Figures 4A–C**). These data have indicated that prophylactic administration of sorafenib does not modify T cell subsets in peripheral immune organs. However, in the pancreas, the percentage and number of IFN-γ-producing Th1 cell were

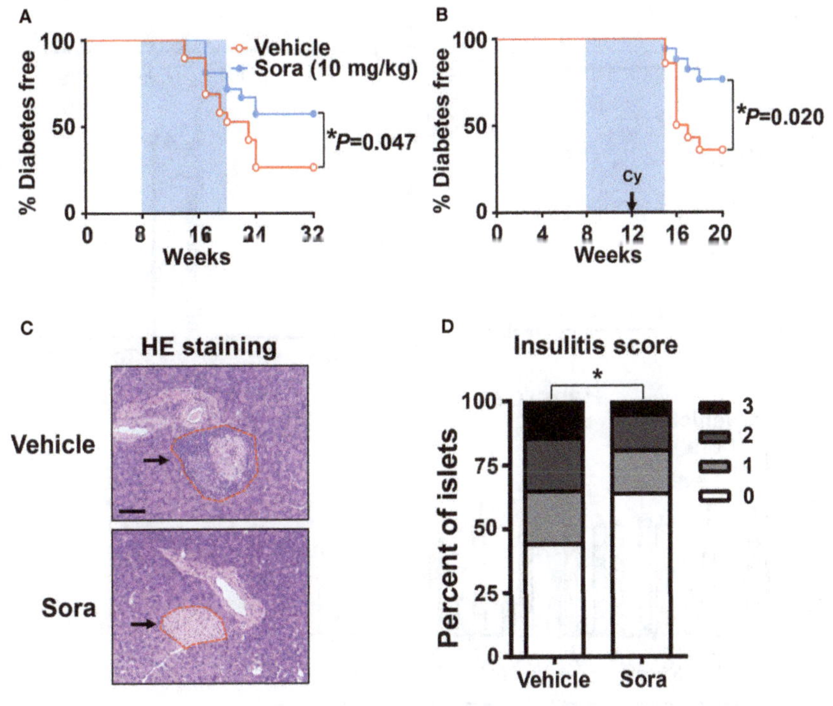

FIGURE 2 | Sorafenib prevents the development of autoimmune diabetes in NOD mice. **(A)** Diabetes incidence of female NOD mice having been treated (gavage) daily with vehicle (n = 19) or sorafenib (10 mg/kg, n = 21) for 12 weeks (blue shaded area). **(B)** Diabetes incidence of female NOD mice having been treated daily with vehicle (n = 14) or sorafenib (10 mg/kg, n = 17) for 7 weeks. Cyclophosphamide (Cy, 300 mg/kg) was injected i.p., 4 weeks after beginning of sorafenib treatment. Statistical significance: $^*P < 0.05$ versus vehicle by long-rank test. **(C)** Representative images of HE staining for pancreatic sections from 14-week-old prediabetic NOD mice having been treated daily with sorafenib (10 mg/kg) or vehicle for 6 weeks, Cy (300 mg/kg) was injected i.p., 4 weeks after beginning of sorafenib treatment, the arrows point to the islet in pancreas. (scale bar indicates 100 μm). **(D)** Insulitis scores from 14-week-old prediabetic NOD mice, data are combined from two independent experiments. $^*P < 0.05$, χ^2 test.

dramatically reduced by sorafenib administration, while the percentage and number of other CD4$^+$ T cell subsets (Th2, Th17 and Treg cells) and CD8$^+$ T cell subsets (Tc1 and Tc2 cells) were unchanged (**Figures 3A–F**). In addition, the mRNA levels of Th1 cell marker genes (*Tbet*) and proinflammatory cytokines (*IFN-γ, IL-1β, TNF-α*) were notably decreased in pancreas of sorafenib-treated mice when compared with vehicle-treated mice, but the mRNA levels of marker genes for Th2 (*Gata3*), Th17 (*Rorc*), Treg (*Foxp3*), and Tfh (*Bcl6*) cells and cytokine (*IL-21*) regulating Th1/Th17 cell differentiation were not different between the two groups (**Figure 3G**). To determine whether the inhibitory effect of sorafenib on Th1 differentiation is specific in pancreas, we investigated the effects of sorafenib on Th1 activation in mesenteric lymph node (MLN) and spleen of *E. coli*-infected

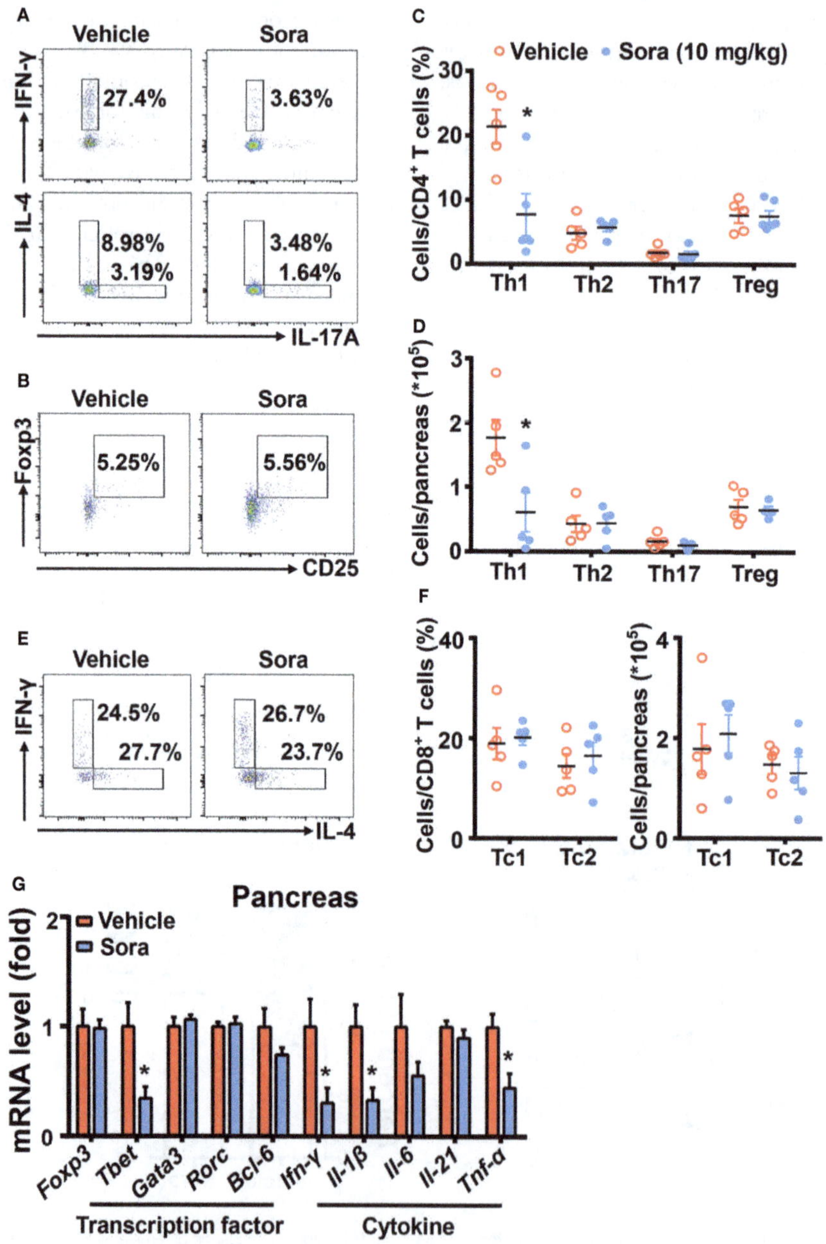

FIGURE 3 | Sorafenib decreases inflammatory Th1 cells in the pancreas of prediabetic NOD mice. Flow cytometry analysis of the frequency and number **(A–D)** of Th1, Th2, Th17 cells and Tregs in pancreas from vehicle-treated or sorafenib-treated prediabetic NOD mice. Flow cytometry analysis of the frequency and number **(E, F)** of Tc1 and Tc2 cells in pancreas from vehicle-treated or sorafenib-treated prediabetic NOD mice. **(G)** RT-PCR analysis of transcription factors (Foxp3, Tbet, Gata3, Rorc and Bcl-6) and cytokines (Ifn-γ, Il-1β, Il-6, Il-21 and Tnf-α) in pancreas from vehicle-treated or sorafenib-treated prediabetic NOD mice. Sora, sorafenib. Data represent means ± s.e.m. and data were pooled from 2 or more independent experiments. n = 5-7 mice per group in each experiment. Statistical significance: $^*P < 0.05$ versus vehicle by t-test.

C57BL/6J mice, an animal model of Th1 activation (26). The flow data showed that sorafenib effectively inhibited *E. coli*-induced Th1 cell activation in both MLN and spleen (**Supplementary Figures 5A–C**). Thus, it is likely that sorafenib, as an inhibitor of Th1 cell differentiation, induces Th1 deficiency and immunosuppression in the tissues accumulated with Th1 cells.

Sorafenib Reverses Autoimmune Diabetes in NOD Mice

In addition to defining its prevention role, we also tested whether sorafenib can reverse type 1 diabetes in NOD mice. Once diagnosed with diabetes, the mice were divided into three groups, including vehicle, low dose (10 mg/kg/day) and high dose (50 mg/kg/day) sorafenib groups. A low dose of sorafenib (10 mg/kg/day) did not reduce hyperglycemia in NOD mice with diabetes (data not shown). However, a high dose of sorafenib (50 mg/kg/day) significantly ameliorated hyperglycemia in diabetic NOD mice after one to three weeks of treatment (**Figures 4A–C**). The flow data showed that sorafenib did not alter the $CD4^+$ T cell subsets such as Th1, Th2, Th17 cell and Tregs populations in the peripheral immune organs, PLN and spleen (**Supplementary Figures 6A–C**). In the pancreas, the frequency and number of

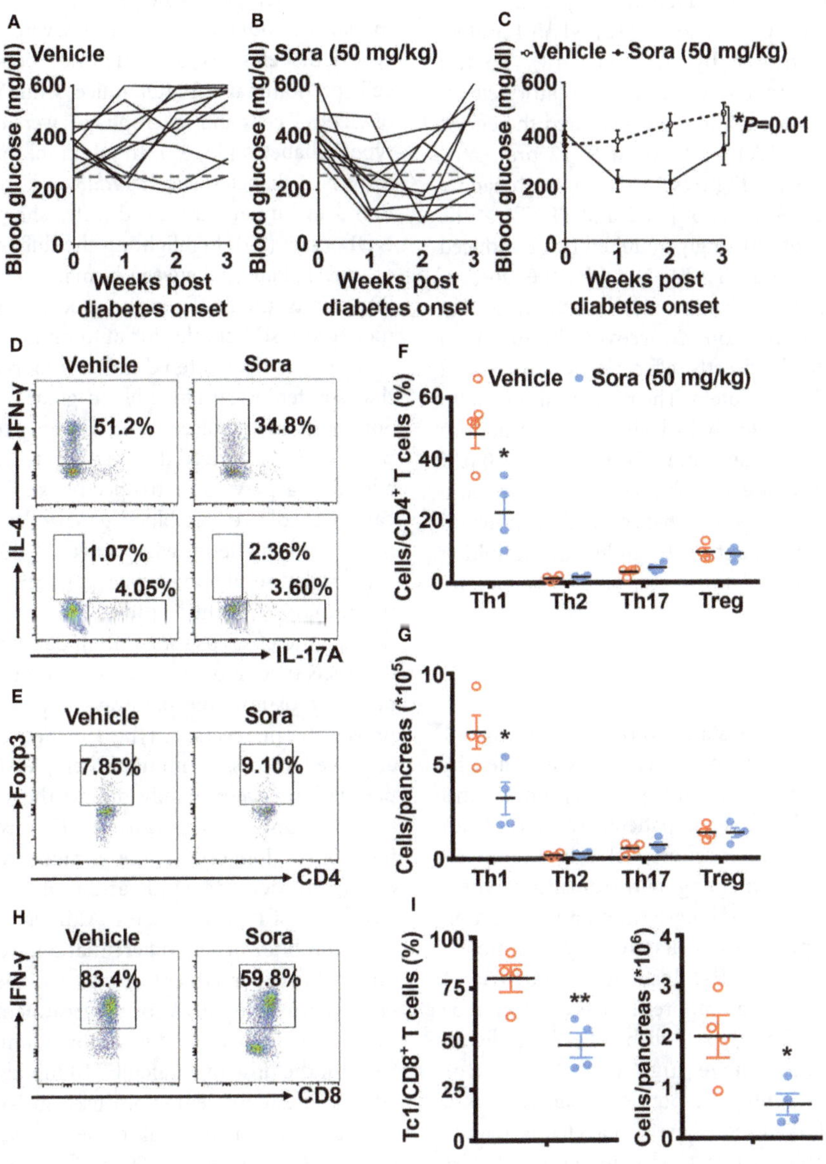

FIGURE 4 | Sorafenib reverses autoimmune diabetes in NOD mice. The trend of blood glucose **(A–C)** from vehicle-treated (n = 11) and sorafenib-treated (50 mg/kg, n = 10) new-onset diabetic NOD mice (diagnosed by two consecutive readings of blood glucose>250 mg/dl). Flow cytometry analysis of the frequency and number **(D–G)** of Th1, Th2, Th17 cells and Tregs in pancreas from vehicle-treated or sorafenib-treated diabetic NOD mice. Flow cytometry analysis of the frequency and number **(H, I)** of Tc1 cells in pancreas from vehicle-treated or sorafenib-treated diabetic NOD mice. Sora, sorafenib. Data represent means ± s.e.m. N = 4 mice per group in each experiment. Statistical significance: $^*P < 0.05$, $^{**}P < 0.01$ versus vehicle by t-test.

Th2, Th17 and Treg cells were also unchanged, but Th1 and Tc1 cells were significantly decreased in the group of sorafenib-treated diabetic NOD mice (**Figures 4D–I**). These results suggest that sorafenib may create a less-inflammatory environment in pancreas of diabetic NOD mice, which leads to the functional recovery of islet beta cells and eventually the remission of autoimmune diabetes.

Sorafenib Indirectly Inhibits the Activation of JAK2/STAT4 Pathway in IL-12-Induced Th1 Cell Differentiation

STAT4 is a transcription factor that mediates IL-12 induced Th1 cell differentiation (6). Disruption of STAT4 activation in NOD mice reduced Th1 type cytokine production and prevented the development of spontaneous type 1 diabetes (10). STAT4 protein is phosphorylated and activated by JAK2 (17, 18). To test whether JAK2 and STAT4 are involved in the inhibitory effects of sorafenib on Th1 cell differentiation, we measured the effects of sorafenib on JAK2 and STAT4 activity in IL-12 pretreated naive $CD4^+$ T cells. As shown in **Figures 5A–F**, sorafenib had no effects on protein and mRNA levels of JAK2 and STAT4 at the concentration of 1-5 μM, but it strongly inhibited IL-12-induced phosphorylations of JAK2 and STAT4. Notably, the dose of sorafenib that inhibited JAK2 activation matched the dose that inhibited Th1 cell differentiation. Moreover, in order to determine whether sorafenib directly affects JAK2, we tested the effect of sorafenib on JAK2 protein. The results from *in-vitro* kinase assay showed that sorafenib had almost no inhibitory effects on JAK2 activity at a concentration from 1 μM to 10 μM (**Figure 5G**), indicating an indirect inhibitory effect of sorafenib on JAK2. Thus, these results suggested that sorafenib suppresses IL-12-induced Th1 cell differentiation by indirectly inhibiting JAK2/STAT4 axis activation.

DISCUSSION

To date, insulin therapy is still the standard treatment for type 1 diabetes. In most cases, blood glucose was well controlled by precise insulin administration, but hypoglycemia and complications are inevitable in some patients (27–29). With the unremitting efforts of researchers, islet or stem cell transplantation is explored as an emerging treatment for type 1 diabetes patients (30, 31). However, long-term immune rejection and islet autoantigen-specific T cells destroy the newly transplanted islet or stem cells, leading to failure of transplantation (32). Currently, a comprehensive cure for type 1 diabetes is not available. Since type 1 diabetes is basically an autoimmune disease, many have high expectations for controlling the excessive immune response in pancreas as a means for curing type 1 diabetes. Type 1 diabetes is mainly mediated by pathogenic autoreactive T cells, among which Th1 cells play a key role in the pathogenesis of type 1 diabetes (4, 5). Utilizing an *in-vitro* cell culture model, we found that sorafenib can effectively block IL-12-induced Th1 cell differentiation in a dose-dependent manner without affecting the viability of T cell in both mice and humans. This finding suggests that sorafenib may be able to fight type 1 diabetes, which is characterized by the over-expansion of Th1 cells in pancreas. Indeed, sorafenib administration prevented and reversed autoimmune type 1 diabetes in NOD mice by decreasing Th1 cells accumulation and expression of inflammatory cytokines in pancreas. Thus, sorafenib may have the potential to protect against type 1 diabetes by improving the immuno-environment in the pancreas.

The NOD mouse model is the most popular animal model of type 1 diabetes. However, it has some limitations for treatment assessment. In NOD mice, about 60%-80% female and 20%-30% male mice spontaneously develop type 1 diabetes, while the sexual discrepancy is not existed in human (33). The insulitis in diabetic NOD mice was more severe than that in patients with type 1 diabetes (34, 35). High numbers of $CD4^+$ T cells and B cells predominate in NOD mice, while relatively small numbers of $CD8^+$ T cells and macrophages were observed in patients with type 1 diabetes (36, 37). In addition, multiple susceptibility loci for type 1 diabetes, such as *Idd*3 and *Idd*5 loci, which have been found in human, are not directly shown to be dysregulated in NOD mice (33), highlighting the difference in the pathogenesis of type 1 diabetes between humans and NOD mice. Despite its limitations, the NOD mouse model is currently the sole animal model to test therapies for autoimmune diabetes *in vivo*.

Importantly, scattered clinical reports have provided evidence that sorafenib can affect blood glucose in malignancy patients. Sorafenib was reported to significantly reduce blood glucose in a patient with advanced diabetic hepatocellular carcinoma (38). In addition, a previous retrospective study showed that sorafenib can markedly reduce blood glucose levels in both diabetic and nondiabetic patients with cancers (39). These clinical studies suggest that sorafenib may have the ability to affect blood glucose in humans. Further studies are warranted to explore the therapeutic effect of sorafenib in patients with type 1 diabetes.

Since type 1 diabetes is an immune-mediated disease, the targeting of immune pathways is a continued focus on either preventing or reversing type 1 diabetes. Currently, there are no approved successful immunotherapies for type 1 diabetes, and past failures were mainly due to the various side effects from systemic immunosuppression (1). Given the comprehensive function of Th1 cells in the immune system, the potential side effects hinder the application of anti-Th1 therapy in the treatment of type 1 diabetes. Although sorafenib was identified as an inhibitor of Th1 differentiation, we believe it is quite a safe option for the treatment of type 1 diabetes. First, sorafenib has been approved by FDA for the treatment of multiple cancers for more than 15 years and has shown limited side effects (40, 41). Second, the dose of sorafenib (10 mg/kg/day for prevention and 50 mg/kg/day for remission) used in NOD mice to treat type 1 diabetes is lower or equal to the generally effective dose for the treatment of cancer (30-50 mg/kg/day) in animal models (42, 43), suggesting that the dose used to treat diabetes may be lower than the current clinical dose for cancer, which also means lower side effects. Third, our *in vivo* data showed that in NOD mice sorafenib decreased Th1 cells and inhibited inflammation

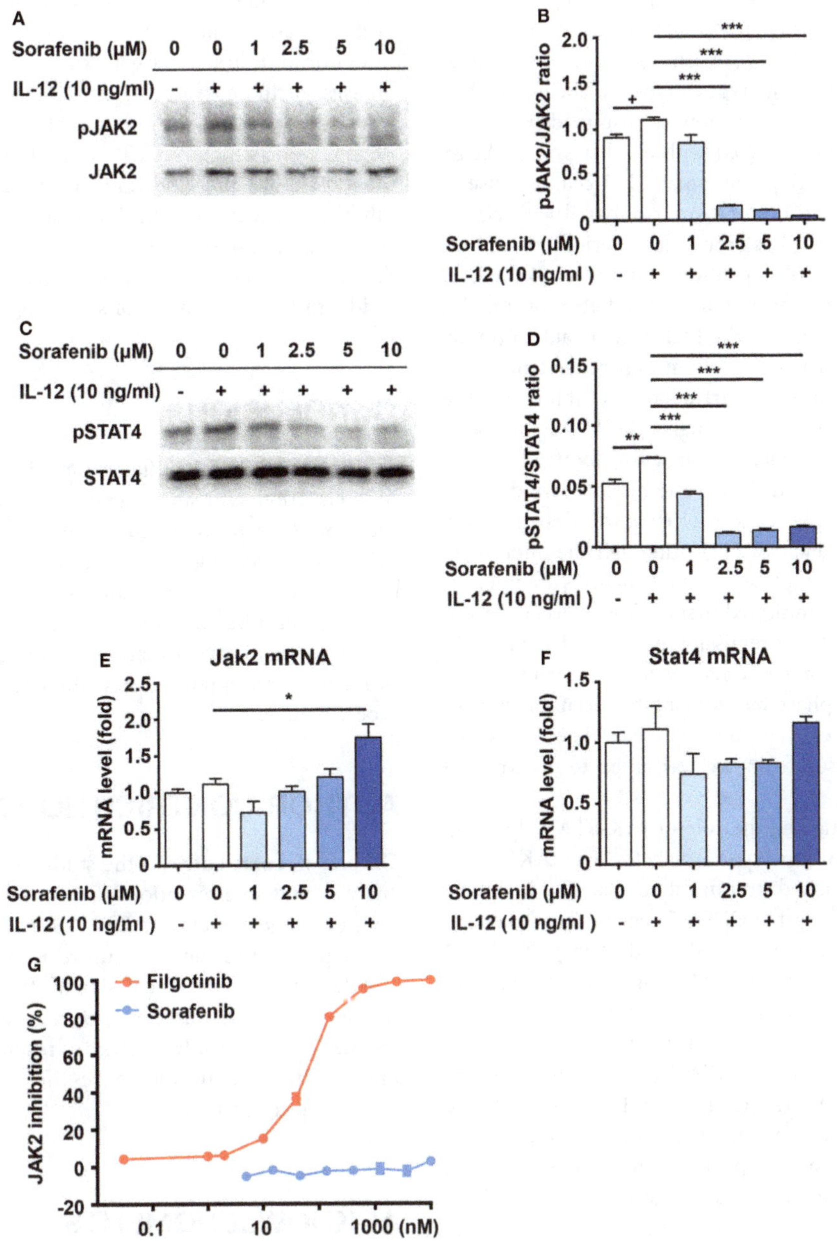

FIGURE 5 | Sorafenib indirectly inhibits phosphorylations of JAK2 and STAT4. Immunoblots and quantitation of pJAK2 **(A, B)** and pSTAT4 **(C, D)** in naive CD4$^+$ T cells, which were stimulated with IL-12 in medium containing different concentration sorafenib as indicated. Quantitation of phosphorylated JAK2 and STAT4 normalized to total JAK2 and STAT4. RT-PCR analysis of JAK2 and STAT4 in naive CD4$^+$ T cells, which were stimulated with IL-12 in medium containing different concentration sorafenib **(E, F)** as indicated. **(G)** The inhibition ratio of filgotinib and sorafenib on JAK2 activity. Data are representative of 3 independent experiments. Data represent means ± s.e.m. Statistical significance: $^+P < 0.1$, $^*P < 0.05$, $^{**}P < 0.01$ or $^{***}P < 0.001$. T-test used for statistical analysis.

specifically in the pancreas, but not in peripheral immune organs (**Figures 3A–C** and **Supplementary Figures 4A, B**), suggesting that sorafenib may not have significant effects on systemic immunity in certain condition. Notably, sorafenib repressed Th1 activation in spleens and MLNs of bacteria-infected mice. Since Th1 cells play a critical role in fighting bacterial infection, sorafenib may not be suitable to be used in patients with infectious diseases.

To date, the treatment of type 1 diabetes is still in a dilemma. Successful interventions at any stage of type 1 diabetes will be a breakthrough. Our study found that a low dose of sorafenib (10 mg/kg/day) has the ability to prevent (**Figures 2A, B**) but cannot reverse type 1 diabetes in NOD mice. However, high dose of sorafenib (50 mg/kg/day) treatment induces the remission of established type 1 diabetes (**Figures 4A–C**) in NOD mice, which may due to the suppression of Th1 and Tc1 cells in pancreas.

This result indicates a therapeutic effect of sorafenib on autoimmune diabetes. We think sorafenib can be applied to treat type 1 diabetes, particularly under certain conditions. Sorafenib may be used for the treatment of latent autoimmune diabetes in adults (LADA), a subtype of type 1 diabetes which is characterized by a slower progression to insulin dependence. Patients with LADA were enriched with a subclass of GAD65 IgG1 autoantibodies, reflecting a dominant Th1 cell response to GAD65 in the pancreas (44). Moreover, compared with classic type 1 diabetes, LADA has a less functional deterioration of beta cells and a slower decline of C-peptide serum level (45). GAD autoantibody has been reported as a predictor of insulin requirement in LADA patients. The higher GAD autoantibody titers indicated the higher risk of early insulin dependence (46). Therefore, sorafenib may be particularly suitable for the treatment of LADA patients with higher GAD autoantibody titers. Another possible application area for sorafenib is the honeymoon phase of type 1 diabetes, a remission period where insulin usage can be sharply reduced or even withdrawn during the treatment of type 1 diabetes (47). Although the underlying mechanisms of honeymoon phase of type 1 diabetes are unclear, some clinical studies have indicated that the lower level of serum IFN-γ was associated with the remission of type 1 diabetes (48–50), suggesting that the sorafenib may be used to maintain and extend the honeymoon phase by reducing the accumulation of IFN-γ producing Th1 cells in the pancreas. These possible clinical applications of sorafenib are warranted to be explored in future studies.

Recent studies investigated the role of JAK-STAT signaling pathway in the pathogenesis of type 1 diabetes. The JAK1/JAK2 inhibitor AZD1480 reversed autoimmune diabetes in newly diagnosed mice by blocking the $CD8^+$ T cell-mediated damage of beta cells (51). A case report showed that JAK1/JAK2 inhibitor ruxolitinib normalized blood-glucose levels and discontinued exogenous insulin in a patient with type 1 diabetes caused by STAT1 gain-of-function (52). A recent review summarized the roles of STAT (STAT1, STAT3 and STAT5b) monogenic mutations in type 1 diabetes. These mutations are associated with an increased susceptibility to type 1 diabetes due to the perturbation of Th17/Treg equilibrium (53). These findings suggest that JAK/STAT inhibitor is a potential therapy for type 1 diabetes. IL-12/JAK2/STAT4 signaling has been defined as an essential way for Th1 cell differentiation (17, 18). In our study, we found that sorafenib significantly suppressed IL-12-induced activations of JAK2 and STAT4 in a dose-dependent manner (**Figures 5A–D**), suggesting that sorafenib is a new JAK2 inhibitor. To further explore whether sorafenib directly affects JAK2, we examined the effect of sorafenib on JAK2 activity in an *in-vitro* kinase assay. The classic JAK2 inhibitor, filgotinib, almost completely inhibited JAK2 activity at concentrations as low as 0.6 μM (**Figure 5G**), indicating that the assay system worked very well. In this *in-vitro* kinase assay, sorafenib had little inhibitory effects on JAK2 activity at a concentration of 10 μM. However, this concentration of sorafenib was sufficient to inhibit the IL-12-induced phosphorylation of JAK2 in T cells. (**Figures 5A, B**). This result suggested that sorafenib cannot directly target JAK2, and may indirectly inhibit IL-12-induced JAK2 activation by targeting an unknown factor. Sorafenib is a multiple kinase inhibitor and directly targets Raf and several receptor tyrosine kinases, including vascular endothelial growth factor receptor (VEGFR), platelet derived growth factor receptor (PDGFR), FLT-3, c-Kit, p38 and RET (40). Although we cannot exclude the possibility that the known sorafenib targets mediate its inhibitory effects on JAK2 activation, it is more likely that sorafenib suppresses the IL-12-induced JAK2 activation through its unidentified target. Further studies are warranted to identify the new target of sorafenib.

CONCLUSION

In summary, we identified sorafenib as an inhibitor of Th1 differentiation and an indirect inhibitor of JAK2 and found that sorafenib prevents and reverses type 1 diabetes in NOD mice by decreasing the accumulation of Th1 cells and the expression of inflammatory cytokines in pancreas. Our findings emphasize the importance of Th1 cells in the pathogenesis of type 1 diabetes and suggest that sorafenib may prove to be an important new therapy for clinical treatment in type 1 diabetes.

AUTHOR CONTRIBUTIONS

QZ and JS contributed to the study design, acquisition of data, analysis and interpretation of results, as well as drafting and revision of the manuscript. DW, XS, YLX, and HZ contributed to the acquisition of the data and revision of the manuscript. YX and ZZ contributed to the design of study, analysis of results and revision of the manuscript. TD contributed to the conception and design of the study, analysis of results and the revision of the manuscript. All authors gave their approval for the final manuscript to be published.

ACKNOWLEDGMENTS

We are grateful to Wanyu Hu, Xiyan Liao, Wufuer ■ Aini, Yujin Ding, Hui Zhou and Zhixia Li for their technical supports in our project.

SUPPLEMENTARY MATERIAL

Supplementary Figure 1 | The effects of 34 FDA-approved TKIs on IL-12-induced Th1 cell differentiation. **(A)** Cell counts using trypan blue exclusion to assess viable cells and **(B, C)** flow cytometry analysis of Th1 cells in naïve splenic CD4+ T cells stimulated with IL-12 in medium containing 10 μM of individual FDA-approved TKI as indicated. Data represent means ± s.e.m; $^*P < 0.05$ or $^{**}P < 0.01$ versus vehicle by t-test.

Supplementary Figure 2 | Gating strategy for flow cytometry analysis of T cells. **(A)** Gating of naïve CD4+ T cells in mouse splenocyte (upper panel); the purity of sorted naïve CD4+ T cells (down panel). **(B)** Gating of Th1 cells in mouse CD4+ T cells.

(C) Gating of naïve CD4+ T cells in human PBMC (upper panel); the purity of sorted naïve CD4+ T cells (down panel). **(D)** Gating of Th1 cells in human CD4+ T cells. PBMC, peripheral blood mononuclear cells.

Supplementary Figure 3 | Sorafenib does not alter IFN-γ expression in Th1 cell. **(A, B)** Flow cytometry analysis of IFN-γ + Th1 cells treated with different concentrations of sorafenib (μM) as indicated.

Supplementary Figure 4 | Sorafenib does not alter T cell subsets in peripheral immune tissues of prediabetic NOD mice. Flow cytometry analysis of the frequency of Th1, Th2, and Th17 cells in PLN **(A)** and splenic **(B)** CD4+ T cells from vehicle-treated or sorafenib-treated NOD mice. **(C)** Flow cytometry analysis of the frequency of Tregs in PLN and splenic CD4+ T cells, respectively. Sora, sorafenib; PLN, pancreatic lymph nodes. Data represent means ± s.e.m. and data were pooled from 2 or more independent experiments. n = 5-7 mice per group in each experiment.

Supplementary Figure 5 | Sorafenib decreases activate Th1 cells in MLN and spleen of E. coli-infected mice. **(A)** Image of E coli on Luria-Bertani Agar plates from vehicle-treated or sorafenib-treated C57BL/6J mice injected with PBS or E.coli (1*107 CFU). Flow cytometry analysis of the frequency of Th1 cells in MLN **(B)** and splenic **(C)** CD4+ T cells from the three groups mice as indicated. Sora, sorafenib; MLN, mesenteric lymph node. Data represent means ± s.e.m.. n = 4 mice per group in this experiment. Statistical significance: *P <0.05 or **P <0.01 versus vehicle by t-test.

Supplementary Figure 6 | Sorafenib does not alter T-cell subsets in peripheral immune tissues of diabetic NOD mice. Flow cytometry analysis of the frequency of Th1, Th2, and Th17 cells in PLN **(A)** and splenic **(B)** $CD4^+$ T cells from vehicle-treated or sorafenib-treated diabetic NOD mice. **(C)** Flow cytometry analysis of the frequency of Tregs in PLN and splenic $CD4^+$ T cells, respectively. Sora, sorafenib; PLN, pancreatic lymph nodes. Data represent means ± s.e.m. n = 4 mice per group in each experiment.

REFERENCES

1. Warshauer JT, Bluestone JA, Anderson MS. New Frontiers in the Treatment of Type 1 Diabetes. *Cell Metab* (2020) 31(1):46–61. doi: 10.1016/j.cmet.2019.11.017
2. Todd JA. Etiology of Type 1 Diabetes. *Immunity* (2010) 32(4):457–67. doi: 10.1016/j.immuni.2010.04.001
3. Adorini L. Interleukin 12 and Autoimmune Diabetes. *Nat Genet* (2001) 27 (2):131–2. doi: 10.1038/84732
4. Katz JD, Benoist C, Mathis D. T Helper Cell Subsets in Insulin-Dependent Diabetes. *Science* (1995) 268(5214):1185–8. doi: 10.1126/science.7761837
5. Esensten JH, Lee MR, Glimcher LH, Bluestone JA. T-Bet-Deficient NOD Mice Are Protected From Diabetes Due to Defects in Both T Cell and Innate Immune System Function. *J Immunol* (2009) 183(1):75–82. doi: 10.4049/jimmunol.0804154
6. Murphy KM, Ouyang W, Farrar JD, Yang J, Ranganath S, Asnagli H, et al. Signaling and Transcription in T Helper Development. *Annu Rev Immunol* (2000) 18:451–94. doi: 10.1146/annurev.immunol.18.1.451
7. Trembleau S, Penna G, Bosi E, Mortara A, Gately MK, Adorini L. Interleukin 12 Administration Induces T Helper Type 1 Cells and Accelerates Autoimmune Diabetes in NOD Mice. *J Exp Med* (1995) 181(2):817–21. doi: 10.1084/jem.181.2.817
8. Rothe H, O'Hara C.OMMAJr RM, Martin S, Kolb H. Suppression of Cyclophosphamide Induced Diabetes Development and Pancreatic Th1 Reactivity in NOD Mice Treated With the Interleukin (IL)-12 Antagonist IL-12(P40)2. *Diabetologia* (1997) 40(6):641–6. doi: 10.1007/s001250050728
9. Nitta Y, Kawamoto S, Tashiro F, Aihara H, Yoshimoto T, Nariuchi H, et al. IL-12 Plays a Pathologic Role at the Inflammatory Loci in the Development of Diabetes in NOD Mice. *J Autoimmun* (2001) 16(2):97–104. doi: 10.1006/jaut.2000.0469
10. Yang Z, Chen M, Ellett JD, Fialkow LB, Carter JD, McDuffie M, et al. Autoimmune Diabetes Is Blocked in Stat4-Deficient Mice. *J Autoimmun* (2004) 22(3):191–200. doi: 10.1016/j.jaut.2003.08.006
11. Morahan G, Huang D, Ymer SI, Cancilla MR, Stephen K, Dabadghao P, et al. Linkage Disequilibrium of a Type 1 Diabetes Susceptibility Locus With a Regulatory IL12B Allele. *Nat Genet* (2001) 27(2):218–21. doi: 10.1038/84872
12. Hubbard SR, Till JH. Protein Tyrosine Kinase Structure and Function. *Annu Rev Biochem* (2000) 69:373–98. doi: 10.1146/annurev.biochem.69.1.373
13. Manning G, Whyte DB, Martinez R, Hunter T, Sudarsanam S. The Protein Kinase Complement of the Human Genome. *Science* (2002) 298(5600):1912–34. doi: 10.1126/science.1075762
14. Ferguson FM, Gray NS. Kinase Inhibitors: The Road Ahead. *Nat Rev Drug Discovery* (2018) 17(5):353–77. doi: 10.1038/nrd.2018.21
15. Levitzki A. Protein Kinase Inhibitors as a Therapeutic Modality. *Acc Chem Res* (2003) 36(6):462–9. doi: 10.1021/ar0201207
16. Roskoski RJR. Properties of FDA-Approved Small Molecule Protein Kinase Inhibitors: A 2020 Update. *Pharmacol Res* (2020) 152:104609. doi: 10.1016/j.phrs.2019.104609
17. Watford WT, Hissong BD, Bream JH, et al. Signaling by IL-12 and IL-23 and the Immunoregulatory Roles of STAT4. *Immunol Rev* (2004) 202:139–56. doi: 10.1111/j.0105-2896.2004.00211.x
18. Zundler S, Neurath MF. Interleukin-12: Functional Activities and Implications for Disease. *Cytokine Growth Factor Rev* (2015) 26(5):559–68. doi: 10.1016/j.cytogfr.2015.07.003
19. Karaghiosoff M, Neubauer H, Lassnig C, Kovarik P, Schindler H, Pircher H, et al. Partial Impairment of Cytokine Responses in Tyk2-Deficient Mice. *Immunity* (2000) 13(4):549–60. doi: 10.1016/S1074-7613(00)00054-6
20. Pignata C, Sanghera JS, Cossette L, Pelech SL, Ritz J. Interleukin-12 Induces Tyrosine Phosphorylation and Activation of 44-Kd Mitogen-Activated Protein Kinase in Human T Cells. *Blood* (1994) 83(1):184–90. doi: 10.1016/S1074-7613(00)00054-6
21. Reinhardt RL, Liang HE, Locksley RM. Cytokine-Secreting Follicular T Cells Shape the Antibody Repertoire. *Nat Immunol* (2009) 10(4):385–93. doi: 10.1038/ni.1715
22. Harada M, Makino S. Promotion of Spontaneous Diabetes in Non-Obese Diabetes-Prone Mice by Cyclophosphamide. *Diabetologia* (1984) 27(6):604–6. doi: 10.1007/BF00276978
23. Atlan-Gepner C, Bouabdallah R, Valero R, Coso D, Vialettes B. A Cyclophosphamide-Induced Autoimmune Diabetes. *Lancet* (1998) 352 (9125):373–4. doi: 10.1016/S0140-6736(05)60474-6
24. Brode S, Raine T, Zaccone P, Cooke A. Cyclophosphamide-Induced Type-1 Diabetes in the NOD Mouse Is Associated With a Reduction of CD4+CD25+Foxp3+ Regulatory T Cells. *J Immunol* (2006) 177(10):6603–12. doi: 10.4049/jimmunol.177.10.6603
25. Louvet C, Szot GL, Lang J, Lee MR, Martinier N, Bollag G, et al. Tyrosine Kinase Inhibitors Reverse Type 1 Diabetes in Nonobese Diabetic Mice. *Proc Natl Acad Sci USA* (2008) 105(48):18895–900. doi: 10.1073/pnas.0810246105
26. Nagayama M, Yano T, Atarashi K, Tanoue T, Sekiya M, Kobayashi Y, et al. TH1 Cell-Inducing Escherichia Coli Strain Identified From the Small Intestinal Mucosa of Patients With Crohn's Disease. *Gut Microbes* (2020) 12(1):1788898. doi: 10.1080/19490976.2020.1788898
27. Action to Control Cardiovascular Risk in Diabetes Study, G, Gerstein HC, Miller ME, Byington RP, Goff DC Jr, Bigger JT, et al. Effects of Intensive Glucose Lowering in Type 2 Diabetes. *N Engl J Med* (2008) 358(24):2545–59. doi: 10.1056/NEJMoa0802743
28. Group AC, Patel A, MacMahon S, Chalmers J, Neal B, Billot L, et al. Intensive Blood Glucose Control and Vascular Outcomes in Patients With Type 2 Diabetes. *N Engl J Med* (2008) 358(24):2560–72. doi: 10.1056/NEJMoa0802987
29. Duckworth W, Abraira C, Moritz T, Reda D, Emanuele N, Reaven PD, et al. Glucose Control and Vascular Complications in Veterans With Type 2 Diabetes. *N Engl J Med* (2009) 360(2):129–39. doi: 10.1056/NEJMoa0808431
30. Shapiro AM, Lakey JR, Ryan EA, Korbutt GS, Toth E, Warnock GL, et al. Islet Transplantation in Seven Patients With Type 1 Diabetes Mellitus Using a Glucocorticoid-Free Immunosuppressive Regimen. *N Engl J Med* (2000) 343 (4):230–8. doi: 10.1056/NEJM200007273430401
31. Voltarelli JC, Couri CE, Stracieri AB, Oliveira MC, Moraes DA, Pieroni F, et al. Autologous Nonmyeloablative Hematopoietic Stem Cell Transplantation in Newly Diagnosed Type 1 Diabetes Mellitus. *JAMA* (2007) 297(14):1568–76. doi: 10.1001/jama.297.14.1568
32. Sneddon JB, Tang Q, Stock P, Bluestone JA, Roy S, Desaiet T, et al. Stem Cell

Therapies for Treating Diabetes: Progress and Remaining Challenges. *Cell Stem Cell* (2018) 22(6):810–23. doi: 10.1016/j.stem.2018.05.016
33. Anderson MS, Bluestone JA. The NOD Mouse: A Model of Immune Dysregulation. *Annu Rev Immumnol* (2005) 23:447–85. doi: 10.1146/annurev.immunol.23.021704.115643
34. Sherry NA, Kushner JA, Glandt M, Kitamura T, Brillantes AB, Herold KC, et al. Effects of Autoimmunity and Immune Therapy on Beta-Cell Turnover in Type 1 Diabetes. *Diabetes* (2006) 55(12):3238–45. doi: 10.2337/db05-1034
35. Coppieters KT, Dotta F, Amirian N, Campbell PD, Kay TW, Atkinson MA, et al. Demonstration of Islet-Autoreactive CD8 T Cells in Insulitic Lesions From Recent Onset and Long-Term Type 1 Diabetes Patients. *J Exp Med* (2012) 209(1):51–60. doi: 10.1084/jem.20111187
36. Willcox A, Richardson SJ, Bone AJ, Foulis AK, Morgan NG. Analysis of Islet Inflammation in Human Type 1 Diabetes. *Clin Exp Immunol* (2009) 155 (2):173–81. doi: 10.1111/j.1365-2249.2008.03860.x
37. Reed JC, Herold KC. Thinking Bedside at the Bench: The NOD Mouse Model of T1DM. *Nat Rev Endocrinol* (2015) 11(5):308–14. doi: 10.1038/nrendo.2014.236
38. Holstein A, Kovacs P, Beil W. Severe Hypoglycemia Due to Possible Interaction Between Glibenclamide and Sorafenib in a Patient With Hepatocellular Carcinoma. *Curr Drug Saf* (2013) 8(2):148–52. doi: 10.2174/15748863113089990027
39. Agostino NM, Chinchilli VM, Lynch CJ, Koszyk-Szewczyk A, Gingrich R, Sivik J, et al. Effect of the Tyrosine Kinase Inhibitors (Sunitinib, Sorafenib, Dasatinib, and Imatinib) on Blood Glucose Levels in Diabetic and Nondiabetic Patients in General Clinical Practice. *J Oncol Pharm Pract* (2011) 17(3):197–202. doi: 10.1177/1078155210378913
40. Wilhelm S, Carter C, Lynch M, Lowinger T, Dumas J, Smith RA, et al. Discovery and Development of Sorafenib: A Multikinase Inhibitor for Treating Cancer. *Nat Rev Drug Discov* (2006) 5(10):835–44. doi: 10.1038/nrd2130
41. Jean GW, Mani RM, Jaffry A, Khan SA. Toxic Effects of Sorafenib in Patients With Differentiated Thyroid Carcinoma Compared With Other Cancers. *JAMA Oncol* (2016) 2(4):529–34. doi: 10.1001/jamaoncol.2015.5927
42. Horwitz E, Stein I, Andreozzi M, Nemeth J, Shoham A, Pappo O, et al. Human and Mouse VEGFA-Amplified Hepatocellular Carcinomas Are Highly Sensitive to Sorafenib Treatment. *Cancer Discovery* (2014) 4(6):730–43. doi: 10.1158/2159-8290.CD-13-0782
43. Wang C, Vegna S, Jin H, Benedict B, Lieftink C, Ramirez C, et al. Inducing and Exploiting Vulnerabilities for the Treatment of Liver Cancer. *Nature* (2019) 574(7777):268–72. doi: 10.1038/s41586-019-1607-3
44. Hillman M, Torn C, Thorgeirsson H, Landin-Olsson M. Igg4-Subclass of Glutamic Acid Decarboxylase Antibody Is More Frequent in Latent Autoimmune Diabetes in Adults Than in Type 1 Diabetes. *Diabetologia* (2004) 47(11):1984–9. doi: 10.1007/s00125-004-1558-5
45. Hernandez M, Mollo A, Marsal JR, Esquerda A, Capel I, Puig-Domingo M, et al. Insulin Secretion in Patients With Latent Autoimmune Diabetes (LADA): Half Way Between Type 1 and Type 2 Diabetes: Action LADA 9. *BMC Endocr Disord* (2015) 15:1. doi: 10.1186/1472-6823-15-1
46. Zampetti S, Campagna G, Tiberti C, Songini M, Arpi ML, Simone GD, et al. High GADA Titer Increases the Risk of Insulin Requirement in LADA Patients: A 7-Year Follow-Up (NIRAD Study 7). *Eur J Endocrinol* (2014) 171:697–704. doi: 10.1530/EJE-14-0342
47. van Belle TL, Coppieters KT, von Herrath MG. Type 1 Diabetes: Etiology, Immunology, and Therapeutic Strategies. *Physiol Rev* (2011) 91(1):79–118. doi: 10.1152/physrev.00003.2010
48. Alizadeh BZ, Hanifi-Moghaddam P, Eerligh P, Slik AR, Kolb H, Kharagjitsingh AV, et al. Association of Interferon-Gamma and Interleukin 10 Genotypes and Serum Levels With Partial Clinical Remission in Type 1 Diabetes. *Clin Exp Immunol* (2006) 145(3):480–4. doi: 10.1111/j.1365-2249.2006.03172.x
49. Karges B, Durinovic-Bello I, Heinze E, Debatin KM, Boehm B, Karges W. Immunological Mechanisms Associated With Long-Term Remission of Human Type 1 Diabetes. *Diabetes Metab Res Rev* (2006) 22(3):184–9. doi: 10.1002/dmrr.600
50. Schloot NC, Hanifi-Moghaddam P, Aabenhus-Andersen N, Alizadeh BZ, Saha MT, Knip M, et al. Association of Immune Mediators at Diagnosis of Type 1 Diabetes With Later Clinical Remission. *Diabetes Med* (2007) 24 (5):512–20. doi: 10.1111/j.1464-5491.2007.02096.x
51. Trivedi PM, Graham KL, Scott NA, Jenkins MR, Majaw S, Sutherland RM, et al. Repurposed JAK1/JAK2 Inhibitor Reverses Established Autoimmune Insulitis in NOD Mice. *Diabetes* (2017) 66(6):1650–60. doi: 10.2337/db16-1250
52. Chaimowitz NS, Ebenezer SJ, Hanson IC, Anderson M, Forbes LR. STAT1 Gain of Function, Type 1 Diabetes, and Reversal With JAK Inhibition. *N Engl J Med* (2020) 383(15):1494–6. doi: 10.1056/NEJMc2022226
53. Fabbri M, Frixou M, Degano M, Fousteri G. Type 1 Diabetes in STAT Protein Family Mutations: Regulating the Th17/Treg Equilibrium and Beyond. *Diabetes* (2019) 68(2):258–65. doi: 10.2337/db18-0627

16

Cholinergic Stimulation Prevents the Development of Autoimmune Diabetes: Evidence for the Modulation of Th17 Effector Cells via an IFNγ-Dependent Mechanism

Junu A. George[1], Ghada Bashir[2], Mohammed M. Qureshi[1], Yassir A. Mohamed[2], Jamil Azzi[3], Basel K. al-Ramadi[2] and Maria J. Fernández-Cabezudo[1]**

[1] Department of Biochemistry, College of Medicine and Health Sciences, United Arab University, Al-Ain, UAE, [2] Department of Medical Microbiology & Immunology, College of Medicine and Health Sciences, United Arab University, Al-Ain, UAE, [3] Renal Division, Transplantation Research Center, Brigham and Women's Hospital, Harvard Medical School, Boston, MA, USA

***Correspondence:**
Basel K. al-Ramadi
ramadi.b@uaeu.ac.ae;
Maria J. Fernández-Cabezudo
mariac@uaeu.ac.ae

Type I diabetes (T1D) results from T cell-mediated damage of pancreatic β-cells and loss of insulin production. The cholinergic anti-inflammatory pathway represents a physiological link connecting the central nervous and immune systems *via* vagus nerve, and functions to control the release of proinflammatory cytokines. Using the multiple low-dose streptozotocin (MLD-STZ) model to induce experimental autoimmune diabetes, we investigated the potential of regulating the development of hyperglycemia through administration of paraoxon, a highly specific acetylcholinesterase inhibitor (AChEI). We demonstrate that pretreatment with paraoxon prevented hyperglycemia in STZ-treated C57BL/6 mice. This correlated with a reduction in T cell infiltration into pancreatic islets and preservation of the structure and functionality of β-cells. Gene expression analysis of pancreatic tissue revealed that increased peripheral cholinergic activity prevented STZ-mediated loss of insulin production, this being associated with a reduction in IL-1β, IL-6, and IL-17 proinflammatory cytokines. Intracellular cytokine analysis in splenic T cells demonstrated that inhibition of AChE led to a shift in STZ-induced immune response from a predominantly disease-causing IL-17-expressing Th17 cells to IFNγ-positive Th1 cells. Consistent with this conclusion, inhibition of AChE failed to prevent STZ-induced hyperglycemia in IFNγ-deficient mice. Our results provide mechanistic evidence for the prevention of murine T1D by inhibition of AChE and suggest a promising strategy for modulating disease severity.

Keywords: neuroimmunology, inhibition of AChE, acetylcholine, IFNγ, Th17, type I diabetes

INTRODUCTION

Type 1 diabetes (T1D) is a T cell-mediated autoimmune disease in which insulin-producing β cells of the pancreatic islets of Langerhans are selectively destroyed. The onset of the hyperglycemia is preceded by a preclinical phase of insulitis, characterized by infiltration by T and B lymphocytes, myeloid cells, and NK cells into the pancreatic islets. Although the etiology of T1D remains incompletely understood, development of disease is influenced by genetic and environmental factors, including viral infections, food antigens, toxins, and stress. The autoimmune response is initiated in genetically pre-disposed individuals when physiological islet remodeling (1), viral infections, or inflammatory cytokines (2) induce the death of β cells. The release of β cell-specific antigens induces the activation of inflammatory T cells, leading to insulitis and, ultimately, β cell destruction. Several experimental models have been developed to study T1D, including spontaneous [biobreeding rats (BB); non-obese diabetic mice (NOD)] and chemically induced disease [multiple low-dose streptozotocin (MLD-STZ); alloxan] (3). In the MLD-STZ mouse model, many studies have shown that the destruction of β cells and development of hyperglycemia resembles the development of T1D in humans in being mediated by inflammatory T cells (both CD4 and CD8) and regulated by inflammatory cytokines (4–7). Moreover, this model has the advantage over the NOD model in that it induces only autoimmune diabetes and not any other systemic autoimmune disease.

It is well established that the nervous system plays a role in the regulation of immune responses and vice versa (8). The capacity of the cholinergic system to modulate immune responses has been amply demonstrated (9–11). Structurally, it has been shown that the major cholinergic parasympathetic nerve, the vagus nerve, innervates many organs, including GI tract, pancreas, and lymphoid tissues where nerve terminals form synaptic contacts with lymphoid cells. Muscarinic and nicotinic acetylcholine receptors (AChR) are known to be expressed on many cell types of the immune system, including lymphocytes, macrophages, and dendritic cells (12–14), suggesting that acetylcholine (ACh) may act as a neuroimmunomodulator in interactions between the nervous and immune systems. T lymphocytes express muscarinic (mAChR) and nicotinic acetylcholine receptors (nAChR) and synthesize ACh and acetylcholinesterase (AChE) (10). Functional studies have demonstrated that ACh stimulation of T cells through the α7 subunit of nAChR reduces mitogen-induced proliferation and secretion of proinflammatory cytokines (15). Likewise, activation of α7 nAChR on macrophages inhibits the secretion of TNF-α (9). In contrast, stimulation through mAChR induces the secretion of proinflammatory cytokines (16). These findings gave rise to the concept of the cholinergic anti-inflammatory pathway or inflammatory reflex (17), amply demonstrated to counteract endotoxemia-induced inflammation (18–20). In this reflex pathway, the presence of inflammatory molecules in the periphery stimulate the afferent vagus nerve that relay the signal to the brain which regulates, through the efferent vagus nerve, the production of proinflammatory cytokines (21). Our group previously demonstrated that inhibition of AChE promotes survival of mice following a lethal oral infection with *Salmonella*, highlighting the physiological significance of this pathway in mucosal immunity (11). Furthermore, cholinergic stimulation has been shown to decrease the severity of inflammatory conditions, such as experimental autoimmune encephalitis (EAE) (15), experimental autoimmune myasthenia gravis (22), and Alzheimer's disease (23).

Several lines of evidence from human studies as well as animal models of spontaneous (NOD mice) and chemically induced (MLD-STZ) T1D indicate the crucial role played by Th17 cells in the pathogenesis of autoimmune diabetes (24–33). In addition to IL-17A, the signature cytokine produced by the Th17 lymphocyte subset, these cells also secrete a host of other inflammatory mediators including IL-17F, IL-21, IL-22, TNFα, GM-CSF, and IL-6 (34), which collectively drive the associated immunopathology. In contrast, induction of IFNγ in NOD mice protected against diabetes development by suppressing Th17 activity and inhibiting IL-17 production (24, 35). Therefore, IL-17 and IFNγ appear to play diverse and often cross-regulatory functions during the development of T1D. Given the central role of T cells and macrophages in the development of T1D and the existence of cholinergic innervation in the pancreas, we investigated the potential immunomodulatory effect of AChE inhibition on the development of diabetes using the MLD-STZ mouse model. Using paraoxon as a systemic AChE inhibitor (11), we demonstrate that cholinergic activation prevents the development of hyperglycemia by inhibiting pancreatic islet inflammation and β cell loss. Moreover, inhibition of AChE prevents the differentiation of naïve $CD4^+$ T cells into IL-17-producing Th17 cells and, instead, promotes their differentiation to IFNγ-secreting Th1 cells. Interestingly, inhibition of AChE fails to modulate streptozotozin (STZ)-induced hyperglycemia in IFNγ-deficient ($IFN\gamma^{-/-}$) mice, demonstrating the crucial role played by IFNγ in ACh-mediated inhibition of the autoimmune response against islet β cells. Our findings provide a rationale for a new strategy in the development of anti-diabetic therapies.

MATERIALS AND METHODS

Experimental Animals

C57BL/6 mice were purchased from Harlan Olac (Bicester, United Kingdom) and bred in the animal facility of the College of Medicine and Health Sciences, UAE University. $IFN\gamma^{-/-}$ mice were purchased from Jackson laboratories (USA) and generously provided by Dr Mariam Al-Shamsi at our institution. Female mice aged 8–10 weeks (weight range 20–22 g) were used for the experiments. All studies involving animals were carried out in accordance with, and after approval of, the animal research ethics committee of the College of Medicine and Health Sciences, UAE University.

Chemicals

Paraoxon (Sigma, St. Louis, MO, USA), an organophosphorous compound, is a highly specific, irreversible, inhibitor of AChE (11). A stock solution (10 mmol/l) was prepared in acetone. Working solution for intraperitoneal (i.p.) injection was prepared *ex tempore* in pyrogen-free saline to a concentration of 80 nmol/ml. The final acetone concentration in the paraxon solution used for i.p. injection was ~108 μM. Each mouse received 40 nmol/day of paraoxon or saline in 0.5 ml volume. STZ (Sigma) was prepared *ex tempore* in citrate buffer (pH 4.5) and used i.p. at 60 mg/kg/day per mouse, unless otherwise indicated.

Diabetes Induction

To induce autoimmune diabetes, the MLD-STZ model was used (3). C57BL/6 and $IFN\gamma^{-/-}$ mice were administered five consecutive daily doses of STZ; control mice received citrate buffer. At different time points post-STZ administration, blood was drawn from the tail vein to determine glucose levels using *One-Touch-ultra-strip* (Lifescan, Zurich, Switzerland). Hyperglycemia was defined as non-fasting blood glucose >200 mg/dl.

Experimental Protocol

Twenty age-matched mice were randomly assigned into two groups (10 animals per group). Group I served as control and received daily i.p. injection of sterile saline for 3 weeks. Group II mice received daily injection of paraoxon for 3 weeks. Mice were weighed weekly, at which time blood was also collected and analyzed for AChE activity. At the end of treatment, each group was divided randomly into two subgroups, A and B. Groups IA (Saline) and IIA (paraoxon) received daily injections of citrate buffer while groups IB (Saline/STZ) and IIB (paraoxon/STZ) received daily injection of STZ for five consecutive days. Pancreas, spleen, and serum were collected from mice sacrificed (ether exposure) at days 10 and 18, post-STZ administration. In some experiments, mice were followed for survival for up to 60 days.

AChE Activity of Red Blood Cells

The detailed procedure for determining AChE enzyme activity in red blood cells (RBC) has been described (36). Briefly, freshly drawn, diluted, venous blood samples were incubated with DTNB (10 mM) and ethopropazine (6 mM) for 20 min at 37°C prior to addition of acetylthiocholine. The change in the absorbance of DTNB was measured at 436 nm. The AChE activity was calculated using an absorption coefficient of TNB^- at 436 nm ($\varepsilon = 10.6\ mM^{-1}\ cm^{1}$). The values were normalized to the hemoglobin (Hb) content (determined as cyanmethemoglobin) and expressed as mU/μM/Hb (37). All enzyme activities were expressed as percentage of the baseline activity (100%).

Histology and Immunohistochemistry of Pancreatic Tissue

Excised pancreata were processed for histological analysis following established protocol (38, 39). Tissue sections were stained with hematoxylin and eosin (H&E), and images were captured using Olympus BX53 microscope equipped with digital camera DP26 (Tokyo, Japan). Indirect immunostaining for insulin was performed using guinea pig polyclonal antibody (Dako, Carpinteria, CA, USA) followed by FITC-conjugated donkey anti-guinea pig IgG (Jackson ImmunoResearch, West Grove, PA, USA). A three-step staining protocol was utilized to detect infiltrating T cells and macrophages. For T lymphocytes, CD3-specific rabbit polyclonal Ab (Dako) was used followed by biotinylated sheep anti-rabbit Ig (AbD Serotec, Hercules, CA, USA) and finally streptavidin-FITC (eBioscience, San Diego, CA, USA). For macrophages, we used rat F4/80 mAb (BMA Biomedicals, Switzerland) followed by streptavidin-HRP and DAB (Dako). Slides with fluorescence were counter-stained with propidium iodide (BD Biosciences, USA) and then examined and photographed under a Nikon C1 laser scanning confocal microscope. Slides stained with DAB were counter-stained with hematoxylin and visualized and photographed with an Olympus BX53. Histological quantification of $CD3^+$ and $F4/80^+$ cells was done on two to four non-consecutive sections per animal and using four to five mice per experimental group. All islets found in each section were included in the quantification, which was carried out in a blinded fashion.

Antibodies and Flowcytometry

Analysis of spleen cells was carried out using a multi-color FACS analysis, following a standard procedure (39, 40). Cells were stained with a combination of directly conjugated mAbs, washed, and analyzed using FACSCanto II (BD Biosciences, San Jose, CA, USA). The antibodies used were CD3-FITC, CD4-APC, and CD8-APC-Cy7 (Biolegend, San Diego, CA, USA), CD19-PE-Cy7 and CD11c-PE (eBioscience), and CD11b-PE-Cy7 (BD Biosciences). Non-viable cells staining positive with 7AAD dye (eBioscience) were excluded from the analysis. Data collected on 50,000 cells were analyzed using FACSDiva software (BD Biosciences).

Intracellular Cytokine Analysis

Spleen single cell suspensions were prepared and 2×10^6 cells/ml were seeded in 24 well plates and stimulated with PMA (100 ng/ml)/Ionomycin (1 μg/ml) for 4 h at 37°C in the presence of brefeldin A (GolgiPlug; BD*cytofix/cytoperm plus*™ solution kit, BD Biosciences). After stimulation, cells were first stained with CD4-APC and CD8-APC-Cy7 antibodies (Biolegend), resuspended in fixation/permeabilization solution and finally stained with anti-IL-17A-PE and anti-IFNγ-PE-Cy7 antibodies (eBioscience) and run using FACSCanto II (BD Biosciences). Data collected from 50,000 cells were analyzed using FACSDiva software (BD Biosciences).

Quantitative RT-PCR

qRT-PCR was carried out as previously described (40) on RNA extracted from spleen and pancreas from each animal. After RNA extraction and purification, cDNA was synthesized using Taqman reverse transcription reagents (Applied Biosystems, Foster City, CA, USA) following manufacturer's protocol. TaqMan primers and probes were used to study the expression of the inflammatory markers IL-1β, IL-6, IL-12p40, IL-17A, IFNγ, and insulin (Applied Biosystems), and IL-23 and TNFα (Metabion, Germany) (**Table 1**). Transcript levels of target genes were normalized

TABLE 1 | List of primers.

Gene	Taqman gene ID/sequence
IL-1β	Mm00434228-m1
IL-6	Mm00446190-m1
IL-12p40	Mm00434174-m1
IL-17F	Mm00521423-m1
IFN-γ	Mm01168134-m1
Insulin	Mm00731595-gh
TNFα (Metabion)	F: 5′-CCT CCC TCT CAT CAG TTC TAT-3′ R: 5′-CTA GTT GGT TGT CTT TGA GAT CC-3′ Probe: 5′-6-Fam-ACA AGC CTG TAG CCC ACG TCG TAG-BHQ-1-3′
IL-23p19 (Metabion)	F: 5′-CATGCTAGCCTGGAACG-3′ R: 5′-GATCCTTTGCAAGCAGAA-3′ Probe: 5′-6-Fam-TGACCCACAAGGACTCAAGGACA BHQ-1-3′

according to the dCq method to respective mRNA levels of the housekeeping gene HPRT.

Insulin and Cytokine Determination

Serum samples were assayed for insulin (Alpco diagnostics, Salem, NH, USA) level by sandwich ELISA and performed according to the manufacturer's instructions. Assay sensitivity was 188 pg/ml.

Statistical Analysis

Statistical significance between control and treated groups was analyzed using the unpaired, two-tailed Student's *t*-test, using the statistical program of GraphPad Prism version 6 software. For multiple comparisons, we used One-way ANOVA with *post hoc* Tukey's test (GraphPad Prism). Two-way ANOVA with Bonferroni post-test was used to analyze repeated measures data, as indicated. Survival analysis was performed by Kaplan–Meier survival curves and log-rank test, using the same GraphPad Prism program. Differences between experimental groups were considered significant when p values were <0.05.

RESULTS

MLD-STZ-Induced Hyperglycemia

Studies were first carried out to optimize the STZ dose necessary to induce hyperglycemia (blood glucose >200 mg/dl) in C57BL/6 mice. Animals were divided into three groups, each receiving either 40, 50, or 60 mg/kg dose of STZ for five consecutive days. As can be seen, the percentage of mice developing hyperglycemia was 0, 50, and 100% by day 21 post administration of STZ at 40, 50, or 60 mg/kg, respectively (Image 1 in Supplementary Material). Hence, for all subsequent studies, a dose of 60 mg/kg STZ was used.

Acetylcholinesterase Inhibition Prevents Hyperglycemia and Preserves Insulin Production

In order to investigate the potential effect of AChE inhibition on experimental diabetes, C57BL/6 mice were pretreated daily with paraoxon or saline for 3 weeks, and then given MLD-STZ (or saline), as described in the Section "Materials and Methods" and followed for the development of hyperglycemia. No changes in glucose levels were observed in control mice (saline or paraoxon only experimental groups) (**Figure 1A**). Saline-pretreated mice that received STZ developed progressive hyperglycemia, first evident at 7 days post-STZ administration, and that continued for up to 51 days (**Figures 1A,B**). All animals in this group were diabetic by day 18 post STZ administration (**Figure 1B**). In contrast, despite an initial mild elevation in blood glucose levels observed at day 7, mice pretreated with paraoxon prior to STZ were resistant to the development of hyperglycemia (**Figure 1B**). This remained evident for up to 51 days following STZ administration, the maximum period of observation (**Figure 1B**).

Serum insulin levels were determined on day 10 (**Figure 1C**) and 18 (**Figure 1D**) post STZ injection. Similar levels of serum insulin were observed in saline- and paraoxon-treated control mice at both time points (**Figures 1C,D**). Interestingly, for STZ-treated mice, while serum insulin was at normal level at day 10 post administration (**Figure 1C**), the level dropped significantly by day 18 to ~64% of control (**Figure 1D**). In contrast, no reduction in serum insulin was observed in mice pretreated with paraoxon followed by STZ (**Figure 1D**). The levels of serum insulin of paraoxon/STZ-treated mice tended to be higher than saline control at days 10 and 18 post STZ injection (2.6-fold and 1.6-fold increase, respectively; **Figures 1C,D**) with the difference being statistically significant at the latter date. Moreover, differences in serum insulin levels between saline/STZ and paraoxon/STZ groups at day 18 were highly significant and inversely correlated with serum glucose levels (compare **Figures 1A,D**).

Insulin mRNA expression was also analyzed in pancreatic tissue at day 18 post-STZ treatment (**Figure 1E**). A dramatic 10.6-fold increase in insulin expression was observed in paraoxon-treated mice compared with saline control (**Figure 1E**). In sharp contrast, STZ treatment (saline/STZ group) led to a 12-fold reduction in the level of insulin mRNA relative to saline control. In mice pretreated with paraoxon prior to STZ (paraoxon/STZ group), insulin mRNA levels were essentially similar to those observed in saline control group (**Figure 1E**). Immunohistochemical analysis of insulin-producing β cells in pancreatic tissue revealed a gradual loss of insulin positivity in STZ-treated mice (saline/STZ group), which was evident starting at day 10 following STZ administration and continued up to day 60 (**Figure 1F**). In contrast, mice pretreated with paraoxon (paraoxon/STZ group) showed evidence of islet preservation and protection from STZ-induced loss of β cells, albeit not total, up to day 60 (**Figure 1F**). These results demonstrate that inhibition of AChE increases the expression of insulin mRNA in pancreatic cells and prevents STZ-induced hyperglycemia.

Inhibition of AChE Prevents Insulitis and Destruction of Islets Induced by MLD-STZ

Hematoxylin and eosin staining of pancreatic tissue showed highly infiltrated islets in saline/STZ group at days 10 and 18 post-STZ administration (**Figure 2A**). Pretreatment with paraoxon reduced islet cell infiltration at day 10 (paraoxon/STZ group) and, by day 18, the pancreatic islets appeared completely healthy with no evidence of insulitis (**Figure 2A**). No infiltrating cells were observed in islets of saline or paraoxon control groups (**Figures 2A–E**). Immunohistological analysis of the islets at days 10 and 18 revealed the presence of $CD3^+$ T cells (**Figure 2B**) and $F4/80^+$ myeloid cells (**Figure 2C**) in STZ-treated mice. However, the degree of T cell infiltration was significantly reduced in mice pretreated with paraoxon (**Figures 2B,D**). At day 10, T cells were distributed uniformly throughout the islets of both saline/STZ and paraoxon/STZ groups. At day 18, however, only a few T cells located primarily in the periphery of the islets could be observed in paraoxon/STZ mice, while in saline/STZ group these cells were uniformly distributed within the islets (**Figure 2B**). Administration of STZ also induced a significant increase in intra-islet recruitment of macrophages, regardless of the pretreatment received (**Figures 2C,E**). No significant differences were found between saline and paraoxon control groups (**Figure 2E**).

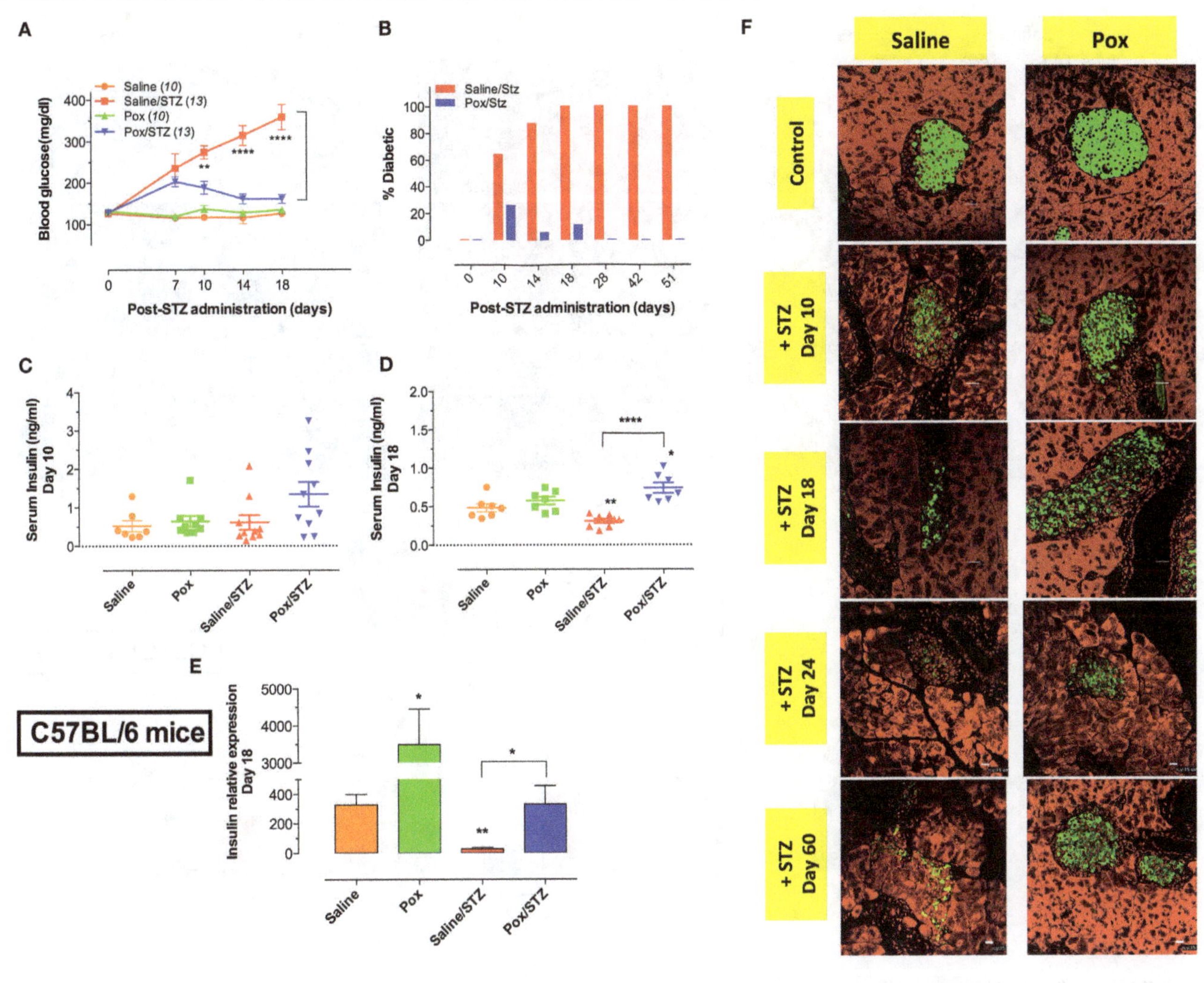

FIGURE 1 | Administration of AChE inhibitor modulates the development of STZ-induced diabetes. C57BL/6 mice pretreated with paraoxon (Pox) or Saline for 3 weeks were challenged with 60 mg/kg/day of STZ for five consecutive days. **(A)** Blood glucose concentrations in tail blood samples were measured at indicated time points. Mice with blood glucose measurements >200 mg/dl were considered diabetic. Data are pooled from three independent experiments and the total number of mice is shown in parenthesis for each group. Two-way ANOVA with Bonferroni post-test was used for statistical analysis. **(B)** Percentage of diabetic animals in mice pretreated with saline or paraoxon followed by MLD-STZ challenge over an observation period of 51 days. Data are pooled from six independent experiments (22–25 mice per group up to day 18 post-STZ and 9 mice per group for later time points). **(C,D)** Serum insulin levels were determined at day 10 **(C)** and day 18 **(D)** post-STZ administration. **(E)** mRNA expression of pancreatic insulin in mice sacrificed at day 18 post-STZ treatment. Each data point represents the mean ± SEM of the values obtained from four to six animals per group. Student's *t*-test was used for graphs **(C–E)**. Asterisks above bars denote statistically significant differences between the indicated experimental groups and saline-control group. Asterisks above brackets denote significance between the indicated experimental groups (*$p < 0.05$, **$p \leq 0.01$, ***$p \leq 0.001$, ****$p \leq 0.0001$). **(F)** Light confocal micrographs (×40) of pancreatic islets of C57BL/6 mice pretreated with saline/STZ or Pox/STZ showing immunofluorescence of insulin-containing β cells. Total follow-up period was 60 days. Photos are representative of two individual experiments (four mice/group/experiment). Bar in the figures indicates 25 μm.

Next, we investigated mRNA expression of proinflammatory cytokines in pancreatic tissue at day 18 post-STZ (**Figures 2F,G**). STZ administration led to a significant increase (3.1-fold) in IFNγ mRNA expression compared with saline controls (**Figure 2F**). Interestingly, mice pretreated with paraoxon alone also exhibited a 2.4-fold increase in pancreatic IFNγ expression compared with controls. In contrast, mice pretreated with paraoxon followed by STZ showed similar levels of IFNγ expression to those receiving paraoxon alone (detectable in only 2/6 mice examined; **Figure 2F**). Expression of pancreatic IL-1β was also assessed in the different experimental groups. The highest level of IL-1β expression was observed in saline/STZ group (**Figure 2G**). In contrast, IL-1β expression levels dropped significantly in paraoxon (2.5-fold) and paraoxon/STZ (2.7-fold) experimental groups compared with saline/STZ group (**Figure 2G**). For pancreatic IL-23, expression was almost undetectable in saline and paraoxon groups, was maximal in saline/STZ group and decreased by >50% in paraoxon/STZ-treated mice compared with saline/STZ group; however, this difference was not statistically significant (**Figure 2H**). Analysis of pancreatic TNFα expression revealed only background levels

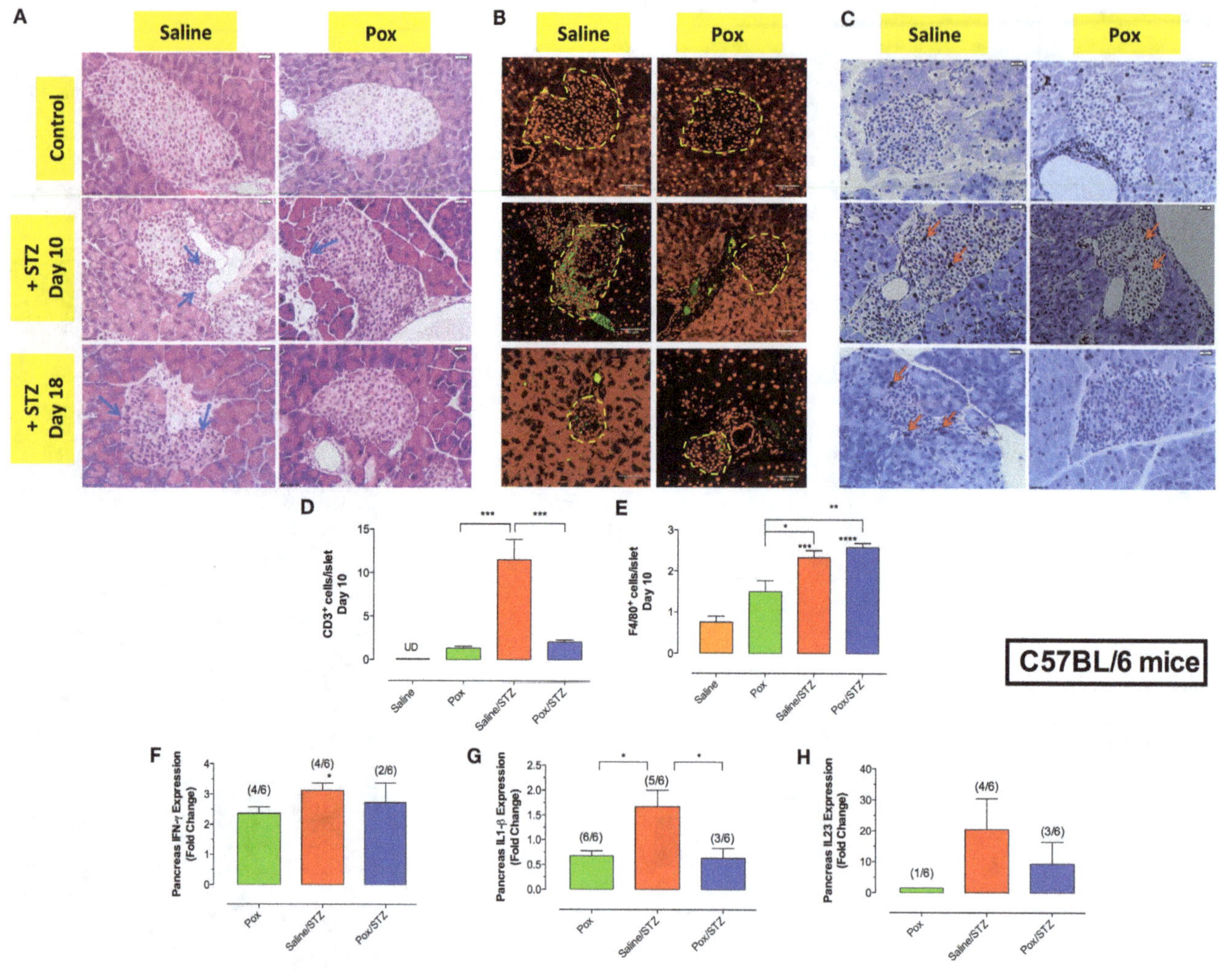

FIGURE 2 | Inhibition of AChE reduces STZ-mediated insulitis. **(A)** Representative images of H&E stained pancreatic islets from the four different experimental groups sacrificed at day 10 or 18 post-STZ administration. Arrows indicate infiltrating inflammatory cells (bar = 20 μm). **(B,C)** Pancreatic sections were stained with anti-CD3 **(B)** or F4/80 **(C)** antibodies, as described in Section "Materials and Methods" to detect T cells and macrophages, respectively. Dashed lines delineate pancreatic islets. Representative images (40x) from two independent experiments (four mice/group/experiment) are shown. Arrows indicate representative cells. Bars in the figures indicate 50 μm in CD3 staining and 20 μm in F4/80 staining. **(D,E)** Quantitative estimation of the number of T cells **(D)** and macrophages **(E)** per islet in pancreatic section of different treatment groups sacrificed at day 10 post-STZ administration. Data are shown as the mean ± SEM of the number of positive cells per high power field. **(F–H)** Relative expression levels of IFN-γ **(F)** and IL-1β **(G)** and IL-23p19 **(H)** mRNA, expressed as fold change compared to saline controls, isolated from pancreas of mice sacrificed day 18 post-STZ administration. Each data point represents the mean ± SEM of the values obtained in that group. Since cytokine expression was not detectable in every mouse of each group, the ratio of the animals positive for each cytokine is also shown. Fractions above the bars indicate the number of mice with positive value/total number of mice in the group. One-way ANOVA was used for statistical analysis in Figures A–E. Asterisks above bars denote statistically significant differences between the indicated experimental groups and saline-control group. Asterisks above brackets denote significance between the indicated experimental groups (*$p < 0.05$; **$p \leq 0.01$; ***$p \leq 0.001$).

with no significant differences among the experimental groups (data not shown). Moreover, no cytokines could be detected in pancreatic tissue at day 10 post-STZ treatment in any of the groups (data not shown).

Inhibition of AChE Reduced Splenic Proinflammatory Cytokines and Th17 Effector Cells

Next, we explored the effect of AChE inhibition on the peripheral immune response in STZ-treated mice. Immunophenotyping revealed no gross differences in the percentage of major spleen cell populations among the four different experimental groups at either day 10 or 18 post STZ administration (Images 2 and 3 in Supplementary Material), the only exception being a small but significant decrease in the frequency of CD8+ T cells in the paraoxon/STZ group compared with saline/STZ-treated mice at day 10 post-STZ administration (Images 2 and 3 in Supplementary Material). Given the role of IL-17 and Th17 cells in autoimmune diabetes and their counter regulation by IFNγ (27, 41), mRNA expression levels of IFNγ and IL-17 were determined in spleen cells. Moderate upregulation of IFNγ expression was observed in mice pretreated with AChE inhibitor (paraoxon and paraoxon/STZ groups) compared with saline control (**Figure 3A**), with the differences being statistically significant between saline/STZ and paraoxon/STZ groups. Conversely, while administration of STZ led to a 4.7-fold increase in IL-17 expression compared with saline control animals (**Figure 3B**), pretreatment with paraoxon abrogated the IL-17 response (paraoxon/STZ group; **Figure 3B**). These results suggest that inhibition of AChE led to an increase in IFN-γ production and a reduction in STZ-induced IL-17. Further analysis revealed a reduction in the expression of IL-6 and IL-23, cytokines involved in the differentiation of Th17 cells, in groups receiving paraoxon compared with saline group (**Figures 3C,D**). Moreover, compared with control animals, IL-6 expression was upregulated in saline/STZ group (**Figure 3C**). On the other hand, expression levels of IL-12, an IFNγ-promoting cytokine, were found to be upregulated in paraoxon-treated groups compared with saline control (2.7-fold and 1.8-fold increase in paraoxon and paraoxon/STZ groups, respectively; **Figure 3E**). Significant differences in IL-12 expression were observed between paraoxon-treated mice compared with the saline or saline/STZ group (**Figure 3E**). No significant differences were observed in the expression of TNFα and IL-1β proinflammatory cytokines among experimental groups (data not shown). These findings suggest that inhibition of AChE may prevent STZ-induced hyperglycemia by modulating the balance between Th1 and Th17 development.

To assess this directly, we determined the percentage of IL-17$^+$ and IFNγ$^+$ splenic T cells at day 18 post-STZ administration. *Ex vivo* stimulation with PMA/ionomycin followed by intracellular cytokine staining revealed that pretreatment with paraoxon induced a moderate increase in the percentage of IFNγ$^+$CD4$^+$

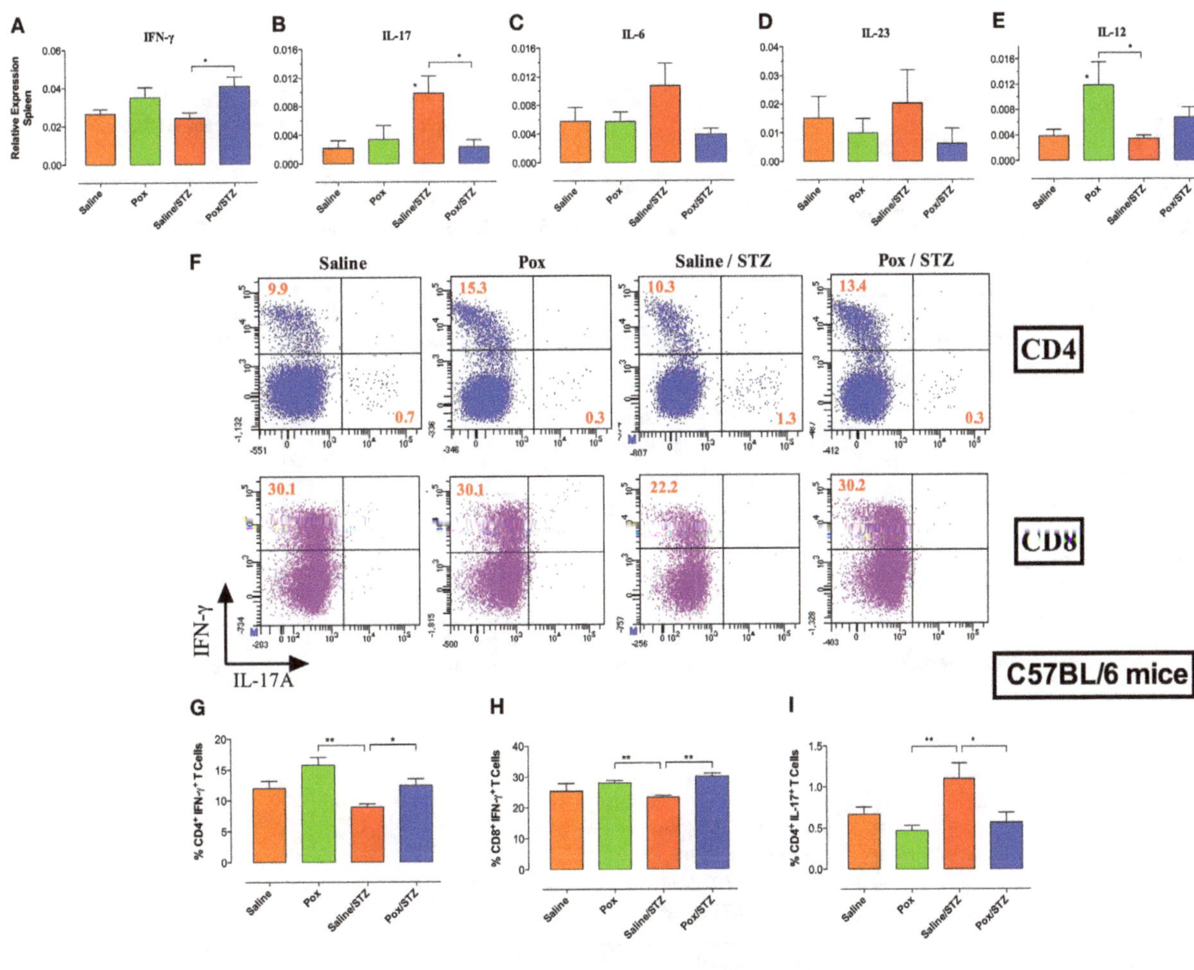

FIGURE 3 | Inhibition of AChE suppresses STZ-induced Th17 cells and promotes IFNγ-secreting Th1 differentiation. C57BL/6 mice pretreated with paraoxon (Pox)/Saline for 3 weeks were administered STZ/vehicle for five consecutive days and sacrificed 18 days later. **(A–E)** Relative mRNA expression levels of IFNγ **(A)**, IL-17F **(B)**, IL-6 **(C)**, IL-23p19 **(D)**, and IL-12p40 **(E)** isolated from whole spleen. Each value represents the mean ± SEM of data collected from three independent experiments (7–10 mice/group). One-way ANOVA was used for the statistical analysis for **(A–E)** graphs. Asterisks above bars denote statistically significant differences between the indicated experimental groups and saline-control group. Asterisks above brackets denote significance between the indicated experimental groups (*$p < 0.05$). **(F–I)** Intracellular cytokine analysis. Splenocytes were stimulated *ex vivo* with PMA/ionomycin and analyzed for CD4 and CD8 positivity and IFNγ and IL-17 content. Each experimental group included three mice. **(F)** Representative results of individual mice are shown, and are representative of two independent experiments. Percentages of CD4$^+$IFNγ$^+$ **(G)**, CD8$^+$IFNγ$^+$ **(H)**, and CD4$^+$IL-17A$^+$ **(I)** T cells are depicted in the graphs. Values represent the mean ± SEM of six mice per group. Student's *t*-test was used for data analysis of Figures G–I. Asterisks denote statistically significant differences between the indicated groups (*$p < 0.05$, **$p \leq 0.01$).

cells (**Figure 3F**). Saline/STZ group exhibited significant reduction in percentage of IFNγ^+CD4$^+$ and IFNγ^+CD8$^+$, but increased percentage of IL-17$^+$CD4$^+$, T cells compared with paraoxon and paraoxon/STZ group (**Figures 3F–I**). Percentage of CD4$^+$IL-17$^+$ cells in saline/STZ group was significantly increased compared with paraoxon-treated groups (2.4-fold and 2-fold that of paraoxon and paraoxon/STZ groups, respectively) (**Figures 3F,I**). Expression of IL-17 was detected mainly in CD4$^+$, but not CD8$^+$ T cells (**Figure 3F**). These results support the idea that inhibition of AChE leads to a preferential induction of a Th1 response that suppresses STZ-driven Th17 cell differentiation.

Inhibition of AChE Fails to Prevent STZ-Induced Hyperglycemia in IFN$\gamma^{-/-}$ Mice

To further elucidate the role of IFNγ in the development of hyperglycemia, we utilized the same MLD-STZ model to induce diabetes in IFN$\gamma^{-/-}$ mice. Administration of paraoxon induced 50–60% inhibition in AChE activity in both wild-type (WT) C57BL/6 as well as IFN$\gamma^{-/-}$ mice (**Figures 4A,D**). Importantly, pretreatment with paraoxon protected against STZ-triggered hyperglycemia in WT (**Figure 4B**) but not in IFN$\gamma^{-/-}$ mice (**Figure 4E**). WT mice developed hyperglycemia 7–10 days post STZ administration and this continued up to 7 weeks later (**Figure 4B**). In contrast, no hyperglycemia was observed in paraoxon-pretreated WT mice after STZ injection (**Figure 4B**). It is intriguing to point out that paraoxon pretreatment in IFN$\gamma^{-/-}$ mice did appear to protect against onset of hyperglycemia during the first 10 days following STZ administration (**Figure 4E**). Subsequently, however, paraoxon-pretreated IFN$\gamma^{-/-}$ mice became hyperglycemic and, by day 49, their blood glucose levels reached 500 mg/dl, identical to saline-pretreated mice (**Figure 4E**). A moderate degree of weight loss (10–15%) is commonly observed in mice treated with AChE inhibitors (36, 42), and this was observed in both WT and

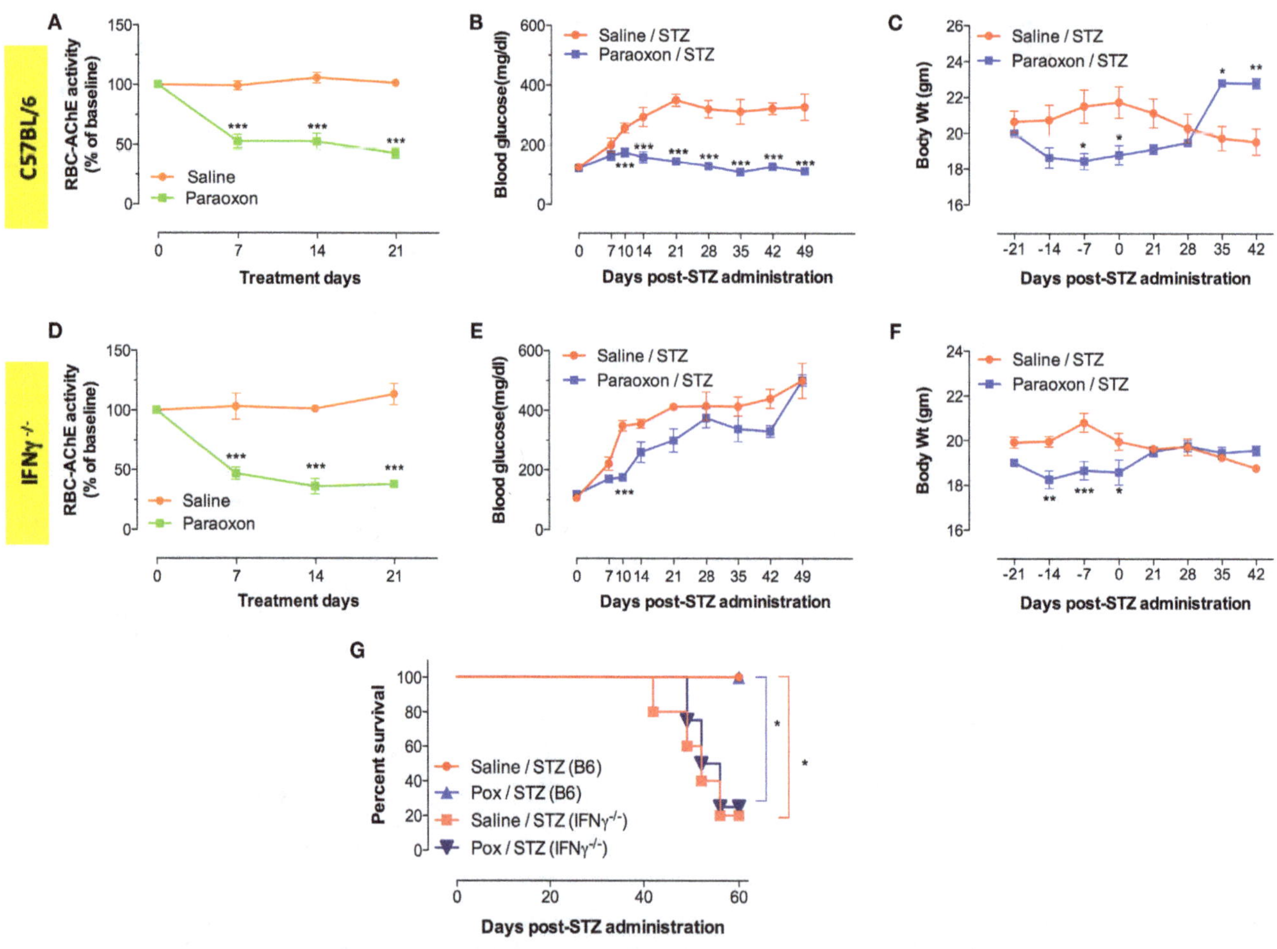

FIGURE 4 | IFNγ is required for amelioration of STZ-induced hyperglycemia. Transient reduction in RBC-AChE activity in C57BL/6 **(A)** and IFN$\gamma^{-/-}$ **(D)** mice during the course of paraoxon administration. All enzyme activities are expressed as percentage of the baseline activity (100%). Blood glucose levels in C57BL/6 **(B)** and IFN$\gamma^{-/-}$ **(E)** mice were measured at indicated time points post STZ treatment. Changes in body weights in C57BL/6 **(C)** and IFN$\gamma^{-/-}$ **(F)** mice during paraoxon treatment and up to 42 days post-STZ administration. The mean values ± SEM are depicted in all graphs. Two-way ANOVA with Bonferroni post-test was used for the statistical analysis of **(A–F)**. Asterisks denote statistically significant differences between the two groups at each time point (*$p < 0.05$, **$p \leq 0.01$, ***$p \leq 0.001$, ****$p \leq 0.0001$). **(G)** Survival was followed for up to 60 days after STZ administration. Kaplan–Meier and log-rank test was used for analysis. All results represent cumulative data of two independent experiments. Asterisks denote statistically significant differences between the indicated groups (*$p < 0.05$).

IFNγ$^{-/-}$ mice particularly during the 3-week (day −21 to day 0) paraoxon pretreatment period (**Figures 4C,F**). Following the end of paraoxon pretreatment period, the animals' weights gradually normalized and by day 28 were identical to saline-pretreated mice (**Figures 4C,F**). As WT mice developed hyperglycemia due to STZ, they begin to loose weight and this was clearly evident by day 35 post STZ injection (**Figure 4C**). However, paraoxon-pretreated WT mice exhibited no further loss of weight after STZ and, in fact, their weights were higher than saline/STZ group at days 35 and 42 post STZ (**Figure 4C**). In contrast, although IFNγ$^{-/-}$ mice also recovered their initial weight after paraoxon treatment, they did not exhibit further weight gain after STZ administration due to their hyperglycemic state (**Figures 4E,F**). Finally, we also assessed long term survival in STZ-injected mice (C57BL/6 and IFNγ$^{-/-}$) following pretreatment with either saline or paraoxon (**Figure 4G**). Irrespective of the treatment, no deaths were recorded in C57BL/6 mice up to 60 days post STZ administration. In sharp contrast, only about 20% of IFNγ$^{-/-}$ mice, whether pretreated with saline or paraoxon, survived by day 60 post-STZ (**Figure 4G**). This is most likely due to the higher levels of hyperglycemia observed in these mice (**Figure 4E**). These findings confirm the important role that IFNγ plays in cholinergic pathway-mediated inhibition of diabetes development in the MLD-STZ model.

AChE Inhibition Does Not Prevent STZ-Mediated Islet β Cell Damage in IFNγ$^{-/-}$ Mice

Next, we analyzed the status of insulin-producing cells in pancreatic tissue of IFNγ$^{-/-}$ mice at days 10 and 18 post STZ administration. Compared with saline controls, saline/STZ group showed a reduction in insulin-producing β cells by day 10 post STZ injection, and this became more pronounced at day 18 post STZ (**Figure 5A**). Pretreatment with paraoxon appeared to delay the loss of insulin-positive β cells. Moreover, paraoxon-treated

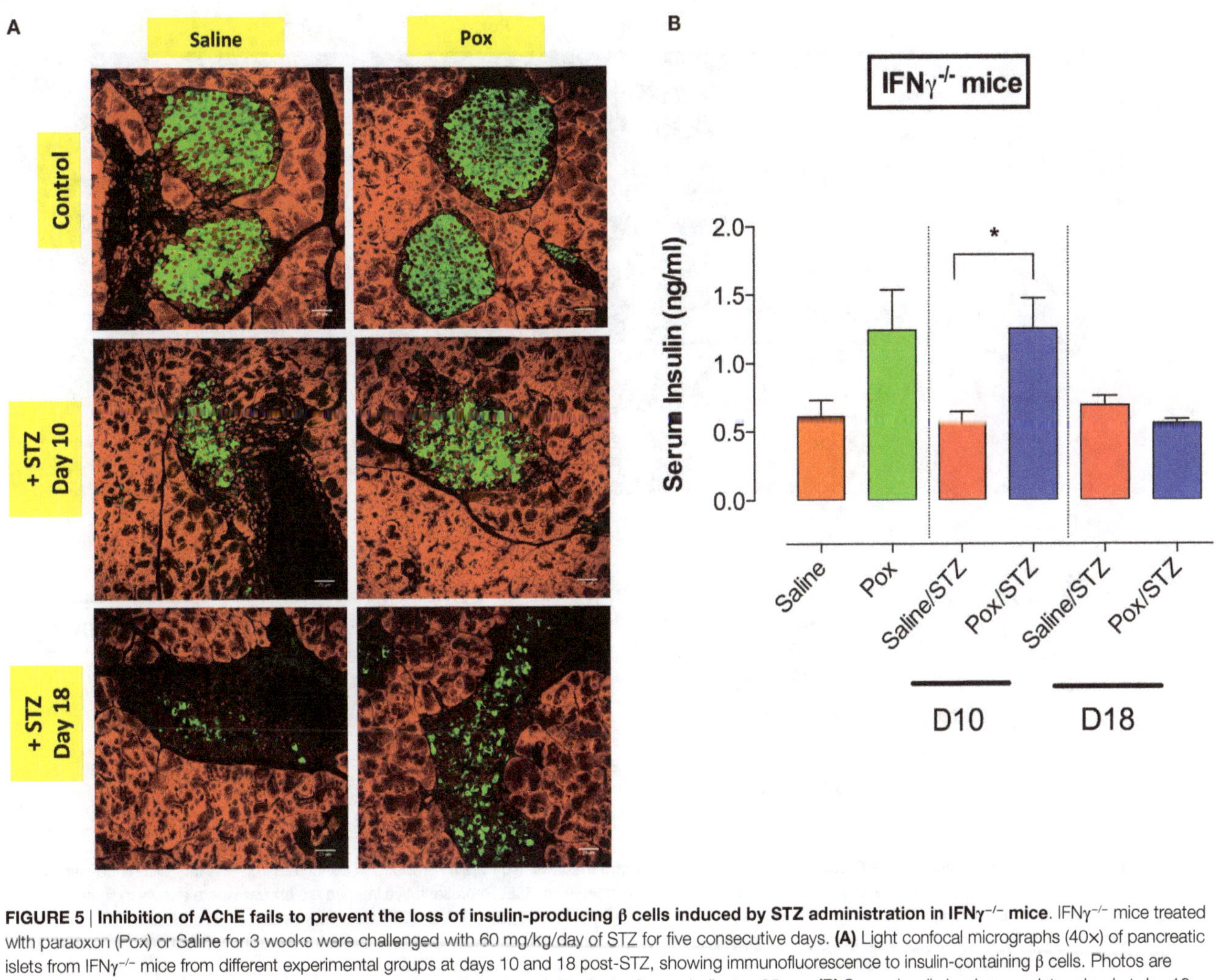

FIGURE 5 | Inhibition of AChE fails to prevent the loss of insulin-producing β cells induced by STZ administration in IFNγ$^{-/-}$ mice. IFNγ$^{-/-}$ mice treated with paraoxon (Pox) or Saline for 3 weeks were challenged with 60 mg/kg/day of STZ for five consecutive days. **(A)** Light confocal micrographs (40x) of pancreatic islets from IFNγ$^{-/-}$ mice from different experimental groups at days 10 and 18 post-STZ, showing immunofluorescence to insulin-containing β cells. Photos are representative of two individual experiments (four mice/group/experiment). Bar in the figures indicates 25 μm. **(B)** Serum insulin levels were determined at day 10 and 18 post-STZ administration. Student's *t*-test was used for the statistical analysis. Asterisks denote statistically significant differences between experimental groups ($^{*}p < 0.05$).

IFNγ$^{-/-}$ mice exhibited higher levels of serum insulin compared with saline control (**Figure 5B**; paraoxon group). No reduction in serum insulin was observed in paraoxon/STZ-treated mice during the first 10 days post-STZ administration (paraoxon/STZ group). However, by day 18, serum insulin levels dropped to become similar to the ones in the saline/STZ group (**Figure 5B**). These data suggest that IFNγ does not play a role in the initial control of STZ-induced hyperglycemia.

Hematoxylin and eosin staining of pancreatic tissue of IFNγ$^{-/-}$ mice showed highly infiltrated islets in the saline/STZ group at day 10 and 18 post STZ administration (**Figure 6A**; left middle and bottom panels). In contrast, pancreatic islets from paraoxon/STZ group exhibited mild infiltration at day 10, but by day 18 all islets appeared infiltrated although to a lesser extent than in saline/STZ group (**Figure 6A**; right middle and bottom panels). No apparent cell infiltration could be observed in islets of saline or paraoxon control groups (**Figure 6A**; top panels). Immunohistological analysis of the islets at day 10 and 18 revealed the presence of fewer CD3$^+$ T cells than in WT mice, with highest levels being detected in saline/STZ group (**Figures 6B,D**). Pretreatment with paraoxon reduced by >60% the extent of T cell infiltration (paraoxon/STZ group) compared to saline/STZ group (**Figure 6D**). Staining with F4/80 mAb revealed a similar extent of macrophage infiltration in all four experimental groups (**Figures 6C,E**).

Inhibition of AChE Leads to a Partial Alteration in Th17 Cell Ratio in the Absence of IFNγ

As expected, intracellular staining of splenocytes of IFNγ$^{-/-}$ mice showed no CD4$^+$IFNγ$^+$ or CD8$^+$IFNγ$^+$ T cells (**Figure 7A**). AChE inhibition induced a partial but not statistically significant reduction in the percentage of CD4$^+$IL-17$^+$ cells (paraoxon group). STZ

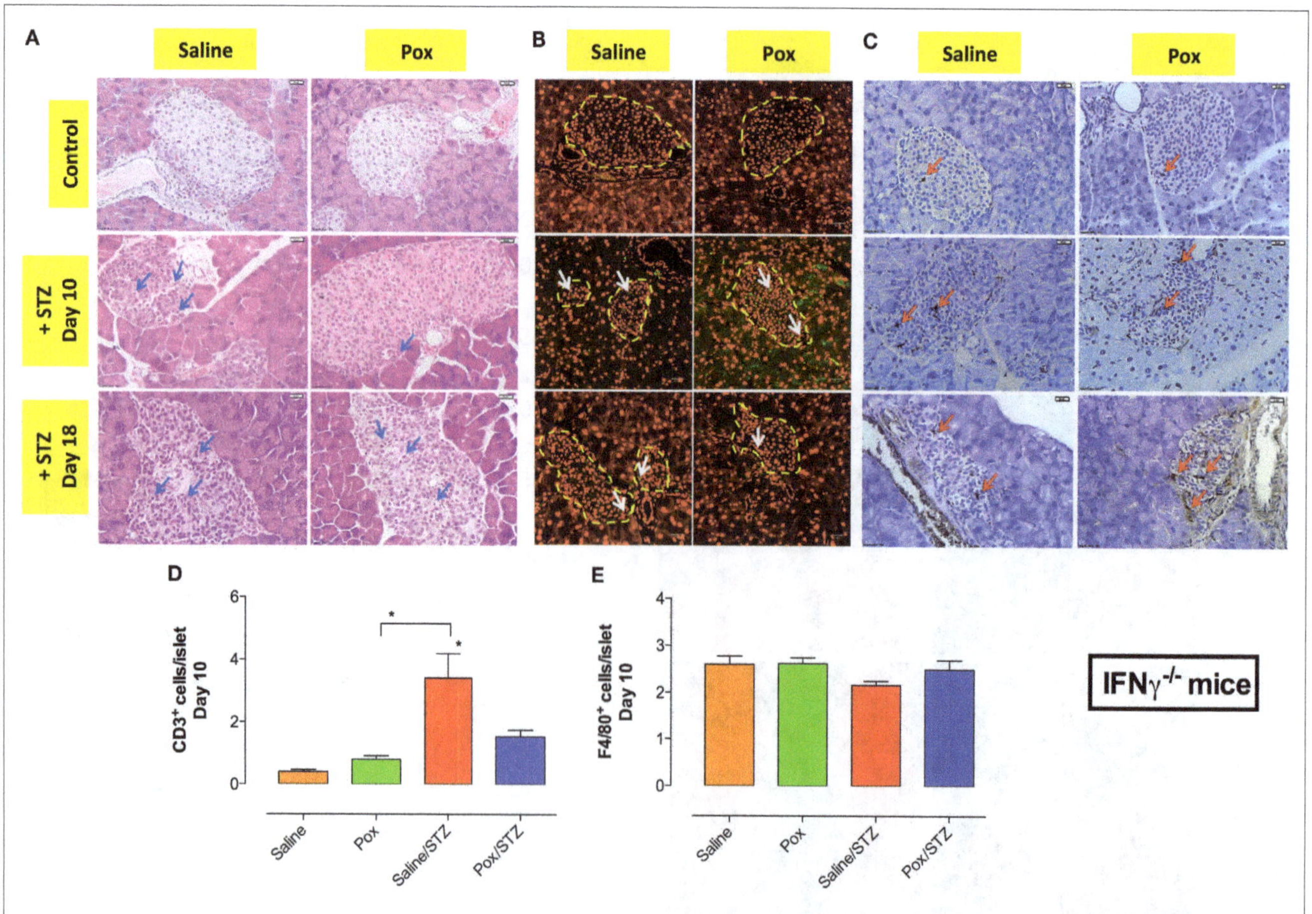

FIGURE 6 | In IFNγ$^{-/-}$ mice, inhibition of AChE does not prevent STZ-induced insulitis. (A) Paraffin embedded pancreata from the four different experimental groups, sacrificed at day 10 or 18 post-STZ administration, were sectioned and stained with H&E. Representative images are shown where arrows indicate infiltrating inflammatory cells (bar = 20 μm). Pancreatic sections were also stained with anti-CD3 **(B)** or F4/80 **(C)** antibodies, as described in Section "Materials and Methods" to detect T cells and macrophages, respectively. Dashed lines delineate pancreatic islets. Representative images (40×) from two independent experiments (four mice/group/experiment) are shown. Arrows indicate representative cells. Bars in the figures indicate 50 μm in CD3 staining and 20 μm in F4/80 staining. Quantitative estimation of the number of T cells **(D)** and macrophages **(E)** per islet in pancreatic section of different treatment groups sacrificed at day 10 post-STZ administration. Data are shown as the mean ± SEM of the number of positive cells per high power field. One-way ANOVA was used for the statistical analysis **(D,E)**. Asterisks above bars denote statistically significant differences between the indicated experimental groups and saline-control group. Asterisks above brackets denote significance between the indicated experimental groups ($^*p < 0.05$).

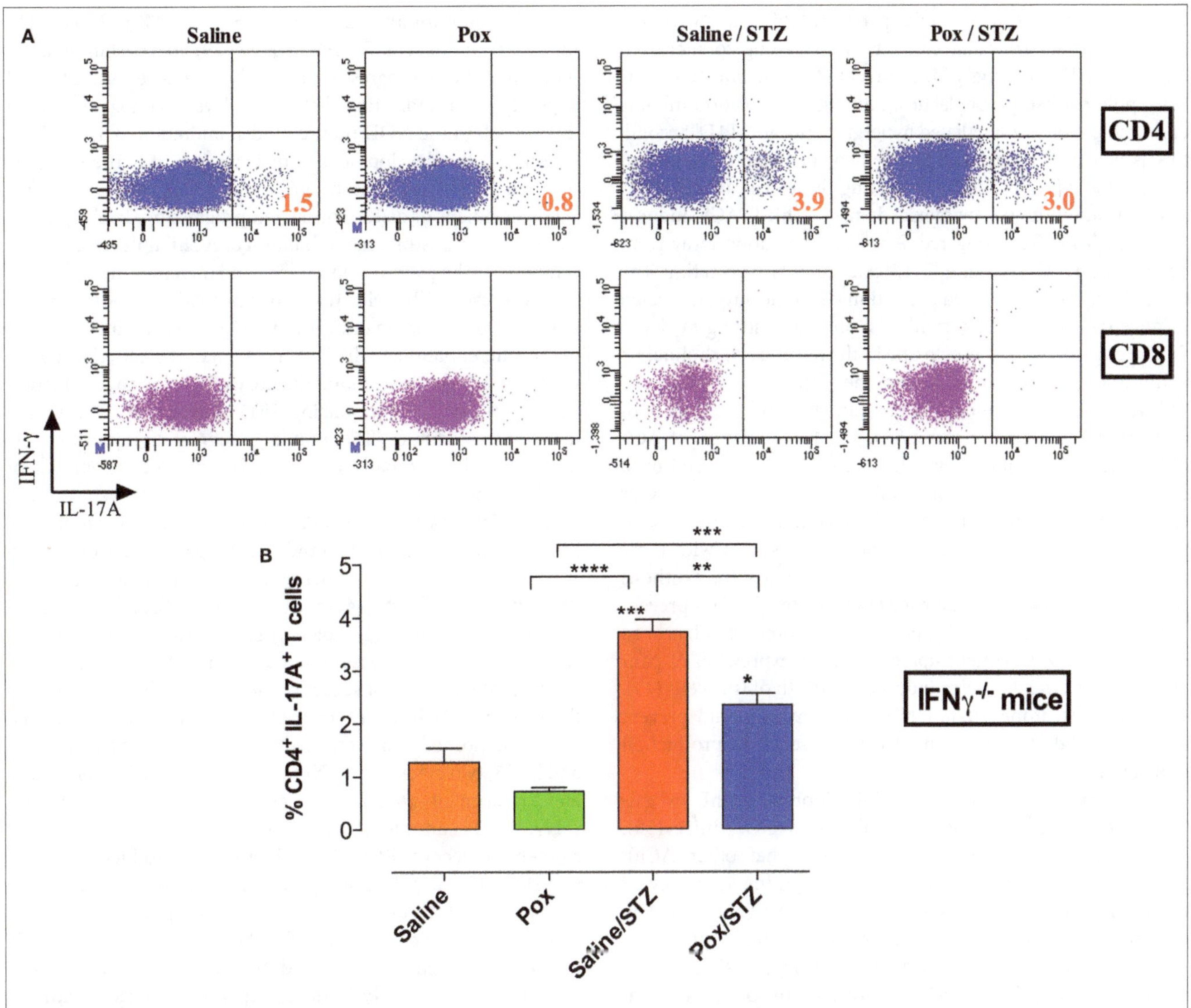

FIGURE 7 | Inhibition of AChE in the absence of IFNγ production leads to a partial decrease in Th17 differentiation. IFNγ$^{-/-}$ mice treated with paraoxon (Pox) or Saline for 3 weeks were administered STZ or vehicle for five consecutive days and sacrificed 18 days later. Spleens were obtained and single cell suspensions prepared. Splenocytes were stimulated with PMA/ionomycin and analyzed for CD4/CD8 positivity and IFNγ/IL-17 content **(A)**. Each experimental group included three mice. Results of individual mice are shown and are representative of two independent experiments. **(B)** Percentages of CD4$^+$IL-17A$^+$ T cells are depicted. Values represent the mean ± SEM of three mice per group. Data analysis was done by Student's *t*-test. Asterisks above bars denote statistically significant differences between the indicated experimental groups and saline-control group. Asterisks above brackets denote significance between the indicated experimental groups (*$p < 0.05$, **$p \leq 0.01$, ***$p \leq 0.001$, ****$p \leq 0.0001$).

administration induced the differentiation of CD4$^+$IL-17$^+$ cells in saline/STZ group (mean ± SEM = 3.7 ± 0.2%; **Figures 7A,B**) which represents a 2.9-fold increase in comparison to saline controls. For paraoxon/STZ-treated mice, the percentage of CD4$^+$IL-17$^+$ cells was slightly, but significantly, reduced (2.3 ± 0.2%) compared to saline/STZ group but was still significantly higher than that of saline and acetylcholinesterase inhibitor (AChEI) groups (**Figures 7A,B**). Nevertheless, the presence of a significant level of CD4$^+$IL-17$^+$ T cells in paraoxon/STZ-treated IFNγ$^{-/-}$ mice is in sharp contrast to the findings in WT mice where similar treatment reduced the ratio of CD4$^+$IL-17$^+$ T cells to background levels (**Figure 3F**). These results highlight the immunomodulatory effect of the cholinergic pathway and the important role of IFNγ in preventing the development of STZ-induced diabetes.

DISCUSSION

Several studies have revealed the importance of the parasympathetic nervous system in regulating immune responses in infectious (9, 11) as well as autoimmune disease models (15, 22). The purpose of this study was to explore the effect of AChE inhibition on the onset and development of T1D induced by MLD-STZ administration. Cholinergic stimulation was induced through the utilization of an irreversible specific inhibitor of AChE, the primary ACh-hydrolyzing enzyme, thus leading to increased ACh levels. The findings of the current study demonstrate four main points. First, prophylactic cholinergic stimulation inhibits development of STZ-mediated hyperglycemia and T1D. Second, this is achieved by direct enhancement of insulin production by pancreatic β cells and by protecting these cells against STZ-induced autoimmune, cytotoxic damage. Third, ACh induces a shift in MLD/STZ-triggered T cell differentiation away from pathogenic IL-17-secreting Th17 cells to IFN-γ-secreting Th1 cells. Finally, ACh-mediated protection is significantly attenuated in mice deficient in IFNγ synthesis, providing strong evidence for the critical role of this cytokine in the response to cholinergic pathway activation in this autoimmune model.

The vagus nerve innervates the pancreas and controls both endocrine and exocrine secretions (43, 44). Secretion of ACh *via* vagus nerve stimulation acts on mAChRs expressed on β cells and upregulates the production of insulin (45–48). Our results showing that inhibition of AChE induced an increase in pancreatic insulin mRNA expression are consistent with these previous findings. The induced increase in insulin synthesis could compensate for the damage triggered by STZ and prevent the initial development of hyperglycemia. Moreover, it has been shown that STZ treatment upregulated the expression of pancreatic AChE, which in turn induced the death of islet cells (49). Therefore, the prophylactic inhibition of AChE could prevent STZ-induced destruction of β cells and preserve the production of insulin.

A recent study reported that inhibition of AChE by galantamine delayed the onset of diabetes in NOD mice (50). Moreover, we have preliminary evidence that other AChE inhibitors, such as galantamine and rivastigmine, also prevent the development of hyperglycemia in the MLD-STZ model (data not shown). Increased cholinergic activity through vagus nerve stimulation also plays an important role in suppressing pancreatic inflammation (51). Previously, we and others reported that peripheral administration of an AChE inhibitor resulted in protective anti-inflammatory manifestations at both the mucosal as well as systemic levels (11, 52). Herein, our results show that inhibition of AChE in STZ-treated mice leads to reduced islet infiltration by $CD3^+$ T cells and significantly lower levels of pancreatic IL-1β and splenic IL-6 and IL-17 mRNA expression. Therefore, our data suggest that cholinergic pathway activation influences the development of hyperglycemia in the MLD-STZ model by acting at both local (pancreas) and systemic immune system levels.

IFNγ was initially considered the cytokine responsible for the pathogenesis of autoimmune diabetes (53, 54). This view changed with the demonstration that IFNγ-deficient NOD mice were still susceptible to insulitis and diabetes, albeit with delayed onset (55). Moreover, splenocytes from diabetic $IFN\gamma^{-/-}$ NOD mice could fully transfer disease to naïve mice, suggesting the involvement of other T cell subpopulations. Th-17 cells have been described as potent inducers of autoimmune tissue inflammation. An expansion of pathogenic Th17 cells and excess IL-17 production have been implicated in murine and human T1D (24, 25, 31, 32) and other autoimmune diseases (56, 57). In STZ-induced T1D, mice deficient in IL-17R (28) or IL-17 (29) are resistant to STZ-induced diabetes progression and exhibit reduced insulitis and hyperglycemia, indicating that IL-17 plays a pathogenic role in this model. In the NOD mouse model, inhibition of Th17/IL-17 suppressed the development of diabetes (24, 25). The interplay between Th17 and Th1 at the effector phase appears to be a critical determinant of disease onset and progression. In the present study, we demonstrate that inhibition of AChE upregulates IFNγ synthesis in the pancreas and spleen and increases the frequency of IFNγ-positive Th1 cells. Taken together with the findings showing reduced expression of IL-6 and IL-1β, two cytokines involved in the differentiation of Th17 from memory cells (58), cholinergic pathway-induced immunomodulatory effects led to a reduction in the ratio of IL-17-producing Th17 cells and IL-17 cytokine levels in treated mice. These findings suggest an important role for the cholinergic pathway in regulating the development of autoimmune diabetes.

The spleen is a major secondary lymphoid organ where antigen presentation, T cell activation and clonal expansion can take place. It is known that the vagus nerve does not innervate the spleen directly. Instead, the vagus nerve terminates in the celiac ganglion from which the adrenergic splenic nerve projects, innervating the spleen through the release of noradrenaline. Within the spleen, noradrenaline acts on a subset of memory T cells and stimulate the release of ACh from these cells (59). Our data demonstrate that inhibition of AChE reduced the expression of splenic IL-6 and IL-23, two cytokines with critical roles in Th17 development and pathogenicity (60), and upregulated expression of IL-12 and IFNγ. IL-12 is an important immunoregulatory cytokine, being a potent inducer of IFNγ while inhibiting the production of IL-6 and IL-23 (35, 61). Increasing evidence suggests that IFNγ has modulatory effects on immune cells, including IL-17-producing Th17 cells. The development of Th17 cells from naïve cells is potently inhibited by IFNγ and IL-4 (27, 62). The presence of higher levels of IFNγ in the spleen would interfere with the differentiation of naïve T cells into Th17 cells (63), reducing the availability of pathogenic Th17 cells to migrate to the pancreas. Our findings are consistent with earlier studies suggesting an inhibitory role for IFNγ in the development of Th17 cells and T1D in NOD mice (24, 27). At the level of target tissue (pancreas), inhibition of AChE led to a reduction in IL-1β and IFNγ expression, two proinflammatory cytokines known to induce apoptosis in the pancreatic β cells (64). These findings support the idea that IFNγ in diabetes may have dual functionalities, a pathogenic role at the level of pancreas and a protective role at the level of spleen (24).

A few studies have addressed the direct effect of cholinergic stimulation on isolated immune cell populations. Nicotine, a cholinergic agonist of nAChR, was shown to increase the production of IL-12 by macrophages and DCs *in vitro* (65, 66). Both mAChR and nAChR are known to be expressed on T cells, with muscarinic stimulation leading to enhanced IL-10 and IL-17 production while nicotinergic stimulation upregulating IFNγ and inhibiting IL-17 (67). Therefore, cholinergic stimulation could act directly on T cells to stimulate IFNγ production or indirectly through DCs and macrophages increasing the production of IL-12. The fact that we observed a partial reduction in IL-17-expressing $CD4^+$ T cells in paraoxon/STZ-treated $IFN\gamma^{-/-}$ mice suggests that IL-12 could regulate Th17 activation independent of IFNγ. In addition to Th17 cells, IL-17-producing $CD8^+$ T cells (Tc17) are also induced in the MLD-STZ diabetes model (28). Interestingly, the increased frequency of Tc17 cells was only evident early after STZ administration (day 6) but normalized by day 11 post-STZ (28). In our current study, we could not detect any significant presence of Tc17 cells in any of the experimental groups, most likely due the earliest time point being at day 10 post STZ. Nevertheless, a small but significant decrease in total $CD8^+$ T cells was noted at day 10 in paraoxon/STZ-treated mice in comparison to the saline/STZ group (Image 2 in Supplementary Material). Therefore, it is possible that administration of AChE inhibitors could also influence disease development by preventing the activation and differentiation of $CD8^+$ T cells and Tc17 cells. Furthermore, there is evidence suggesting that IL-12 could enhance the suppressive activity of Tregs, thereby contributing indirectly to the control of pathogenic autoimmune T cells (68). Further studies are needed to investigate the exact mechanism by which AChE inhibition mitigates against the development of pathogenic Th17 cells in autoimmune diabetes.

In conclusion, the findings in the present report demonstrate that inhibition of AChE reduces the incidence of STZ-induced T1D and provides, for the first time, mechanistic evidence that this is achieved through the inhibition of pathogenic Th17 cells. Furthermore, the data demonstrate a pivotal role for IFNγ in mediating the observed protective effect. The possibility of modulating disease severity by therapeutic administration of AChE inhibitors is currently under investigation. Taken together, these results suggest a promising strategy for preventing T1D and other autoimmune diseases.

PRIOR PRESENTATION

Parts of the study were presented in abstract form at the 102nd Annual Meeting of the American Association of Immunologists, New Orleans, LA, USA. May, 2015.

AUTHOR CONTRIBUTIONS

JG performed all animal experiments and analyzed data. GB performed all histological experiments and analyzed data. MQ helped with obtaining some of the data. YM provided valuable support for all molecular studies. JA contributed to the discussion and reviewed the final manuscript. Ba-R designed the study, analyzed data, and wrote the final manuscript. MF-C designed the study, supervised the project, and wrote the final manuscript.

ACKNOWLEDGMENTS

We wish to thank Mr. Saeed Tariq for his invaluable assistance with the confocal microscopy. We also like to thank Prof. Eric Mensah-Brown for his advice on the STZ murine model and Ms. Amna Al-Zaabi and Mr Sheikh Azimullah for their initial work on this project. This work was funded by a grant from the Scientific Research Council, UAE University, United Arab Emirates (NRF-21M074) and by Sheikh Hamdan Medical Research Grants Award, United Arab Emirates (MRG-22/2011-2012) to MF-C.

REFERENCES

1. Kassem SA, Ariel I, Thornton PS, Scheimberg I, Glaser B. Beta-cell proliferation and apoptosis in the developing normal human pancreas and in hyperinsulinism of infancy. *Diabetes* (2000) 49:1325–33. doi:10.2337/diabetes.49.8.1325
2. Eizirik DL, Colli ML, Ortis F. The role of inflammation in insulitis and beta-cell loss in type 1 diabetes. *Nat Rev Endocrinol* (2009) 5:219–26. doi:10.1038/nrendo.2009.21
3. Rees DA, Alcolado JC. Animal models of diabetes mellitus. *Diabet Med* (2005) 22:359–70. doi:10.1111/j.1464-5491.2005.01499.x
4. Like AA, Rossini AA. Streptozotocin-induced pancreatic insulitis: new model of diabetes mellitus. *Science* (1976) 193:415–7. doi:10.1126/science.180605
5. Herold KC, Montag AG, Fitch FW. Treatment with anti-T-lymphocyte antibodies prevents induction of insulitis in mice given multiple doses of streptozocin. *Diabetes* (1987) 36:796–801. doi:10.2337/diabetes.36.7.796
6. Cockfield SM, Ramassar V, Urmson J, Halloran PF. Multiple low dose streptozotocin induces systemic MHC expression in mice by triggering T cells to release IFN-gamma. *J Immunol* (1989) 142:1120–8.
7. Herold KC, Vezys V, Koons A, Lenschow D, Thompson C, Bluestone JA. CD28/B7 costimulation regulates autoimmune diabetes induced with multiple low doses of streptozotocin. *J Immunol* (1997) 158:984–91.
8. Salamone G, Lombardi G, Gori S, Nahmod K, Jancic C, Amaral MM, et al. Cholinergic modulation of dendritic cell function. *J Neuroimmunol* (2011) 236:47–56. doi:10.1016/j.jneuroim.2011.05.007
9. Borovikova LV, Ivanova S, Zhang M, Yang H, Botchkina GI, Watkins LR, et al. Vagus nerve stimulation attenuates the systemic inflammatory response to endotoxin. *Nature* (2000) 405:458–62. doi:10.1038/35013070
10. Kawashima K, Fujii T. The lymphocytic cholinergic system and its contribution to the regulation of immune activity. *Life Sci* (2003) 74:675–96. doi:10.1016/j.lfs.2003.09.037
11. Fernandez-Cabezudo MJ, Lorke DE, Azimullah S, Mechkarska M, Hasan MY, Petroianu GA, et al. Cholinergic stimulation of the immune system protects against lethal infection by *Salmonella enterica* serovar Typhimurium. *Immunology* (2010) 130:388–98. doi:10.1111/j.1365-2567.2009.03238.x
12. Kawashima K, Yoshikawa K, Fujii YX, Moriwaki Y, Misawa H. Expression and function of genes encoding cholinergic components in murine immune cells. *Life Sci* (2007) 80:2314–9. doi:10.1016/j.lfs.2007.02.036
13. Saeed RW, Varma S, Peng-Nemeroff T, Sherry B, Balakhaneh D, Huston J, et al. Cholinergic stimulation blocks endothelial cell activation and leukocyte recruitment during inflammation. *J Exp Med* (2005) 201:1113–23. doi:10.1084/jem.20040463
14. Sato KZ, Fujii T, Watanabe Y, Yamada S, Ando T, Kazuko F, et al. Diversity of mRNA expression for muscarinic acetylcholine receptor subtypes and neuronal nicotinic acetylcholine receptor subunits in human mononuclear leukocytes and leukemic cell lines. *Neurosci Lett* (1999) 266:17–20. doi:10.1016/S0304-3940(99)00259-1
15. Nizri E, Hamra-Amitay Y, Sicsic C, Lavon I, Brenner T. Anti-inflammatory properties of cholinergic up-regulation: a new role for acetylcholinesterase inhibitors. *Neuropharmacology* (2006) 50:540–7. doi:10.1016/j.neuropharm.2005.10.013

16. Razani-Boroujerdi S, Behl M, Hahn FF, Pena-Philippides JC, Hutt J, Sopori ML. Role of muscarinic receptors in the regulation of immune and inflammatory responses. *J Neuroimmunol* (2008) 194:83–8. doi:10.1016/j.jneuroim.2007.11.019
17. Tracey KJ. The inflammatory reflex. *Nature* (2002) 420:853–9. doi:10.1038/nature01321
18. de Jonge WJ, van der Zanden EP, The FO, Bijlsma MF, van Westerloo DJ, Bennink RJ, et al. Stimulation of the vagus nerve attenuates macrophage activation by activating the Jak2-STAT3 signaling pathway. *Nat Immunol* (2005) 6:844–51. doi:10.1038/ni1229
19. Huston JM, Ochani M, Rosas-Ballina M, Liao H, Ochani K, Pavlov VA, et al. Splenectomy inactivates the cholinergic antiinflammatory pathway during lethal endotoxemia and polymicrobial sepsis. *J Exp Med* (2006) 203:1623–8. doi:10.1084/jem.20052362
20. Rosas-Ballina M, Ochani M, Parrish WR, Ochani K, Harris YT, Huston JM, et al. Splenic nerve is required for cholinergic antiinflammatory pathway control of TNF in endotoxemia. *Proc Natl Acad Sci U S A* (2008) 105:11008–13. doi:10.1073/pnas.0803237105
21. Pavlov VA, Tracey KJ. The vagus nerve and the inflammatory reflex – linking immunity and metabolism. *Nat Rev Endocrin* (2012) 8:743–54. doi:10.1038/nrendo.2012.189
22. Brenner T, Hamra-Amitay Y, Evron T, Boneva N, Seidman S, Soreq H. The role of readthrough acetylcholinesterase in the pathophysiology of myasthenia gravis. *FASEB J* (2003) 17:214–22. doi:10.1096/fj.02-0609com
23. Desai AK, Grossberg GT. Diagnosis and treatment of Alzheimer's disease. *Neurology* (2005) 64:S34–9. doi:10.1212/WNL.64.12_suppl_3.S34
24. Jain R, Tartar DM, Gregg RK, Divekar RD, Bell JJ, Lee HH, et al. Innocuous IFNgamma induced by adjuvant-free antigen restores normoglycemia in NOD mice through inhibition of IL-17 production. *J Exp Med* (2008) 205:207–18. doi:10.1084/jem.20071878
25. Emamaullee JA, Davis J, Merani S, Toso C, Elliott JF, Thiesen A, et al. Inhibition of Th17 cells regulates autoimmune diabetes in NOD mice. *Diabetes* (2009) 58:1302–11. doi:10.2337/db08-1113
26. Mensah-Brown EP, Shahin A, Al-Shamisi M, Wei X, Lukic ML. IL-23 leads to diabetes induction after subdiabetogenic treatment with multiple low doses of streptozotocin. *Eur J Immunol* (2006) 36:216–23. doi:10.1002/eji.200535325
27. Lee IF, Wang X, Hao J, Akhoundsadegh N, Chen L, Liu L, et al. B7-H4.Ig inhibits the development of type 1 diabetes by regulating Th17 cells in NOD mice. *Cell Immunol* (2013) 282:1–8. doi:10.1016/j.cellimm.2013.03.005
28. Yaochite JN, Caliari-Oliveira C, Davanso MR, Carlos D, Malmegrim KC, Cardoso CR, et al. Dynamic changes of the Th17/Tc17 and regulatory T cell populations interfere in the experimental autoimmune diabetes pathogenesis. *Immunobiology* (2013) 218:338–52. doi:10.1016/j.imbio.2012.05.010
29. Tong Z, Liu W, Yan H, Dong C. Interleukin-17A deficiency ameliorates streptozotocin-induced diabetes. *Immunology* (2015) 146:339–46. doi:10.1111/imm.12512
30. Bradshaw EM, Raddassi K, Elyaman W, Orban T, Gottlieb PA, Kent SC, et al. Monocytes from patients with type 1 diabetes spontaneously secrete proinflammatory cytokines inducing Th17 cells. *J Immunol* (2009) 183:4432–9. doi:10.4049/jimmunol.0900576
31. Ferraro A, Socci C, Stabilini A, Valle A, Monti P, Piemonti L, et al. Expansion of Th17 cells and functional defects in T regulatory cells are key features of the pancreatic lymph nodes in patients with type 1 diabetes. *Diabetes* (2011) 60:2903–13. doi:10.2337/db11-0090
32. Honkanen J, Nieminen JK, Gao R, Luopajarvi K, Salo HM, Ilonen J, et al. IL-17 immunity in human type 1 diabetes. *J Immunol* (2010) 185:1959–67. doi:10.4049/jimmunol.1000788
33. Marwaha AK, Crome SQ, Panagiotopoulos C, Berg KB, Qin H, Ouyang Q, et al. Cutting edge: increased IL-17-secreting T cells in children with new-onset type 1 diabetes. *J Immunol* (2010) 185:3814–8. doi:10.4049/jimmunol.1001860
34. Korn T, Bettelli E, Oukka M, Kuchroo VK. IL-17 and Th17 Cells. *Annu Rev Immunol* (2009) 27:485–517. doi:10.1146/annurev.immunol.021908.132710
35. Zhang J, Huang Z, Sun R, Tian Z, Wei H. IFN-gamma induced by IL-12 administration prevents diabetes by inhibiting pathogenic IL-17 production in NOD mice. *J Autoimmun* (2012) 38:20–8. doi:10.1016/j.jaut.2011.11.017
36. Fernandez-Cabezudo MJ, Azimullah S, Nurulain SM, Mechkarska M, Lorke DE, Hasan MY, et al. The organophosphate paraoxon has no demonstrable effect on the murine immune system following subchronic low dose exposure. *Int J Immunopathol Pharmacol* (2008) 21:891–901.
37. van KE, Zijlstra WG. Standardization of hemoglobinometry. II. The hemiglobincyanide method. *Clin Chim Acta* (1961) 6:538–44. doi:10.1016/0009-8981(61)90145-0
38. al-Ramadi BK, Fernandez-Cabezudo MJ, El-Hasasna H, Al-Salam S, Bashir G, Chouaib S. Potent anti-tumor activity of systemically-administered IL2-expressing Salmonella correlates with decreased angiogenesis and enhanced tumor apoptosis. *Clin Immunol* (2009) 130:89–97. doi:10.1016/j.clim.2008.08.021
39. Ramadi KB, Mohamed YA, Al-Sbiei A, Almarzooqi S, Bashir G, Al Dhanhani A, et al. Acute systemic exposure to silver-based nanoparticles induces hepatotoxicity and NLRP3-dependent inflammation. *Nanotoxicology* (2016) 10(8):1061–74. doi:10.3109/17435390.2016.1163743
40. Kaimala S, Mohamed YA, Nader N, Issac J, Elkord E, Chouaib S, et al. Salmonella-mediated tumor regression involves targeting of tumor myeloid suppressor cells causing a shift to M1-like phenotype and reduction in suppressive capacity. *Cancer Immunol Immunother* (2014) 63:587–99. doi:10.1007/s00262-014-1543-x
41. Dardalhon V, Korn T, Kuchroo VK, Anderson AC. Role of Th1 and Th17 cells in organ-specific autoimmunity. *J Autoimmun* (2008) 31:252–6. doi:10.1016/j.jaut.2008.04.017
42. Satapathy SK, Ochani M, Dancho M, Hudson LK, Rosas-Ballina M, Valdes-Ferrer SI, et al. Galantamine alleviates inflammation and other obesity-associated complications in high-fat diet-fed mice. *Mol Med* (2011) 17:599–606. doi:10.2119/molmed.2011.00083
43. Woods SC, Porte D Jr. Neural control of the endocrine pancreas. *Physiol Rev* (1974) 54:596–619.
44. Holst JJ, Schwartz TW, Knuhtsen S, Jensen SL, Nielsen OV. Autonomic nervous control of the endocrine secretion from the isolated, perfused pig pancreas. *J Auton Nerv Syst* (1986) 17:71–84. doi:10.1016/0165-1838(86)90045-7
45. Van der Zee EA, Buwalda B, Strubbe JH, Strosberg AD, Luiten PG. Immunocytochemical localization of muscarinic acetylcholine receptors in the rat endocrine pancreas. *Cell Tissue Res* (1992) 269:99–106. doi:10.1007/BF00384730
46. Ahren B. Autonomic regulation of islet hormone secretion – implications for health and disease. *Diabetologia* (2000) 43:393–410. doi:10.1007/s001250051322
47. Gilon P, Henquin JC. Mechanisms and physiological significance of the cholinergic control of pancreatic beta-cell function. *Endocr Rev* (2001) 22:565–604. doi:10.1210/er.22.5.565
48. Gautam D, Han SJ, Hamdan FF, Jeon J, Li B, Li JH, et al. A critical role for beta cell M3 muscarinic acetylcholine receptors in regulating insulin release and blood glucose homeostasis in vivo. *Cell Metab* (2006) 3:449–61. doi:10.1016/j.cmet.2006.04.009
49. Zhang B, Yang L, Yu L, Lin B, Hou Y, Wu J, et al. Acetylcholinesterase is associated with apoptosis in beta cells and contributes to insulin-dependent diabetes mellitus pathogenesis. *Acta Biochim Biophys Sin (Shanghai)* (2012) 44:207–16. doi:10.1093/abbs/gmr121
50. Hanes WM, Olofsson PS, Kwan K, Hudson LK, Chavan SS, Pavlov VA, et al. Galantamine attenuates type 1 diabetes and inhibits anti-insulin antibodies in non-obese diabetic mice. *Mol Med* (2015) 21(1):702–8. doi:10.2119/molmed.2015.00142
51. van Westerloo DJ, Giebelen IA, Florquin S, Bruno MJ, Larosa GJ, Ulloa L, et al. The vagus nerve and nicotinic receptors modulate experimental pancreatitis severity in mice. *Gastroenterology* (2006) 130:1822–30. doi:10.1053/j.gastro.2006.02.022
52. Pavlov VA, Parrish WR, Rosas-Ballina M, Ochani M, Puerta M, Ochani K, et al. Brain acetylcholinesterase activity controls systemic cytokine levels through the cholinergic anti-inflammatory pathway. *Brain Behav Immun* (2009) 23:41–5. doi:10.1016/j.bbi.2008.06.011
53. Campbell IL, Kay TW, Oxbrow L, Harrison LC. Essential role for interferon-gamma and interleukin-6 in autoimmune insulin-dependent diabetes in NOD/Wehi mice. *J Clin Invest* (1991) 87:739–42. doi:10.1172/JCI115055
54. Debray-Sachs M, Carnaud C, Boitard C, Cohen H, Gresser I, Bedossa P, et al. Prevention of diabetes in NOD mice treated with antibody to murine IFN gamma. *J Autoimmun* (1991) 4:237–48. doi:10.1016/0896-8411(91)90021-4

55. Hultgren B, Huang X, Dybdal N, Stewart TA. Genetic absence of gamma-interferon delays but does not prevent diabetes in NOD mice. *Diabetes* (1996) 45:812–7. doi:10.2337/diab.45.6.812

56. Honorati MC, Meliconi R, Pulsatelli L, Cane S, Frizziero L, Facchini A. High in vivo expression of interleukin-17 receptor in synovial endothelial cells and chondrocytes from arthritis patients. *Rheumatology (Oxford)* (2001) 40:522–7. doi:10.1093/rheumatology/40.5.522

57. Tzartos JS, Friese MA, Craner MJ, Palace J, Newcombe J, Esiri MM, et al. Interleukin-17 production in central nervous system-infiltrating T cells and glial cells is associated with active disease in multiple sclerosis. *Am J Pathol* (2008) 172:146–55. doi:10.2353/ajpath.2008.070690

58. Lee YK, Mukasa R, Hatton RD, Weaver CT. Developmental plasticity of Th17 and Treg cells. *Curr Opin Immunol* (2009) 21:274–80. doi:10.1016/j.coi.2009.05.021

59. Rosas-Ballina M, Olofsson PS, Ochani M, Valdes-Ferrer SI, Levine YA, Reardon C, et al. Acetylcholine-synthesizing T cells relay neural signals in a vagus nerve circuit. *Science* (2011) 334:98–101. doi:10.1126/science.1209985

60. Lee Y, Awasthi A, Yosef N, Quintana FJ, Xiao S, Peters A, et al. Induction and molecular signature of pathogenic TH17 cells. *Nat Immunol* (2012) 13:991–9. doi:10.1038/ni.2416

61. Trinchieri G. Interleukin-12 and the regulation of innate resistance and adaptive immunity. *Nat Rev Immunol* (2003) 3:133–46. doi:10.1038/nri1001

62. Park H, Li Z, Yang XO, Chang SH, Nurieva R, Wang YH, et al. A distinct lineage of CD4 T cells regulates tissue inflammation by producing interleukin 17. *Nat Immunol* (2005) 6:1133–41. doi:10.1038/ni1261

63. Kim KW, Cho ML, Park MK, Yoon CH, Park SH, Lee SH, et al. Increased interleukin-17 production via a phosphoinositide 3-kinase/Akt and nuclear factor kappaB-dependent pathway in patients with rheumatoid arthritis. *Arthritis Res Ther* (2005) 7:R139–48. doi:10.1186/ar1454

64. Thomas HE, Angstetra E, Fernandes RV, Mariana L, Irawaty W, Jamieson EL, et al. Perturbations in nuclear factor-kappaB or c-Jun N-terminal kinase pathways in pancreatic beta cells confer susceptibility to cytokine-induced cell death. *Immunol Cell Biol* (2006) 84:20–7. doi:10.1111/j.1440-1711.2005.01397.x

65. Lau PP, Li L, Merched AJ, Zhang AL, Ko KW, Chan L. Nicotine induces proinflammatory responses in macrophages and the aorta leading to acceleration of atherosclerosis in low-density lipoprotein receptor(-/-) mice. *Arterioscler Thromb Vasc Biol* (2006) 26:143–9. doi:10.1161/01.ATV.0000193510.19000.10

66. Jin HJ, Li HT, Sui HX, Xue MQ, Wang YN, Wang JX, et al. Nicotine stimulated bone marrow-derived dendritic cells could augment HBV specific CTL priming by activating PI3K-Akt pathway. *Immunol Lett* (2012) 146:40–9. doi:10.1016/j.imlet.2012.02.015

67. Qian J, Galitovskiy V, Chernyavsky AI, Marchenko S, Grando SA. Plasticity of the murine spleen T-cell cholinergic receptors and their role in in vitro differentiation of naive CD4 T cells toward the Th1, Th2 and Th17 lineages. *Genes Immun* (2011) 12:222–30. doi:10.1038/gene.2010.72

68. Sela U, Park CG, Park A, Olds P, Wang S, Steinman RM, et al. Dendritic cells induce a subpopulation of IL-12Rbeta2-expressing treg that specifically consumes IL-12 to control Th1 responses. *PLoS One* (2016) 11:e0146412. doi:10.1371/journal.pone.0146412

17

Lymphotoxins Serve as a Novel Orchestrator in T1D Pathogenesis

Shi-Wei Liu[1†], Fei Sun[2†], Shan-Jie Rong[2], Ting Wang[2] and Cong-Yi Wang[2*]*

[1] Department of Endocrinology, Shanxi Bethune Hospital, Shanxi Academy of Medical Sciences, Tongji Shanxi Hospital, Third Hospital of Shanxi Medical University, Taiyuan, China, [2] Department of Respiratory and Critical Care Medicine, The Center for Biomedical Research, National Health Commission (NHC) Key Laboratory of Respiratory Diseases, Tongji Hospital, Tongji Medical College, Huazhong University of Sciences and Technology, Wuhan, China

Correspondence:
Cong-Yi Wang
wangcy@tjh.tjmu.edu.cn
Ting Wang
wangting@tjh.tjmu.edu.cn

[†]These authors have contributed equally to this work

Type 1 diabetes (T1D) stems from pancreatic β cell destruction by islet reactive immune cells. Similar as other autoimmune disorders, there is no curative remedy for T1D thus far. Chronic insulitis is the hallmark of T1D, which creates a local inflammatory microenvironment that impairs β cell function and ultimately leads to β cell death. Immune regulation shows promise in T1D treatment by providing a time window for β cell recovery. However, due to the complex nature of T1D pathogenesis, the therapeutic effect of immune regulation is often short-lasting and unsatisfying in monotherapies. Lymphotoxins (LTs) were first identified in 1960s as the lymphocyte-producing cytokine that can kill other cell types. As a biological cousin of tumor necrosis factor alpha (TNFα), LTs play unique roles in T1D development. Herein in this review, we summarized the advancements of LTs in T1D pathogenesis. We particularly highlighted their effect on the formation of peri-islet tertiary lymphoid organs (TLOs), and discussed their synergistic effect with other cytokines on β cell toxicity and autoimmune progression. Given the complex and dynamic crosstalk between immune cells and β cells in T1D setting, blockade of lymphotoxin signaling applied to the existing therapies could be an efficient approach to delay or even reverse the established T1D.

Keywords: type 1 diabetes (T1D), lymphotoxins, tertiary lymphoid organ (TLO), immune regulation, insulitis

INTRODUCTION

Type 1 diabetes (T1D) is a prototypical autoimmune disease featured by islet β cell destruction along with absolute insulin deficiency and uncontrolled autoreactive immune attack (1). Genetic factors contribute to T1D susceptibility and play a pivotal part in disease initiation and progression. In general, the polymorphisms conferring T1D risk predominantly locate within loci that are either associated with β cell functionality (e.g., *Mda5, Ptpn2, Usp18* and *Glis3*) or linked to autoimmune responses (e.g., *HLA, IL-2, IL-2rα, Ctla4* and *Stat3*) (2, 3). These findings laid a foundation for the existence of a vicious crosstalk between immune cells and β cells, which forms a positive feedback

Abbreviations: T1D, type 1 diabetes; LT, lymphotoxin; TNFα, tumor necrosis factor alpha; TLO, tertiary lymphoid organ; LTi, lymphoid tissue inducer; ILC, innate lymphoid cell; HVEM, herpes virus entry mediator; NOD, nonobese diabetic; HEV, high endothelial venule; GSIS, glucose stimulated insulin secretion; LEC, lymphatic endothelial cell; SHM, somatic hypermutation.

loop hard to be halted by the existing therapeutics in clinical settings (4). Moreover, environmental perturbations (such as viral infections, exposure of toxic pollutants, microbiota alteration, diet, exercise and lifestyle changes) linked to epigenetic machineries (e.g., DNA methylation, histone or protein post-translational modifications, and non-coding RNAs) modulate the initiation, progression and remission process of T1D (5, 6). Altogether, these etiological cues make T1D a chronic and complex disease.

The immune factors are crucial in mediating the crosstalk between immune cells and β cells. Particularly, inflammatory cytokines produced by dendritic cells (DCs), macrophages, natural killer (NK) cells, T cells and B cells could act on β cells and impair β cell function by eliciting endoplasmic reticulum (ER) stress, oxidative stress and mitochondrial dysfunction (7). $CD4^+$ helper T cells (Th) and $CD8^+$ cytotoxic T cells (CTLs) are the major subsets responsible for islet destruction (8). Effector Th cells (Teffs) directly secrete IFN-γ, IL-1β and other soluble mediators such as nitric oxide (NO) to induce β cell death (9), or indirectly motivate CTLs to release granzymes and perforin to exert the killing effect (10). Teffs contain several distinct subpopulations, among which Th1 and Th17 play the most critical role. Th1 cells are the well-recognized β cell destroyers due to their capacity of producing massive type 1 cytokines (e.g., IFN-γ, TNF-α, IL-12 and so on) (11). In contrast, the pathogenicity of Th17 is controversial (12, 13). It is generally accepted that Th17 cells polarized by IL-6, IL-23 and IL-1β *in vitro* are pathogenic (termed as pTh17), and diabetogenic Th17 cells display characteristics resembling those of Th1 cells (11, 12). Therefore, the Th1 derived cytokines, IL-1β, IFN-γ and TNFα, constitute the classical trio frequently used to induce β cell dysfunction *in vitro* (14). Likewise, stressed or damaged β cells actively secret cytokines and chemokines to propagate the self-attacking program. Notably, β cells serve as the main source of CXCL10, and the highest CXCL10 expression has been noted at the time of diagnosis rather than the chronic phase of T1D development (15, 16). Concurrently, CXCR3, the receptor for CXCL10, is detected on islet-infiltrating lymphocytes of recent-onset T1D patients. Blockade of the CXCL10/CXCR3 axis with neutralizing antibody reduced T1D incidence in mice, and hopefully, a persistent remission of T1D could be achieved once anti-CD3 therapy is combined (17). Collectively, these studies highlight the complex interaction between immune cells and β cells, which alternatively explain why monotherapies targeting on a single molecule or signaling pathway are unsatisfying in T1D treatment.

Tumor necrosis factor superfamily members (TNFSF), through binding to their corresponding receptors (TNFRSF), affect both immune system and function of β cells. The TNFSF/TNFRSF axes regulate basic biological processes such as cell survival, differentiation, activation, and immune cell development by utilizing different sets of downstream adaptors (18, 19). Specifically, TNFRSF with cytoplasmic death domain (DD) recruits TRADD and FADD, initiating apoptotic pathway *via* the activation of Caspases (20). TNFRSF with non-death domain in the cytoplasmic tail recruits TRAF 1-6 (21), which in turn activates serine/threonine kinases such as MAPK, AKT and NF-κB, and induces the expression of cyclins and inflammatory cytokines. There are over 20 TNFSF/TNFRSF pairs in the superfamily, and many of them are critically engaged with T1D pathogenesis. Based on the action mode, they can be classified into two groups. One group contains members capable of inducing β cell apoptosis through FasL/Fas, TNFα/TNFR1 (13, 22) and TRAIL/TRAILR, while the other group function through immune modulation, which includes OX40L/OX40, CD40L/CD40, CD70/CD27, 4-1BBL/4-1BB, RANKL/RANK, BAFF/BAFFR, GITRL/GITR etc. (23). However, this simplified dichotomy does not mean each TNFSF/TNFRSF pair has only confined regulatory function. For instance, TNFR1 expressing on β cells is related to the initiation of apoptotic pathway, while its expression in regulatory T (Treg) cells affects Treg suppressive capacity (24, 25). Lymphotoxins (LTs) belong to the TNFSF superfamily and are potent immune factors to mediate the crosstalk between immune cells and β cells. Herein, we intend to summarize the advancement of lymphotoxins in T1D pathogenesis. Discussion would be focused on the related mechanisms in the formation of tertiary lymphoid organs (TLOs), induction of β cell dysfunction and enhancement of autoimmune responses during T1D development.

LTS AND THEIR COGNATE RECEPTORS IN T1D PATHOGENESIS

LTs share approximately 35% sequence homology with TNFα, and they are evolutionarily correlated and employ the same receptors (TNFR1 and TNFR2) (26). However, LTs differ from TNFα in many aspects, including the source of producing cell types, the working mechanism, and the resulting biological consequences. LTs, consisting of LTA (TNFSF1, also known as TNFβ) and LTB (TNFSF3), are produced by lymphoid tissue inducer (LTi), Th1, CD8 T cells, NK cells, B cells, and innate lymphoid cells (ILCs) (27–29). LTs exist in the form of LTα3, which is a soluble homotrimer that binds to TNFR1, TNFR2, HVEM (herpes virus entry mediator, minor binding) and signals through the canonical NF-κB pathway (30); or in the form of LTα1β2, which is a membrane-bound heterotrimer that binds to LTβR and activates alternative NF-κB pathway (31). The LT receptors display distinct expression patterns and a division of labor. TNFR1 and TNFR2 are present on most cell types, mediating the processes of apoptosis, inflammation and immune activation, while LTβR is predominantly expressed on monocytes, DCs, follicular DCs (FDCs), endothelial cells, epithelial cells and lymphoid stromal cells, contributing to the ectopic formation of TLOs (32). These unique features of LT-LT receptor signaling render LTs a pleiotropic player in the process of infection, autoimmunity, development of tumor and many other immune related disorders.

The LT genes situate in the MHC cluster, mapped between class III and class I genes and near the TNFα locus. From the perspective of evolution, LTA, LTB and TNFα probably arise from the process of gene duplication. Genetic studies suggest that the TNFα polymorphisms (308 A/G and 857 T/C in particular) confer T1D risk (33). Although the LTA genetic polymorphism has been linked to T1D (34), the supporting evidence is unsolid (35). Moreover, blockade of LT-LT receptor signaling has been proven effective to prevent T1D in mice. Studies in nonobese diabetic (NOD) mice (a mouse model of human T1D) with TNFR1 deficiency abrogated T1D progression (36). Adoptive transfer of either splenocytes or TCR transgenic CD8 T cells demonstrated the existence of two distinct diabetogenic pathways: one is TNFR1 independent which is predominantly caused by the cytotoxic effect of CD8 T cell; the other is TNFR1 dependent which relies on the impact of TNFα and LT (36). In particular, pregnant NOD mice treated with LT-beta receptor immunoglobulin fusion protein (LTbetaR-Ig) on embryonic day 11 (E11) and E14 generated offspring absent of insulitis and free of diabetes at 12-month of age (37). Similarly, embryonic expression of LTbetaR-Ig blocked the development of diabetes in NOD mice. However, the protective effect wanes once the concentration of chimeric LTbetaR-Ig declines (38). Taken together, these studies demonstrated convincing evidence supporting the implication of LTs in T1D pathogenesis.

LTS IN THE DEVELOPMENT OF PERI-ISLET TLO

In the pancreas, artificial over-expression of chemokines including CCL19, CCL21 or CXCL13 in the pancreatic islets, together with the presence of IL-2 family cytokines, induce LTα1β2 expression on naïve T cells and mimic the neogenic process of TLO (39, 40). Ectopic development of TLO is a controlled multistep event that involves the recruitment of circulating immune cells (step 1), which is mediated by the CCL19/CCL21-CCR7 or CXCL13-CXCR5 axes; and the clustering of recruited cells (step 2), which relies partially on the IL-7Rα dependent LTα1β2 signals delivered by $CD4^{+}CD3^{-}IL\text{-}7R\alpha^{hi}$ LTi cells (41) **(Figure 1)**.

Under the context of persistent insulitis, formation of TLO in the pancreas is a key immuno-pathologic feature (42). Chronic inflammatory lesions developed in the pancreas of RIP-LT mice (LT transgenic expression controlled by the rat insulin promoter) manifest intact cellular composition (e.g., T cells, B cells, plasma cells, and antigen-presenting cells), compartmentalized T and B cell regions, primary and secondary follicles, high endothelial venules (HEVs), and the ability to undergo immunoglobulin (Ig) class switch upon antigen challenge (43). Those observed characteristics support the formation of organized lymphoid tissue within the pancreas following sustained autoimmune insult. Moreover, LTβR is upregulated in aged NOD pancreas to promote the local formation of TLO once it's ligated to TNFSF14 (LIGHT). In support of this notion, NOD mice with transgenic TNFSF14 expression in the islets develop spontaneous T1D even when pancreatic draining lymph nodes are absent (44).

It is worthy of note that TLOs could exist in a distinct immune state and largely differ between mice and humans. For example, unlike the transgenic TNFSF14 NOD mice, the Ins2-CCL21 transgenic NOD mice do not develop autoimmune diabetes due to the formation of "regulatory TLOs" around 4-week-old of age, which contain immunosuppressive Tregs (45). In sharp contrast, Tregs are essentially absent from human pancreatic TLOs and the formation of reticular fibers is not associated with CCL21. Particularly, studies in 21 donors exhibited TLOs diagnosed with clinical onset of T1D and insulitis, 12 of whom developed disease at younger age as compared to those lacking TLOs (46). Evidence also supports the formation of "inflammatory TLOs" under T1D setting, since administration of LTbetaR-Ig neutralizes the function of LTs, disassembles the established TLO and prevents T1D development at both early and late stage (47). Therefore, LT induced TLO remains a good interventional option for T1D treatment.

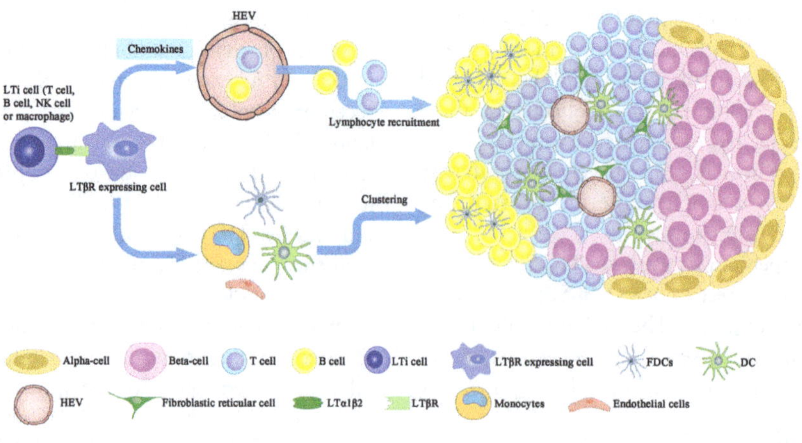

FIGURE 1 | LT signaling participates in the formation of peri-islet TLO. Neogenesis of peri-islet TLO is orchestrated by the interaction between LTα1β2 expressing cells, including LTi, NK, B cells and activated T cells, and the LTβR expressing cells (FDCs, DCs, monocytes and stromal cells). This interaction induces islet infiltration of lymphocytes, which are then clustered into organized TLOs and contribute to β cell destruction. LTi, lymphoid tissue inducer; FDC, follicular dendritic cells; HEV, high endothelial vessels.

LTS IN CYTOKINE INDUCED B CELL TOXICITY

Once tested alone, the murine IFN-γproduces a mild dose-dependent lysis of islet cells, while human IFN-γ, murine IFN-α/β, IL-1, TNFα and LT have no effect. However, the combinations of TNFα (or LT) plus IL-1, TNFα (or LT) plus IFN-γ, and IL-1 plus IFN-γ exhibit synergistic cytotoxic effects, demonstrating a requirement of multiple cytokines for β cell destruction in T1D setting (48). As for glucose stimulated insulin secretion (GSIS), the hallmark of β cell functional capacity, it is suppressed by the treatment of TNFα or IFN-γ rather than by the stimulation of LT or IL-6, but synergistic effect on the suppression of GSIS between LT and IL-1β was observed (49). In another set of experiments, a half-maximal inhibition of GSIS after 7 days of culture was performed. The authors found that 100pg/ml of IL-1β is equivalent to 1000pg/ml of IL-1α in terms of inhibition of GSIS, while 25ng/ml of TNFα, 40ng/ml of LT or 25ng/ml of IFN-γ alone are not effective to impair GSIS or induce morphologic damage to islets (50). Taken together, although the toxicity of LTs in the pancreatic β cells is limited, they may, however, paly a subordinate role in the direct killing of β cells (**Figure 2**).

THE REGULATORY ROLE OF LTS IN IMMUNE RESPONSES

LTs are traditionally regarded as pro-inflammatory cytokines, but their role in the induction of inflammation is relatively weak as compared to that of TNFα. Indeed, pancreatic over-expression of TNFα resulted in overwhelming insulitis with majority of islets manifested infiltration. On the contrary, predominant peri-insulitis was observed in LTA transgenic mice, and LTA over-expression did not cause the reduction of insulin content nor led to the development of diabetes. These data suggest that LT alone is insufficient to initiate an inflammatory response strong enough to induce β cell destruction (51, 52). LTs may only possess a minor and ancillary effect on β cell toxicity (53). Distinct from most other cell types, islet β cells are not stimulated to express HLA class II by IFN-γ. However, IFN-γ in combination with either TNFα or LT induces HLA class II expression in β cells, which may enhance the antigen-presenting function of β cells and subsequent CD4 T cell activation (4, 54).

Surprisingly, LTs also display an unexpected anti-inflammatory function. Under the setting of islet allo-transplantation, circulating Treg cells firstly arrive in the allograft and then access into the draining lymph nodes *via* the afferent lymphatic vessel, thereby suppressing the overactive immune response. The lymphatic trans-endothelial migration process is essential for the suppressive function of Treg cells. Specifically, Treg surface LTα1β2 binds to LTβR expressed on the lymphatic endothelial cells (LECs), which then activates the non-canonical NF-κB signaling pathway and promotes the expression of adhesion molecules such as VCAM-1, thereby facilitating Treg trans-endothelial migration. Deficiency or blockade of LT abrogates Treg migration and accelerates islet allograft rejection (55). Furthermore, under the inflammatory condition of islet transplantation, activation of TLR2 on Treg cells augments LTα1β2-LTβR signaling and enhances the permissiveness of lymphatic vessel, thereby directing leukocytes out of tissue and promoting resolution of inflammation (56). Collectively, the immune regulatory function of LTs exhibits an opposing effect (**Figure 2**). The pro-inflammatory or anti-inflammatory effect of LTs might hinge on the cell types affected, which warrants future investigations.

CONCLUSION AND PERSPECTIVES

LTs are multifunctional cytokines involved in T1D pathogenesis *via* promoting the formation of peri-islet TLOs, by which they synergize with other inflammatory mediators to enhance autoimmune responses and β cell destruction. It is worthy of note that LT alone manifests a relatively weak effect on β cell destruction. In this case, its contribution to T1D pathogenesis was almost neglected since the *in vivo* concentration of lymphotoxin is much lower than the dosage adopted in the *in vitro* studies. However, its impact on the formation of TLOs play a crucial role in autoimmune initiation and progression in T1D settings.

A critical feature for LTs is that they could exhibit both pro- and anti-inflammatory function. Previous studies demonstrated the role of LTs in stimulating immune responses. For instance, in LTA

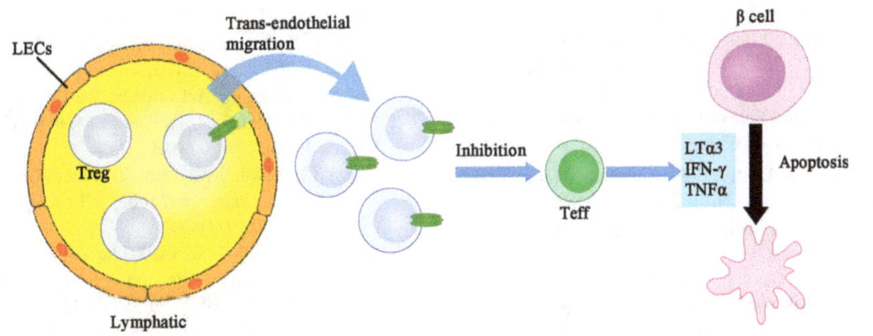

FIGURE 2 | The direct immune regulatory function of LTs. LTs exert dual immune regulatory roles. One the one hand, LTα1β2 expressing Treg cells have more active trans-endothelial migration which facilitates their suppression of islet infiltrating Teff cells. On the other, LTα3 assists in the direct killing of β cells, although the toxicity of LTα3 alone is limited. LEC, lymphatic endothelial cells; Treg, regulatory T cells; Teff, effector T cells.

deficient mice, CD8 T cells fail to up-regulate activation or memory markers coupled with lower level of IL-12 receptor expression and impaired cytotoxic function (57). Blockade of membrane LT inhibits CD8 T cell mediated rejection of intestinal allograft, indicating that it could be a feasible target to prevent allograft rejection (58). Moreover, LTs not only regulate DC and CD4 T cell homeostasis at steady state, but are essential for maintaining the symbiotic relationship between the hosts and their microbiota (59). LTα1β2 expressed on Treg cells alters the permeability of lymphatic vessel and promotes the resolution of inflammatory response, which represents a novel aspect of Treg suppressive function. Nonetheless, as the relevant studies are focused on the islet transplantation model, whether such mechanism can be applied to Treg cells under the context of T1D settings and other autoimmune diseases is yet an open question.

Ectopic lymphoid neogenesis is a characteristic pathological event observed in tissues with chronic inflammation. During the process of insulitis, TLOs form around the islets and resemble the function of pancreatic draining lymph nodes. Administration of LTbetaR-Ig impedes TLO formation or disintegrates already formed TLOs, thereby alleviating the progression of T1D (47). However, B lymphocytes may not be significantly affected by TLO disassembly. Specifically, after blockade of chemoattractant CXCL13 to destroy the organization TLOs in the islets, B cells located in the "chaotic milieu" are comparable to those presented in the "organized TLOs" in terms of BCR diversity and the occurrence of somatic hypermutation (SHM) (60). Moreover, FTY-720 treatment aimed at maintaining TLO integrity also exhibited a protective effect on T1D, although the possibility of FTY-720 mediated blockade of the exit of lymphocytes from the pancreatic draining lymph nodes into the pancreatic tissue could not be excluded (61).

In summary, blockade of LT signaling could be a useful supplement in the early intervention of T1D. Given the complex nature of crosstalk between immune cells and β cells under T1D setting, blockade of LT signaling applied to the existing therapies could be an efficient approach to delay or even reverse the established T1D.

AUTHOR CONTRIBUTIONS

S-WL and FS wrote the manuscript; S-JR gave valuable suggestions and made critical revisions. TW and C-YW conceptualized and supervised the preparation of this manuscript. All authors contributed to the article and approved the submitted version.

REFERENCES

1. Bluestone JA, Herold K, Eisenbarth G. Genetics, Pathogenesis and Clinical Interventions in Type 1 Diabetes. *Nature* (2010) 464(7293):1293–300. doi: 10.1038/nature08933
2. Bakay M, Pandey R, Grant SFA, Hakonarson H. The Genetic Contribution to Type 1 Diabetes. *Curr Diabetes Rep* (2019) 19(11):116. doi: 10.1007/s11892-019-1235-1
3. Santin I, Eizirik DL. Candidate Genes for Type 1 Diabetes Modulate Pancreatic Islet Inflammation and Beta-Cell Apoptosis. *Diabetes Obes Metab* (2013) 15(Suppl 3):71–81. doi: 10.1111/dom.12162
4. Li Y, Sun F, Yue TT, Wang FX, Yang CL, Luo JH, et al. Revisiting the Antigen-Presenting Function of Beta Cells in T1D Pathogenesis. *Front Immunol* (2021) 12:690783. doi: 10.3389/fimmu.2021.690783
5. Dedrick S, Sundaresh B, Huang Q, Brady C, Yoo T, Cronin C, et al. The Role of Gut Microbiota and Environmental Factors in Type 1 Diabetes Pathogenesis. *Front Endocrinol (Lausanne)* (2020) 11:78. doi: 10.3389/fendo.2020.00078
6. Zullo A, Sommese L, Nicoletti G, Donatelli F, Mancini FP, Napoli C, et al. Epigenetics and Type 1 Diabetes: Mechanisms and Translational Applications. *Transl Res* (2017) 185:85–93. doi: 10.1016/j.trsl.2017.05.002
7. Jacobsen LM, Newby BN, Perry DJ, Posgai AL, Haller MJ, Brusko TM, et al. Immune Mechanisms and Pathways Targeted in Type 1 Diabetes. *Curr Diabetes Rep* (2018) 18(10):90. doi: 10.1007/s11892-018-1066-5
8. Tsai S, Shameli A, Santamaria P. CD8+ T Cells in Type 1 Diabetes. *Adv Immunol* (2008) 100:79–124. doi: 10.1016/S0065-2776(08)00804-3
9. Kurohane Kaneko Y, Ishikawa T. Dual Role of Nitric Oxide in Pancreatic Beta-Cells. *J Pharmacol Sci* (2013) 123(4):295–300. doi: 10.1254/jphs.13R10CP
10. Thomas HE, Kay TW. Beta Cell Destruction in the Development of Autoimmune Diabetes in the Non-Obese Diabetic (NOD) Mouse. *Diabetes Metab Res Rev* (2000) 16(4):251–61. doi: 10.1002/1520-7560(200007/08)16:4<251::AID-DMRR126>3.0.CO;2-C
11. Yue T, Sun F, Wang FX, Yang CL, Luo JH, Rong SJ, et al. MBD2 Acts as a Repressor to Maintain the Homeostasis of the Th1 Program in Type 1 Diabetes by Regulating the STAT1-IFN-Gamma Axis. *Cell Death Differ* (2022) 29(1):218–29. doi: 10.1038/s41418-021-00852-6
12. Haskins K, Cooke A. CD4 T Cells and Their Antigens in the Pathogenesis of Autoimmune Diabetes. *Curr Opin Immunol* (2011) 23(6):739–45. doi: 10.1016/j.coi.2011.08.004
13. Li CR, Mueller EE, Bradley LM. Islet Antigen-Specific Th17 Cells can Induce TNF-Alpha-Dependent Autoimmune Diabetes. *J Immunol* (2014) 192 (4):1425–32. doi: 10.4049/jimmunol.1301742
14. Wachlin G, Augstein P, Schröder D, Kuttler B, Klöting I, Heinke P, et al. IL-1beta, IFN-Gamma and TNF-Alpha Increase Vulnerability of Pancreatic Beta Cells to Autoimmune Destruction. *J Autoimmun* (2003) 20(4):303–12. doi: 10.1016/S0896-8411(03)00039-8
15. Javeed N, Her TK, Brown MR, Vanderboom P, Rakshit K, Egan AM, et al. Pro-Inflammatory Beta Cell Small Extracellular Vesicles Induce Beta Cell Failure Through Activation of the CXCL10/CXCR3 Axis in Diabetes. *Cell Rep* (2021) 36(8):109613. doi: 10.1016/j.celrep.2021.109613
16. Antonelli A, Ferrari SM, Corrado A, Ferrannini E, Fallahi P. CXCR3, CXCL10 and Type 1 Diabetes. *Cytokine Growth Factor Rev* (2014) 25(1):57–65. doi: 10.1016/j.cytogfr.2014.01.006
17. Christen U, Kimmel R. Chemokines as Drivers of the Autoimmune Destruction in Type 1 Diabetes: Opportunity for Therapeutic Intervention in Consideration of an Optimal Treatment Schedule. *Front Endocrinol (Lausanne)* (2020) 11:591083. doi: 10.3389/fendo.2020.591083
18. Dostert C, Grusdat M, Letellier E, Brenner D. The TNF Family of Ligands and Receptors: Communication Modules in the Immune System and Beyond. *Physiol Rev* (2019) 99(1):115–60. doi: 10.1152/physrev.00045.2017
19. Holbrook J, Lara-Reyna S, Jarosz-Griffiths H, McDermott M. Tumour Necrosis Factor Signalling in Health and Disease. *F1000Res* (2019) 8. doi: 10.12688/f1000research.17023.1
20. Andera L. Signaling Activated by the Death Receptors of the TNFR Family. *BioMed Pap Med Fac Univ Palacky Olomouc Czech Repub* (2009) 153(3):173–80. doi: 10.5507/bp.2009.029
21. Arron JR, Walsh MC, Choi Y. TRAF-Mediated TNFR-Family Signaling. *Curr Protoc Immunol* (2002) Chapter 11:Unit11.9D. doi: 10.1002/0471142735.im1109ds87
22. Lee LF, Xu BH, Michie SA, Beilhack GF, Warganich T, Turley S, et al. The Role of TNF-Alpha in the Pathogenesis of Type 1 Diabetes in the Nonobese Diabetic Mouse: Analysis of Dendritic Cell Maturation. *Proc Natl Acad Sci USA* (2005) 102(44):15995–6000. doi: 10.1073/pnas.0508122102
23. So T, Ishii N. The TNF-TNFR Family of Co-Signal Molecules. *Adv Exp Med Biol 2019* (1189), 53–84. doi: 10.1007/978-981-32-9717-3_3
24. Thomas HE, Graham KL, Chee J, Thomas R, Kay TW, Krishnamurthy B, et al. Proinflammatory Cytokines Contribute to Development and Function of

Regulatory T Cells in Type 1 Diabetes. *Ann NY Acad Sci* (2013) 1283:81–6. doi: 10.1111/j.1749-6632.2012.06797.x

25. Chee J, Angstetra E, Mariana L, Graham KL, Carrington EM, Bluethmann H, et al. TNF Receptor 1 Deficiency Increases Regulatory T Cell Function in Nonobese Diabetic Mice. *J Immunol* (2011) 187(4):1702–12. doi: 10.4049/jimmunol.1100511
26. Paul NL, Ruddle NH. Lymphotoxin. *Annu Rev Immunol* (1988) 6:407–38. doi: 10.1146/annurev.iy.06.040188.002203
27. Gramaglia I, Mauri DN, Miner KT, Ware CF, Croft M. Lymphotoxin Alphabeta is Expressed on Recently Activated Naive and Th1-Like CD4 Cells But is Down-Regulated by IL-4 During Th2 Differentiation. *J Immunol* (1999) 162(3):1333–8.
28. Vanderkerken M, Baptista AP, De Giovanni M, Fukuyama S, Browaeys R, Scott CL, et al. ILC3s Control Splenic cDC Homeostasis via Lymphotoxin Signaling. *J Exp Med* (2021) 218(5). doi: 10.1084/jem.20190835
29. Withers DR, Kim MY, Bekiaris V, Rossi SW, Jenkinson WE, Gaspal F, et al. The Role of Lymphoid Tissue Inducer Cells in Splenic White Pulp Development. *Eur J Immunol* (2007) 37(11):3240–5. doi: 10.1002/eji.200737541
30. Suna S, Sakata Y, Shimizu M, Nakatani D, Usami M, Matsumoto S, et al. Lymphotoxin-Alpha3 Mediates Monocyte-Endothelial Interaction by TNFR I/NF-kappaB Signaling. *Biochem Biophys Res Commun* (2009) 379(2):374–8. doi: 10.1016/j.bbrc.2008.12.064
31. Dejardin E. The Alternative NF-KappaB Pathway From Biochemistry to Biology: Pitfalls and Promises for Future Drug Development. *Biochem Pharmacol* (2006) 72(9):1161–79. doi: 10.1016/j.bcp.2006.08.007
32. Weinstein AM, Storkus WJ. Therapeutic Lymphoid Organogenesis in the Tumor Microenvironment. *Adv Cancer Res* (2015) 128:197–233. doi: 10.1016/bs.acr.2015.04.003
33. Wen PF, Wang XS, Zhang M, Cen H, Pan HF, Ye QL, et al. Associations Between TNF Gene Polymorphisms (-308 A/G, -238 A/G, -1031 C/T and -857 T/C) and Genetic Susceptibility to T1D: A Meta-Analysis. *Endocrine* (2014) 46(3):435–44. doi: 10.1007/s12020-014-0172-7
34. Vendrell J, Ercilla G, Gutierrez C, Gomis R, Goday A, Fernandez J, et al. A Tumor Necrosis Factor Beta-Gene Polymorphism Associated With Islet Cell Antibodies in Newly Diagnosed Type I Diabetic Patients. *Diabetes Care* (1994) 17(8):944–5. doi: 10.2337/diacare.17.8.944
35. Noble JA, Valdes AM, Lane JA, Green AE, Erlich HA. Linkage Disequilibrium With Predisposing DR3 Haplotypes Accounts for Apparent Effects of Tumor Necrosis Factor and Lymphotoxin-Alpha Polymorphisms on Type 1 Diabetes Susceptibility. *Hum Immunol* (2006) 67(12):999–1004. doi: 10.1016/j.humimm.2006.10.002
36. Kägi D, Ho A, Odermatt B, Zakarian A, Ohashi PS, Mak TW, et al. TNF Receptor 1-Dependent Beta Cell Toxicity as an Effector Pathway in Autoimmune Diabetes. *J Immunol* (1999) 162(8):4598–605.
37. Levisetti MG, Suri A, Frederick K, Unanue ER. Absence of Lymph Nodes in NOD Mice Treated With Lymphotoxin-Beta Receptor Immunoglobulin Protects From Diabetes. *Diabetes* (2004) 53(12):3115–9. doi: 10.2337/diabetes.53.12.3115
38. Ettinger R, Munson SH, Chao CC, Vadeboncoeur M, Toma J, McDevitt HO. A Critical Role for Lymphotoxin-Beta Receptor in the Development of Diabetes in Nonobese Diabetic Mice. *J Exp Med* (2001) 193(11):1333–40. doi: 10.1084/jem.193.11.1333
39. Luther SA, Bidgol A, Hargreaves DC, Schmidt A, Xu Y, Paniyadi J, et al. Differing Activities of Homeostatic Chemokines CCL19, CCL21, and CXCL12 in Lymphocyte and Dendritic Cell Recruitment and Lymphoid Neogenesis. *J Immunol* (2002) 169(1):424–33. doi: 10.4049/jimmunol.169.1.424
40. Luther SA, Lopez T, Bai W, Hanahan D, Cyster JG. BLC Expression in Pancreatic Islets Causes B Cell Recruitment and Lymphotoxin-Dependent Lymphoid Neogenesis. *Immunity* (2000) 12(5):471–81. doi: 10.1016/S1074-7613(00)80199-5
41. Luther SA, Ansel KM, Cyster JG. Overlapping Roles of CXCL13, Interleukin 7 Receptor Alpha, and CCR7 Ligands in Lymph Node Development. *J Exp Med* (2003) 197(9):1191–8. doi: 10.1084/jem.20021294
42. Astorri E, Bombardieri M, Gabba S, Peakman M, Pozzilli P, Pitzalis C. Evolution of Ectopic Lymphoid Neogenesis and in Situ Autoantibody Production in Autoimmune Nonobese Diabetic Mice: Cellular and Molecular Characterization of Tertiary Lymphoid Structures in Pancreatic Islets. *J Immunol* (2010) 185(6):3359–68. doi: 10.4049/jimmunol.1001836
43. Kratz A, Campos-Neto A, Hanson MS, Ruddle NH. Chronic Inflammation Caused by Lymphotoxin is Lymphoid Neogenesis. *J Exp Med* (1996) 183 (4):1461–72. doi: 10.1084/jem.183.4.1461
44. Lee Y, Chin RK, Christiansen P, Sun Y, Tumanov AV, Wang J, et al. Recruitment and Activation of Naive T Cells in the Islets by Lymphotoxin Beta Receptor-Dependent Tertiary Lymphoid Structure. *Immunity* (2006) 25 (3):499–509. doi: 10.1016/j.immuni.2006.06.016
45. Gonzalez Badillo FE, Zisi Tegou F, Abreu MM, Masina R, Sha D, Najjar M, et al. CCL21 Expression in Beta-Cells Induces Antigen-Expressing Stromal Cell Networks in the Pancreas and Prevents Autoimmune Diabetes in Mice. *Diabetes* (2019) 68(10):1990–2003. doi: 10.2337/db19-0239
46. Korpos É, Kadri N, Loismann S, Findeisen CR, Arfuso F, Burke GW 3rd, et al. Identification and Characterisation of Tertiary Lymphoid Organs in Human Type 1 Diabetes. *Diabetologia* (2021) 64(7):1626–41. doi: 10.1007/s00125-021-05453-z
47. Wu Q, Salomon B, Chen M, Wang Y, Hoffman LM, Bluestone JA, et al. Reversal of Spontaneous Autoimmune Insulitis in Nonobese Diabetic Mice by Soluble Lymphotoxin Receptor. *J Exp Med* (2001) 193(11):1327–32. doi: 10.1084/jem.193.11.1327
48. Pukel C, Baquerizo H, Rabinovitch A. Destruction of Rat Islet Cell Monolayers by Cytokines. Synergistic Interactions of Interferon-Gamma, Tumor Necrosis Factor, Lymphotoxin, and Interleukin 1. *Diabetes* (1988) 37(1):133–6. doi: 10.2337/diab.37.1.133
49. Kawahara DJ, Kenney JS. Species Differences in Human and Rat Islet Sensitivity to Human Cytokines. Monoclonal Anti-Interleukin-1 (IL-1) Influences on Direct and Indirect IL-1-Mediated Islet Effects. *Cytokine* (1991) 3(2):117–24. doi: 10.1016/1043-4666(91)90031-8
50. Mandrup-Poulsen T, Bendtzen K, Dinarello CA, Nerup J. Human Tumor Necrosis Factor Potentiates Human Interleukin 1-Mediated Rat Pancreatic Beta-Cell Cytotoxicity. *J Immunol* (1987) 139(12):4077–82.
51. Picarella DE, Kratz A, Li CB, Ruddle NH, Flavell RA. Transgenic Tumor Necrosis Factor (TNF)-Alpha Production in Pancreatic Islets Leads to Insulitis, Not Diabetes. Distinct Patterns of Inflammation in TNF-Alpha and TNF-Beta Transgenic Mice. *J Immunol* (1993) 150(9):4136–50.
52. Picarella DE, Kratz A, Li CB, Ruddle NH, Flavell RA. Insulitis in Transgenic Mice Expressing Tumor Necrosis Factor Beta (Lymphotoxin) in the Pancreas. *Proc Natl Acad Sci USA* (1992) 89(21):10036–40. doi: 10.1073/pnas.89.21.10036
53. Hirai H, Kaino Y, Ito T, Kida K. Analysis of Cytokine mRNA Expression in Pancreatic Islets of Nonobese Diabetic Mice. *J Pediatr Endocrinol Metab* (2000) 13(1):91–8. doi: 10.1515/JPEM.2000.13.1.91
54. Pujol-Borrell R, Todd I, Doshi M, Bottazzo GF, Sutton R, Gray D, et al. HLA Class II Induction in Human Islet Cells by Interferon-Gamma Plus Tumour Necrosis Factor or Lymphotoxin. *Nature* (1987) 326(6110):304–6. doi: 10.1038/326304a0
55. Brinkman CC, Iwami D, Hritzo MK, Xiong Y, Ahmad S, Simon T, et al. Treg Engage Lymphotoxin Beta Receptor for Afferent Lymphatic Transendothelial Migration. *Nat Commun* (2016) 7:12021. doi: 10.1038/ncomms12021
56. Piao W, Xiong Y, Li L, Saxena V, Smith KD, Hippen KL, et al. Regulatory T Cells Condition Lymphatic Endothelia for Enhanced Transendothelial Migration. *Cell Rep* (2020) 30(4):1052–62.e5. doi: 10.1016/j.celrep.2019.12.083
57. Kumaraguru U, Davis IA, Deshpande S, Tevethia SS, Rouse BT. Lymphotoxin Alpha-/- Mice Develop Functionally Impaired CD8+ T Cell Responses and Fail to Contain Virus Infection of the Central Nervous System. *J Immunol* (2001) 166(2):1066–74. doi: 10.4049/jimmunol.166.2.1066
58. Guo Z, Wang J, Meng L, Wu Q, Kim O, Hart J, et al. Cutting Edge: Membrane Lymphotoxin Regulates CD8(+) T Cell-Mediated Intestinal Allograft Rejection. *J Immunol* (2001) 167(9):4796–800. doi: 10.4049/jimmunol.167.9.4796
59. Upadhyay V, Fu YX. Lymphotoxin Signalling in Immune Homeostasis and the Control of Microorganisms. *Nat Rev Immunol* (2013) 13(4):270–9. doi: 10.1038/nri3406
60. Henry RA, Kendall PL. CXCL13 Blockade Disrupts B Lymphocyte Organization in Tertiary Lymphoid Structures Without Altering B Cell Receptor Bias or Preventing Diabetes in Nonobese Diabetic Mice. *J Immunol* (2010) 185(3):1460–5. doi: 10.4049/jimmunol.0903710
61. Penaranda C, Tang Q, Ruddle NH, Bluestone JA. Prevention of Diabetes by FTY720-Mediated Stabilization of Peri-Islet Tertiary Lymphoid Organs. *Diabetes* (2010) 59(6):1461–8. doi: 10.2337/db09-1129

18

Tracking of an Oral *Salmonella*-Based Vaccine for Type 1 Diabetes in Non-Obese Diabetic Mice

*Jacques C. Mbongue[1], Ali Alhoshani[2], Jeffrey Rawson[1], Pablo A. Garcia[1], Nelson Gonzalez[1], Kevin Ferreri[1], Fouad Kandeel[1] and Mohamed I. Husseiny[1,3]**

[1] Department of Translational Research and Cellular Therapeutics, Diabetes and Metabolism Research Institute, Beckman Research Institute, City of Hope National Medical Center, Duarte, CA, United States, [2] Department of Pharmacology and Toxicology, College of Pharmacy, King Saud University, Riyadh, Saudi Arabia, [3] Faculty of Pharmacy, Zagazig University, Zagazig, Egypt

***Correspondence:**
Mohamed I. Husseiny
melsayed@coh.org

Type 1 diabetes (T1D) arises secondary to immune-driven destruction of pancreatic β-cells and manifests as insulin-deficient hyperglycemia. We showed that oral vaccination with live attenuated *Salmonella*, which simultaneously delivers autoantigens and a TGFβ expression vector to immune cells in the gut mucosa, provides protection against the progression of T1D in non-obese diabetic (NOD) mice. In this study we employed the Sleeping Beauty (SB) transposon system that is composed of a transposase and transposon encoding the td-Tomato to express red fluorescent protein (RFP) to permanently mark the cells that take up the *Salmonella* vaccine. After animal vaccination, the transposon labeled-dendritic cells (DCs) with red fluorescence appeared throughout the secondary lymphoid tissues. Furthermore, Sleeping Beauty containing *tgfβ1* gene (SB-tgfβ1) co-expressed TGFβ and RFP. The labeled DCs were detected predominantly in Peyer's patches (PP) and mesenteric lymph nodes (MLN) and expressed CD103 surface marker. CD103$^+$ DCs induced tolerogenic effects and gut homing. TGFβ significantly increased programmed death-ligand-1 (PDL-1 or CD274) expression in the DCs in the MLN and PP of treated mice. Also, TGFβ increased cytotoxic T-lymphocyte-associated protein-4 (CTLA-4) levels in CD4$^+$ cells in MLN and PP. Interestingly, DCs increased in all lymphatic organs of mice vaccinated with oral live *Salmonella*-based vaccine expressing preproinsulin (PPI), in combination with TGFβ, IL10, and subtherapeutic-doses of anti-CD3 mAb compared with vehicle-treated mice. These DCs are mostly tolerogenic in MLN and PP. Furthermore the DCs obtained from vaccine-treated but not vehicle-treated mice suppressed *in vitro* T cell proliferation. These data suggest that the MLN and the PP are a central hub for the beneficial anti-diabetic effects of an oral *Salmonella*-based vaccine prevention of diabetes in rodents.

Keywords: *Salmonella*-based vaccine, sleeping beauty, transposons, Type 1 Diabetes, CD103$^+$DC, TGFβ, tolerogenic dendritic cells

INTRODUCTION

Type 1 diabetes (T1D) results from auto-reactive killing of the pancreatic islet insulin-producing β-cells (1). Studies have shown that pre-proinsulin (PPI) is an initial autoantigen in non-obese diabetic (NOD) mice (2) and humans (3–5) promoting dysfunctional autoimmunity. Using oral antigen-specific vaccines of live attenuated (non-pathogenic) *Salmonella typhimurium* diabetic autoantigens have been delivered to mice (6, 7). Non-specific immune response in NOD mice was reported when an infection was induced with attenuated *S. typhimurium* (8–10). When orally administered, *Salmonella* moves from the gut to the gut-associated lymphoid tissues (GALT) of antigen presenting cells (APCs), resulting in formation of *Salmonella*-containing vacuoles (SCV) (11–13). *Salmonella* has two Type 3 Secretion Systems (T3SS) to invade and disseminate in organs (14). The T3SS encoded by *Salmonella* Pathogenicity Island 1 (SPI1-T3SS) is expressed by extracellular bacteria and is required for the invasion of non-phagocytic cells. The T3SS encoded by *Salmonella* Pathogenicity Island 2 (SPI2-T3SS) is expressed by intracellular *Salmonella* and is required for intracellular replication and systemic pathogenesis (15). The genes of SPI2-T3SS are induced inside the SCV and express specific antigens in GALT APCs. This has promoted the development of anti-cancer vaccines and a T1D vaccine (6, 10–12, 16–18). Fusion of heterologous antigens to specific SPI2-T3SS proteins causes them to be presented to lymphocytes within the gut mucosa (12, 19, 20). This minimizes and/or bypasses intestinal lumen antigen expression and subsequent degradation of the same. *Salmonella* can also deliver plasmids to host APCs and this feature has led to generation of DNA vaccines (21, 22). A novel diabetes vaccine enabled direct expression of tolerogenic cytokines like TGFβ and IL10 and induced tolerance to diabetic auto-antigens (10, 23). These APCs process and produce the antigens which migrate to other organs in the gut and stimulate the immune cells (9, 24).

Initial uptake of *Salmonella* vaccine by GALT-associated DCs helped promote oral tolerance (25). Antigens arising in the large bowel were transported to the GALT by migrating $CD103^+$ DCs (25, 26). Tolerogenic dendritic cells (tolDCs) are especially active at suppressing immune activation (27–30). These effects are mediated through tolerogenic APC that induce T cell anergy, T cell apoptosis as well as induction of Tregs and type 1 regulatory T cells (Tr1) (28–35). $CD103^+$ DCs induced tolerance and gut homing, protecting against colitis in mice. Also, reduction in celiac disease was attributed to the activity of $CD11c^+CD103^+$ DCs in rodents (36–38). We hypothesized that tolerogenic $CD103^+$ DCs are intimately involved in the sampling and trafficking of the *Salmonella* antigen in NOD mice (37, 39–41). To identify the initial cell population mediating the oral vaccine effect, we developed a novel approach to label the cells that take up the *Salmonella* vaccine. It uses a transposon system known as Sleeping Beauty (SB;) (42) which is composed of Sleeping Beauty transposase and a transposon encoding the td-Tomato red fluorescent protein-expressing gene which permanently inserts into the genome of vertebrate animals (43, 44). Treating mice with *Salmonella* containing both plasmids enables passing of the plasmids to the host cells resulting in permanent marking of the cells. Using this approach permitted tracking and characterization of the cells mediating the vaccine effect. Here, we define the cells that uptake *Salmonella* and are essential for mediating the vaccine effect and characterize these cells as tolerogenic DCs based on the expression of regulatory molecules and secretion of cytokines.

MATERIALS AND METHODS

Preparation of *Salmonella* Strain and Plasmid Construction

Salmonella typhimurium MvP728 (Δ*htrA*/Δ*purD*) has function as an oral vaccine vector (10, 23, 45). Bacteria were cultured in Luria-Bertani (LB) with or without chloramphenicol and/or carbenicillin (50 μ g/ml).

The pSBbi-RP (#60513) (42) and pCMV(CAT)T7-SB100 (#34879) (46) plasmids for the Sleeping Beauty transposon system were from Addgene and kindly donated from the Kowarz and Izsvak Laboratories. The two plasmids were transformed into competent double mutant *S. typhimurium* MvP728 using electroporation (Bio Rad) after which sensitivity to carbenicillin and chloramphenicol was employed for selection.

Mouse *tgfb1* sequence was amplified from pCMV6-Entry-*tgfb1* (Origene, MR227339) using forward primer 5′-CCATGGATGCCGCCCTCGGG-3′ and 5′-AAGCTTTTAAACCTTATCGTCGTCATCCTTG-3′ reverse primer. The PCR fragment was cloned using TOPO TA cloning kit (Thermo fisher, 450641) and confirmed by sequencing. Next, the *tgfb1* sequence was cut by *NcoI*/*Hin*dIII then subcloned into *NcoI*/*Hin*dIII digested pSBbi-RP plasmid to yield pSBbi-RP-TGFβ (**Figure 1A**). The pSBbi-RP-TGFβ and pCMV(CAT)T7-SB100 plasmids were transformed into *Salmonella* as described (47).

In vitro Infection

The murine RAW264.7 macrophage cell line was obtained from the American Type Culture Collection (ATCC no.-TIB-71). The cells were plated in 24-well plates (5×10^4 cells per well) and were allowed to attach overnight at 37°C in an atmosphere of 5% CO_2. Overnight cultures of *Salmonella* containing pCMV(CAT)T7-SB100 and pSBbi-RP or pSBbi-RP-TGFβ were diluted and added to the cells growing in 24 well tissue culture plates at a multiplicity of infection of about 20. The bacteria were centrifuged onto the cells at $500 \times g$ for 5 min. The plates were placed in an incubator for 25 min at 37°C for uptake of bacteria. Wells were washed three times with PBS and then incubated for 1 h in media containing 100 μg/ml of gentamicin to kill extracellular bacteria. Subsequent growth media were supplemented with 10 μg/ml of gentamicin for the remainder of the experiment. Given that pSBbi-RP confers resistance to puromycin, RAW 264.7 macrophages that incorporated the transposon were positively selected by the addition of puromycin (2 μg/ml). Cultures were treated with *Salmonella*-expressing both pSBbi-RP or pSBbi-RP-TGFβ and pCMV(CAT)T7-SB100 and cultured from 7 to 60 days for expression analysis. A ZEISS inverted LSM700 microscope was employed to obtain images that were processed with ZEN-lite digital imaging software (CarlZeiss, Oberkochen, Germany) for processing. The expression of TGFβ by macrophages was analyzed in cell lysate or culture supernatant by Western blot analysis.

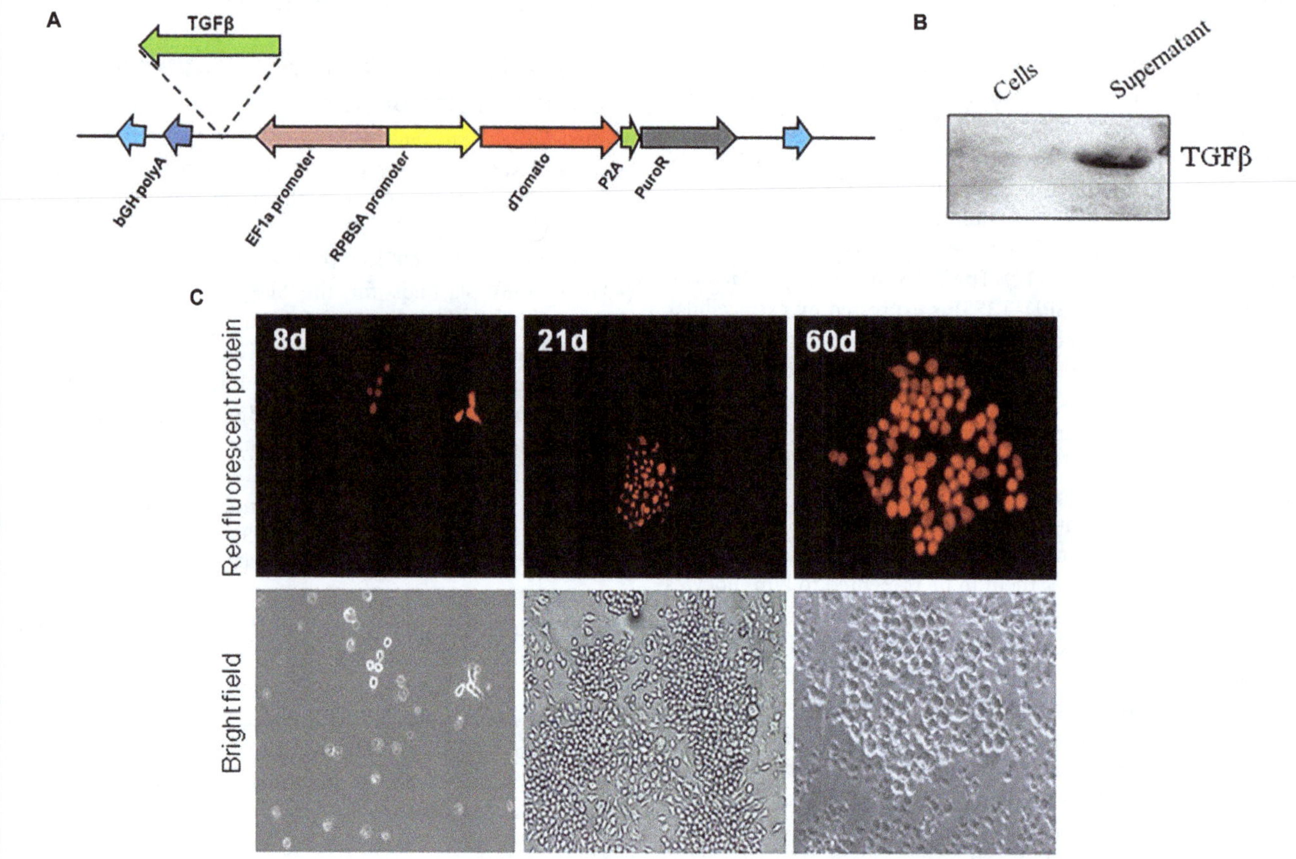

FIGURE 1 | *In vitro* expression of Sleeping Beauty transposon in RAW 264.7 macrophages. **(A)** Plasmid (pSBbi-RP-TGFβ) construct for transposon coding for Td-Tomato and a puromycin resistance gene. The location for insertion of the mouse TGFβ on the plasmid is shown. *In vitro* infection of RAW 264.7 macrophages with *Salmonella*-carrying both the Sleeping Beauty Transposon plasmid pSBbi-RP or pSBbi-RP-TGFβ and transposase plasmid pCMV (CAT) T7 SB-100. **(B)** Western blot of cell lysate and supernatant performed 60 days after bacterial infection of macrophages using a DDK tag for TGFβ. **(C)** Expression of red fluorescent protein at 8, 21, and 60 days post-infection. Fluorescent images were acquired on a ZEISS inverted LSM700 microscope at 20x.

Animal Experiments

Seven-week-old female NOD/ShiLtJ mice (Jackson Laboratory, Bar Harbor, ME, United States) were housed in pathogen-free conditions. City of Hope has been fully accredited by the Association for Assessment and Accreditation of Laboratory Animal Care International (AAALAC). The study was approved by the Institutional Animal Care and Use Committee of City of Hope (IACUC# 11032).

Eight-week-old NOD mice were vaccinated on days 0 and 7 by oral gavage with 10^7 CFU/mouse in a total volume of 200 μl of 5% sodium bicarbonate as described (10, 23, 45). Furthermore, vaccinated animals were treated with hamster anti-CD3 mAb for five consecutive days (days 0–4; 2.5 μ g i.p./mouse).

Flow Cytometry

Single cell suspensions of spleen, pancreatic lymph nodes (PLN), mesenteric lymph nodes (MLN), and Peyer's patches (PP) were digested in collagenase D (1 mg/ml) at week 4 post-vaccination. Cells were stained directly with the following conjugated antibodies: MHC-II FITC anti-mouse I-Ak (Aβk), APC anti-mouse CD11c, Brilliant Violet 605 anti-mouse CD103, PE anti-mouse CD80, Brilliant Violet 711 anti-mouse CD86 and matching isotype controls. Cells were also stained with anti-mouse CD11b PE/Cy7, BV650 anti-mouse/human CD45R/B220, BV510 anti- mouse Ly-6G/Ly-6C (Gr-1) and matching isotype controls. Signal height and width were used to exclude doublets. Dead cells were excluded using Fixable Live/Dead Yellow Stain (Invitrogen), according to the manufacturer's protocol. All antibodies and isotypes were obtained from Biolegend (San Diego, United States). A BD Fortessa flow cytometer (BD Biosciences) and FlowJo software gated on isotype controlled single DAPI-negative cell populations was used for FACS.

In vitro Proliferation Assay and Cytokine Assay

Responder T cells (Tresp) were generated and isolated from spleens of NOD mice (3 mice) immunized with insulin peptide B9-23 (100 μg) and emulsified in complete Freund adjuvant (CFA). After 11 days $CD4^+CD25^-$ Tresp cells were isolated from pooled splenocytes using negative selection for $CD4^+$ followed by negative selection for $CD25^+$ using a $CD4^+CD25^+$ regulatory T Cell Isolation Kit (Miltenyi Biotec, 130-091-041) and then

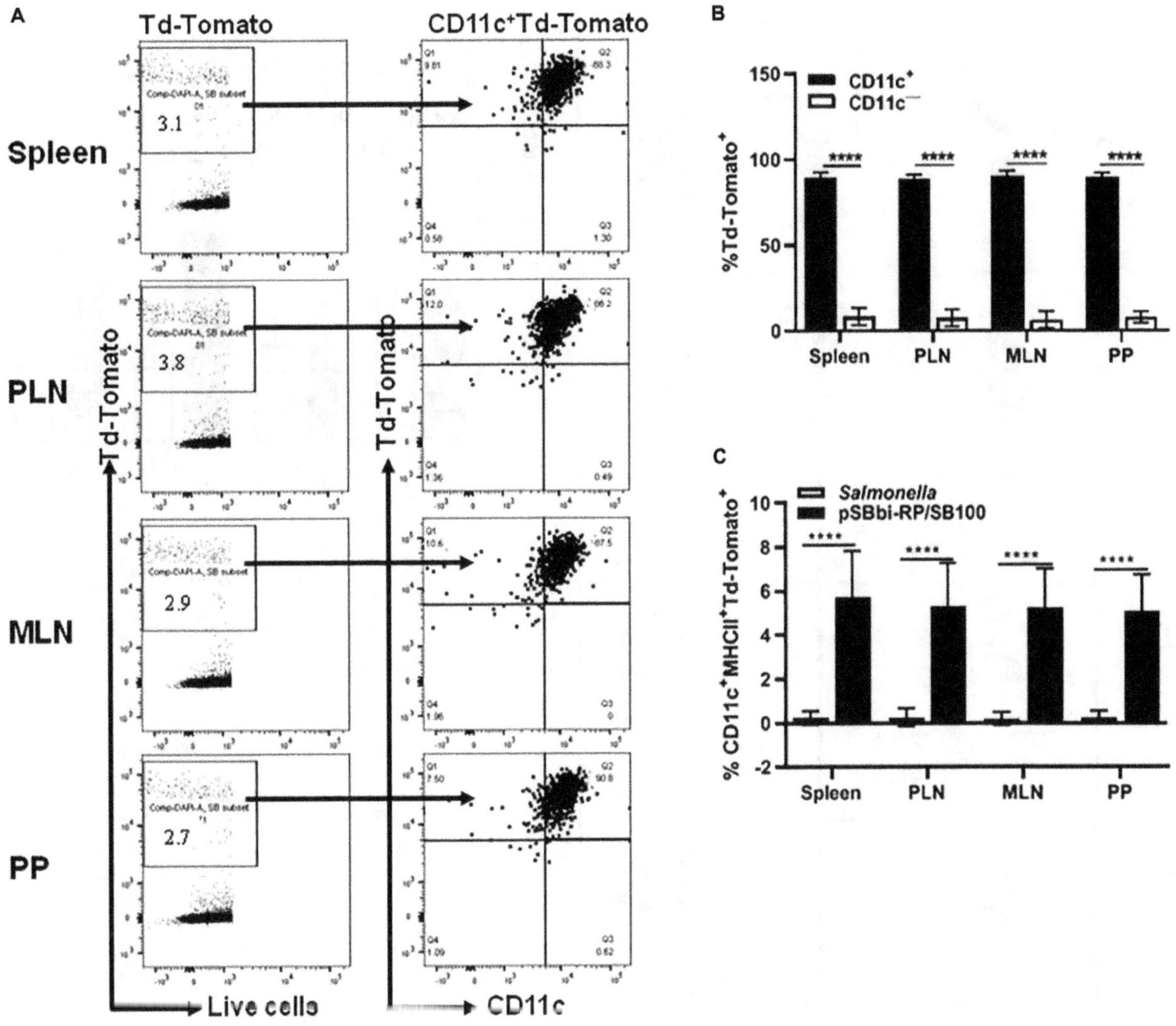

FIGURE 2 | *In vivo* detection of the red fluorescent protein in different organs of vaccinated NOD mice. NOD mice were given a single oral dose of *Salmonella*-containing plasmid (pSBbi-RP/SB100, $n = 10$) compared to *Salmonella* only ($n = 10$). Four weeks post-vaccination, red fluorescent protein was detected in different organs. **(A)** Representative FACS plots gated the frequency of live red-labeled $CD11c^+$ and $CD11c^-$ cells in the spleens, pancreatic lymph nodes (PLN), mesenteric lymph nodes (MLN), and Peyer's patches (PP) of mice from each group. **(B)** Quantification of the percentages of the $CD11c^+$ and $CD11c^-$ red-labeled cells in all organs. **(C)** Quantification of the percentages of red-labeled $CD11c^+MHCII^+$ in total live cells isolated from the spleen, PLN, MLN, and PP. The data shown are as the average with standard deviation (SD) obtained from two independent experiments. Statistical analysis using two-way ANOVA shows significance between groups ($^{****}p < 0.0001$).

labeled with 1:1000 of 5 mM Cell Trace Violet (CTV) (48). $CD4^+CD25^+$ Treg cells were isolated from pooled splenocytes of non-vaccinated NOD mice (5 mice) using negative selection for $CD4^+$ followed by positive selection for $CD25^+$ using a $CD4^+CD25^+$ regulatory T Cell Isolation Kit (Miltenyi Biotec, 130-091-041). Dendritic cells (DCs) were isolated from pooled splenocytes (5 mice) isolated from either vaccinated or non-vaccinated mice using PE-conjugated CD11c antibody (Miltenyi, 130-110-701) followed by anti-PE microbeads (Miltenyi Biotec, 130-091-041). The Tresp cells (1×10^5 cells/well) were co-cultured in 96-well round bottom plates with or without 1×10^5 Treg cells isolated from non-vaccinated mice using different ratios of DCs isolated from either vaccinated or non-vaccinated mice in the presence of insulin peptide B9-23 (10 μg/ml). After 3 days, the proliferation of CD4 responder T cells positive for CTV and with surface expression of CD44 and CD69 (signifying cell activation) was analyzed by gating on proliferated cells using FlowJo software 10.4.

Cell free supernatants were collected for detection of IL10, TGFβ, IFNγ, and TNFα using Mouse Quantikine ELISA Kits (R&D Systems) according to the manufacturer's instructions.

Gene Expression

RNA isolated from sorted $CD11c^+$ and $CD3^+CD4^+$ cells obtained from splenocytes, PLN, MLN, and PP were isolated using the DirectZol kit (Zymo Research). Between 3 and 5×10^5 cells were sorted with 80 to 90% viability. RNA concentration was measured with a Nanodrop 2000 (Thermo

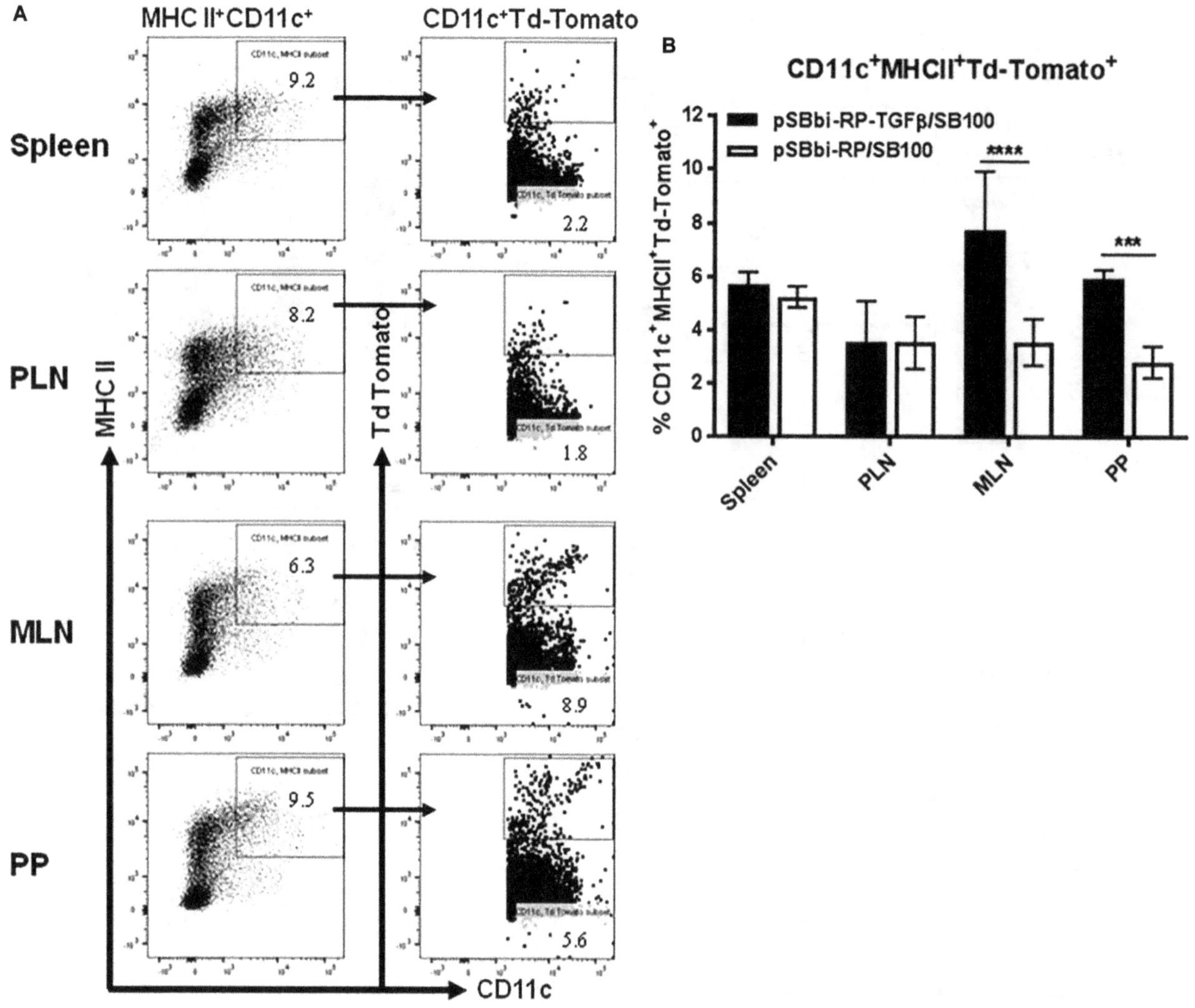

FIGURE 3 | Vaccine-delivered TGFβ alters levels of DCs in secondary lymphoid tissues. NOD mice were given a single oral dose of *Salmonella* (pSBbi-RP-TGFβ/SB100, $n = 10$) or *Salmonella* (pSBbi-RP/SB100, $n = 10$). Four weeks post-vaccination, red fluorescent protein was detected in DCs of different organs. **(A)** Representative FACS plots gated the frequency of $MHCII^+CD11c^+Td\text{-}Tomato^+$ cells in the spleens, PLN, MLN, and PP of mice from each group. **(B)** Quantification of the percentages of $MHCII^+CD11c^+Td\text{-}Tomato^+$ cells in the spleen, PLN, MLN, and PP. The data shown are the average with SD from two independent experiments. Statistical analysis using two-way ANOVA shows significance between *Salmonella* (pSBbi-RP-TGFβ/SB100) and *Salmonella* (pSBbi-RP/SB100) groups (***$p < 0.001$, ****$p < 0\ 0001$).

Scientific). A 260/280 ratio of 1.8 to 2.00 was considered for RNA purity. Total RNA (500 ng) was used for cDNA synthesis using the qScript cDNA SuperMix kit (Quantabio). qPCR analysis was performed using TaqMan gene expression assays (Applied Biosystem) according to the manufacturer's protocol. qRT-PCR was done with ABI Fast 7500 software (Applied Biosystems, ABI). Primers and probes were purchased from Applied Biosystems: CD274 (Mm03048248_ml), and CTLA4 (Mm00486849_ml). Relative changes in mRNA were calculated using the ΔΔCt method. Ct values of target genes were calculated relative to a reference control gene (TATA box binding protein, Tbp (Mm01277042_ml) using the following formula $\Delta Ct = Ct_{Target}\text{-}Ct_{Reference}$. Expression level = $2^{-\Delta Ct}$.

Statistical Analyses

Two-way ANOVA were used for analysis of the percentage of positive cells between groups and to compare cell populations after FACS analysis. A $p < 0.05$ was considered significant. Statistical analysis was performed using GraphPad Prism 8 software.

RESULTS

In vitro Expression of Sleeping Beauty

RAW 264.7 macrophages were infected *in vitro* with *S. typhimurium* carrying both Sleeping Beauty Td-Tomato transposon plasmid (pSBbi-RP) and the transposase plasmid

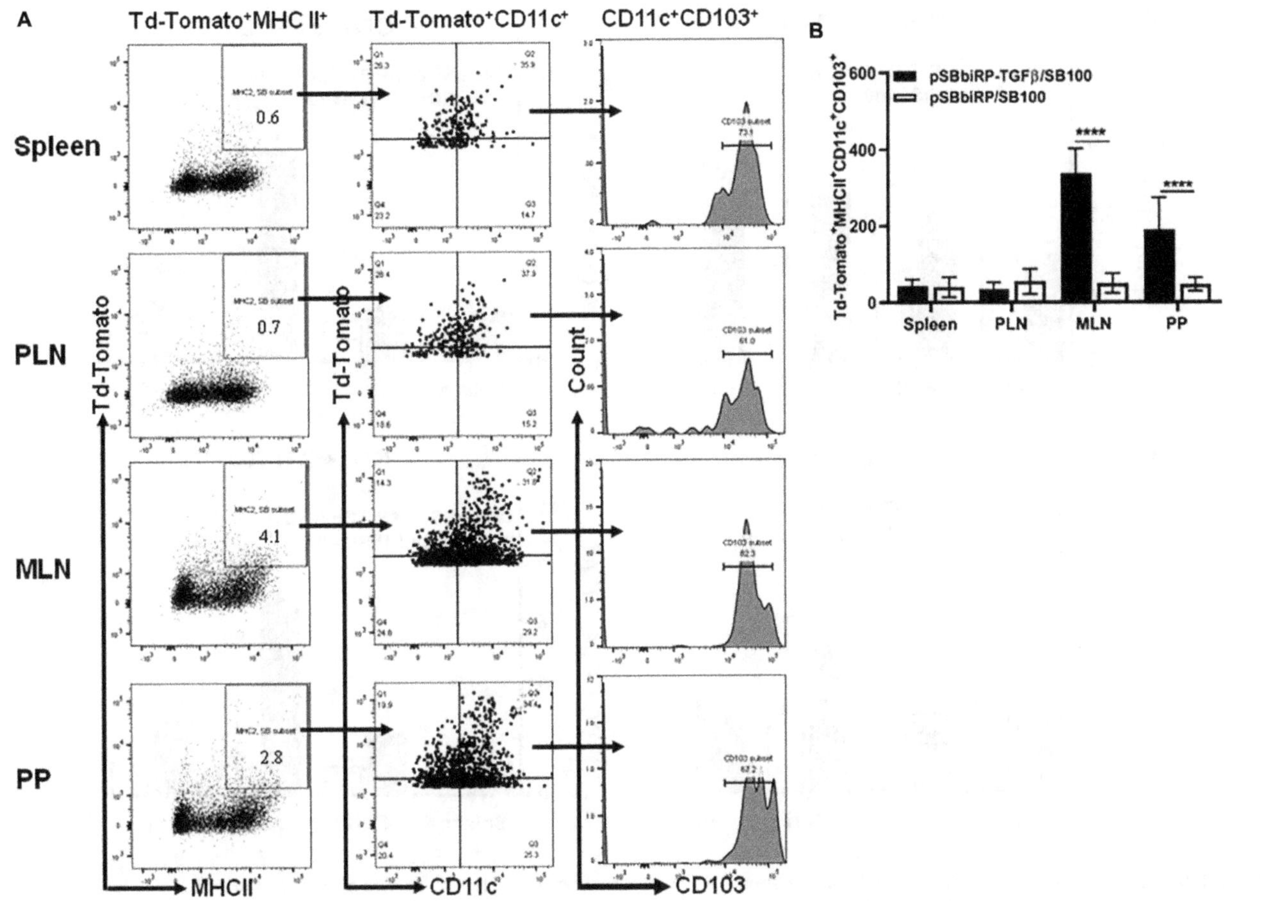

FIGURE 4 | Vaccine-delivered TGFβ alters levels of gut DCs. NOD mice were given a single oral dose of *Salmonella* (pSBbi-RP-TGFβ/SB100, $n = 10$) or *Salmonella* (pSBbi-RP/SB100, $n = 10$). Four weeks post-vaccination, red fluorescent protein was detected in DCs of different organs. **(A)** Representative FACS plots gated the frequency of the live red-labeled MHCII$^+$CD11c$^+$CD103$^+$ cells in the spleens, PLN, MLN, and PP of mice from each group. **(B)** Quantification of the numbers of MHCII$^+$CD11c$^+$CD103$^+$ in red-labeled cells in the spleen, PLN, MLN, and PP. The data shown are the average with SD from two independent experiments. Statistical analysis using two-way ANOVA shows significance between *Salmonella* (pSBbi-RP-TGFβ/SB100) and *Salmonella* (pSBbi-RP/SB100) groups (****$p < 0.0001$).

pCMV(CAT)T7-SB100 (SB100) (**Figure 1A**). The expression of TGFβ was detected in supernatant only after infection of macrophages with pSBbi-RP-TGFβ and pCMV(CAT)T7-SB100 (**Figure 1B**), implying that TGFβ was secreted after expression by host cells under the control of the CMV promoter.

Additionally the expression of RFP after infection of RAW macrophages was detected. RAW macrophages infected with the pSBbi-RP transposon, but not the pCMV(CAT)T7-SB100 transposase plasmid, were negatively selected by the addition of 2 μg/ml of puromycin. pCMV(CAT)T7-SB100 which codes for transposase conferred long-term resistance to puromycin in RAW macrophages as well as permanent expression of RFP. The presence of red colonies was seen consistently at 7–8 days post-infection (**Figure 1C**). The expression of the RFP appeared to be permanent as the fluorescent colonies grown for more than 60 days post-infection continued to show signal (**Figure 1C**).

In vivo Labeling of Antigen-Presenting Cells

Although *Salmonella*-mediated labeling of RAW cells occurred *in vitro*, it was not known whether this cell labeling would occur *in vivo*. Mice were administered a single dose of *Salmonella*-containing both transposon (pSBbi-RP) and transposase (SB100) plasmids. Four weeks later, flow cytometry demonstrated red fluorescent cells in the PP, MLN, PLN, and spleen of inoculated NOD mice. Characterization showed that the majority of red-labeled cells were CD11c$^+$ indicating that they were indeed DCs (**Figure 2A**). However, a minority of red-labeled cells were found to be other than DCs (**Figure 2B**). Further characterization of red-labeled DCs showed that they were MHCII$^+$ APCs (**Figure 2C**). Overall, red-labeled MHCII$^+$CD11c$^+$ DCs comprised 5 to 10% of total live cells in the secondary lymphoid tissues (**Figure 2C**).

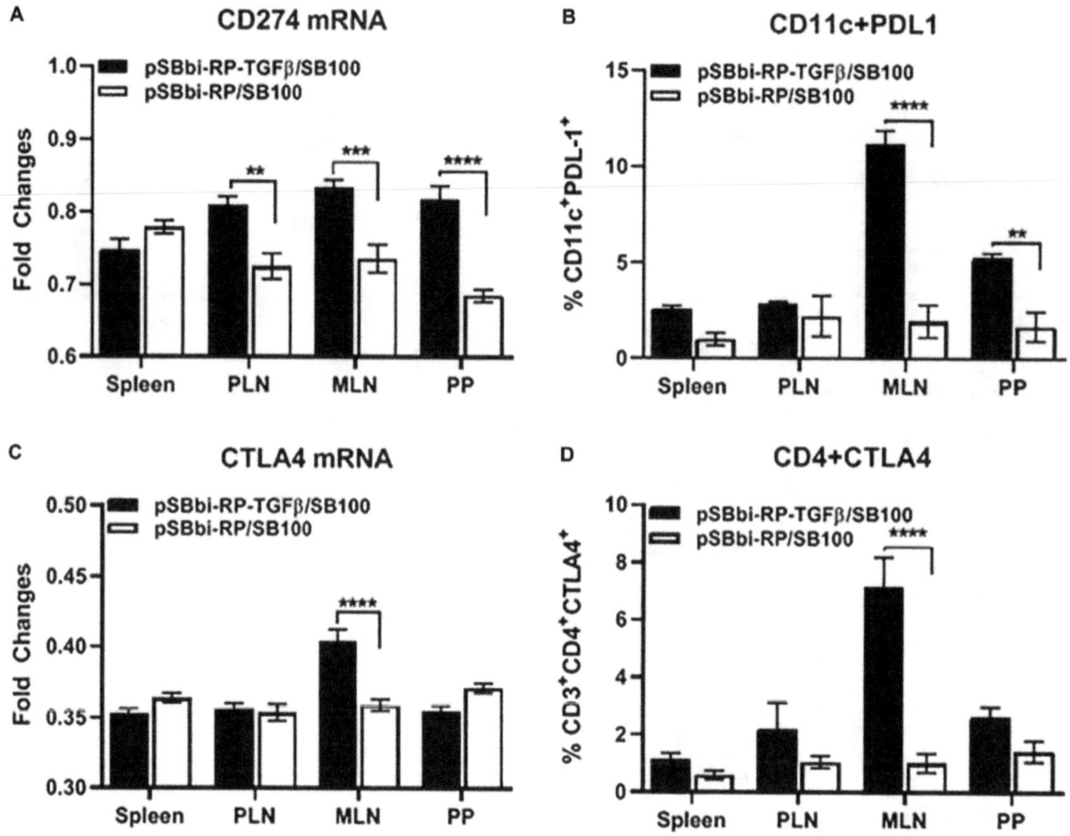

FIGURE 5 | Endogenous TGFβ alters PDL-1 and CTLA4 expression in secondary lymphoid tissues. NOD mice were given a single oral dose of *Salmonella* (pSBbi-RP-TGFβ/SB100) or *Salmonella* (pSBbi-RP/SB100). Four weeks post-vaccination, the fold changes in gene expression of **(A)** CD274 (PDL-1) in sorted CD11c cells and **(C)** CTLA4 in sorted CD4 cells isolated from specified organs was determined. Percentage of $CD11c^+$ cells expressing PDL-1 **(B)** or $CD4^+$ cells expressing CTLA4 **(D)** were quantified in the spleen, PLN, MLN, and PP. The data shown are the average with SD from two independent experiments. Statistical analysis using two-way ANOVA shows significance between *Salmonella* (pSBbi-RP-TGFβ/SB100) and *Salmonella* (pSBbi-RP/SB100) groups (**$p < 0.01$, ***$p < 0.001$, ****$p < 0.0001$).

TGFβ Induces Higher Levels of DCs

An important component of the T1D *Salmonella*-based vaccine is the combination of diabetic autoantigens with TGFβ. TGFβ is used as an immunomodulator and is expressed by the host cells under the CMV promoter. To investigate the effect of TGFβ on the red-labeled cell populations, the mouse *tgfβ1*-coding region was inserted into the pSBbi-RP transposon plasmid upstream of the EF1a promoter to create pSBbi-RP-TGFβ (**Figure 1A**) that express both TFGβ and RFP. Mice were given the *Salmonella*-containing both pSBbi-RP-TGFβ and transposase (SB100) orally and compared with animals receiving the *Salmonella*-containing the pSBbi-RP/SB100 plasmids. Incorporation of the pSBbi-RP-TGFβ transposon into the host cell genome conferred both red fluorescent labeling and host cell secretion of mouse TGFβ. Four weeks after administration of *Salmonella*, labeled cells were found to be red fluorescent $MHCII^+CD11c^+$ DCs which subsequently migrated to the spleen, MLN, PLN, and PP (**Figures 3A,B**). However, in this situation the presence of TGFβ appeared to induce a significant increase in the number of red fluorescent $MHCII^+CD11c^+$ DCs in the PP and MLN (two-way ANOVA, $p < 0.001$, $p < 0.0001$, **Figure 3B**) compared to mice given *Salmonella* lacking the mouse *tgfβ1*-coding region.

TGFβ-Induces Gut $CD103^+$ DCs

The $MHCII^+CD11c^+CD103^+$ populations in mice administered *Salmonella*-containing pSBbi-RP-TGFβ/SB100 plasmids with and without TGFβ were assessed 4 weeks after inoculation (**Figure 4A**). Interestingly, very few red fluorescent DCs from mice given vaccine lacking TGFβ were $CD103^+$. However, mice given vaccine with TGFβ showed a significant increase in PP and MLN of red-labeled DCs that were also $CD103^+$ (two-way ANOVA, $p < 0.0001$, **Figure 4B**).

Salmonella-Delivered TGFβ Increases PDL-1 and CTLA-4 Expression Levels in Secondary Lymphoid Tissues

Cells from animals given *Salmonella*-containing pSBbi-RP-TGFβ/SB100 plasmids with and without TGFβ were compared. The $CD11c^+$ DCs and $CD4^+$ T-cells from splenocytes, MLN, PLN and PP were sorted for qRT-PCR analysis. Programmed

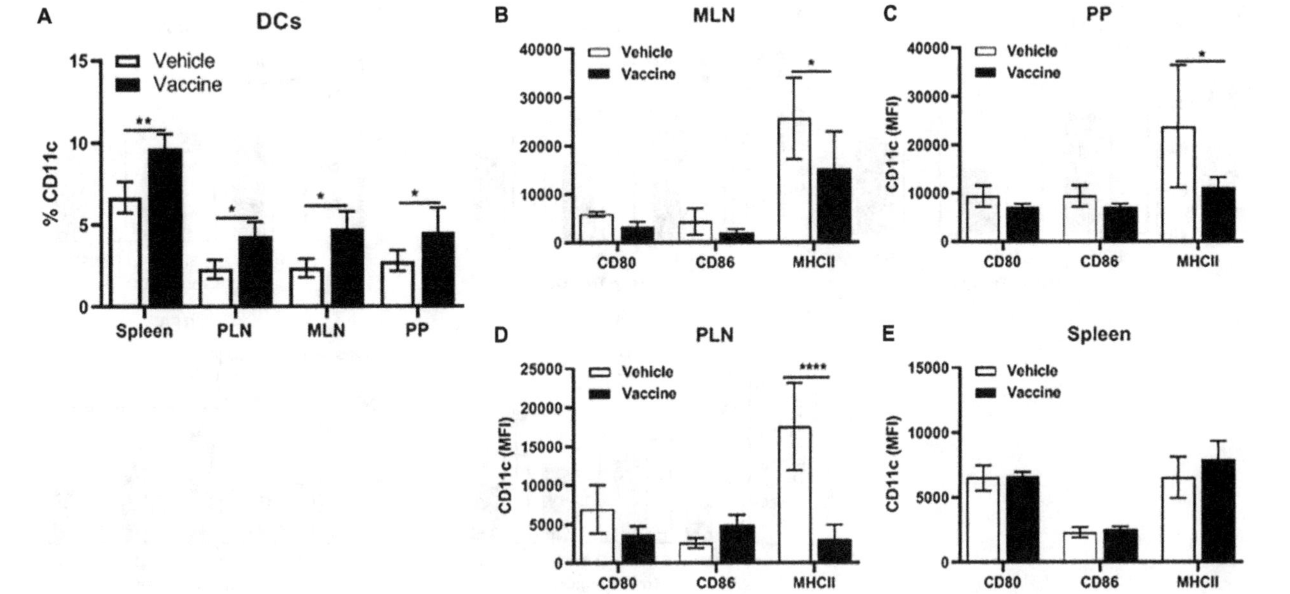

FIGURE 6 | A *Salmonella*-based vaccine increase DCs in lymphoid organs. NOD mice were injected with 2.5 μg/mouse of anti-CD3 mAb for 5 days followed by 2 doses of oral vaccine containing PPI + TGFβ + IL10 ($n = 5$). Four weeks post-vaccination, DCs were analyzed in different organs by FACS analysis. **(A)** Quantification of the percentage of CD11c$^+$ in total live cells of the spleen, PLN, MLN, and PP. **(B)** MLN, **(C)** PP, **(D)** PLN, and **(E)** spleen expression of CD80, CD86, and MHCII was measured in DCs from each organ. The data shown are the average with SD from two independent experiments. Statistical analysis using two-way ANOVA shows significance between vaccine and vehicle treated groups (*$p < 0.05$, **$p < 0.01$, ****$p < 0.0001$).

death-ligand-1 (PDL-1or CD274) expression was significantly increased in DCs in PLN, MLN, and PP but not the spleen of NOD mice treated with TGFβ-containing plasmid (two-way ANOVA, $p = 0.001$, $p = 0.0003$, $p > 0.0001$) compared with the plasmid without TGFβ (**Figure 5A**). Furthermore the percentage of DCs expressing PDL-1 measured by flow cytometry was significantly elevated in MLN and PP but not spleen and PLN of mice treated with TGFβ-containing plasmid (two-way ANOVA, $p < 0.0001$, $p = 0.002$) compared with the plasmid without TGFβ (**Figure 5B**). Interestingly, cytotoxic T-lymphocyte-associated protein-4 (CTLA-4) expression was significantly increased in CD4$^+$ T-cells in MLN of mice treated with TGFβ-containing plasmid (two-way ANOVA, $p < 0.0001$) compared with the plasmid without TGFβ (**Figure 5C**). FACS also showed that CTLA-4 is significantly elevated on the surface of CD4$^+$ T cells in the MLN mice treated with TGFβ-containing plasmid (two-way ANOVA, $p < 0.0001$) compared with the plasmid without TGFβ (**Figure 5D**).

A *Salmonella*-Based Vaccine Increases the DCs in Lymphoid Organs

Pre-diabetic NOD mice were vaccinated with *Salmonella*-based vaccine (PPI + TGFβ + IL10 + anti-CD3) to quantify the percentage of DCs in the spleen, PLN, MLN, and PP. **Figure 6A** shows the frequency of CD11c$^+$ DCs was 5 to 10% of the total number of live cells in all detected lymphoid organs. The percentage of DCs was significantly increased in all organs isolated from vaccine-treated mice compared to vehicle (two-way ANOVA, $p < 0.01$, $p < 0.05$). Additionally, we could not detect any differences between vaccine or vehicle treated mice in the percentage of cell populations that were characterized as B220$^+$GR-1$^-$ (B cells, **Supplementary Figure S1A**) and CD11b$^+$GR-1$^+$ as polymorph nuclear macrophages (PMN, **Supplementary Figure S1B**) in the spleens, PLN, MLN, and PP.

Moreover, CD11c$^+$ DCs from vaccinated mice showed lowered expression of the MHCII molecule and co-stimulatory molecules CD80, and CD86 in cells from MLN (**Figure 6B**), PP (**Figure 6C**) and PLN (**Figure 6D**) compared to DCs from these lymphoid organs from vehicle-treated mice. In contrast, CD11c$^+$ DCs from the spleen from vaccinated mice (**Figure 6E**) showed no difference in the level of expression of MHCII, CD80 and CD86 compared to DCs from vehicle-treated mice.

Importance of DCs for *Salmonella*-Based Vaccine Therapy

We next evaluated whether the DCs in vaccine-treated NOD mice were tolerogenic. As responder T cells, we used CD4$^+$CD25$^-$ T cells isolated from spleens of normoglycemic B9-23 vaccinated NOD mice. We found that CD4$^+$CD25$^+$ Treg cells from vehicle-treated mice efficiently suppressed proliferation and activation of responder T cells when combined with equal amount of DCs from vaccinated mice but did not alter proliferation when cultured with DCs from vehicle-treated animals (**Figure 7A**). As well, these tolerogenic DCs lowered expression of activation markers CD44 (**Figure 7B**) and CD69 (**Figure 7C**). Additionally DCs from vaccine-treated mice, when combined with Tregs, efficiently increased regulatory cytokines such as IL10 (**Figure 7D**) and TGFβ (**Figure 7E**) and

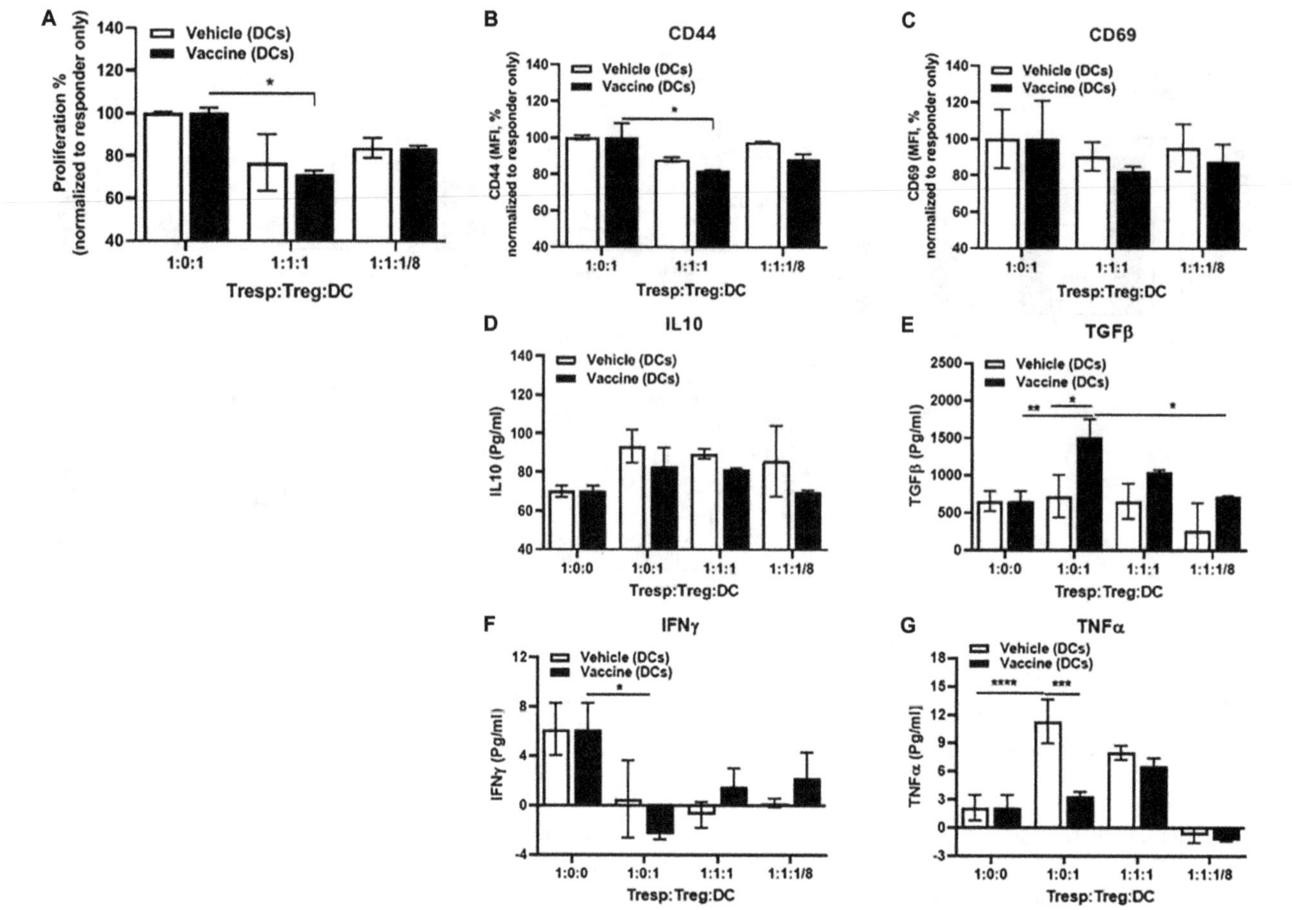

FIGURE 7 | DCs mediated *in vitro Salmonella*-based anti-inflammatory effects. Female 8-week-old NOD mice were treated with 2.5 μg/mouse of anti-CD3 mAb via i.p. injection for 5 days followed by 2 doses of oral combined vaccines. Splenocytes were harvested from the indicated group at day 30 post-vaccination. $CD4^{+}CD25^{-}$ Tresp cells isolated from splenocytes of B9-23 vaccinated mice were dye-labeled, co-cultured with $CD4^{+}CD25^{+}$ Treg cells isolated from non-vaccinated mice, and DCs from vaccinated or non-vaccinated mice for 3 days with insulin peptide B9-23 (10 μg/ml). **(A)** Proliferation of Tresp was measured by flow cytometry of dye dilution and shown as the percentage of Tresp normalized to Tresp only culture. **(B)** Activation of Tresps, shown as MFI of CD44 expression or **(C)** CD69 normalized to Tresp-only culture. ELISA for regulatory **(D)** IL-10, and **(E)** TGFβ. ELISA for inflammatory **(F)** IFNγ, and **(G)** TNFα. The data shown are the average with SD from two independent experiments. Statistical analysis was performed using two-way ANOVA (*$p < 0.05$, **$p < 0.01$, ***$p < 0.001$, ****$p < 0.0001$).

decreased the inflammatory cytokines such as IFNγ (**Figure 7F**) and TNFα (**Figure 7G**). In contrast DCs from vehicle-treated mice, when combined with Tregs decreased the regulatory cytokines IL10 (**Figure 7D**) and TGFβ (**Figure 7E**) and increased the inflammatory cytokines IFNγ (**Figure 7F**) and TNFα (**Figure 7G**). Finally, when we decreased the number of DCs to a ratio of 1:8, the suppressor activity of Tregs decreased indicating that the DCs from vaccinated animals were important to the suppressor activity of the Tregs.

DISCUSSION

Recently we developed an oral vaccine using live attenuated *Salmonella* that prevented and reverted the onset T1D in NOD mice (45). This vaccine was a combination of PPI + TGFβ + IL10 and anti-CD3 mAb. We showed that the vaccine increased Tregs and Tr1 cells in vaccinated mice (23, 45). To understand how *Salmonella* prevented diabetes, it was important to first identify the cell populations that interact with the microorganism and to investigate the role of *Salmonella*-delivered TGFβ in creation of a tolerogenic micro-environment in NOD mice. On oral administration, *Salmonella* gains access to the individual via DCs that phagocytosis the bacteria, through SPI1-T3SS-mediated invasion of other cells or by GALT cells. Indeed, these several mechanisms likely contribute to wider spread of the bacteria beyond the gut. In specialized lymphatic organs such as PP and MLN, the bacteria is mostly intracellular, its survival and replication dependent on the function of SPI2-T3SS (49).

Transposable elements are naturally occurring vehicles and are used for transgenesis and mutagenesis. The Sleeping Beauty transposon shows efficient transposition in a wide range of vertebrate cells, including humans (50, 51, 52). The current study employed attenuated *Salmonella* as a vehicle to deliver the transposon plasmid expressing a detectable fluorescent protein to host cells and allowed tracking of *Salmonella*-bearing host cells throughout the GALT. Secondary lymphoid organs provide the specialized microenvironment necessary for generating an immune-specific response. DCs, while present in low numbers, are distributed widely and beyond lymphatic tissues. Because DCs work very efficiently at controlling T cells, they are critical to turning on or off immune responses (53). We found that the DCs labeled after oral administration of *Salmonella* were present in all lymphoid tissues examined, consistent with results from others.

Previous studies have shown that tolerance to oral antigens is mediated by CD103^{+} DCs in the lamina propria (39, 41, 54–56). CD103^{+} DCs are unique to the gut. Transforming growth factor receptor 1 (TGFβR1) has a cell-intrinsic role in the development of these cells. Together, these published data suggested that MHCII^{+}CD11c^{+}CD103^{+} cells mediate the regulatory effects of the *Salmonella*-based vaccine. In keeping with this, TGFβ promoted the upregulation of DC cell surface CD103 in animals administered the vaccine. In the intestinal tract, CD103^{+} DCs carry acquired antigens to the local lymph nodes where they encounter CD8^{+} T cells (57). By promoting naïve T cell transformation to regulatory Foxp3^{+} T cells, DCs promote immune suppression (39, 54, 56). Our results demonstrate that *Salmonella*-delivered TGFβ recruits CD103^{+} DCs in the MLN and PP. These data suggest that *Salmonella*-autoantigen driven education of the naïve T-cells into iTregs or Trl occurs specifically in these secondary lymph nodes (45). Our data further indicate that TGFβ is involved in the trafficking and control of CD103^{+} DCs, concentrating their function within MLN and PP.

Additionally, it appears that TGFβ has an impact on PDL-1 and CTLA-4 expression in NOD mice. PD-L1 suppresses the immune system in cancer and autoimmune disease (58). Endogenous ligand-receptor pathways, such as the PD-L1/PD-1, limit T cell antigen activation and promote regulatory T cell survival (58, 59). Similarly, CTLA-4 limits T cell activation in part by blunting CD28 co-activation (60). Indeed, some data suggests that variation in the CTLA-4 gene may promote autoimmunity (61–64). Our data suggest that TGFβ increases PDL-1 and CTLA-4 at the lymphoid sites where CD103^{+} DCs are found to be elevated consistent with a tolerogenic microenvironment. As some time differentiation of naïve T cells into nTregs or Trl occurs in the MLN and the PP (31, 34, 54, 56, 65) and these lymphoid sites appear to be the central hub for *Salmonella* vaccine activity.

Some studies characterized semi-mature phenotype DCs that are thought to be most effective in inducing tolerance in autoimmune diseases (66, 67). In this study, our combined therapy increased DCs in all lymphatic tissues of vaccinated mice. Additionally, these DCs expressed low levels of co-stimulatory molecules. Moreover, *in vitro* proliferation assays conformed that the DCs from vaccinated mice were essential for suppressor activity of Tregs by decreasing proliferation and activation of effector T cells. Furthermore, these DCs secreted less inflammatory cytokines such as TNFα, and IFNγ while secreting increased tolerogenic cytokines such as IL10 and TGFβ .

Together, the data herein suggest the oral vaccine could be an effective immunotherapy to reestablish tolerance to self-antigens and of value to individuals with T1D. The vaccine may also find use in the treatment of other autoimmune disorders. Using *Salmonella* offers several advantages over other methods of drug delivery. First, oral delivery exploits the natural tolerogenic functions of the GALT system. Second, oral delivery is a patient-friendly treatment approach. Third, inclusion of TGFβ and possibly other tolerogenic cytokines should improve the efficacy of the vaccine. Fourth, protection of the antigen from degradation while it traverses the digestion system is important. Lastly for clinical relevance, a vaccine for typhoid fever that uses the *Salmonella typhi* Ty21a strain is approved by the FDA.

AUTHOR CONTRIBUTIONS

JM, KF, and MH conceived and designed the experiments. JM, AA, JR, PG, NG, and MH performed the experiments. KF and MH analyzed the data. JM, FK, and MH wrote the manuscript.

ACKNOWLEDGMENTS

We extend our gratitude to Dr. Eric Kowarz and Dr. Zsuzsanna Izsvak for their kind donations of the Sleeping Beauty transposon system plasmids. We thank Jacob Cobb, City of Hope, for his technical assistance and acknowledge the expert assistance provided by the Analytical Cytometry Core facility at the Beckman Research Institute of City of Hope.

REFERENCES

1. Atkinson MA. The pathogenesis and natural history of type 1 diabetes. *Cold Spring Harb Perspect Med.* (2012) 2:a007641 doi: 10.1101/cshperspect.a007641
2. Nakayama M, Beilke JN, Jasinski JM, Kobayashi M, Miao D, Li M, Coulombe MG. Priming and effector dependence on insulin B:9–23 peptide in NOD islet autoimmunity. *J Clin Invest.* (2007) 117:1835–43.
3. Achenbach P, Koczwara K, Knopff A, Naserke H, Ziegler AG, Bonifacio E. Mature high-affinity immune responses to (pro)insulin anticipate the autoimmune cascade that leads to type 1 diabetes. *J Clin Investigat.* (2004) 114:589–97.
4. Kronenberg D, Knight RR, Estorninho M, Ellis RJ, Kester MG, De Ru A, Eichmann M. Circulating preproinsulin signal peptide-specific CD8 T cells restricted by the susceptibility molecule HLA-A24 are expanded at onset of type 1 diabetes and kill beta-cells. *Diabetes.* (2012) 61:1752–59.
5. Skowera A, Ellis RJ, Varela-Calvino R, Arif S, Huang GC, Van-Krinks C, Zaremba A, Rackham C. CTLs are targeted to kill beta cells in patients with type 1 diabetes through recognition of a glucose-regulated preproinsulin epitope (vol 118, pg 3390, 2008). *J Clin Investigat.* (2009) 119:2843–43.
6. Cheminay C, Hensel M. Rational design of *Salmonella* recombinant vaccines. *Int J Med Microbiol.* (2008) 298:87–98. doi: 10.1016/j.ijmm.2007.08.006
7. Cheminay C, Mohlenbrink A, Hensel M. Intracellular *Salmonella* inhibit antigen presentation by dendritic cells. *J Immunol.* (2005) 174:2892–99.
8. Raine T, Zaccone P, Mastroeni P, Cooke A. *Salmonella typhimurium* infection in nonobese diabetic mice generates immunomodulatory dendritic cells able to prevent type 1 diabetes. *J Immunol.* (2006) 177:2224–33.
9. Ashkar AA, Reid S, Verdu EF, Zhang K, Coombes BK. Interleukin-15 and NK1.1+ cells provide innate protection against acute *Salmonella enterica* serovar Typhimurium infection in the gut and in systemic tissues. *Infect Immun.* (2009) 77:214–22.

10. Husseiny MI, Rawson J, Kaye A, Nair I, Todorov I, Hensel M, Kandeel F, Ferreri K. An oral vaccine for type 1 diabetes based on live attenuated *Salmonella*. *Vaccine*. (2014) 32:2300–7.
11. Xiong G, Husseiny MI, Song L, Erdreich-Epstein A, Shackleford GM, Seeger RC, Jackel D, Hensel M, Metelitsa LS. Novel cancer vaccine based on genes of *Salmonella* pathogenicity island 2. *Int J Cancer*. (2010) 126:2622–34.
12. Husseiny MI, Hensel M. Evaluation of an intracellular-activated promoter for the generation of live *Salmonella* recombinant vaccines. *Vaccine*. (2005) 23:2580–90.
13. Xu X, Husseiny MI, Goldwich A, Hensel M. Efficacy of intracellular activated promoters for generation of *Salmonella*-based vaccines. *Infect Immun*. (2010) 78:4828–38.
14. Hansen-Wester I, Hensel M. *Salmonella* pathogenicity islands encoding type III secretion systems. *Microbes Infect*. (2001) 3:549–59.
15. Galan JE. *Salmonella* interactions with host cells: type III secretion at work. *Annu Rev Cell Dev Biol*. (2001) 17:53–86.
16. Figueira R, Holden DW. Functions of the *Salmonella* pathogenicity island 2 (SPI-2) type III secretion system effectors. *Microbiol SGM*. (2012) 158:1147–61.
17. Haga T, Kumabe S, Ikejiri A, Shimizu Y, Li H, Goto Y, Matsui H, Miyata H, Miura T. *In vitro* and *in vivo* stability of plasmids in attenuated *Salmonella enterica* serovar typhimurium used as a carrier of DNA vaccine is associated with its replication origin. *Exp Anim Tokyo*. (2006) 55:405–9.
18. Laniewski P, Jagusztyn-Krynicka EK. Subunit vaccine construction using *Salmonella enterica* cells as a carrier of heterologous genes. *Postep Mikrobiol*. (2013) 52:281–94.
19. Abrahams GL, Hensel M. Manipulating cellular transport and immune responses: dynamic interactions between intracellular *Salmonella enterica* and its host cells. *Cell Microbiol*. (2006) 8:728–37.
20. Holzer SU, Hensel M. Divergent roles of *Salmonella* pathogenicity island 2 and metabolic traits during interaction of *S. enterica* serovar typhimurium with host cells. *PLoS One*. (2012) 7:e33220. doi: 10.1371/journal.pone.0033220
21. Chen H, Schifferli DM. Construction, characterization, and immunogenicity of an attenuated *Salmonella enterica* serovar typhimurium pgtE vaccine expressing fimbriae with integrated viral epitopes from the spiC promoter. *Infect Immun*. (2003) 71:4664–73.
22. Kong W, Brovold M, Koeneman BA, Clark-Curtiss J, Curtiss R. Turning self-destructing *Salmonella* into a universal DNA vaccine delivery platform. *P Natl Acad Sci USA*. (2012) 109:19414–19.
23. Husseiny MI, Du W, Mbongue J, Lenz A, Rawson J, Kandeel F, Ferreri K. Factors affecting *Salmonella*-based combination immunotherapy for prevention of type 1 diabetes in non-obese diabetic mice. *Vaccine*. (2018) 36:8008–18
24. Hu Q, Coburn B, Deng W, Li Y, Shi X, Lan Q, Wang B, Coombes BK, Finlay BB. *Salmonella enterica* serovar Senftenberg human clinical isolates lacking SPI-1. *J Clin Microbiol*. (2008) 46:1330–36. doi: 10.3389/fmicb.2014.00781
25. Chistiakov DA, Bobryshev YV, Kozarov E, Sobenin IA, Orekhov AN. Intestinal mucosal tolerance and impact of gut microbiota to mucosal tolerance. *Front Microbiol*. (2014) 5:781.
26. Pabst O, Bernhardt G, Forster R. The impact of cell-bound antigen transport on mucosal tolerance induction. *J Leuk Biol*. (2007) 82:795–800. doi: 10.1189/jlb.0307144
27. Hill M, Cuturi MC. Negative vaccination by tolerogenic dendritic cells in organ transplantation. *Curr Opin Organ Tran*. (2010) 15:738–43.
28. Raker VK, Domogalla MP, Steinbrink K. Tolerogenic dendritic cells for regulatory T cell induction in man. *Front Immunol*. (2015) 6:569. doi: 10.3389/fimmu.2015.00569
29. Gregori S, Tomasoni D, Pacciani V, Scirpoli M, Battaglia M, Magnani CF, Hauben E, Roncarolo MG. Differentiation of type 1 T regulatory cells (Tr1) by tolerogenic DC-10 requires the IL-10-dependent ILT4/HLA-G pathway (vol 116, pg 935, 2010). *Blood*. (2011) 118:5060–60.
30. Wakkach A, Fournier N, Brun V, Breittmayer JP, Cottrez F, Groux H. Characterization of dendritic cells that induce tolerance and T regulatory 1 cell differentiation *in vivo*. *Immunity*. (2003) 18:605–17.
31. Brockmann L, Gagliani N, Steglich B, Giannou AD, Kempski J, Pelczar P, Geffken M. IL-10 receptor signaling is essential for T(R)1 cell function *in vivo*. *J Immunol*. (2017) 198:1130–41.
32. Roncarolo MG, Gregori S, Bacchetta R, Battaglia M. Tr1 cells and the counter-regulation of immunity: natural mechanisms and therapeutic applications. *Int Health Dis*. (2014) 380:39–68. doi: 10.1007/978-3-662-43492-5_3
33. Saito H, Tsurikisawa N, Tsuburai T, Oshikata C, Akiyama K. The proportion of regulatory T cells in the peripheral blood reflects the relapse or remission status of patients with Churg-Strauss syndrome. *Int Arch Allerg Immunol*. (2011) 155(Suppl. 1):46–52. doi: 10.1159/000327265
34. Yu H, Gagliani N, Ishigame H, Huber S, Zhu S, Esplugues E, Herold KC, Wen L, Flavell RA. Intestinal type 1 regulatory T cells migrate to periphery to suppress diabetogenic T cells and prevent diabetes development. *Proc Natl Acad Sci USA*. (2017) 114:10443–8.
35. Sakaguchi S, Yamaguchi T, Nomura T, Ono M. Regulatory T cells and immune tolerance. *Cell* (2008) 133:775–87.
36. Beitnes AC, Raki M, Lundin KE, Jahnsen J, Sollid LM, Jahnsen FL. Density of CD163$^+$ CD11c$^+$ dendritic cells increases and CD103$^+$ dendritic cells decreases in the coeliac lesion. *Scand J Immunol*. (2011) 74:186–94.
37. Annacker O, Coombes JL, Malmstrom V, Uhlig HH, Bourne T, Johansson-Lindbom B, Agace WW. Essential role for CD103 in the T cell-mediated regulation of experimental colitis. *J Exp Med*. (2005) 202:1051–61.
38. Iliev ID, Mileti E, Matteoli G, Chieppa M, Rescigno M. Intestinal epithelial cells promote colitis-protective regulatory T-cell differentiation through dendritic cell conditioning. *Mucosal Immunol*. (2009) 2:340–50.
39. Schulz O, Jaensson E, Persson EK, Liu XS, Worbs T, Agace WW, Pabst O. Intestinal CD103(+), but not CX3CR1(+), antigen sampling cells migrate in lymph and serve classical dendritic cell functions. *J Exp Med*. (2009) 206:3101–14.
40. Yrlid U, Cerovic V, Milling S, Jenkins CD, Klavinskis LS, MacPherson CG. A distinct subset of intestinal dendritic cells responds selectively to oral TLR7/8 stimulation. *Eur J Immunol*. (2006) 36:2639–48.
41. Milling S, Yrlid U, Cerovic V, MacPherson G. Subsets of migrating intestinal dendritic cells. *Immunol Rev*. (2010) 234:259–67.
42. Kowarz E, Loscher D, Marschalek R. Optimized sleeping beauty transposons rapidly generate stable transgenic cell lines. *Biotechnol J*. (2015) 10:647–53.
43. Plasterk RH. Molecular mechanisms of transposition and its control. *Cell*. (1993) 74:781–6.
44. Plasterk RH. The ins and outs of transposition. Molecular mechanisms of transposition and its control, sponsored by the European molecular biology organization, roscoff, France, June 24–28, 1990. *New Biol*. (1990) 2: 787–92.
45. Mbongue JC, Rawson J, Garcia PA, Gonzalez N, Cobb J, Kandeel F, Ferreri K, Husseiny MI. Reversal of new onset type 1 diabetes by oral *Salmonella*-based combination therapy and mediated by regulatory T-cells in NOD mice. *Front Immunol*. (2019) 10:320.
46. Mates L, Chuah MK, Belay E, Jerchow B, Manoj N, Acosta-Sanchez A, Grzela DP, Schmitt A. Molecular evolution of a novel hyperactive sleeping beauty transposase enables robust stable gene transfer in vertebrates. *Nat Genet*. (2009) 41:753–61.
47. Husseiny MI, Wartha F, Hensel M. Recombinant vaccines based on translocated effector proteins of *Salmonella* pathogenicity Island 2. *Vaccine*. (2007) 25:185–93.
48. Takiishi T, Korf H, Van Belle TL, Robert S, Grieco FA, Caluwaerts S, Galleri L. Reversal of autoimmune diabetes by restoration of antigen-specific tolerance using genetically modified *Lactococcus lactis* in mice. *J Clin Invest*. (2012) 122:1717–25.
49. Jantsch J, Chikkaballi D,Hensel M. Cellular aspects of immunity to intracellular *Salmonella enterica*. *Immunol Rev*. (2011) 240:185–95.
50. Grabundzija I, Wang J, Sebe A, Erdei Z, Kajdi R, Devaraj A, Steinemann D. Sleeping Beauty transposon-based system for cellular reprogramming and targeted gene insertion in induced pluripotent stem cells. *Nucleic Acids Res*. (2013) 41:1829–47.
51. Sumiyoshi T, Holt NG, Hollis RP, Ge S, Cannon PM, Crooks GM, Kohn DB. Stable transgene expression in primitive human CD34$^+$ hematopoietic stem/progenitor cells, using the Sleeping Beauty transposon system. *Hum Gene Ther*. (2009) 20:1607–26.
52. Singh H, Huls H, Kebriaei P, Cooper LG. A new approach to gene therapy using sleeping beauty to genetically modify clinical-grade T cells to target CD19. *Immunol Rev*. (2014) 257:181–90.

53. Banchereau J, Steinman RM. Dendritic cells and the control of immunity. *Nature.* (1998) 392:245–52.
54. Badami E, Sorini C, Coccia M, Usuelli V, Molteni L, Bolla AM, Scavini M, Mariani A, King C, Bosi E, Falcone M. Defective differentiation of regulatory FoxP3(+) T cells by small-intestinal dendritic cells in patients with type 1 diabetes. *Diabetes.* (2011) 60:2120–4.
55. Johansson-Lindbom B, Svensson M, Pabst O, Palmqvist C, Marquez G, Forster R, Agace WW. Functional specialization of gut $CD103^{+}$ dendritic cells in the regulation of tissue-selective T cell homing. *J Exp Med.* (2005) 202: 1063–73.
56. Siddiqui KRR, Powrie F. CD103(+) GALT DCs promote Foxp3(+) regulatory T cells. *Mucosal Immunol.* (2008) 1:S34–8.
57. Farache J, Koren I, Milo I, Gurevich I, Kim KW, Zigmond E, Furtado GC, Lira SA, Shakhar G. Luminal bacteria recruit CD103(+) dendritic cells into the intestinal epithelium to sample bacterial antigens for presentation. *Immunity.* (2013) 38:581–95.
58. Dai S, Jia R, Zhang X, Fang Q, Huang L. The PD-1/PD-Ls pathway and autoimmune diseases. *Cell Immunol.* (2014) 290:72–9.
59. Chemnitz JM, Parry RV, Nichols KE, June CH, Riley JL. SHP-1 and SHP-2 associate with immunoreceptor tyrosine-based switch motif of programmed death 1 upon primary human T cell stimulation, but only receptor ligation prevents T cell activation. *J Immunol.* (2004) 173:945–54.
60. Devarajan P, Chen ZB. Autoimmune effector memory T cells: the bad and the good. *Immunol Res.* (2013) 57:12–2.
61. Klocke K, Sakaguchi S, Holmdahl R, Wing K. Induction of autoimmune disease by deletion of CTLA-4 in mice in adulthood. *Eur J Immunol.* (2016) 46:770.
62. Salomon B, Bluestone JA. Complexities of CD28/B7: CTLA-4 costimulatory pathways in autoimmunity and transplantation. *Annu Rev Immunol.* (2001) 19:225–52.
63. Fife BT, Bluestone JA. Control of peripheral T-cell tolerance and autoimmunity via the CTLA-4 and PD-1 pathways. *Immunol Rev.* (2008) 224:166–82. doi: 10.1111/j.1600-065X.2008.00662.x
64. Romo-Tena J, Gomez-Martin D, Alcocer-Varela J. CTLA-4 and autoimmunity: New insights into the dual regulator of tolerance. *Autoimmun Rev.* (2013) 12:1171–6. doi: 10.1016/j.autrev.2013.07.002
65. Geem D, Ngo V, Harusato A, Chassaing B, Gewirtz AT, Newberry RD, Denning TL. Contribution of mesenteric lymph nodes and GALT to the intestinal $Foxp3^{+}$ regulatory T-cell compartment. *Cell Mol Gastroenterol Hepatol.* (2016) 2:274–80.
66. Menges M, Rossner S, Voigtlander C, Schindler H, Kukutsch NA, Bogdan C, Erb K, Schuler G, Lutz MB. Repetitive injections of dendritic cells matured with tumor necrosis factor alpha induce antigen-specific protection of mice from autoimmunity. *J Exp Med.* (2002) 195:15–21.
67. Lutz MB, Schuler G. Immature, semi-mature and fully mature dendritic cells: which signals induce tolerance or immunity? *Trends Immunol.* (2002) 23:445–9.

19

GAD65 Antibody Epitopes and Genetic Background in Latent Autoimmune Diabetes in Youth (LADY)

Yiman Peng[1], Xia Li[1], Yufei Xiang[1], Xiang Yan[1], Houde Zhou[1], Xiaohan Tang[1], Jin Cheng[1], Xiaohong Niu[2], Jing Liu[3], Qiuhe Ji[4], Linong Ji[5], Gan Huang[1] and Zhiguang Zhou[1]*

[1] National Clinical Research Center for Metabolic Diseases, Key Laboratory of Diabetes Immunology (Central South University), Ministry of Education, and Department of Metabolism and Endocrinology, The Second Xiangya Hospital of Central South University, Changsha, China, [2] Department of Endocrinology, Heji Hospital Affiliated to Changzhi Medical College, Changzhi, China, [3] Department of Endocrinology, Gansu Provincial Hospital, Lanzhou, China, [4] Department of Endocrinology, Xijing Hospital, Fourth Military Medical University, Xi an, China, [5] Department of Endocrinology and Metabolism, Peking University People's Hospital, Beijing, China

***Correspondence:**
Gan Huang
huanggan007@csu.edu.cn

Epitope-specific GAD65Abs and *HLA-DR-DQ* gene assays help improve the value of risk stratification in autoimmune diabetes mellitus and protect islet function. Identification and early intervention are important for latent autoimmune diabetes in youth (LADY). The aims of this study were to investigate 1) the frequencies of the epitope-specific GAD65Abs and *HLA-DR-DQ* genes in LADY and 2) the association between *HLA-DR-DQ* genes and epitope-specific GAD65Abs. Higher frequencies of GAD65-CAb and multiepitope GAD65Abs were observed in young type 1 diabetes, LADY, and old type 1 diabetes subjects than those in latent autoimmune diabetes in adult (LADA) patients. The frequencies of the specific susceptible HLA haplotype *DR3*, total susceptible HLA haplotypes, and high-risk genotypes were higher in type 1 diabetes and LADY patients than those in LADA patients. In contrast, type 1 diabetes and LADY patients had lower frequencies of low/no genetic risk genotypes *(DRX/X)* than those of LADA patients. Logistic regression analysis suggested that the susceptible HLA haplotypes were risk factors for glutamic acid decarboxylase antibody (GADA) multiepitope positivity in autoimmune diabetes mellitus. LADY may be more severe than LADA, and LADY seemed to be a transitional type of type 1 diabetes and LADA. GADA epitope and *HLA-DR-DQ* gene assays are important for risk stratification in autoimmune diabetes mellitus and protection of islet function.

Keywords: glutamic acid decarboxylase autoantibody, GAD epitopes, HLA, type 1 diabetes (T1D), latent autoimmune diabetes in adults (LADA), latent autoimmune diabetes in youth

INTRODUCTION

Autoimmune diabetes mellitus (ADM) is a group of highly heterogeneous autoimmune diseases characterized by autoimmune mediation and destruction of islet beta cells. In general, type 1 diabetes (T1D) is characterized by islet autoantibody positivity, juvenile onset, and the requirement for insulin therapy. In addition, subjects with phenotypic type 2 diabetes and islet antibody positivity, which has been described as "type 1.5 diabetes" (T1.5DM) or "latent autoimmune diabetes in adults (LADA)", are non-insulin dependent for at least 6 months after onset (1). Importantly, studies have reported that 10%–75% of Caucasians and 11.7% of Chinese juvenile-onset phenotypes may have "latent autoimmune diabetes in youth (LADY)" (2, 3). Patients with LADY have a younger age of onset than those with LADA, and clinically, islet function and C-peptide levels decline more rapidly in LADY than in LADA. To date, there has been limited research on LADY, and it has not yet received attention from the international community.

Islet autoantibodies are a hallmark of ADM. The major diabetes-related autoantibodies include glutamic acid decarboxylase antibody (GADA), tyrosine phosphatase (IA-2A), zinc transporter 8 autoantibody (ZnT8A), and insulin autoantibody (IAA) (4). GADA is dominant in Western and Chinese newly diagnosed diabetes patients. Moreover, GADA has been used to screen individuals with ADM (5, 6). Epitope-specific assays of GADA may improve the clinical diagnostic specificity of diabetes patients (7).

GAD65Ab is heterogeneous with respect to its epitope specificity. Previous studies have shown the different binding patterns of GADA in T1D and LADA patients. Compared with that in T1D patients, the percentage of GAD65-NAb (N-terminal of the GAD65 protein) is significantly higher in LADA patients, while the frequency of GAD65-CAb (C-terminal of the GAD65 protein) is significantly lower in LADA patients. LADA patients with GAD65-M+Cabs (C-terminal and middle region of the GAD65 protein) have clinical features similar to those of T1D patients, and GAD65-CAb appears to confer a higher risk of the development of lower serum C-peptide levels and the requirement for insulin therapy (8–11). Schlosser et al. (12) suggested that the autoimmune response might undergo intramolecular epitope spreading progression from the N-terminal fragment to the middle fragment of GAD65 in predisposed subjects and that GAD65-CAb may be associated with the failure of islet beta cell function during disease progression.

HLA-DRB1-DQA1 genes confer the highest risk of the occurrence of diabetes (13), and susceptible HLA genes vary among different ethnicities (14). For example, the susceptible haplotype *DRB1*0901-DQA1*0302-DQB1*0303 (DR9)* is more common in Chinese patients than in Caucasian patients. Furthermore, there are discrepancies in terms of susceptible HLA genotypes and haplotypes between T1D and LADA patients. For example, in Chinese patients, *DR3/DR3, DR3/DR9*, and *DR9/DR9* are T1D-associated high-risk genotypes, whereas only *DR9/DR9* is related to LADA. The haplotype *DRB1*0901-DQA1*05-DQB1*0201*, which confers the highest risk of T1D, is not associated with LADA. Susceptible haplotypes, including *DRB1*0301-DQA1*0501-DQB1*0201 (DR3), DRB1*0405-DQA1*0303-DQB1*0401 (DR4), and DRB1*0901-DQA1*0302-DQB1*0303 (DR9)*, were found to be the common high-risk susceptible HLA haplotypes in T1D and LADA (15).

To date, the epitope specificity of GAD65Abs and the *HLA-DRB1-DQA1-DQB1* risk in LADY remain completely unknown, especially in large-scale research. Here, we hypothesize that LADY is a transitional type of LADA and T1D in terms of the GADA epitope and *HLA-DRB1-DQA1-DQB1* genes. We investigated the association between the *HLA-DR-DQ* genes and epitope-specific GAD65Abs. These studies could provide helpful information for understanding the pathogenesis of LADY.

MATERIALS AND METHODS

Subjects

A total of 17,536 newly diagnosed diabetes mellitus patients aged 15–79 years old were recruited for this cross-sectional study from April 2015 to October 2017 (**Figure 1**). Patients from 46 different hospitals in 25 major cities were recruited consecutively to launch the "Diagnosis and Treatment Optimization of Autoimmune Diabetes in Chinese Adults" project funded by the National Key R&D Program of China (2013BAI09B12). Research staff at each participating hospital underwent standardized training on all procedures and data collection methods (16).

Type 1 Diabetes Patients

The inclusion criteria for T1D subjects were as follows: 1) diagnosis of diabetes (World Health Organization criteria of 1999) (17) at ≥15 years of age; 2) disease duration <1 year; 3) acute onset and presence of diabetic ketosis or ketoacidosis; 4) positivity for GADA; and 5) insulin dependency at the time of diagnosis. The exclusion criteria were patients with LADY, LADA, type 2 diabetes, or a malignancy and those who were pregnant.

Latent Autoimmune Diabetes in Youth, Latent Autoimmune Diabetes in Adults, and Type 2 Diabetes Patients

The inclusion criteria for LADY, LADA, and type 2 diabetes subjects were as follows: 1) diagnosis of diabetes (World Health

---

Abbreviations: ADM, Autoimmune diabetes mellitus; DBP, Diastolic blood pressure; FBS, Fasting blood glucose; FCP, Fasting C-peptide; GADA, GAD autoantibodies; GAD-C, C-terminal of the GAD65 protein; GAD-M, Middle region of the GAD65 protein; GAD-N, N-terminal of the GAD65 protein; GAD65, 65-kDa isoform of GAD; GAD67, 67-kDa isoform of GAD; HDL-C, High-density lipoprotein cholesterol; IAA, Insulin autoantibodies; IA-2A, Protein tyrosine phosphatase autoantibodies; LADA, Latent autoimmune diabetes in adults; LADY, Latent autoimmune diabetes in youth; LDL-C, Low-density lipoprotein cholesterol; PCP, 2-h postprandial C-peptide; SBP, Systolic blood pressure; TC, Total cholesterol; TG, Triglycerides; ZnT8A, Zinc transporter 8 autoantibodies.

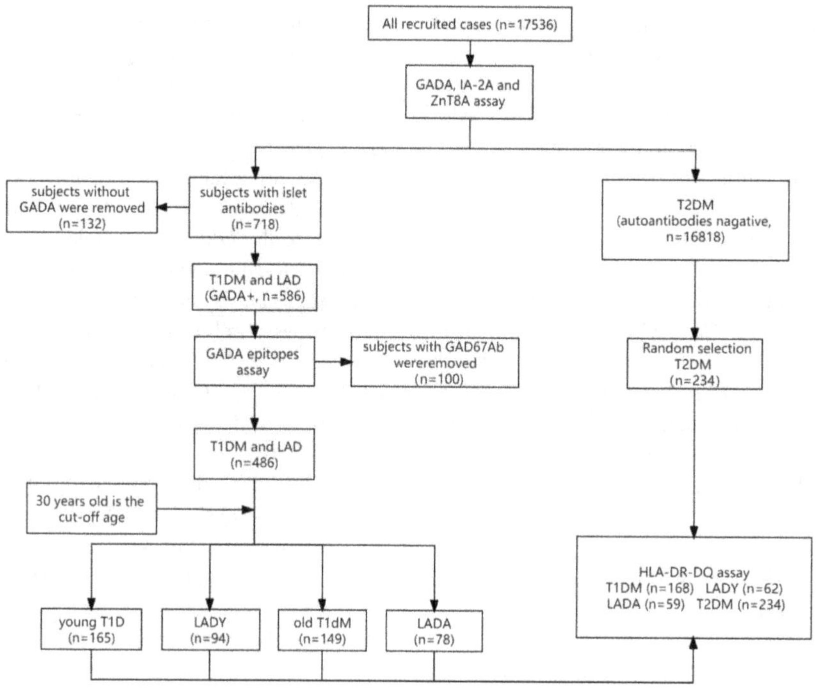

FIGURE 1 | Flowchart of sampling, grouping, assaying and genotyping.

Organization criteria of 1999) (17) at ≥15 years of age; 2) disease duration <1 year; 3) no ketoacidosis in the first 6 months after diagnosis of diabetes; and 4) insulin independence for at least 6 months after onset. If subjects fulfilled the above criteria, those who were autoimmune antibody (GADA, IA-2A, or ZnT8A) positive and <30 years old were diagnosed with LADY, those who were autoimmune antibody (GADA, IA-2A, or ZnT8A) positive and ≥30 years old were diagnosed with LADA, and subjects who were negative for all islet autoantibodies were diagnosed with type 2 diabetes. Patients with T1D, gestational diabetes mellitus, or malignancy and those who were pregnant were excluded. In general, LADY is distinguished from T1D by a period of at least 6 months after the onset of diabetes during which insulin is not required, LADY differs from type 2 diabetes by positivity for GADA, and 30 years old was used as the cutoff age to distinguish LADY from LADA (1).

There were 165 young T1D, 94 LADY, 149 old T1D, and 78 LADA subjects who were GADA positive assayed for epitope-specific GAD65Abs. Furthermore, 168 T1D, 62 LADY, 59 LADA, and 234 type 2 diabetes subjects were genotyped for *HLA-DRB1*, *HLA-DQA1*, and *HLA-DQB1* by direct DNA sequencing. GADA epitopes and *HLA-DRB1-DQA1-DQB1* were assayed in 289 patients, which comprised 97 young T1D, 62 LADY, 71 old T1D, and 59 LADA patients. This study was approved by the ethics committee of the Second Xiangya Hospital of Central South University, and all participants or their guardians provided written informed consent.

Physical characteristics (sex, age, height, and body weight) were recorded by professional researchers. Fasting blood was used for the measurement of fasting blood glucose (FBS), HbA1c, and fasting C-peptide (FCP). Postprandial blood samples were used to test 2-h postprandial plasma glucose (PPG) and 2-h postprandial C-peptide (PCP).

GADA, IA-2A, and ZnT8A Assays

GADA, IA-2A, and ZnT8A were measured by radioligand binding assay in duplicate as previously described (18, 19). The cutoff values of positivity for GADA and IA-2A were 18.0 U/ml and 3.3 U/ml in World Health Organization units, and ZnT8A was positive with an antibody index of 0.011 according to the 99th percentile observed in the healthy controls. The healthy control group consisted of 405 volunteers (264 men and 141 women, mean age: 37.8 years) with normal response to the 75-g oral glucose tolerance test; they had no family history of diabetes, autoimmune diabetes, or any other chronic diseases; and they were selected for establishing the cutoff values of GADA, IA-2A, and ZnT8A assays (19, 20). The sensitivity and specificity in our laboratory were 82% and 96.7% for GADA, 76% and 100% for IA-2A, and 76% and 100% for ZnT8A, respectively, according to the Islet Autoantibody Standardization Program (IASP) 2020.

Epitope Analysis of GAD65Ab

The epitopes of GAD65Ab were analyzed as previously described (8). The GAD65/67 chimeric constructs were responsible for the expression of fusion proteins of the N-terminal region ($GAD65_{1-95}$/$GAD67_{102-593}$), the middle region ($GAD67_{1-243}$/$GAD65_{235-444}$/$GAD67_{453-593}$), or the C-terminal region ($GAD67_{1-452}$/$GAD65_{445-585}$). The levels of epitope-specific GAD65Ab were expressed as relative indices according to the 99th percentile observed in 100 local healthy controls (58 men and 42 women; mean age: 36.5 years). The cutoff values were 0.06 for the GAD67-Ab assay, 0.05 for the GAD65-NAb and GAD65-MAb assays, and 0.03 for the GAD65-CAb assay.

HLA-DR-DQ Genetic Analysis

Genomic DNA was extracted from peripheral blood nucleated cells. The genotypes for *HLA-DRB1*, *HLA-DQA1*, and *HLA-DQB1* were determined by direct DNA sequencing *via* amplification of the second exon of each gene, and *DR-DQ* haplotypes were constructed by the PHASE program as described previously (15). Multiplex PCR amplifications of three HLA loci (*HLA-DRB1*, *HLA-DQA1*, and *HLA-DQB1*) were performed for all patients. For each donor, all HLA amplicons were pooled in a single well in approximately equimolar amounts. The samples from each individual were prepared using the Nextera XT protocol, pooled, and sequenced on a MiSeq instrument with a 2 × 250-bp paired-end cartridge (Illumina). The susceptible HLA haplotypes were *DR3 (DRB1*0301-DQA1*0501-DQB1*0201), DR4 (DRB1*0405-DQA1*0303-DQB1*0401), DRB1*0405-DQA1*0301-DQB1*0302*, and DR9 (*DRB1*0901-DQA1*0303-DQB1*0302*) (15, 21–23). The genotypes with a high genetic risk included *DR3/3, DR3/9*, and *DR9/9* (15).

Statistical Analysis

All statistical analyses were performed using SPSS (version 26; SPSS). Two-sided *p*-values <0.05 were considered statistically significant. Data are presented as the mean ± SD or medians (25th–75th percentile). Categorical variables were compared using Fisher's exact test or a χ^2 test as appropriate. Continuous variables were compared using one-way ANOVA. Nonparametric tests were performed by the Mann–Whitney assay. Binary logistic regression was performed to investigate possible *HLA-DQ-DR* factors for epitope-specific GAD65Abs. A *p*-value <0.05 was considered statistically significant.

RESULTS

Patterns of Epitope-Specific GAD65Abs in Young Type 1 Diabetes, Latent Autoimmune Diabetes in Youth, Old Type 1 Diabetes, and Latent Autoimmune Diabetes in Adult Patients

We used three different fragments (C-terminal, middle region, and N-terminal) to detect the GADA epitopes. Of the 586 GADA-positive patients, 100 subjects with GAD67Abs were removed to eliminate confounding factors. GAD65 epitope analysis was performed on 165 young T1D patients, 94 LADY patients, 149 old T1D patients, and 78 LADA patients. No reactivity to any of the epitopes of GAD65 was detected in 24.8%, 26.6%, 23.5%, and 41.0% of samples from young T1D patients, LADY patients, old T1D patients, and LADA patients, respectively. Further epitope analysis results are shown in **Table 1**. Compared with that in LADA subjects, the frequency of GAD65-CAb was higher in young T1D, LADY, and old T1D subjects (57.6% vs. 33.3%, $p < 0.001$; 48.9% vs. 33.3%, $p < 0.05$; and 58.4% vs. 33.3%, $p < 0.001$, respectively), and the frequency of GAD65-MAb was higher in young T1D and LADY subjects than that in LADA subjects (60.0% vs. 42.3%, $p < 0.05$; 66.0% vs. 42.3%, $p < 0.01$, respectively), whereas the frequency of GAD65-NAb was higher in LADA subjects than that in young T1D subjects (20.5% vs. 7.3%, $p < 0.01$). There was no significant difference among young T1D, LADY, and old T1D subjects in the percentage of the three different epitope-specific GAD65Abs (GAD65-CAb, GAD65-Mab, and GAD65-NAb).

Frequency of GAD65Abs That Bind Different Numbers of Epitopes of GAD65 in Young Type 1 Diabetes, Latent Autoimmune Diabetes in Youth, Old Type 1 Diabetes, and Latent Autoimmune Diabetes in Adult Patients

GADA binding to different GAD65 epitopes (N-terminal, middle region, and C-terminal) in the different groups is shown in **Table 1** and **Figure 2**. A total of 44.2% (73/165) of young T1D patients, 45.7% (43/94) of LADY patients, 43.6% (65/149) of old T1D patients, and 26.9% (21/78) of LADA patients reacted to at least two regions of GAD65. Noticeably, young T1D, LADY, and old T1D patients showed higher levels of reactivity against multiple epitopes of GAD65 than the levels of LADA patients (44.2% vs. 26.9%, $p < 0.05$; 45.7% vs. 26.9%, $p < 0.05$; and 43.6% vs. 26.9%, $p < 0.05$, respectively). There was no significant difference among young T1D, LADY, and old T1D patients in the frequency of GAD65Ab that binds different numbers of epitopes of GAD65.

Clinical Characteristics of Young Type 1 Diabetes, Latent Autoimmune Diabetes in Youth, Old Type 1 Diabetes, and Latent Autoimmune Diabetes in Adult Patients

As shown in **Table 2**, the levels of FCP were higher in LADY and LADA subjects than those in young T1D and old T1D subjects; furthermore, compared with levels in LADA patients, LADY patients had lower levels of FCP. The level of PCP manifested a similar trend; compared with levels in young T1D and old T1D patients, LADY and LADA patients had a higher level of PCP, but there was no significant difference between LADY and LADA patients in the level of PCP. GADA titers were significantly different only between old T1D and LADA patients [old T1D vs. LADA: 376.8 (118.4–902.6) vs. 180.4 (50.3–450.3) U/ml, $p < 0.01$].

HLA-DR-DQ Haplotype and Genotype Frequency Analysis

As shown in **Table 3**, the frequency of the susceptible HLA haplotype DR3 was higher in T1D and LADY patients than that in LADA patients (T1D vs. LADA: 16.7% vs. 6.8%, $p < 0.01$; LADY vs. LADA: 26.6% vs. 6.8%, $p < 0.001$). Similarly, the frequencies of total susceptible HLA haplotypes were significantly higher in T1D and LADY patients than that in

TABLE 1 | Prevalence of epitope-specific GAD65Ab in young T1DM, old T1DM, LADY, and LADA patients.

GADA reactivities to epitopes of GAD65	Young T1DM (n = 165)	LADY (n = 94)	Old T1DM (n = 149)	LADA (n = 78)	*p*-value
C-terminal	57.6% (95)	48.9% (46)	58.4% (87)	33.3% (26) †††§***	0.001
N-region	7.3% (12)	12.8% (12)	12.8% (19)	20.5% (16) ††	0.031
M-terminal	60.0% (99)	66.0% (62)	54.4% (81)	42.3% (33) †§§	0.012
Positive for 1 epitope	30.9% (51)	27.7% (26)	32.9% (49)	32.1% (25)	0.855
Positive for at least 2 epitopes	44.2% (73)	45.7% (43)	43.6% (65)	26.9% (21) †§*	0.040

Data are expressed as % (n).
GADA, glutamic acid decarboxylase antibody.
When compared with young T1DM patients, † $p < 0.05$, †† $p < 0.01$, ††† $p < 0.001$.
When compared with LADY patients, § $p < 0.05$, §§ $p < 0.01$.
When compared with old T1DM patients, * $p < 0.05$, *** $p < 0.001$.
T1DM, type 1 diabetes mellitus; LADY, latent autoimmune diabetes in youth; LADA, latent autoimmune diabetes in adults.

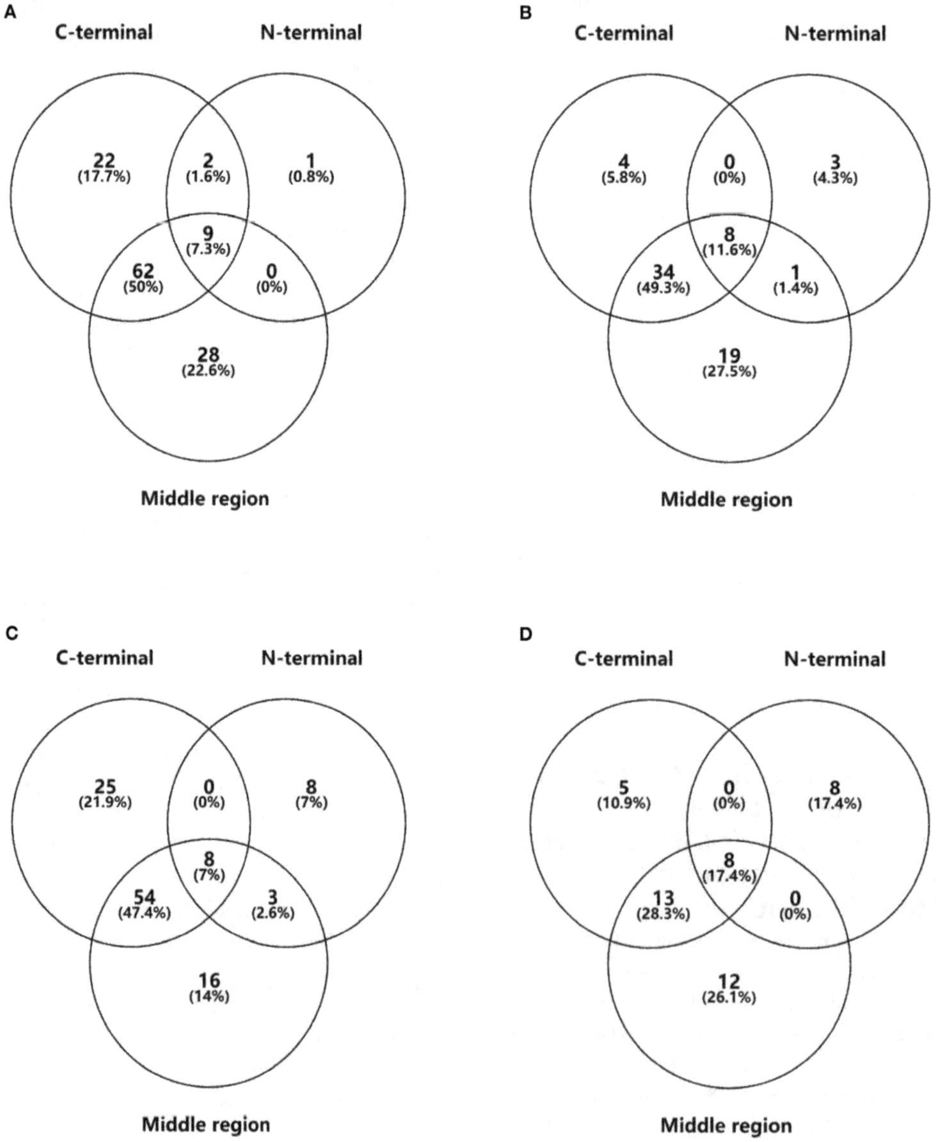

FIGURE 2 | The distribution of GADA binding to different epitopes of GAD65 in young T1DM **(A)**, LADY **(B)**, old T1DM **(C)**, and LADA **(D)** patients. Data are expressed as n (%).

TABLE 2 | Comparison of clinical features of patients with young T1DM, LADY, old T1DM, and LADA.

Variable	Young T1DM (n = 165)	LADY (n = 94)	Old T1DM (n = 149)	LADA (n = 78)	*p*-value
Age (years)	23 ± 4	25 ± 4†	47 ± 11†††§§§	52 ± 12†††§§§**	<0.001
Female/male	72/93	33/61	53/96	36/42	0.231
BMI (kg/m^2)	19.8 ± 3.5	21.3 ± 3.6††	22.0 ± 3.7†††	22.5 ± 3.3†††§	<0.001
SBP (mmHg)	116 ± 13	116 ± 14	120 ± 15††§	123 ± 13†††§§	<0.001
DBP (mmHg)	74 ± 9	74 ± 9	77 ± 11†	79 ± 10††§§	0.004
FBS (mmol/L)	9.8 ± 4.7	9.2 ± 4.3	9.7 ± 4.1	9.6 ± 4.2	0.746
HbA$_{1C}$ (mmol/mol)	105.6 ± 37.8	100.5 ± 38.2	98.8 ± 33.1	88.9 ± 31.9††	0.008
HbA$_{1C}$ (%)	11.8 ± 3.5	11.3 ± 3.5	11.2 ± 3.0	10.3 ± 2.9††	0.008
FCP (pmol/L)	120 (60–202)	230 (143–380) †††	122 (53–239) §§§	423 (223–655) †††§***	<0.001
PCP (pmol/L)	190 (96–395)	490 (289–815) †††	208 (114–463) §§§	1,070 (442–1747) †††***	<0.001
TG (mmol/L)	0.94 (0.72–1.49)	1.10 (0.79–1.74)	1.03 (0.70–1.65)	1.37 (0.93–2.07) ††	0.013
TC (mmol/L)	4.30 ± 1.22	4.48 ± 1.39	4.46 ± 1.61	4.64 ± 1.22	0.379
LDL-C (mmol/L)	2.58 ± 0.91	2.79 ± 1.08	2.61 ± 1.04	2.74 ± 1.34	0.386
HDL-C (mmol/L)	1.21 (0.99–1.48)	1.11 (0.96–1.40)	1.17 (0.97–1.50)	1.16 (0.96–1.42)	0.341
GAD65Ab (U/ml)	269.2 (97.2–757.2)	267.7 (84.5–600.5)	376.8 (118.4–902.6)	180.4 (50.3–450.3) **	0.007

Data are presented as the mean ± SD, median (IQR), or ratio.

SBP, systolic blood pressure; DBP, diastolic blood pressure; FBS, fasting blood glucose; FCP, fasting C peptide; PCP, 2-h postprandial C peptide; TG, triglycerides; TC, total cholesterol; HDL-C, HDL cholesterol; LDL-C, LDL cholesterol.

When compared with young T1DM patients, † $p < 0.05$, †† $p < 0.01$, ††† $p < 0.001$.

When compared with LADY patients, § $p < 0.05$, §§ $p < 0.01$, §§§ $p < 0.001$.

*When compared with old T1DM patients, ** $p < 0.01$, *** $p < 0.001$.*

T1DM, type 1 diabetes mellitus; LADY, latent autoimmune diabetes in youth; LADA, latent autoimmune diabetes in adults.

LADA patients (T1D vs. LADA: 58.6% vs. 37.3%, $p < 0.001$; LADY vs. LADA: 64.5% vs. 37.3%, $p < 0.001$). Moreover, the frequencies of high-risk genotypes were higher in T1D and LADY patients than that in LADA patients (T1D vs. LADA: 25.0% vs. 10.2%, $p < 0.05$; LADY vs. LADA: 35.5% vs. 10.2%, $p < 0.01$). In contrast, T1D and LADY patients had lower frequencies of low/no genetic risk genotypes (*DRX/X*) than the frequencies of LADA patients (T1D vs. LADA: 14.9% vs. 40.7%, $p < 0.001$; LADY vs. LADA: 14.5% vs. 40.7%, $p < 0.01$). Unexpectedly, LADY patients had a higher frequency of the susceptible haplotype *DR3* than that of T1D patients (26.6% vs. 16.7%, $p < 0.05$). There were no significant differences between LADY and T1D patients in the frequencies of total susceptible HLA haplotypes, high-risk genotypes, and low/no genetic risk genotypes (*DRX/X*). There was no difference in HLA genes between LADA and type 2 diabetes patients.

Correlation Between the *HLA-DR-DQ* Genes and Epitope-Specific GAD65Ab

Because the appearance, positivity, and affinity of GADA are related to the *HLA-DR-DQ* genes, as reported in previous studies (24–27), we tried to investigate the association between epitope-specific GAD65Abs (GAD65-CAb, GAD65-Mab, and GAD65-NAb) and the *HLA-DR-DQ* gene. As shown in **Table 4**, the susceptible HLA haplotype was a risk factor for GAD65Ab multiepitope positivity ($r = 1.900$; $p < 0.05$). Among the susceptible HLA haplotypes shared by T1D and LADA patients, *DR3* conferred the highest genetic susceptibility (15).

TABLE 3 | The frequency of susceptible HLA haplotypes and genotypes among T1DM, LADY, LADA, and T2DM subjects.

Variable	T1DM	LADY	LADA	T2DM	*p*-value
n	168	62	59	234	N/A
Onset age	32 ± 13	25 ± 4†††	54 ± 11†††§§§	36 ± 15§§§***	<0.001
Female/male	67/101	23/39	28/31	82/152	0.339
DR3	16.7 (56)	26.6 (33) †	6.8 (8) ††§§§	5.8 (27) †††§§§	<0.001
DR4	12.5 (42)	11.3 (14)	7.6 (9)	4.5 (21) †††§§	<0.001
*DRB1*04:05-DQA1*03:01-DQB1*03:02*	0.3 (1)	0.8 (1)	1.7 (2)	0.2 (1)	0.181
DR9	29.2 (98)	25.8 (32)	21.2 (25)	18.8 (88) ††	0.006
Total susceptible haplotypes	58.6 (197)	64.5 (80)	37.3 (44) †††§§§	29.3 (137) †††§§§	<0.001
DR3/3, DR-3/9, DR-9/9 (high genetic risk)	25.0 (42)	35.5 (22)	10.2 (6) †§§	5.1 (12) †††§§§	<0.001
DRX/X (no/low genetic risk)	14.9 (25)	14.5 (9)	40.7 (24) †††§§	51.3 (120) †††§§§	<0.001

Data are presented as the mean ± SD or % (n).

†Compared with T1DM $p < 0.05$, †† Compared with T1DM $p < 0.01$, ††† Compared with T1DM $p < 0.001$.

§§Compared with LADY $p < 0.01$, §§§ Compared with LADY $p < 0.001$.

Compared with LADA $p < 0.05$, * Compared with LADA $p < 0.001$.*

*DR3, DRB1*03:01-DQA1*05:01-DQB1*02:01; DR4, DRB1*04:05-DQA1*03:03-DQB1*04:01; DR9, DRB1*09:01-DQA1*03:02-DQB1*03:03; Total susceptible haplotypes, DR3+DR4+ DRB1*04:05-DQA1*03:01-DQB1*03:02+DR9; X, other than DR3, DR4, DRB1*04:05-DQA1*03:01-DQB1*03:02, and DR9; LADY, latent autoimmune diabetes in youth; LADA, latent autoimmune diabetes in adults; T1DM, type 1 diabetes mellitus; T2DM, type 2 diabetes mellitus.*

TABLE 4 | Association of the frequency of GADA binding to multiple epitopes of GAD65 with the frequencies of *HLA-DR-DQ* haplotypes and genotypes.

Variable	OR (95% CI)	*p*-value
DR3	1.76 (1.04–2.99)	0.035*
DR4	1.22 (0.69–2.16)	0.499
DR9	0.81 (0.50–1.31)	0.384
Susceptible haplotypes	1.90 (1.02–3.54)	0.043*
DR3/DR3, DR3/DR9, and *DR9/DR9*	1.23 (0.71–2.12)	0.457

*DR3, DRB1*03:01-DQA1*05:01-DQB1*02:01; DR4, DRB1*04:05-DQA1*03:03-DQB1*04:01; DR9, DRB1*09:01-DQA1*03:02-DQB1*03:03; susceptible haplotypes, DR3+ DR4+ DR9.*

**Represents p value <0.05, which is statistically significant.*

We further investigated the association between different common susceptible HLA haplotypes and GAD65Ab multiepitope positivity. Logistic regression analysis suggested that patients with *DR3* had a higher risk of GAD65Ab multiepitope positivity ($r = 1.763$; $p < 0.05$). In addition, GAD65-CAb was considered to be related to worse beta-cell function and greater insulin therapy demand (7, 8, 20). We analyzed the association between *HLA-DR-DQ* genes and GAD65-CAb but found no significant association between them (**Table 5**).

DISCUSSION

GADA has been used to screen individuals with autoimmune diabetes. Over the past few decades, reports about the epitope specificity of GAD65Abs in T1D and LADA have increased (8, 11). Autoimmune diabetes is considered to be a continuous spectrum (28). For the first time, we disclosed the epitope-specific GAD65Ab frequencies from young T1D, LADY, old T1D, and LADA patients, but especially in LADY patients. We also found an association between the *HLA-DR-DQ* gene and epitope-specific GAD65Abs. LADY seems to be a transitional type of T1D and LADA. This finding suggests the important value of the identification and early intervention in protecting islet function for LADY. Clinically, it is necessary to protect the islet function of LADY patients as early as possible in the window period. These results provide helpful information for understanding the pathogenesis of LADY.

Compared with T1D patients, a lower frequency of GAD65-CAb and a higher frequency of GAD65-Nab were observed in LADA patients, and the discrepancy in GAD65 epitope patterns between T1D and LADA suggests different immune activities toward islet beta cells. As the results showed, LADY may be more severe than LADA, and the percentage of GAD65-CAb was significantly higher in young T1D, LADY, and old T1D subjects than that in LADA subjects, which reveals the important value of epitope-specific assays in the identification process and islet function protection. Furthermore, compared with those of LADA patients, the levels of FCP were observed to be lower in LADY patients, and GAD65-CAb and multiepitope GAD65Ab positivity were considered to be related to worse islet function (7, 8). In terms of epitope reactivity, young T1D, LADY, and old T1D patients showed higher reactivities to multiple epitopes of GAD65 than did LADA patients, which indicates a stronger or broader immune response. These findings suggested that there may be more severe immune damage progression in young T1D, LADY, and old T1D patients than in LADA patients. Epitope-specific assays of GAD65Abs may be useful in predicting the need for insulin therapy in autoimmune diabetes.

The *DRB1, DQA1*, and *DQB1* loci were highly associated with diabetes susceptibility (3, 15, 29, 30). *HLA-DR-DQ* genes in T1D, LADY, LADA, and type 2 diabetes patients were compared for the first time in this study, especially between LADY and LADA patients. The higher frequencies of total susceptible HLA haplotypes and high-risk genotypes in T1D and LADY manifested an increased HLA genetic susceptibility load compared with that of LADA, which may imply a shared pathogenesis between T1D and LADY, suggesting that the similarity in the frequencies of the epitope-specific GAD65Abs between T1D and LADY subjects may be derived from similar HLA genetic backgrounds. *DR3*, total susceptible haplotypes, and high-risk HLA genotypes were more frequent in LADY than those in LADA, and the discrepancy in HLA genes between LADY and LADA indicated an increased HLA genetic susceptibility load in LADY patients, LADY was likely to be more severe than LADA, and early clinical intervention and different therapeutic strategies to preserve islet function were required for LADY patients.

T1D and LADY subjects had a higher susceptible HLA risk and higher reactivity to GAD65Ab than LADA subjects. An association between HLA genes and the affinity of GAD65Ab has been reported (16, 24, 25). This study investigated the association between *HLA-DR-DQ* genes and the epitope specificity of GAD65Abs, which may be useful in revealing the interaction between HLA and the diabetes autoimmune response. HLA gene risk and GAD65 epitope specificity may accurately stratify the risk of ADM patients. Susceptible HLA haplotypes were a risk factor for GADA multiepitope positivity, especially *DR3*. HLA genes affected GADA multiepitope positivity, which is an immunoreactive process with epitope expansion within the GADA molecule. This finding has an implication similar to that of a previous study by Pöllänen et al. (31). They reported that HLA genes affected positivity for multiple islet autoantibodies, and patients with high-risk HLA genotypes had a greater tendency to be positive for

TABLE 5 | Association of the frequency of GAD65-CAb with the frequencies of *HLA-DR-DQ* haplotypes and genotypes.

Variable	OR (95% CI)	*p*-value
DR3	1.49 (0.88–2.52)	0.139
DR4	1.16 (0.66–2.04)	0.612
DR9	0.90 (0.56–1.44)	0.649
Susceptible haplotypes	1.56 (0.88–2.79)	0.130
DR3/DR3, DR3/DR9, and *DR9/DR9*	1.18 (0.69–2.02)	0.555

*DR3, DRB1*03:01-DQA1*05:01-DQB1*02:01; DR4, DRB1*04:05-DQA1*03:03-DQB1*04:01; DR9, DRB1*09:01-DQA1*03:02-DQB1*03:03; susceptible haplotypes, DR3+ DR4+DR9.*

multiple antibodies than that of patients with moderate-risk HLA genotypes (31). Transitioning from single antibody positivity to multiple antibody positivity reflects an expansion of the immune response between different islet autoantibody molecules. The above two findings revealed that HLA contributed to both the intermolecular and intramolecular expansion of islet autoimmunity.

LADY seems to be more closely related to T1D than LADA. First, the percentage of GAD65-CAb was higher in young T1D, LADY, and old T1D subjects than that in LADA subjects. Second, young T1D, LADY, and old T1D patients showed a higher frequency of multiepitope GAD65Abs than that in LADA patients. Third, the frequencies of total susceptible HLA haplotypes and high-risk genotypes were higher in T1D and LADY subjects than those in LADA subjects, while the frequency of no/low genetic risk genotypes (*DRX/X*) was higher in LADA subjects than those in T1D and LADY subjects. Last, the levels of FCP and PCP were similarly lower in T1D and LADY subjects than those in LADA subjects, which suggested similar islet function in T1D and LADY patients. These findings are of great importance in clinical prevention, judgment, and the use of insulin in LADY patients.

In summary, T1D and LADY patients had more similar HLA-DR-DQ genetic backgrounds and epitope-specific GAD65Abs than LADA patients. The discrepancies in terms of the frequencies of susceptible HLA genes between LADY and LADA may contribute to the different manifestations of epitope-specific GAD65Abs; LADY was likely to be more severe than LADA. This information could be useful for classifying LADY patients and could provide novel insight into understanding the pathology underlying LADY. In addition, the existence of susceptible HLA haplotypes was a risk factor for the frequency of GAD65Ab multiepitope positivity, especially *DR3*, revealing the intricate pathogenesis of autoimmune diabetes in terms of the HLA genetic background and GADA immune response. Whereas the number of individuals with LADY and LADA in this study was relatively small, there was no long-term observation of the level of C-peptide and the frequencies of epitope-specific GAD65Abs, which may be dynamic during the progression of disease. It will be necessary to explore more specific and detailed results in large-scale and follow-up cohort studies to provide novel insight into the pathogenesis of autoimmune diabetes.

AUTHOR CONTRIBUTIONS

YP conducted the experiments, analyzed the data, and wrote the article. GH and ZZ conceived and designed the study. YP and GH analyzed and interpreted the results. XL, YX, XY, HZ, XT, JC, XN, JL, QJ, and LJ researched the data. All the authors critically revised the article and approved the final version. GH is the guarantor of this work and, as such, had full access to all the data in the study and takes responsibility for the integrity of the data and the accuracy of the data analysis.

ACKNOWLEDGMENTS

The authors thank all of the patients, nurses, doctors, investigators, and technicians involved at the 46 participating centers of the National Clinical Research Center for Metabolic Diseases for their efforts in data and sample collection. We thank Prof. Bill Hagopian for providing the recombinant hGAD65 and IA-2 plasmids and Prof. John C. Hutton for providing the recombinant ZnT8 plasmid. We thank Dr. Vito Lampasona and Dr. Ezio Bonifacio for providing the recombinant hGAD65/GAD67 plasmid.

REFERENCES

1. Fourlanos S, Dotta F, Greenbaum CJ, Palmer JP, Rolandsson O, Colman PG, et al. Latent Autoimmune Diabetes in Adults (LADA) Should be Less Latent. *Diabetologia* (2005) 48(11):2206–12. doi: 10.1007/s00125-005-1960-7
2. Wang L, Gao P, Zhang M, Huang Z, Zhang D, Deng Q, et al. Prevalence and Ethnic Pattern of Diabetes and Prediabetes in China in 2013. *Jama* (2017) 317 (24):2515–23. doi: 10.1001/jama.2017.7596
3. Xiang Y, Liu B, Yun C, Zhou P, Li X, Luo S, et al. Frequency, Clinical Features, Inflammatory Cytokines and Genetic Background of Latent Autoimmune Diabetes in Youth in Youth-Onset Type 2 Diabetes: Results From a Nationwide, Multicentre, Clinic-Based, Cross-Sectional Study (LADA China). *Diabetes Obes Metab* (2021) 23(6):1282–91. doi: 10.1111/dom.14336
4. Lampasona V, Liberati D. Islet Autoantibodies. *Curr Diabetes Rep* (2016) 16 (6):53. doi: 10.1007/s11892-016-0738-2
5. Vandewalle CL, Falorni A, Svanholm S, Lernmark A, Pipeleers DG, Gorus FK. High Diagnostic Sensitivity of Glutamate Decarboxylase Autoantibodies in Insulin-Dependent Diabetes Mellitus With Clinical Onset Between Age 20 and 40 Years. The Belgian Diabetes Registry. *J Clin Endocrinol Metab* (1995) 80(3):846–51. doi: 10.1210/jcem.80.3.7883841
6. Liu B, Xiang Y, Liu Z, Zhou Z. Past, Present and Future of Latent Autoimmune Diabetes in Adults. *Diabetes Metab Res Rev* (2020) 36(1): e3205. doi: 10.1002/dmrr.3205
7. Falorni A, Gambelunghe G, Forini F, Kassi G, Cosentino A, Candeloro P, et al. Autoantibody Recognition of COOH-Terminal Epitopes of GAD65 Marks the Risk for Insulin Requirement in Adult-Onset Diabetes Mellitus. *J Clin Endocrinol Metab* (2000) 85(1):309–16. doi: 10.1210/jcem.85.1.6301
8. Jin P, Huang G, Lin J, Luo S, Zhou Z. Epitope Analysis of GAD65 Autoantibodies in Adult-Onset Type 1 Diabetes and Latent Autoimmune Diabetes in Adults With Thyroid Autoimmunity. *Acta Diabetol* (2011) 48 (2):149–55. doi: 10.1007/s00592-010-0250-0
9. Achenbach P, Hawa MI, Krause S, Lampasona V, Jerram ST, Williams AJK, et al. Autoantibodies to N-Terminally Truncated GAD Improve Clinical Phenotyping of Individuals With Adult-Onset Diabetes: Action LADA 12. *Diabetologia* (2018) 61(7):1644–9. doi: 10.1007/s00125-018-4605-3
10. Daw K, Powers AC. Two Distinct Glutamic Acid Decarboxylase Auto-Antibody Specificities in IDDM Target Different Epitopes. *Diabetes* (1995) 44(2):216–20. doi: 10.2337/diab.44.2.216
11. Hampe CS, Kockum I, Landin-Olsson M, Törn C, Ortqvist E, Persson B, et al. GAD65 Antibody Epitope Patterns of Type 1.5 Diabetic Patients are Consistent With Slow-Onset Autoimmune Diabetes. *Diabetes Care* (2002) 25(8):1481–2. doi: 10.2337/diacare.25.8.1481
12. Schlosser M, Banga JP, Madec AM, Binder KA, Strebelow M, Rjasanowski I, et al. Dynamic Changes of GAD65 Autoantibody Epitope Specificities in Individuals at Risk of Developing Type 1 Diabetes. *Diabetologia* (2005) 48 (5):922–30. doi: 10.1007/s00125-005-1719-1
13. Davies JL, Kawaguchi Y, Bennett ST, Copeman JB, Cordell HJ, Pritchard LE, et al. A Genome-Wide Search for Human Type 1 Diabetes Susceptibility Genes. *Nature* (1994) 371(6493):130–6. doi: 10.1038/371130a0

14. Aly TA, Ide A, Jahromi MM, Barker JM, Fernando MS, Babu SR, et al. Extreme Genetic Risk for Type 1A Diabetes. *Proc Natl Acad Sci USA* (2006) 103(38):14074–9. doi: 10.1073/pnas.0606349103
15. Luo S, Lin J, Xie Z, Xiang Y, Zheng P, Huang G, et al. HLA Genetic Discrepancy Between Latent Autoimmune Diabetes in Adults and Type 1 Diabetes: LADA China Study No. 6. *J Clin Endocrinol Metab* (2016) 101 (4):1693–700. doi: 10.1210/jc.2015-3771
16. Tang X, Yan X, Zhou H, Yang X, Niu X, Liu J, et al. Prevalence and Identification of Type 1 Diabetes in Chinese Adults With Newly Diagnosed Diabetes. *Diabetes Metab Syndr Obes* (2019) 12:1527–41. doi: 10.2147/dmso.S202193
17. Padmos RC, Schloot NC, Beyan H, Ruwhof C, Staal FJ, de Ridder D, et al. Distinct Monocyte Gene-Expression Profiles in Autoimmune Diabetes. *Diabetes* (2008) 57(10):2768–73. doi: 10.2337/db08-0496
18. Zhou Z, Xiang Y, Ji L, Jia W, Ning G, Huang G, et al. Frequency, Immunogenetics, and Clinical Characteristics of Latent Autoimmune Diabetes in China (LADA China Study): A Nationwide, Multicenter, Clinic-Based Cross-Sectional Study. *Diabetes* (2013) 62(2):543–50. doi: 10.2337/db12-0207
19. Huang G, Xiang Y, Pan L, Li X, Luo S, Zhou Z. Zinc Transporter 8 Autoantibody (ZnT8A) Could Help Differentiate Latent Autoimmune Diabetes in Adults (LADA) From Phenotypic Type 2 Diabetes Mellitus. *Diabetes Metab Res Rev* (2013) 29(5):363–8. doi: 10.1002/dmrr.2396
20. Huang G, Yin M, Xiang Y, Li X, Shen W, Luo S, et al. Persistence of Glutamic Acid Decarboxylase Antibody (GADA) Is Associated With Clinical Characteristics of Latent Autoimmune Diabetes in Adults: A Prospective Study With 3-Year Follow-Up. *Diabetes Metab Res Rev* (2016) 32(6):615–22. doi: 10.1002/dmrr.2779
21. Kawabata Y, Ikegami H, Kawaguchi Y, Fujisawa T, Shintani M, Ono M, et al. Asian-Specific HLA Haplotypes Reveal Heterogeneity of the Contribution of HLA-DR and -DQ Haplotypes to Susceptibility to Type 1 Diabetes. *Diabetes* (2002) 51(2):545–51. doi: 10.2337/diabetes.51.2.545
22. Lin J, Zhou ZG, Wang JP, Zhang C, Huang G. From Type 1, Through LADA, to Type 2 Diabetes: A Continuous Spectrum? *Ann N Y Acad Sci* (2008) 1150:99–102. doi: 10.1196/annals.1447.036
23. Kawabata Y, Ikegami H, Awata T, Imagawa A, Maruyama T, Kawasaki E, et al. Differential Association of HLA With Three Subtypes of Type 1 Diabetes: Fulminant, Slowly Progressive and Acute-Onset. *Diabetologia* (2009) 52 (12):2513–21. doi: 10.1007/s00125-009-1539-9
24. Mayr A, Schlosser M, Grober N, Kenk H, Ziegler AG, Bonifacio E, et al. GAD Autoantibody Affinity and Epitope Specificity Identify Distinct Immunization Profiles in Children at Risk for Type 1 Diabetes. *Diabetes* (2007) 56(6):1527–33. doi: 10.2337/db06-1715
25. Bender C, Schlosser M, Christen U, Ziegler AG, Achenbach P. GAD Autoantibody Affinity in Schoolchildren From the General Population. *Diabetologia* (2014) 57(9):1911–8. doi: 10.1007/s00125-014-3294-9
26. Krischer JP, Liu X, Vehik K, Akolkar B, Hagopian WA, Rewers MJ, et al. Predicting Islet Cell Autoimmunity and Type 1 Diabetes: An 8-Year TEDDY Study Progress Report. *Diabetes Care* (2019) 42(6):1051–60. doi: 10.2337/dc18-2282
27. Krischer JP, Lynch KF, Schatz DA, Ilonen J, Lernmark Å, Hagopian WA, et al. The 6 Year Incidence of Diabetes-Associated Autoantibodies in Genetically at-Risk Children: The TEDDY Study. *Diabetologia* (2015) 58(5):980–7. doi: 10.1007/s00125-015-3514-y
28. Buzzetti R, Zampetti S, Maddaloni E. Adult-Onset Autoimmune Diabetes: Current Knowledge and Implications for Management. *Nat Rev Endocrinol* (2017) 13(11):674–86. doi: 10.1038/nrendo.2017.99
29. Cucca F, Muntoni F, Lampis R, Frau F, Argiolas L, Silvetti M, et al. Combinations of Specific DRB1, DQA1, DQB1 Haplotypes are Associated With Insulin-Dependent Diabetes Mellitus in Sardinia. *Hum Immunol* (1993) 37(2):85–94. doi: 10.1016/0198-8859(93)90146-r
30. Noble JA, Valdes AM, Cook M, Klitz W, Thomson G, Erlich HA. The Role of HLA Class II Genes in Insulin-Dependent Diabetes Mellitus: Molecular Analysis of 180 Caucasian, Multiplex Families. *Am J Hum Genet* (1996) 59 (5):1134–48.
31. Pöllänen PM, Ryhänen SJ, Toppari J, Ilonen J, Vähäsalo P, Veijola R, et al. Dynamics of Islet Autoantibodies During Prospective Follow-Up From Birth to Age 15 Years. *J Clin Endocrinol Metab* (2020) 105(12):e4638–4651. doi: 10.1210/clinem/dgaa624

20

Tellurium Compounds Prevent and Reverse Type-1 Diabetes in NOD Mice by Modulating α4β7 Integrin Activity, IL-1β and T Regulatory Cells

Tom Eitan Yossipof [1†]***, Ziva Roy Bazak*** [1†]***, Dvora Kenigsbuch-Sredni*** [2]***, Rachel R. Caspi*** [3]***, Yona Kalechman*** [1] ***and Benjamin Sredni*** [1*]

[1] *The Mina & Everard Goodman Faculty of Life Sciences, The Safdiè AIDS and Immunology Research Center, C.A.I.R. Institute, Ramat Gan, Israel,* [2] *Interdisciplinary Department, Bar-Ilan University, Ramat Gan, Israel,* [3] *Laboratory of Immunology, National Eye Institute, National Institutes of Health, Bethesda, MD, United States*

Correspondence:
Benjamin Sredni
srednib@biu.ac.il

[†] *These authors have contributed equally to this work*

The study shows that treatment of NOD mice with either of two tellurium-based small molecules, AS101 [ammonium trichloro(dioxoethylene-o,o')tellurate] or SAS [octa-O-bis-(R,R)-tartarate ditellurane] could preserve β cells function and mass. These beneficial effects were reflected in decreased incidence of diabetes, improved glucose clearance, preservation of body weight, and increased survival. The normal glucose levels were associated with increased insulin levels, preservation of β cell mass and increased islet size. Importantly, this protective activity could be demonstrated when the compounds were administered either at the early pre-diabetic phase with no or initial insulitis, at the pre-diabetic stage with advanced insulitis, or even at the advanced, overtly diabetic stage. We further demonstrate that both tellurium compounds prevent migration of autoimmune lymphocytes to the pancreas, via inhibition of the α4β7 integrin activity. Indeed, the decreased migration resulted in diminished pancreatic islets damage both with respect to their size, β cell function, and caspase-3 activity, the hallmark of apoptosis. Most importantly, AS101 and SAS significantly elevated the number of T regulatory cells in the pancreas, thus potentially controlling the autoimmune process. We show that the compounds inhibit pancreatic caspase-1 activity followed by decreased levels of the inflammatory cytokines IL-1β and IL-17 in the pancreas. These properties enable the compounds to increase the proportion of Tregs in the pancreatic lymph nodes. AS101 and SAS have been previously shown to regulate specific integrins through a unique redox mechanism. Our current results suggest that amelioration of disease in NOD mice by this unique mechanism is due to decreased infiltration of pancreatic islets combined with increased immune regulation, leading to decreased inflammation within the islets. As these tellurium compounds show remarkable lack of toxicity in clinical trials (AS101) and pre-clinical studies (SAS), they may be suitable for the treatment of type-1 diabetes.

Keywords: diabetes, tellurium, integrin, inflammation, IL-1β, Tregs

INTRODUCTION

Type 1 diabetes mellitus (T1D) develops as a result of pancreatic islet β-cells loss, mainly by means of CD4 T cells and other leukocytes action. The autoimmune etiology of T1D is affected by both genetic and environmental factors. Nevertheless, the exact mechanisms of disease initiation remain largely unknown.

There is no proven means to avoid the development of diabetes, nor to control the anti-β-cell autoimmune response after the disease has been diagnosed. Furthermore, the progressive loss of self-tolerance to islet β-cell antigens in human patients and animal models, is one of the most important fundamental contributing factors to T1D development. One of the main primary factors controlling such self-tolerance is the activity of Regulatory T cells (Tregs) (1).

Upon immunological challenge, lymphocytes migrate from the bloodstream into secondary lymphoid tissues such as lymph nodes (LNs) and Peyer's patches. Infiltration of immune cells is essential for organ and antigen-specific adoptive immunity against pathogens and antigens, including autoimmunity.

This migration is controlled in part by adhesion molecules and chemokine receptors on lymphocytes and their ligands on blood vessel high endothelial venules (HEVs) in LNs and Peyer's patches (2–4).

In T1D, activated $CD4^+$ and $CD8^+$ T lymphocytes destroy the insulin-producing β-cells of the pancreatic islets. In recent years it was recognized that B cells in pancreatic LNs are crucial antigen presenting cells (APCs) not only to initiate and optimize priming of naive autoreactive $CD4^+$ T cells by β cell antigens, but also to contribute to epitope spreading of T cell autoimmunity among β cell antigens (5). Furthermore, the α4β7 integrin/MAdCAM-1 pathway has been found crucial for the migration of B cells from the bloodstream into pancreatic lymph nodes (PLN) in NOD mice (6). Importantly, an α4-integrin-VCAM-1 interaction contributes to T cell entry into the pancreatic islets and in the pathogenesis of T1D (7).

AS101 is a potent tellurium-based immunomodulator, which has demonstrated activity for several indications, both *in vitro* and *in vivo*, and has a large number of potential therapeutic applications (8, 9). The compound is non-toxic and is currently undergoing phase II/III testing in patients with cervical tumors, and phase I/II testing for treatment of patients with age-related macular degeneration. Much of the biological activity of AS101 can be attributed to its chemical redox interactions with vicinal thiols in the exofacial domain of VLA-4 (10); these modifications enable this agent to mediate diverse effects including abrogation of acquired drug resistance in acute myelogenous leukemia (10), and improvement of symptoms in experimental autoimmune encephalomyelitis (11) and uveitis (12). The specific redox-modulating activities of AS101 result in a variety of beneficial biological effects, demonstrated in diverse preclinical and clinical studies (13). The anti-inflammatory properties were found to be crucial for the clinical activities of AS101, including the protective effects of AS101 in autoimmune diseases (14–17) and in septic mice (18). The same thiol–redox interactions of AS101 enabled it to exert beneficial effects in a variety of tumor models in mice and humans where AS101 had clear antitumor effects (10, 19, 20).

The second generation tellurium IV compound SAS synthesized by us, has also been shown to possess a unique Te^{IV}-thiol chemistry and exert biological activities similar to those of AS101 (13).

Based on our previous data showing that AS101 inhibits the α4β7 activity in mesenteric lymph node cells of DSS-induced murine colitis (14), we hypothesized that both tellurium compounds may have the potential to suppress the activity of the α4β7 integrin on lymphocytes from NOD mice, and consequently prevent their infiltration into pancreatic LNs, potentially affecting the pathogenesis of T1D.

We demonstrate that AS101 and SAS are able to prevent as well as inverse new onset type 1 diabetes in the NOD mouse model, and exhibit effects on α4β7 activity and lymphocyte migration, as well as inhibition of pancreatic IL-1β and IL-17 production and enrichment of T-regulatory (Treg) cells in the islets. Our data thus suggest that tellurium compounds may have potential in the treatment of type 1 diabetes.

METHODS

Antibodies and Reagents

FITC anti-mouse CD3; PE anti-human/mouse Integrin β7 (Biolegend, San Diego, CA, USA); APC anti-mouse CD45R/B220; anti-Mouse/Rat Foxp3 PE; anti-Mouse CD4 FITC; anti-Mouse CD25 APC; rat IgG2a Isotype Control PE (eBioscience, Carlsbad, CA, USA); Alexa 594 anti-mouse; Alexa 488 anti-rabbit; anti-glucagon; anti-insulin (Innovex Biosciences, Richmond, CA, USA); recombinant mouse MAdCAM-1 Fc chimera (R&D BioSystems, Minneapolis, MN, USA); murine TNF-α (Peprotech, Rocky Hill, NJ, USA); mouse IL-1β, IFNγ, and IL-17 ELISA kits (R&D Biosystems). AS101 and SAS were supplied by M. Albeck, Bar-Ilan University, Ramat-Gan, Israel, and were synthesized at Bar-Ilan University.

Mice

Three to Four week old NOD/ShiLtJ (strain 001976) female mice were purchased from the Jackson Laboratory (Bar Harbor, ME), bred, and housed in individual metabolic cages with unlimited access to food and water. Experiments conformed to approved institutional protocols and were approved by the Institutional Animal Care and Use Committee.

Cells

SVEC-4 murine endothelial cells were obtained from the American Type Culture Collection. Cells were cultured in DMEM containing 10% fetal calf serum at 37°C with 5% CO_2 and 95% air.

Purification of Tregs and T Effector Cells

$CD4^+CD25^+$ Treg were purified from 3 months old NOD mice using a $CD4^+CD25^+$ Treg purification kit (Miltenyi Biotec) according to the manufacturer's instructions, with slight modifications. The CS columns were used for depleting non-T cells, and LS columns were employed to positively select

$CD4^+CD25^+$ cells. Non-CD4 cells were magnetically labeled using a cocktail of biotin-conjugated antibodies recognizing CD8, CD11b, CD45R, CD49b, Ter-119, followed by incubation with anti-biotin micro beads. The labeled cells were then depleted over a column. To attain maximum purity, the CD25 positive selection was performed twice. $CD4^+CD25^-$ T cells were isolated from the CD25-depleted fraction using CD4 microbeads and LS columns.

Cell Migration Assays

Cells (2.5×10^5) were incubated for 1 h in the presence of mobilized MadCAM-1 (100 μg/ml) medium containing MnCl2 (0.25 mM) and various concentrations of SAS or AS101. The cells were washed twice with PBS, and equal numbers of cells were loaded onto 8 mm polycarbonate membrane inserts. The bottom chambers were filled with RPMI-1640 (800 μl) with FBS (20%), containing MadCAM-1 (100 μg/ml) as a chemoattractant. Cell migration was quantified after 24 h by Trypan Blue exclusion test using a hemacytometer.

FACS Analysis

For evaluation of integrin expression on lymphocyte suspensions, single cells from spleens, peripheral LNs, and PLNs from 8 week old NOD mice were stained with FITC-conjugated anti CD3, PE-conjugated anti β7, and APC-conjugated anti B220. Cells were then analyzed on a BD FACSCalibur flow cytometer. The proportion of B and T cells that express the integrin was evaluated on 1×10^4 B220 B or CD3 T cells in the lymphocyte forward scatter/side scatter gate. For evaluation of the proportion of Tregs, lymphocytes from PLNs from 20 w old treated mice were isolated and stained for membranal CD4 (FITC) and CD25 (APC) and nuclear Foxp3 (PE). Cells positive for both CD4 and CD25 were gated, and the expression of Foxp3 on this subpopulation was evaluated. The percentage of $CD4^+CD25^+Foxp3^+$ cells from total lymphocytes was evaluated.

Quantitation of Caspase Activity

Isolated pancreatic extracts from treated mice were prepared in Tris/acetate buffer (pH 7.5) at 30°C. The extracts were centrifuged at 12,000 × *g* for 10 min, and the supernatant was collected. A volume of supernatant equivalent to 100 μg of protein was assayed for caspase-1 or caspase-3 activity using colorimetric caspase-1 and−3 assay kits (R&D Biosystems).

Quantitation of Cytokine Levels

IL-1β, IFNγ, and IL-17 ELISA kits were used for the quantitative measurement of these cytokines in pancreas extracts of treated mice.

Attachment Assay for Evaluation of the α4β7 Activity

For testing attachment to MadCAM-1, 96-well plates were coated with 80 μL of MAdCAM1 (100 μg/ml), or BSA. Cells were incubated in the wells for 2 h in the presence or absence of AS101 or SAS followed by extensive (3x) washing. The proportion of cells that remained attached to the wells was determined by the colorimetric XTT (2,3-bis[2-methoxy-4-nitro-S-sulfophenynl]H-tetrazolium-5-carboxanilide) assay at 450 nm.

For testing attachment to endothelial cells, SVEC-4 endothelial cells were cultured on 6 well plates until 80% confluency. Next, 10 μl of rTNFα (20 ng/ml) was added to the wells to induce MadCAM-1 expression, and then washed. Lymphocytes at 1×10^6/well were then added in the presence or absence of AS101 or SAS and incubated o.n.. Wells were washed with PBS. The remaining attached cells were stained with anti CD3 and anti B220. Endothelial cells are not stained by either antibody (**Supplementary Figure 1**). The proportion of T or B cells in the total cell population was recorded.

Islet Histology

Resected pancreas heads were fixed in 4% formalin and then paraffinized. To prepare histological sections, 5 μM sections were cut from each paraffin block, and stained with hematoxylin-eosin for detection of insulitis.

The level of insulitis was determined according to the following scale: Grade 0 - no insulitis (no infiltration); Grade 1- pre-insulitis (<25% of the islet area infiltrated); Grade 2- mild insulitis (<50% of the islet area infiltrated); Grade 3 – severe insulitis (>50% of the islet area infiltrated).

Immunohistochemistry: Insulin and Glucagon Staining

Fixed paraffin embedded pancreas head sections were deparaffinized and rehydrated. After antigen retrieval, slides were incubated with anti-mouse insulin Ab and anti-glucagon Ab o.n. at 4°C, followed by secondary Alexa 594-conjugated and Alexa 488-conjugated secondary antibodies for 1 h at RT. This was followed by Hoechst staining. Ten slides/mouse were visualized by fluorescence microscopy.

I.P Glucose Tolerance Test

After 12 h fast, mice were administered an i.p bolus of 2 g/kg glucose Blood glucose concentrations were measured by tail bleed at the indicated time points before and after glucose administration. All glucose measurements were performed using a Free Style Freedom (Alameda, CA, USA) glucometer.

Adoptive Transfer

NOD mice (5 w old) were treated with PBS or with 1 mg/kg AS101 every other day. Mice were mated, and treatment continued during gestation and during lactation, until the offspring reached an age of 3 weeks. At that time treatment stopped. Some of the male offspring of treated mothers were irradiated at 6w of age with 550 rads and were injected 24 h later with 20×10^6 splenocytes from diabetic female NOD mice.

Statistics

Data are presented as means ± SE. For comparisons between groups in the *in vitro* and in some *in vivo* studies, we used the one- or two-way ANOVA. For *in vivo* studies (weight, blood glucose, glucose tolerance test, insulitis), ANOVA multiple comparisons with repeated measures

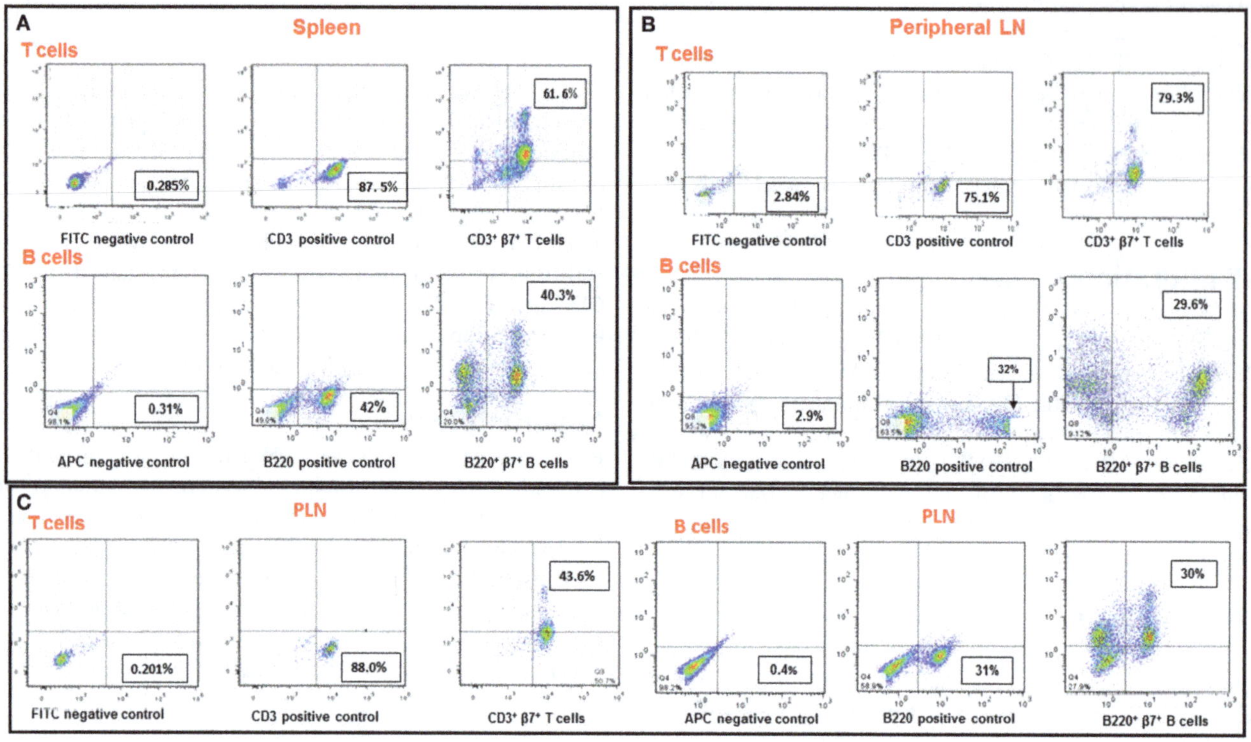

FIGURE 1 | Expression of the β7 integrin subunit on T and B cells in various organs of NOD mice. Single cell suspensions from spleens **(A)**, peripheral LN **(B)**, and PLN **(C)** from 8-week-old NOD mice were stained with FITC-conjugated anti CD3, PE-conjugated anti β7 and APC-conjugated anti B220. $CD3^+\beta7^+$ positive cells represent T cells expressing the β7 integrin subunit. $B220^+\beta7^+$ positive cells represent B cells expressing the β7 integrin subunit. The results represent one experiment representative of three performed.

with Bonferroni corrections, were applied. For analysis of incidence of diabetes and survival, the Kaplan Meier survival analysis tests were applied. The software used for all statistical analysis was IBM SPSS Statistics 21. $p < 0.05$ was considered statistically significant.

RESULTS

AS101 and SAS Attenuate α4β7 Activity in Mononuclear Cells Isolated From NOD Mice

The α4β7 integrin, MAdCAM-1 pathway is essential for infiltration of lymphocytes into pancreatic islets, and for the initiation of T1D in NOD mice (21).Therefore, regulation of this pathway has the potential to ameliorate the course of the disease. For this purpose, we first analyzed β7 integrin expression on T and B cells from various organs of NOD mice. The results shown in **Figure 1** demonstrate that most spleen (**Figure 1A**) and peripheral lymph node (**Figure 1B**) T and B cells express the α4β7 integrin, while about 50% of pancreatic T cells (**Figure 1C**), but most of B cells in this organ still express this integrin. We then analyzed the ability of AS101 and SAS to inhibit the activity of α4β7 on T and B cells from various organs of NOD mice. This was performed by testing the level of attached cells to the α4β7 specific ligand, MADCAM-1. **Figure 2** shows a dose dependent and significant inhibition of the α4β7 integrin activity by both compounds. This was evident in both total spleen cells (**Figure 2A**), peripheral lymph node cells (**Figure 2B**), and pancreatic lymph node cells (**Figure 2C**). Moreover, SAS significantly inhibited the activity of the integrin in sorted T (**Figure 3A**), and B (**Figure 3B**) splenocytes (**Figure 3**).

To further substantiate the inhibitory effect of SAS on integrins, we examined the extent of lymphocyte adhesion, to high endothelial venular ('HEV') cells. MAdCAM-1 is expressed on approximately 95% of HEVs on the lymph nodes of young NOD mice (6). The interaction between MAdCAM-1 on HEVs in PLN and α4β7 on lymphocytes enables their trafficking to PLN. For these experiments, we used the SVEC-4 endothelial cell line which represents HEV cells and highly expresses MADCAM-1 after exposure to TNFα (22). **Figure 4** shows that treatment with SAS significantly inhibits attachment of both T and B cells from NOD mice to endothelial cells, and that the effect is dose-dependent. Collectively, these results suggest that by inhibiting the interaction between α4β7 on T or B lymphocytes from NOD mice, and MADCAM-1 on endothelial cells, AS101 and SAS might affect attachment and penetration of autoreactive T and B cells through pancreatic high endothelial venules, potentially affecting the course of T1D. For this purpose, we used the NOD mouse model of T1D using AS101 and SAS in various concentrations and different timing of administration.

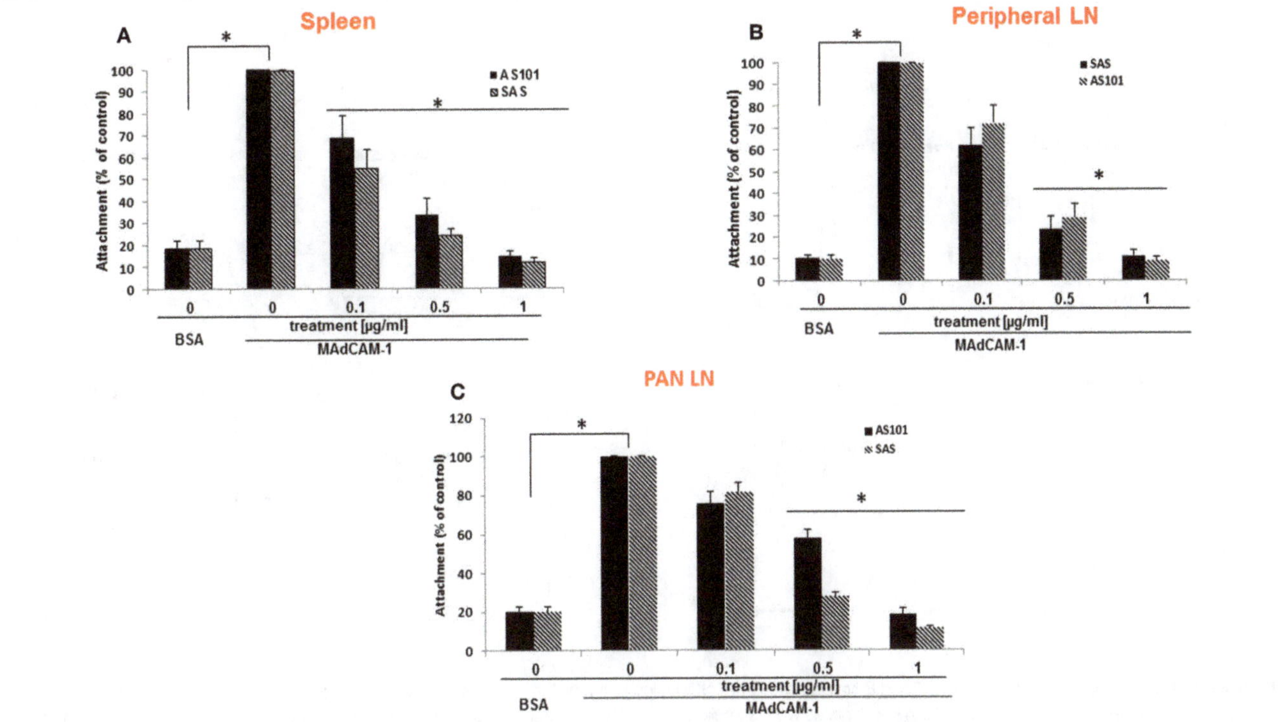

FIGURE 2 | AS101 and SAS inhibit *in vitro* the activity of the α4β7 integrin in various organs of NOD mice. 5×10^5 single cells from spleens **(A)**, peripheral LN **(B)**, and PLN **(C)** from 10 week old NOD mice were cultured on BSA or MAdCAM-1-coated micro wells for 2 h in the presence or absence of different concentrations of SAS or AS101The cells were washed twice and then subjected to XTT reagent according to the manufacturer's instructions. The results represent means±SE of three different experiments. $^*p < 0.001$ decrease vs. MAdCAM-1 without AS101 or SAS (SAS 0).

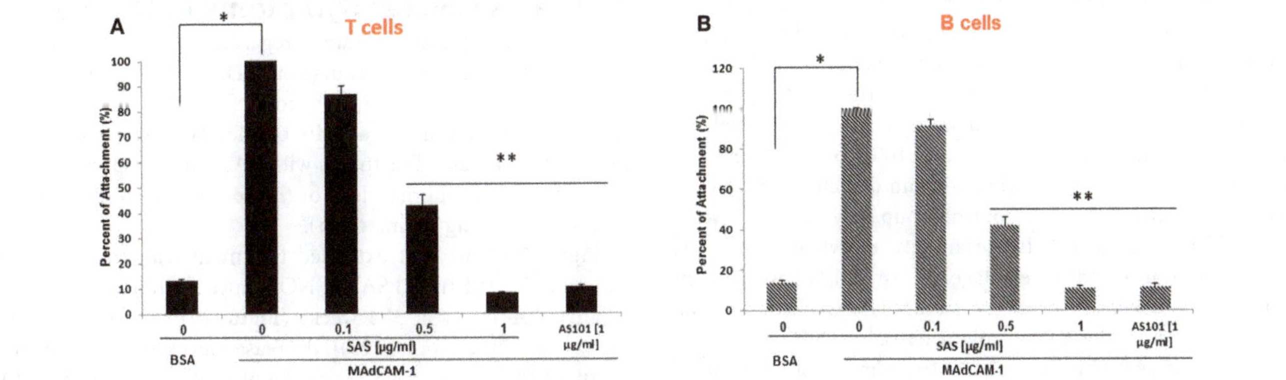

FIGURE 3 | AS101 and SAS inhibit *in vitro* the activity of the a4β7 integrin on both T and B spleen cells of NOD mice. T and B spleen cells from 10 week old mice were sorted by FACS, using anti CD3 or anti B220 antibodies. Single cells (5×10^5) of each lineage (**A**= T cells; **B**= B cells) were cultured on BSA or MAdCAM-1-coated microwells for 2 h in the presence or absence of different concentrations of SAS or 1 μg/ml AS101. The cells were washed twice and then subjected to the XTT reagents according to the manufacturer's instructions. The results represent means ± SE from three different experiments. $^*p < 0.01$; $^{**}p < 0.001$ decrease vs. MAdCAM-1 without AS101 or SAS (SAS 0).

Treatment of NOD Mice With AS101 Alleviates Clinical Symptoms of Diabetes

Figure 5A shows that extended treatment of NOD mice with an optimal dose of AS101 starting at 5–6 weeks (before the development of insulitis), resulted in the delay and prevention of diabetes incidence in a dose-dependent fashion, showing a narrow effective dose range (**Figure 5**). The optimal concentration of AS101 (0.5 mg/kg/injection) prevented disease in 90% of mice. Moreover, sub or supra-optimal concentrations of AS101 marginally delayed the onset of the disease, though these effects did not reach statistical significance This effect was accompanied by increased body weight (**Figure 5B**), and

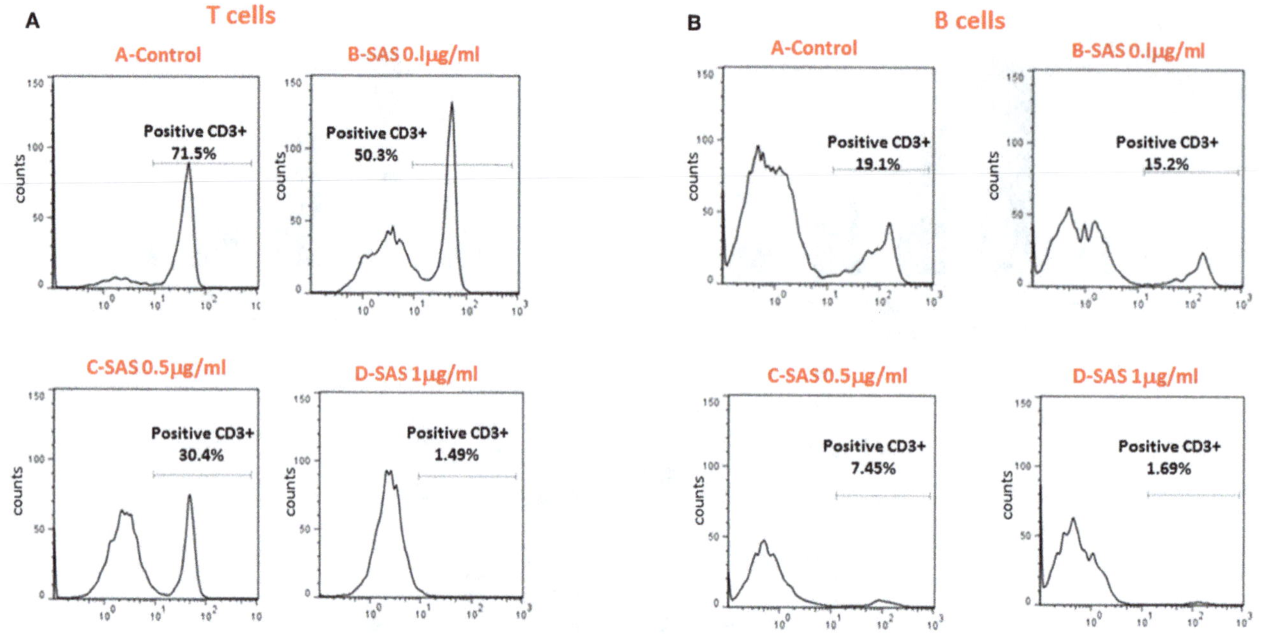

FIGURE 4 | SAS inhibits *in vitro* attachment of T and B lymphocytes from NOD mice to the high endothelial venular ('HEV') cells (SVEC-4). Cells were washed twice. Eighty percent confluent endothelial SVEC cells in 6 well plates were stimulated with TNFα to induce MAdCAM-1 expression. After 10 h, 3×10^6 splenocytes from 10 week old NOD mice were added in the presence or absence of various concentrations of SAS o.n.. Culture plates were washed and the attached cells were removed and stained with FITC-conjugated anti CD3, and APC-conjugated anti B220 antibodies for the detection of attached T **(A)** or B **(B)** cells. The results represent one experiment, representative of three performed.

increased survival (**Figure 5C**) in mice receiving the optimal dose of 0.5 mg/kg. When treatment with AS101 at 0.5 mg/kg/mouse was stopped at 40 weeks of age, no change occurred with respect to percent incidence of diabetes, percent survival, or body weight until at least 52 weeks, suggesting a lasting and significant remission in the course of the disease. The average weight of mice at 52 weeks was 30 ± 77 gr, and 100% of mice surviving at 40 weeks, were also surviving with no diabetes at 52 weeks. None of the mice in the PBS control group survived to 52 weeks of age (data not shown). Importantly, even when AS101 was administered at an advanced stage of insulitis (12 weeks), the incidence of diabetes in treated mice until 40 weeks of age was only 10%, whereas that of control mice reached 90% at that time point (**Figure 6A**). This timing of AS101 administration resulted in preserved body weight (**Figure 6B**) and increased survival (**Figure 6C**). Importantly, even when treatment with AS101 at 0.5 mg/kg/mouse was started at 12 weeks and stopped at 40 weeks, all mice were remained alive, diabetes-free, and maintained their body weight at 52 weeks (average body weight of 26.88 ± 1.01 grams at 52 weeks). None of the mice in the control group were still alive at that time (data not shown). Moreover, not only could AS101 prevent development of diabetes when administered to pre-diabetic mice with different degrees of insulitis, but AS101 increased survival and body weight as well when administered to 14 w old mice that already developed symptoms of diabetes (all untreated NOD mice were diabetic at this time point, not shown) (**Figures 6D,E**).

Treatment of NOD Mice With SAS Alleviates Clinical Symptoms of Diabetes

The encouraging results obtained regarding the beneficial effects of AS101 treatment on the course of T1D led us to investigate the potential effect of the new generation tellurium compound, SAS, shown here to inhibit the activity of α4β7 (**Figures 2–4**), on the intensity of disease. Treatment with SAS was compared to that with AS101 (the optimal dose of the specific batch of AS101 at that time was 1 mg/kg/injection).

Figure 7 shows that extended treatment with the tellurium compounds, AS101 and SAS of NOD mice starting at 5–6 weeks (**Figures 7A–D**) or at 3–4 weeks (**Figures 7E–H**) [initiation of the autoimmune process (23)], decreased levels of blood glucose (**Figures 7A,E**), decreased incidence of diabetes (**Figures 7B,F**), decreased weight loss (**Figures 7C,G**) and eventually increased survival (**Figures 7D,H**) (**Figure 7**). The results show that treatment with the tellurium compounds delay the onset of the disease, and even result in its prevention with increased efficiency when treatment is started earlier.

Pretreatment with AS101 or SAS preserved optimal glucose tolerance (**Figure 8**). Treatment with AS101 and SAS resulted in normal levels of glucose in intraperitoneal glucose tolerance test (IPGTT), either when the test was performed at 12 w of age (**Figure 8A**), or at 20 w (**Figure 8B**), suggesting that preservation of pancreatic islets may have occurred in AS101 or SAS-treated mice early after treatment The fact that in treated mice, 1 h after glucose loading, glucose levels amounted to only

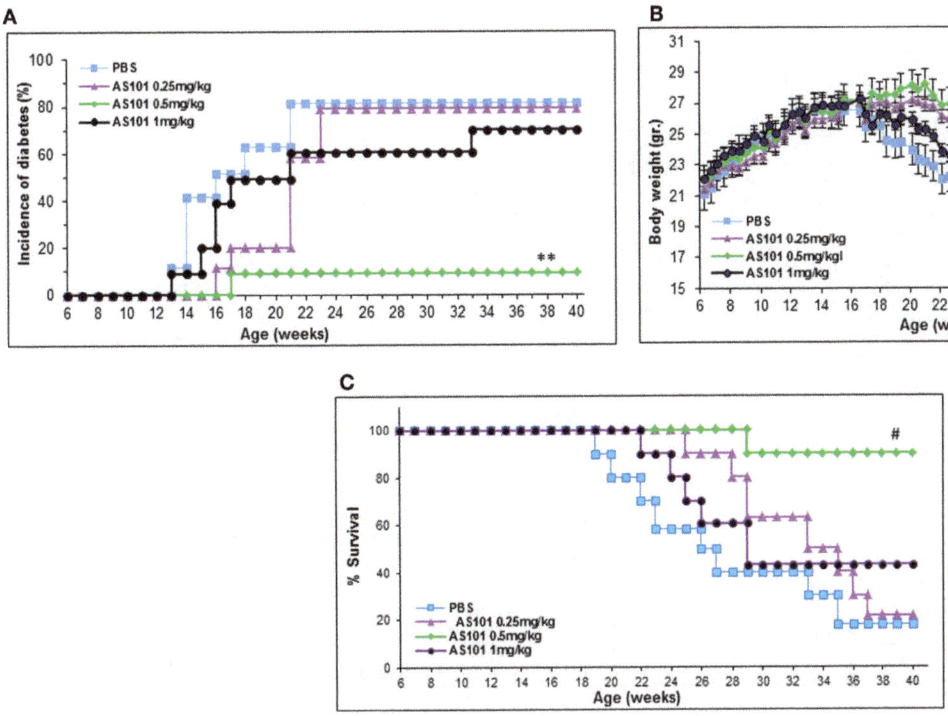

FIGURE 5 | Treatment with AS101 starting at 5–6 weeks of age prevents the development of T1D in NOD mice. AS101 was administered i.p. every other day at different doses to female NOD mice, starting at 5–6 weeks of age, until 40 weeks. The incidence of diabetes (glucose levels at least 200 mg/dL **(A)**, body weight **(B)**, and percent survival **(C)** were monitored. $n = 10$ animals/group. **$p < 0.05$ decrease vs. PBS; *$p < 0.05$ increase vs. PBS; #$p < 0.05$ increase vs. PBS.

~100 mg/dL, considered to be normal levels, suggests that treatment with tellurium compounds prevents islet destruction, enabling normal function of β cells. Indeed, the results show that the level of insulitis was dramatically and significantly decreased in treated mice (**Figures 8C–H**) both with respect to the percentage of infiltrated islets (**Figure 8G**) and the percentage of cells with severe insulitis score (**Figure 8H**). Moreover, the function of the islets was preserved in treated mice, producing normal insulin in pancreatic islets (**Figure 9A**), as compared to mice in a pre-diabetic state. More importantly, in addition to the normal morphology and size of islets of treated mice (**Figure 9B**), caspase-3 activity, the classical hallmark of apoptosis, was significantly decreased compared to control mice, and not significantly different from that of pre-diabetic mice (**Figure 9C**).

AS101 and SAS Attenuate Pancreatic Inflammation and Increase the Frequency of Tregs

In order to gain insight into the mechanism of the beneficial effects of both tellurium compounds in T1D, we first examined whether integrin α4β7 activity in PAN lymph nodes was inhibited following treatment. As can be seen in **Figure 10A**, the integrin activity in PLN lymphocytes from NOD mice treated with the compounds from 3 to 20 w was significantly inhibited. This was manifested by diminished attachment of the cells to the α4β7 specific ligand, MADCAM-1. This inactivation might prevent the infiltration of autoreactive cells to the pancreas.

We next examined protein expression of IL-1β, a key proinflammatory cytokine, which drives several autoimmune diseases. IL-1 is a pleiotropic cytokine, which attenuates $CD4^+CD25^+FoxP3^+$ regulatory T cell function, and allows the $CD4^+CD25^-$ autoreactive effector subset to escape from suppression (24). IL-1β has been previously shown to be inhibited by AS101 in various pre-clinical studies (14, 16, 25). **Figure 10B** shows that both AS101 and SAS significantly inhibited pancreatic IL-1 protein levels at 20 weeks. Furthermore, caspase-1 activity, previously shown to be inhibited by AS101 (16, 25) resulting in decreased IL-1β, was also inhibited in this study in PAN LN by AS101 and SAS-treated mice (**Figure 10C**). Importantly, the pro-inflammatory cytokine IL-17, which is implicated as essential in the development of T1D (26), was also inhibited in treated mice (**Figure 10D**). Furthermore, the Th1 cytokine IFNγ, playing a dominant role in the pathogenesis of autoimmune diabetes (27), was also significantly decreased in SAS and AS101-treated mice (**Figure 10E**). These results prompted us to evaluate the proportion of $CD4^+CD25^+FoxP3^+$ regulatory T cells, known to be affected by these two inflammatory cytokines (IL-1β and IL-17). **Figures 11A–D** shows a significant increase in the proportion of Tregs among PAN LN cells.

The increase in Tregs following treatment by SAS or AS101 prompted us to evaluate if the tellurium compounds affect the α4β7 integrin activity in Tregs vs. T effector cells and to

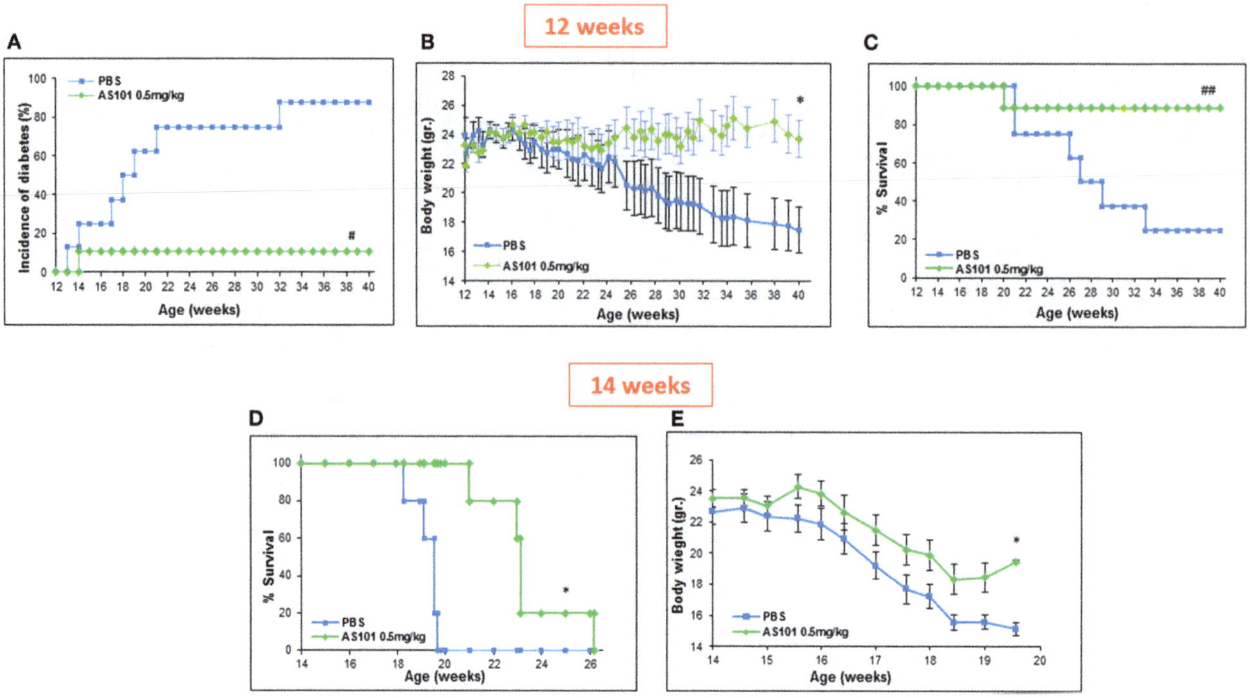

FIGURE 6 | Treatment with AS101 starting at 12 weeks of age prevents the development of T1D in NOD mice. PBS or AS101 at 0.5 mg/kg/injection was administered i.p. every other day at different doses to female NOD mice, starting at 12 weeks of age, until 40 weeks. The incidence of diabetes **(A)**, body weight **(B)**, and percent survival **(C)** were monitored, $n = 10$/group. **(D,E)** AS101 at 0.5 mg/kg/injection was administered i.p. every other day at different doses to female NOD mice, starting at 14 weeks of age. Survival **(D)** and body weight **(E)** of mice was monitored. $n = 5$ mice/group. ##$p < 0.005$ increase vs. PBS. **#**$p < 0.01$ decrease vs. PBS; *$p < 0.05$ increase vs. PBS.

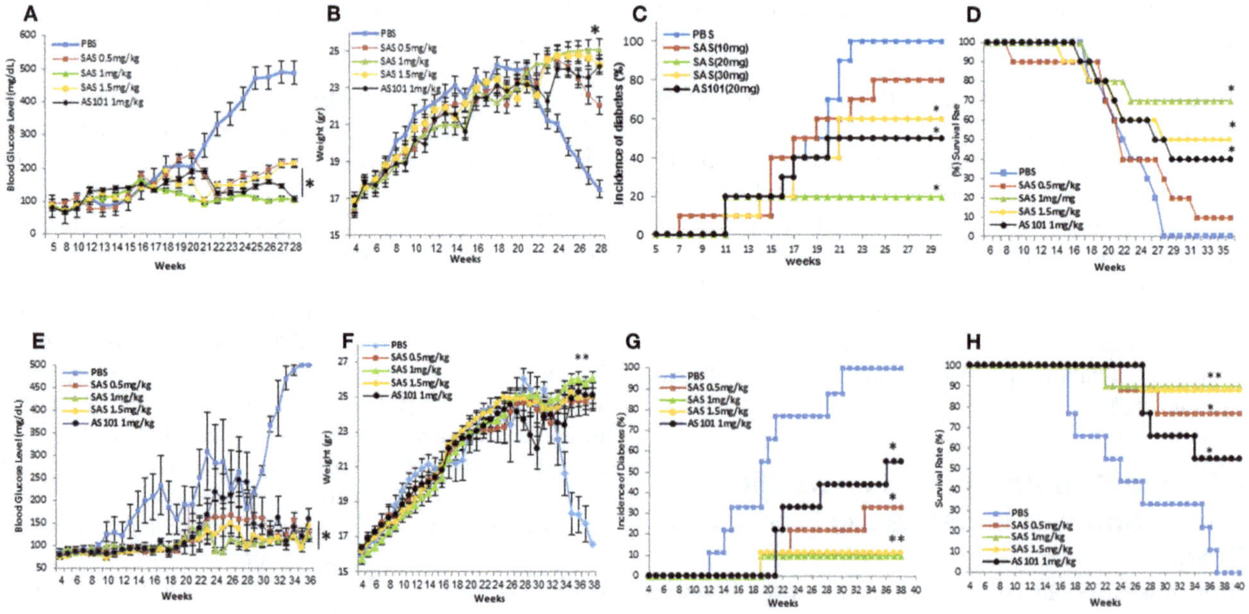

FIGURE 7 | Treatment of NOD mice with SAS or AS101 decreases clinical symptoms of T1D in NOD mice. SAS at different concentrations or AS101 at 1 mg/kg/injection were administered i.p. every other day to female NOD mice, starting at either 5–6 weeks of age **(A–D)**, or at 3 weeks of age **(E-H)** until 30 weeks. Blood glucose levels (*$p < 0.005$ decrease vs PBS) **(A,E)**, body weight (**$p < 0{,}001$; *$p < p < 0.005$ increase vs. PBS) **(B,F)**, percent incidence of diabetes (*$p < 0.005$ decrease vs. PBS; **$p < 0.001$) **(C,G)**, and survival (*$p < 0.005$ increase vs. PBS) **(D,H)** were monitored. $N = 10$ mice/group.

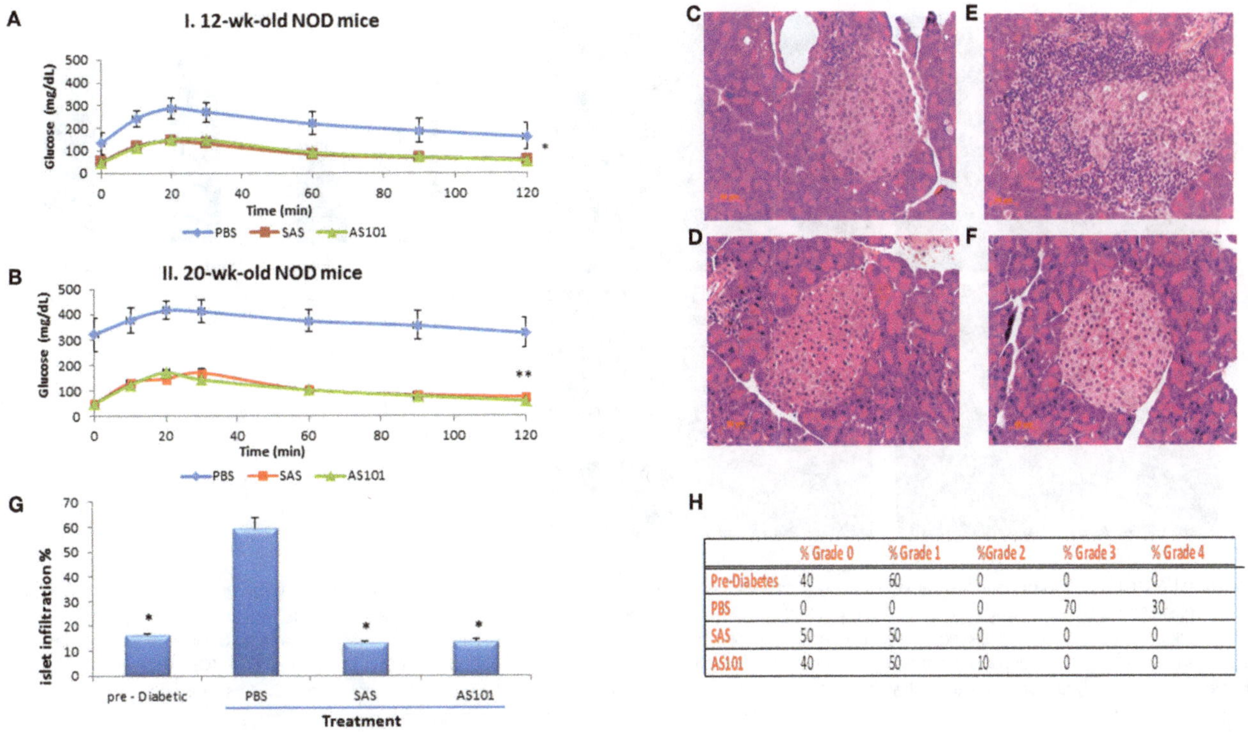

	% Grade 0	% Grade 1	%Grade 2	% Grade 3	% Grade 4
Pre-Diabetes	40	60	0	0	0
PBS	0	0	0	70	30
SAS	50	50	0	0	0
AS101	40	50	10	0	0

FIGURE 8 | Effect of the compounds on islet morphology and insulitis. AS101 or SAS at 1mg/kg/injection were administered i.p. every other day to female NOD mice, starting at 3 weeks of age. At 12 weeks **(A)** (beginning of insulitis) or at 20 weeks **(B)** (severe diabetes)., mice were starved O.N. and injected i.p. with 2gr/kg glucose. Blood glucose levels were monitored at different time points. $^{**}p < 0.01$ vs. PBS; $^{*}p < 0.05$ vs. PBS. $N = 10$/group. **(C–F)** At 20 weeks, pancreatic heads were fixed and stained with H&E. **(C)** Pre-diabetic mice islets at 5w. **(D)** PBS. **(E)** AS101 (1 mg/kg/injection). **(F)** SAS (1 mg/kg/injection). Results show representative data of five mice/group. X200. **(G)** Percent insulitis of 5 mice/group at 20 weeks in comparison to islets from 5 weeks old mice (pre-diabetic). 20 islets/mouse were scored. $^{*}p <$ 0.01 vs. PBS. **(H)** Percentage of infiltrating cells according to the severity of insulitis. Grade 0, No insulitis (no infiltration); Grade 1, Pre-insulitis (<25% of the islet area infiltrated); Grade 2, Mild insulitis (<50% of the islet area infiltrated); Grade 3, Severe insulitis (>50% of the islet area infiltrated); Grade 4, Massive insulitis (total loss of β cell mass).

explore the effects and if this property affects the migration of each subset of cells. **Figures 12A,B** shows that SAS and AS101 inhibits the activity of the α4β7 integrin in both isolated T effector cells (**Figure 12A**) and regulatory cells (**Figure 12B**); nevertheless, the extent of inhibition is higher in T effector cells. Moreover, the α4β7 integrin-dependent migration of both T cell subsets was also inhibited by both compounds, however that of T effector cells was more intense. Furthermore, The extent of control T regulatory cells migration was significantly lower than that of T effector cells (**Figure 12C**). Interestingly, the expression of a4b7 in T regulstoty cells was lower than that of T effector cells (**Figure 12D**). This might explain the lower a4b7-dependent of Tregs and their decreased sensitivity to tellurium compound inhibition.

Finally, we wished to evaluate if offspring of AS101-treated NOD mothers acquire some resistance to T1D development. Female NOD mice were treated with AS101 starting 2 weeks prior to mating, during pregnancy and throughout breast feeding. When the pups were analyzed, they exhibited decreased incidence of diabetes (**Supplementary Figure 1A**) and increased survival (**Supplementary Figure 1B**). Moreover, offspring of treated mothers were relatively more resistant to adoptive transfer of autoreactive cells as expressed by decreased incidence of diabetes (**Supplementary Figure 1C**) and increased survival (**Supplementary Figure 1D**). These results suggest that AS101 can significantly protect the fetus from future diabetes development when the mother is treated during pregnancy. Furthermore, the fetus might acquire both diminished autoreactive cells and increased regulatory mechanisms.

DISCUSSION

The present study presents evidence demonstrating the beneficial effects of the two non-toxic tellurium small molecules AS101 and SAS in a mouse model of T1D. Systemic treatment with these compounds could preserve β cells function and mass. These beneficial effects were reflected in decreased incidence of diabetes, decreased hyperglycemia, improved glucose clearance, preservation of body weight and increased survival. The normal glucose levels were associated with increased insulin levels, preservation of β cell mass and increased islet size compared to controls. Importantly, this protective activity could be demonstrated when the compounds were administered either at the early pre-diabetic phase with either no or early insulitis, at the pre-diabetic stage with advanced insulitis, or even at the

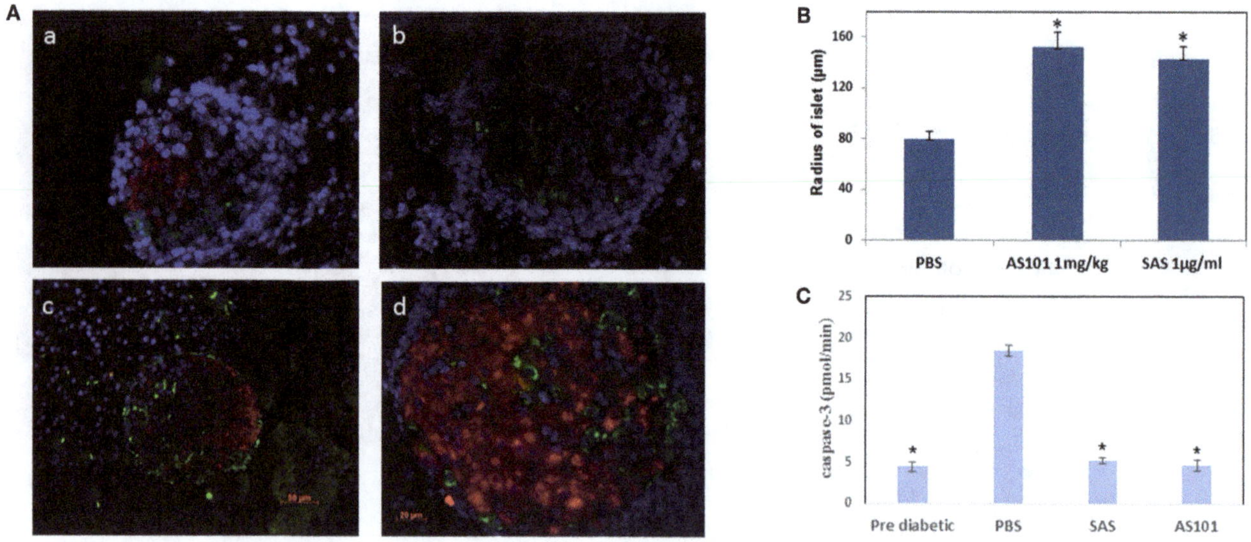

FIGURE 9 | AS101 and SAS prevent islet damage and preserve islet function. **(A)**AS101 or SAS at 1 mg/kg/injection were administered i.p. every other day to female NOD mice, starting at 3 weeks of age. At 20 weeks, pancreatic heads were fixed and stained for insulin (red), glucagon (green), and nuclear staining (blue). Pancreata from 5 week old mice (pre-diabetic) served as a control. (a) Pre-diabetic; (b) PBS; (c) AS101; (d) SAS. The results are representative of 3 mice/group. 10 slides/mouse were visualized. X400. **(B)** Microscopic determination of islet radius. Results represent means ± SE of 5 mice/group. $^{*}p < 0.01$ vs PBS. **(C)** Pancreas cell lysates from 20w old mice were analyzed for caspase-3 activity by colorimetric assay. Results represent means ± SE of 5 mice/group. $^{*}p < 0.01$ vs. all groups.

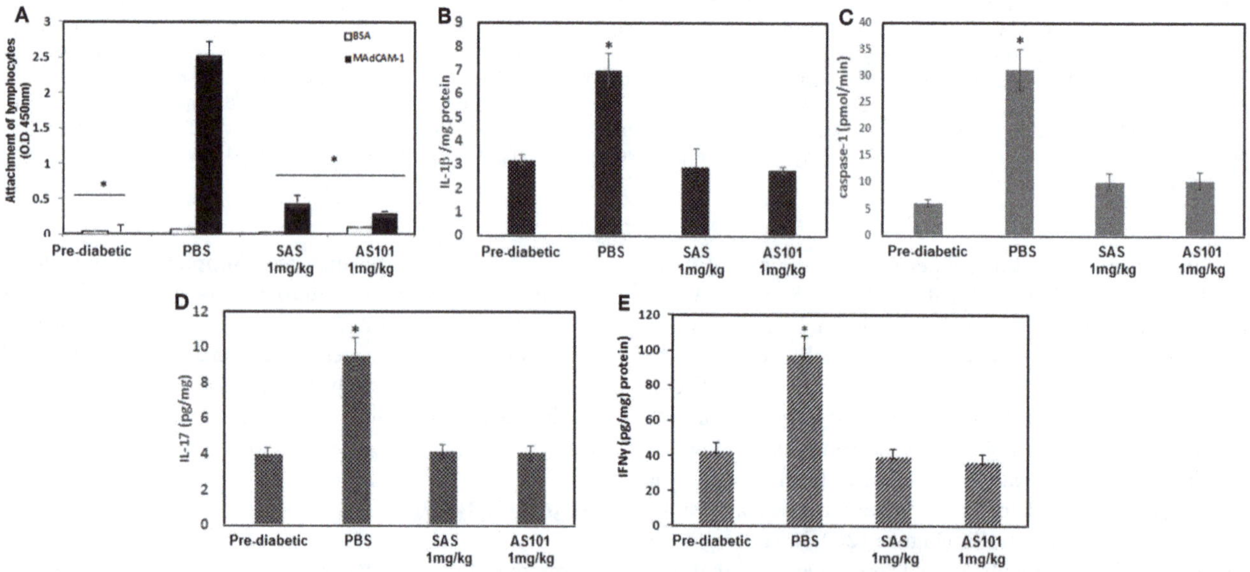

FIGURE 10 | Treatment with AS101 or SAS attenuates α4β7 integrin activity and suppresses inflammatory cytokines in NOD mice. **(A)** AS101 or SAS at 1 mg/kg/injection were administered i.p. every other day to female NOD mice, starting at 3 weeks of age until 20 weeks. Pre-diabetic mice at 5 weeks of age served as controls. Lymphocytes from PAN LN at 5×10^5/well were isolated and incubated in 96 well plates coated with BSA or MAdCAM-1 for 2 h. Nonattached cells were then washed twice, and the adherent cells were subjected to XTT. The results represent means ± SE of 8 mice/group. $^{*}p < 0.01$ vs. MadCAM-1 alone. **(B)** IL-1β protein levels from 20 w old mice. Pancreatic cell lysates were evaluated for IL-1β by ELISA. The results represent means ± SE of 5 mice/group. $^{*}p < 0.01$ vs. PBS. **(C)** At 20 weeks pancreas cell lysates were analyzed for caspase-1 activity by a colorimetric assay, IL-17 **(D)** and IFNγ **(E)** protein levels by ELISA.. The results represent means ± SE of 3 mice/group. $^{*}p < 0.001$ vs. all.

advanced, overtly diabetic stage. Moreover, delaying the onset of diabetes or its prevention was dose-dependent, showing an optimum curve.

Our results suggest that both tellurium compounds prevent migration of autoimmune lymphocytes to the pancreas, i.e., prevent insulitis, by inhibiting α4β7 integrin activity. Indeed,

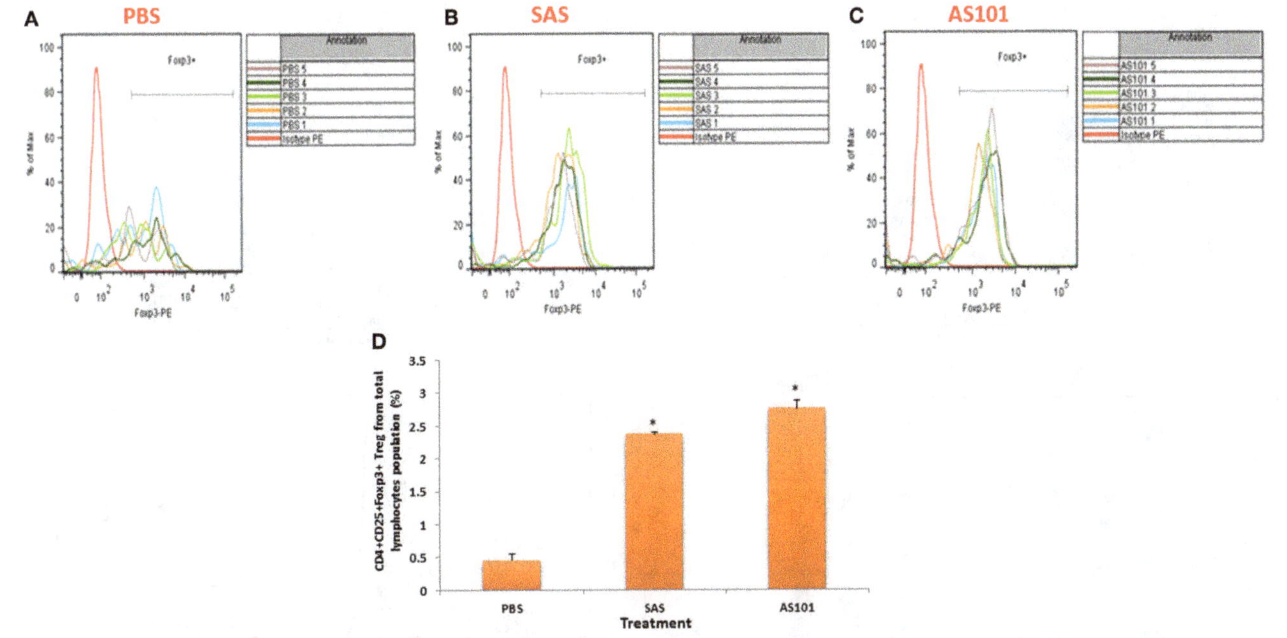

FIGURE 11 | Treatment with AS101 or SAS increases the proportion of T regulatory cells in PLN of NOD mice. AS101 or SAS were administered i.p. at 1 mg/kg/injection every other day to female NOD mice, starting at 3 weeks of age. At 20 weeks lymphocytes from PLN were isolated and stained for CD4, CD25 and Foxp3. **(A)** PBS; **(B)** SAS (1 mg/kg/injection); **(C)** AS101 1mg/kg/injection. Each curve represents cells isolated from different animal $N = 5$/group. **(D)** Evaluation of the proportion of regulatory cells in treated mice. The results represent means ± SE of 5 mice/group.*$p < 0.001$ vs. PBS.

the decreased infiltration resulted in a significantly diminished extent of pancreatic islet damage, both with respect to their size, β cell function (insulin production), and caspase-3 activity, the hallmark of apoptosis. Most importantly AS101 and SAS significantly elevated the frequency of T regulatory cells in the pancreas, thus potentially controlling the autoimmune process.

We have shown in our previous studies that much of the biological activity of AS101 and SAS is directly mediated by their unique chemical interactions with specific cysteine thiol residues. The formation of such TeIV-thiol bonds may induce conformational changes or alter disulfide bond formation in specific proteins, possibly resulting in the loss of their biologic activity, in cases where the thiol residue is essential for a particular function (28, 29). Much of the biological activity of AS101 may be directly attributed to its redox interactions with vicinal thiols in the exofacial of the α4β1 integrinVLA-4 (10), residing within the α but not the β chain of the integrin. We thus suggested that the α4β7 integrin sharing the same α4 chain might be similarly inhibited by the tellurium compounds. This also implies that the specific thiol residues on the α4 chain of the α4β7 integrin are essential for the α4β7 integrin activity. Indeed, we previously showed that AS101 inhibits the α4β7 activity in mesenteric lymph node cells of DSS-induced murine colitis (14). This study shows for the first time that both tellurium compounds suppress the activity of the α4β7 integrin in pancreatic LNs, impacting lymphocyte infiltration into PanLN, and consequently affecting the pathogenesis of T1D.

It was previously shown that the mucosal vascular addressin MAdCAM-1, the ligand for α4β7, is also constitutively expressed at low levels on pancreatic vasculature and, in conjunction with the appearance of lymphocyte infiltrates (insulitis) in pancreatic islets, becomes strongly induced on islet vessels (30–32). Indeed, we show in the present work that both tellurium compounds inhibit the attachment of lymphocytes from pancreatic lymph nodes of NOD mice to either rMAdCAM-1 or to MAdCAM-1 expressed on endothelial cells after exposure to TNFα. This inhibition was demonstrated both *in vitro* and *in vivo*. MAdCAM - 1 is expressed on the surface of endothelial cells in response to secretion of inflammatory cytokines such as to secretion of inflammatory cytokines, including Tumor necrosis alpha (TNF-α) and Interleukin-1 beta (IL-1β). We found that mice successfully treated with AS101 or SAS, showed a significant decrease in pancreatic IL-1β, a cytokine that plays an important role in many autoimmune diseases (33). The decrease in Il-1β suggests that AS101 and SAS prevent insulitis not only by inhibiting the activity of the α4β7 integrin but also possibly by indirectly inhibiting the expression MAdCAM-1 on pancreatic vasculature via inhibition of IL-1β. This cytokine has been previously shown to be inhibited by the tellurium compounds in various preclinical studies due to inhibition of caspase-1 activity (14, 16, 26). Interestingly, we have recently shown that modulation of caspase-1 activity is dependent on VLA-4 inactivation and is mediated through VLA-4 inactivation, and underlies the anti-inflammatory activity of AS101 (16). In line with this, the present study shows a significant decrease in pancreatic caspase-1 activity. The inhibition of α4β7 activity by both Tellurium compounds was most evident both in T effector cells an Treg cells, although that of Tregs was lower. This might

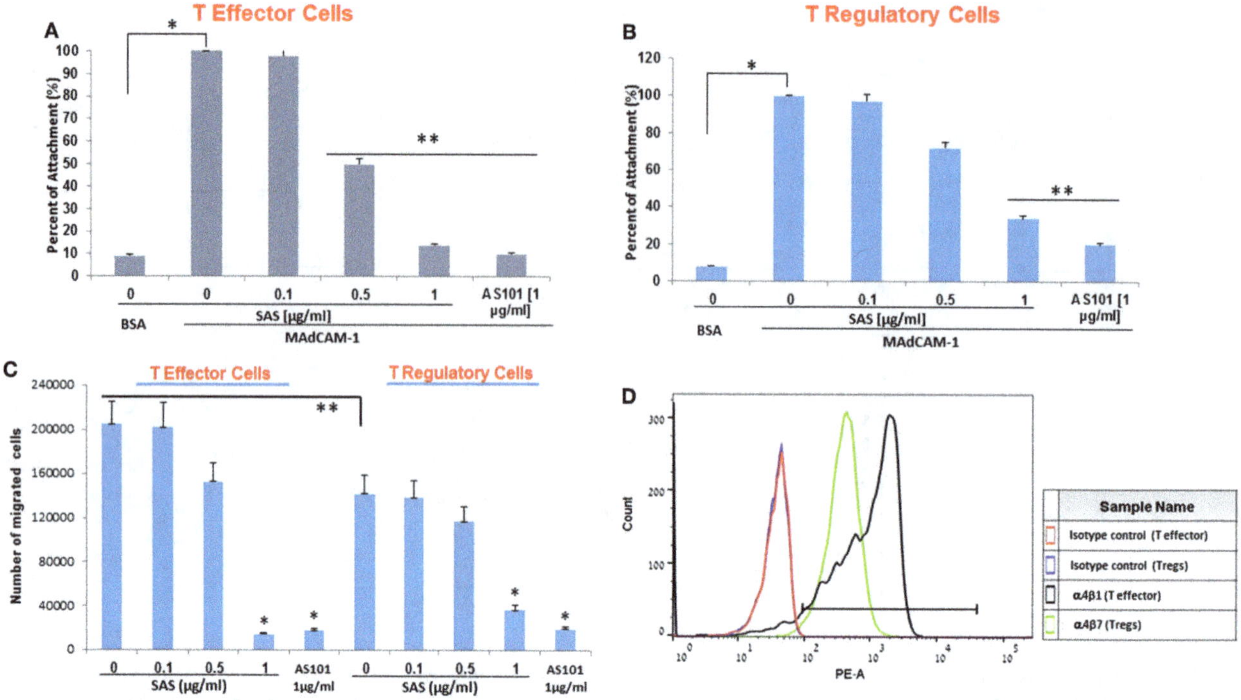

FIGURE 12 | AS101 and SAS inhibit α4β7 integrin activity and α4β7-depenfent migration of T effector cells and Tregs. **(A)** T effector cells and **(B)** T regulatory cells were isolated from spleens of 20w old NOD female mice. Cells at 5×10^5/well were incubated in 96 well plates coated with BSA or MAdCAM-1 for 2 hours. Nonattached cells were then washed twice, and the adherent cells were subjected to XTT. The results represent means ± SE of 4 mice/group. *$p < 0.001$ vs. BSA; **$p < 0.005$ vs. MAdCAM-1 alone (SAS 0), **(C)** T effector cells and T regulatory cells were isolated from spleens of 20w old NOD female mice. Cells (2.5×10^5) were incubated for 1 h in the presence of mobilized MadCAM-1 and various doses of SAS or AS101 and then loaded onto 8 mm polycarbonate membrane inserts. The bottom chambers were filled with FBS (20%) and MadCAM-1 (100 µg/ml) serving as a chemo attractant. Migrated cells were quantified after 24 h. The results represent means±SE of 4 mice/group. *$p < 0.001$ vs control (SAS 0 of the relevant cell subset). **$p < 0.05$ (comparison between controls of both cell subsets). **(D)** Tregs and T effector cells were isolated from spleens of 20w old female NOD mice and stained for the expression of α4β7. The results represent one experiment representative of three performed with 3 mice/group.

be explained by the diminished expression of the a4b7 integrin in Tregs.

It has been previously reported that IL-1β induces proliferation and cytokine production by $CD4^+CD25^+FoxP3^-$ effector/memory T cells, attenuates $CD4^+CD25^+FoxP3^+$ regulatory T cell function, and releases $CD4^+CD25^-$ autoreactive effectors from physiological suppression (24). Thus, inflammation or constitutive overexpression of IL-1β in a genetically predisposed host can promote activation and expansion of autoreactive effector T cells, thereby interfering with the ability of Treg cells to maintain self-tolerance. Thus, inhibition of of IL-1β by AS101 and SAS might explain the upregulation of Tregs by the compounds.

Multiple studies support an essential role of Th17 cells together with defects in T regulatory (Treg) cell function in the development of T1D in both animal models and in humans (34). The decrease in pancreatic Th17 in AS101 or SAS treated mice can be explained in two ways. IL-1β is known to promote IL-17 production by memory $CD4^+$ T cells (35). Hence, its inhibition by the tellurium compounds might affect IL-17 levels. Conversely, the increase in regulatory cells could regulate Th17 cells. The potential pathways through which Treg cells regulate the Th17 cell response have been elucidated in several studies. In mice, $CD4^+$ Treg cells restrain the Th17 immune response via Foxp3 binding to STAT3, a key factor in the initiation of Th17 differentiation (36). Overexpression of Foxp3 results in a strong reduction of IL17A gene expression by inhibiting RORγt-mediated IL-17A mRNA transcription (37). On the other hand, Th17 cells counteract the Treg cells, to expand and allow the development of T1D (26). Thus, the homeostasis between Th17 and Tregs is important in keeping autoimmunity in check. Our results showing a delay of the onset of diabetes by AS101 and SAS combined with their effect on IL-17 and Tregs imply they have the ability to preserve this homeostasis and regulate autoimmunity. Interestingly, although the tellurium compounds inhibited α4β7-dependent migration of both effector cells and Tregs, the proportion of Tregs in PLNs was increased in treated mice. We assume that this this may be explained by our results showing that the extent of inhibition is lower in Tregs as opposed to T effector cells, possibly because of the lower expression of α4β7 on Tregs (**Figure 12D**). Furthermore, even if less Tregs arrived to pancreatic lymph nodes, their number would be much increased with time within their low IL-1β and IL-17 environment.

Several clinically relevant observations emerged from this study:

1. When treatment with AS101 was stopped at 40 weeks of age, no change occurred with respect to incidence of diabetes, survival, or body weight at least until 52 weeks, suggesting that this compound had a long lasting effect on preventing T1D.
2. AS101 could alleviate symptoms of the disease even when treatment was started at relatively advanced stages of the disease (12 or 14 weeks of age). While T1D can be predicted in human patients based on the presence of antibodies recognizing autoantigens, such as insulin, GAD65 (glutamic acid decarboxylase), IA-2 (islet antigen 2), and ZnT8 (islet zinc transporter) (38), there is no known way to prevent or arrest the development of this disease, nor has any treatment been demonstrated that can reduce the anti-β-cell autoimmune response following the diagnosis of diabetes. Therefore, our positive results in the early treatment protocol (starting at 3 weeks of age) are applicable to individuals at risk, in which the disease is predicted by the presence of autoantibodies. Conversely, at more advanced stages of disease, AS101 might enable regeneration of β cells or their preservation. Indeed, it has been previously suggested that β cell regeneration can be induced in animal models provided a sufficient endogenous β cell mass remains (39, 40).
3. The increased resistance to diabetes followed by the increased survival could be transferred to offspring of 5w old female NOD mice treated with AS101 starting 2 weeks prior to gestation, during pregnancy and throughout breast feeding (**Supplementary Figure 1**). These results suggest that AS101 can significantly protect the fetus from future diabetes development when the mother is treated during pregnancy. The fact that decreased incidence of diabetes occurs in offspring of treated mothers undergoing adoptive transfer of autoreactive cells suggests that these offspring acquire from the mother regulatory means to fight the autoimmune cells injected. Thus, not only the fetus but the newborn as well can benefit from treatment of his mother. It has been recently reported that breastfeeding transfers to the infant not only protective antibodies but also maternal immune cells (41). The mechanisms underlying these important results are now the focus of our laboratory studies.

In summary, we introduce in the present study two non-toxic small molecules that, by virtue of their unique mechanism of action, may both prevent trafficking of autoreactive B and T cells to the pancreas and regulate the activity of those that have infiltrated the tissue. As AS101 demonstrated an excellent safety profile in clinical trials for other indications, these compounds may serve as good candidates for the treatment of T1D.

AUTHOR CONTRIBUTIONS

TY and ZB performed and analyzed the experiments. DK-S provided technical assistance. YK, RC, and BS designed the study, discussed the results, and wrote the paper. All the authors discussed the results and commented on the manuscript.

SUPPLEMENTARY MATERIAL

Supplementary Figure 1 | The decreased incidence of diabetes followed by the increased survival can be transferred to offspring of treated female NOD mice. 5 w old female mice were treated with PBS or with various concentrations of AS101. Treatment continued during gestation and pregnancy and during breast feeding until the offspring aged 3 weeks. At that time treatment stopped and female offspring were evaluated for % incidence of diabetes **(A)** and for % survival **(B)** from 10 to 40 weeks. $N = 15$ offspring mice/group. $*p < 0.05$; $**p < 0.005$ vs. PBS. Some of the male offspring of treated mothers were irradiated at 6w of age with 550Gy and were injected 24h later with 20×10^6 splenocytes from diabetic female NOD mice. The incidence of diabetes **(C)** and the percentage of survival **(D)** were monitored until 30 weeks.$*p < 0.05$ vs. PBS. N-9.

REFERENCES

1. Wing K, Sakaguchi S. Regulatory T cells exert checks and balances on self-tolerance and autoimmunity. *Nat Immunol.* (2010) 11:7–13. doi: 10.1038/ni.1818
2. Butcher EC, Picker LJ. Lymphocyte homing and homeostasis. *Science.* (1996) 272:60–6.
3. Campbell DJ, Kim, C.H, Butcher EC. Chemokines in the systemic organization of immunity. *Immunol. Rev.* (2003) 195:58–71.
4. von Andrian UH, Mempel TR. Homing and cellular traffic in lymph nodes. *Nat. Rev. Immunol.* (2003) 3:867–78. doi: 10.1038/nri1222
5. Wong FS, Wen L, Tang M, Ramanathan M, Visintin I, Daugherty J, et al. Investigation of the role of B-cells in type 1 diabetes in the NOD mouse. *Diabetes.* (2004) 53:2581–7. doi: 10.2337/diabetes.53.10.2581
6. Xu B, Cook RE, Michie SA. α4β7 integrin/MAdCAM-1 adhesion pathway is crucial for B cell migration into pancreatic lymph nodes in nonobese diabetic mice. *J. Autoimmun.* (2010) 35:124–9. doi: 10.1016/j.jaut.2010.04.002
7. Baron JL, Reich EP, Visintin I, Janeway, CA Jr. The pathogenesis of adoptive murine autoimmune diabetes requires an interaction between alpha 4-integrins and vascular cell adhesion molecule-1. *J. Clin. Invest.* (1994) 93:1700–8. doi: 10.1172/JCI117153
8. Sredni B, Caspi RR, Klein A, Kalechman Y, Danziger Y, Ben Ya'akov M, et al. New immunomodulating compound (AS-101) with potential therapeutic application. *Nature.* (1987) 330:173–6. doi: 10.1038/330173a0
9. Sredni B, Xu RH, Albeck M, Gafter U, Gal R, Shani A, et al. The protective role of the immunomodulator AS101 against chemotherapy-induced alopecia studies on human and animal models. *Int. J. Cancer.* (1996) 65:97–103.
10. Layani-Bazar A, Skornick I, Berrebi A, Pauker MH, Noy E, Silberman A, et al. Redox modulation of adjacent thiols in VLA-4 by AS101 converts myeloid leukemia cells from a drug-resistant to drug-sensitive state. *Cancer Res.* (2014) 74:3092–103. doi: 10.1158/0008-5472.CAN-13-2159
11. Lee JH, Halperin-Sheinfeld M, Baatar D, Mughal MR, Tae HJ, Kim JW, et al. Tellurium compound AS101 ameliorates experimental autoimmune encephalomyelitis by VLA-4 inhibition and suppression of monocyte and T cell infiltration into the CNS. *Neuromolecular Med.* (2014) 16:292–307. doi: 10.1007/s12017-013-8277-3
12. Bing SJ, Shemesh I, Chong WP, Horai R, Jittayasothorn Y, Silver PB, et al. AS101 ameliorates experimental autoimmune uveitis by regulating Th1 and Th17 responses and inducing Treg cells. *J Autoimmun.* (2019) 100:52–61. doi: 10.1016/j.jaut.2019.02.006
13. Sredni B. Immunomodulating tellurium compounds as anti-cancer agents. *Semin Cancer Biol.* (2012) 22:60–69. doi: 10.1016/j.semcancer.2011.12.003

14. Halpert G, Eitan T, Voronov E, Apte RN, Rath-Wolfson L, Albeck M, et al. Multifunctional activity of a small tellurium redox immunomodulator compound, AS101, on dextran sodium sulfate-induced murine colitis. *J Biol Chem.* (2014) 289:17215–27. doi: 10.1074/jbc.M113.536664
15. Kalechman Y, Gafter U, Da JP, Albeck M, Alarcon-Segovia D, Sredni B. Delay in the onset of systemic lupus erythematosus following treatment with the immunomodulator AS101: association with IL-10 inhibition and increase in TNF-alpha levels. *J Immunol.* (1997) 159:2658–67.
16. Hachmo Y, Kalechman, Y, Skornick I, Gafter U, Caspi RR, Sredni B. The small tellurium compound AS101 ameliorates rat crescentic glomerulonephritis: Association with inhibition of macrophage caspase-1 activity via very late antigen-4 inactivation. *Front Immunol.* (2017) 8:240. doi: 10.3389/fimmu.2017.00240
17. Halpert G, Sredni B. *Autoimmun Rev.* (2014) 13:1230–5. doi: 10.1016/j.autrev.2014.08.003
18. Kalechman Y, Gafter U, Gal R, Rushkin G, Yan D, Albeck M, et al. Anti-IL-10 therapeutic strategy using the immunomodulator AS101 in protecting mice from sepsis-induced death: dependence on timing of immunomodulating intervention. *J Immunol.* (2002) 169:384–92. doi: 10.4049/jimmunol.169.1.384
19. Danoch H, Kalechman Y, Albeck M, Longo DL, Sredni B. Sensitizing B- and T- cell lymphoma cells to paclitaxel/abraxane-induced death by AS101 via inhibition of the VLA-4-IL10-survivin axis. *Mol. Cancer Res.* (2015) 13:411–22. doi: 10.1158/1541-7786.MCR-14-0459
20. Sredni B, Weil M, Khomenok G, Lebenthal I, Teitz S, Mardor Y, et al. Ammonium trichloro(dioxoethylene-o,o')tellurate (AS101) sensitizes tumors to chemotherapy by inhibiting the tumor interleukin 10 autocrine loop. *Cancer Res.* (2004) 64:1843–52.
21. Yang, XD., Sytwu HK, McDevitt HO, Michie SA. Involvement of β7 integrin and mucosal addressin cell adhesion molecule-1 (MAdCAM-1) in the development of diabetes in obese diabetic mice. *Diabetes.* (1997) 46:1542–7.
22. Oshima T, Pavlick KP, Laroux FS, Verma SK, Jordan P, Grisham MB, et al. Regulation and distribution of MAdCAM-1 in endothelial cells *in vitro*. *Am J Physiol Cell Physiol.* (2001) 281:C1096–1105. doi: 10.1152/ajpcell.2001.281.4.C1096
23. Hoglund P, Mintern J, Waltzinger C, Heath W, Benoist C, Mathis D. Initiation of autoimmune diabetes by developmentally regulated presentation of islet cell antigens in the pancreatic lymph nodes. *J Exp Med.* (1999) 189:331–9.
24. O'Sullivan BJ, Thomas HE, Pai S, Santamaria P, Iwakura Y., Steptoe RJ, et al. IL-1 beta breaks tolerance through expansion of CD25+ effector T cells. *J Immunol.* (2006) 176:7278–7. doi: 10.4049/jimmunol.176.12.7278
25. Sredni, Geffen-Aricha R, Duan W, Albeck M, Shalit F, Lander HM, et al. Multifunctional tellurium molecule protects and restores dopaminergic neurons in Parkinson's disease models. *FASEB J.* (2007) 21:1870–83. doi: 10.1096/fj.06-7500com
26. Emamaullee JA, Davis J, Merani S, Toso C, Elliott JF, Thiesen A, et al. Inhibition of Th17 cells regulates autoimmune diabetes in NOD mice. *Diabetes.* (2009) 58:1302–11. doi: 10.2337/db08-1113
27. Sobel D, Ahvazi B, Pontzer C. The role of type I interferon subtypes and interferon-gamma in type I interferon diabetes inhibitory activity in the NOD mouse. *J Interferon Cytokine Res.* (2016) 36:238–46. doi: 10.1089/jir.2014.0232
28. Kalechman. Y, Longo DL, Catane R, Shani A, Albeck M, Sredni B. Synergistic antitumoral effect of paclitaxel (Taxol)+AS101 in a murine model of B16 melanoma: association with ras-dependent signal-transduction pathways. *Int J Cancer.* (2000) 86:281–8.
29. Yosef S, Brodsky M, Sredni B, Albeck A, Albeck M. *ChemMedChem.* (2007) 2:1601–6. doi: 10.1002/cmdc.200700155
30. Hänninen A, Taylor C, Streeter PR, Stark LS, Sarte JM, Shizuru JA, et al. Vascular addressins are induced on islet vessels during insulitis in nonobese diabetic mice and are involved in lymphoid cell binding to islet endothelium. *J Clin Invest.* (1993) 92:2509–15. doi: 10.1172/JCI116859
31. Yang XD, Michie SA, Tisch R, Karin N, Steinman L, McDevitt HO. A predominant role of integrin a4 in the spontaneous development of autoimmune diabetes in nonobese diabetic mice. *Proc Natl Acad Sci USA.* (1994) 91:12604–08. doi: 10.1073/pnas.91.26.12604
32. Hänninen A, Jaakkola I, Jalkanen S. Mucosal addressin is required for the development of diabetes in nonobese diabetic mice. *J Immunol.* (1998) 160:6018–25.
33. Dinarello CA, van der Meer JW. Treating inflammation by blocking interleukin-1 in humans. *Semin. Immunol.* (2013) 25:469–84. doi: 10.1016/j.smim.2013.10.008
34. Li Y, Liu Y, Chu CQ. Th17 cells in type 1 diabetes: Role in the pathogenesis and regulation by gut microbiome. *Mediators Inflamm.* (2015) 2015:638470–77. doi: 10.1155/2015/638470
35. Bradshaw EM, Raddassi K, Elyaman W, Orban T, Gottlieb PA, Kent SC, et al. Monocytes from patients with type 1 diabetes spontaneously secrete proinflammatory cytokines inducing Th17 cells. *J Immunol.* (2009) 183:4432–9. doi: 10.4049/jimmunol.0900576
36. Chaudhry A, Rudra D, Treuting, P, Samstein RM, Liang Y, Kas A, et al. $CD4^+$ regulatory T cells control TH17 responses in a stat3-dependent manner. *Science.* (2009) 326:986–91. doi: 10.1126/science.1172702
37. Ichiyama K, Yoshida H, Wakabayashi Y, Chinen, T., Saeki, K., Nakaya M, et al. Foxp3 inhibits RORγt-mediated IL-17A mRNA transcription through direct interaction with RORγt. *J Biol Chem.* (2008) 283:17003–8. doi: 10.1074/jbc.M801286200
38. Stadinski B, Kappler J, Eisenbarth GS. Molecular targeting of islet autoantigens. *Immunity.* (2010) 32: 446–6. doi: 10.1016/j.immuni.2010.04.008
39. Chong AS, Shen J, Tao J, Yin D, Kuznetsov A, Hara M, et al. Reversal of diabetes in non-obese diabetic mice without spleen cell-derived β cell regeneration. *Science.* (2006) 311:1774–5. doi: 10.1126/science.1123510
40. Pospisilik JA, Martin J, Doty T, Ehses JA, Pamir N, Lynn FC, et al. Dipeptidyl peptidase IV inhibitor treatment stimulates β-cell survival and islet neogenesis in streptozotocin-induced diabetic rats. *Diabetes.* (2003) 52:741–50. doi: 10.2337/diabetes.52.3.741
41. Cabinian A, Sinsimer D, Tang M, Zumba O, Mehta H, Toma A, et al. Transfer of maternal immune cells by breastfeeding: Maternal cytotoxic T lymphocytes present in breast milk localize in the Peyer's patches of the nursed infant. *PLoS ONE.* (2016) 11:e0156762. doi: 10.1371/journal.pone.0156762

Permissions

All chapters in this book were first published Frontiers; hereby published with permission under the Creative Commons Attribution License or equivalent. Every chapter published in this book has been scrutinized by our experts. Their significance has been extensively debated. The topics covered herein carry significant findings which will fuel the growth of the discipline. They may even be implemented as practical applications or may be referred to as a beginning point for another development.

The contributors of this book come from diverse backgrounds, making this book a truly international effort. This book will bring forth new frontiers with its revolutionizing research information and detailed analysis of the nascent developments around the world.

We would like to thank all the contributing authors for lending their expertise to make the book truly unique. They have played a crucial role in the development of this book. Without their invaluable contributions this book wouldn't have been possible. They have made vital efforts to compile up to date information on the varied aspects of this subject to make this book a valuable addition to the collection of many professionals and students.

This book was conceptualized with the vision of imparting up-to-date information and advanced data in this field. To ensure the same, a matchless editorial board was set up. Every individual on the board went through rigorous rounds of assessment to prove their worth. After which they invested a large part of their time researching and compiling the most relevant data for our readers.

The editorial board has been involved in producing this book since its inception. They have spent rigorous hours researching and exploring the diverse topics which have resulted in the successful publishing of this book. They have passed on their knowledge of decades through this book. To expedite this challenging task, the publisher supported the team at every step. A small team of assistant editors was also appointed to further simplify the editing procedure and attain best results for the readers.

Apart from the editorial board, the designing team has also invested a significant amount of their time in understanding the subject and creating the most relevant covers. They scrutinized every image to scout for the most suitable representation of the subject and create an appropriate cover for the book.

The publishing team has been an ardent support to the editorial, designing and production team. Their endless efforts to recruit the best for this project, has resulted in the accomplishment of this book. They are a veteran in the field of academics and their pool of knowledge is as vast as their experience in printing. Their expertise and guidance has proved useful at every step. Their uncompromising quality standards have made this book an exceptional effort. Their encouragement from time to time has been an inspiration for everyone.

The publisher and the editorial board hope that this book will prove to be a valuable piece of knowledge for researchers, students, practitioners and scholars across the globe.

List of Contributors

Teresa Rodriguez-Calvo
Institute of Diabetes Research, Helmholtz Zentrum München, German Research Center for Environmental Health, Munich-Neuherberg, Germany
German Center for Diabetes Research (DZD), Neuherberg, Germany

Gustaf Christoffersson
Science for Life Laboratory, Uppsala University, Uppsala, Sweden
Department of Medical Cell Biology, Uppsala University, Uppsala, Sweden

Christine Bender and Matthias G. von Herrath
Center for Autoimmunity and Inflammation, Type 1 Diabetes Center at La Jolla Institute for Immunology, La Jolla, CA, United States

Roberto Mallone
Université de Paris, Institut Cochin, CNRS, INSERM, Paris, France
Assistance Publique Ho^ pitaux de Paris, Cochin Hospital, Service de Diabe´ tologie et Immunologie Clinique, Paris, France

Sally C. Kent
Department of Medicine, Division of Diabetes, Diabetes Center of Excellence, University of Massachusetts Medical School, Worcester, MA, United States

Eddie A. James
Translatonal Research Program, Benaroya Research Institute, Seattle WA, United States
Department of Translational Research, Benaroya Research Institute at Virginia Mason, Seattle, WA, United States

Brittney N. Newby
Department of Pathology, Immunology and Laboratory Medicine, University of Florida, Gainesville, FL, United States

Timothy A. Wiles, Mylinh Dang, Roger Powell and Thomas Delong
Department of Pharmaceutical Sciences, University of Colorado Skaggs School of Pharmacy and Pharmaceutical Sciences, Aurora, CO, United States

Kathryn Haskins and Rocky L. Baker
Department of Immunology and Microbiology, University of Colorado School of Medicine, Aurora, CO, United States

Anita Hohenstein
Department of Pharmaceutical Sciences, University of Colorado Skaggs School of Pharmacy and Pharmaceutical Sciences, Aurora, CO, United States
Department of Immunology and Microbiology, University of Colorado School of Medicine, Aurora, CO, United States

Laurie G. Landry
Barbara Davis Center for Childhood Diabetes, University of Colorado School of Medicine, Aurora, CO, United States

Maki Nakayama
Department of Immunology and Microbiology, University of Colorado School of Medicine, Aurora, CO, United States
Barbara Davis Center for Childhood Diabetes, University of Colorado School of Medicine, Aurora, CO, United States

Perrin Guyer
Department of Translational Research, Benaroya Research Institute at Virginia Mason, Seattle, WA, United States

Michele L. Semeraro, Lindsey M. Glenn and Margaret A. Morris
Department of Internal Medicine, Strelitz Diabetes Center, Eastern Virginia Medical School, Norfolk, VA, United States

Sefina Arif, Irma Pujol-Autonell, Yogesh Kamra, Evangelia Williams, Norkhairin Yusuf, Clara Domingo-Vila, Yasaman Shahrabi, Emily Pollock, Leena Khatri, Mark Peakman, Timothy Tree and Anna Lorenc
Department of Immunobiology, King's College London, Guy's Hospital, London, United Kingdom

Zachary J. Morse and Marc S. Horwitz
Department of Microbiology and Immunology, University of British Columbia, Vancouver, BC, Canada

Qi You, Yiming Shen, Fengjie Huang, Yiling Wu and Jie Wu
College of Life Science and Technology, China Pharmaceutical University, Nanjing, China

Yuyan Li and Chang Liu
State Key Laboratory of Natural Medicines, China Pharmaceutical University, Nanjing, China

Harvest F. Gu
Center for Pathophysiology, School of Basic Medicine and Clinical Pharmacy, China Pharmaceutical University, Nanjing, China

Yi-Guang Chen
Department of Pediatrics, Medical College of Wisconsin, Milwaukee, WI, United States

Clayton E. Mathews
Department of Pathology, Immunology and Laboratory Medicine, College of Medicine, University of Florida, Gainesville, FL, United States
Department of Pathology, Immunology and Laboratory Medicine, University of Florida, Gainesville, FL, United States

John P. Driver
Department of Animal Sciences, University of Florida, Gainesville, FL, United States

Ranjeny Thomas
University of Queensland Diamantina Institute, Princess Alexandra Hospital, Woolloongabba, QLD, Australia

Josè M. Carballido
Translational Medicine/Preclinical Safety, Novartis Institutes for Biomedical Research, Basel, Switzerland

Johnna D. Wesley
Type 1 Diabetes, Immunology, & Kidney Disease Research, Novo Nordisk Research Center Seattle, Inc., Seattle, WA, United States

Simi T. Ahmed
Strategic Partnerships, The New York Stem Cell Foundation Research Institute, New York, United States

David H. Wagner Jr.
The Program in Integrated Immunology, Department of Medicine, Webb-Waring Center, University of Colorado Anschutz Medical Campus, Aurora, CO, United States

Meghan L. Marré and Jon D. Piganelli
Division of Pediatric Surgery, Department of Surgery, Children's Hospital of Pittsburgh, University of Pittsburgh, Pittsburgh, PA, United States

Saurabh Vig and Arnaud Zaldumbide
Department of Cell and Chemical Biology, Leiden University Medical Center, Leiden, Netherlands

Bruno Guigas
Department of Parasitology, Leiden University Medical Center, Leiden, Netherlands

Joost M. Lambooij
Department of Cell and Chemical Biology, Leiden University Medical Center, Leiden, Netherlands
Department of Parasitology, Leiden University Medical Center, Leiden, Netherlands

Mark A. Wallet, Katherine E. Santostefano, Naohiro Terada and Todd M. Brusko
Department of Pathology, Immunology, and Laboratory Medicine, University of Florida Diabetes Institute, College of Medicine, Gainesville, FL, United States

Mohamed Abu-Farha, Sina Kavalakatt and Jehad Abubaker
Department of Biochemistry and Molecular Biology, Dasman Diabetes Institute, Dasman, Kuwait

Fahd Al-Mulla and Thangavel Alphonse Thanaraj
Department of Genetics and Bioinformatics, Dasman Diabetes Institute, Dasman, Kuwait

Hamad Ali
Department of Genetics and Bioinformatics, Dasman Diabetes Institute, Dasman, Kuwait
Department of Medical Laboratory Sciences, Faculty of Allied Health Sciences, Health Sciences Center, Kuwait University, Jabriya, Kuwait

Mohammed Abdul Ghani
Diabetes Division, University of Texas Health Science Center at San Antonio, San Antonio, TX, United States

Qin Zeng, Jianfeng Song, Dandan Wang, Xiaoxiao Sun, Yalun Xiao, Haowei Zhang and Yang Xiao
National Clinical Research Center for Metabolic Diseases, and Department of Metabolism and Endocrinology, The Second Xiangya Hospital of Central South University, Changsha, China
Key Laboratory of Diabetes Immunology, Ministry of Education, and Metabolic Syndrome Research Center, The Second Xiangya Hospital of Central South University, Changsha, China

Zhiguang Zhou
National Clinical Research Center for Metabolic Diseases, and Department of Metabolism and Endocrinology, The Second Xiangya Hospital of Central South University, Changsha, China
Key Laboratory of Diabetes Immunology, Ministry of Education, and Metabolic Syndrome Research Center, The Second Xiangya Hospital of Central South University, Changsha, China
National Clinical Research Center for Metabolic Diseases, Key Laboratory of Diabetes Immunology (Central South University), Ministry of Education, and Department of Metabolism and Endocrinology, The Second Xiangya Hospital of Central South University, Changsha, China

Tuo Deng
National Clinical Research Center for Metabolic Diseases, and Department of Metabolism and Endocrinology, The Second Xiangya Hospital of Central South University, Changsha, China
Key Laboratory of Diabetes Immunology, Ministry of Education, and Metabolic Syndrome Research Center, The Second Xiangya Hospital of Central South University, Changsha, China
Clinical Immunology Center, The Second Xiangya Hospital of Central South University, Changsha, China

Junu A. George, Mohammed M. Qureshi and Maria J. Fernández-Cabezudo
Department of Biochemistry, College of Medicine and Health Sciences, United Arab University, Al-Ain, UAE

Ghada Bashir, Yassir A. Mohamed and Basel K. al-Ramadi
Department of Medical Microbiology & Immunology, College of Medicine and Health Sciences, United Arab University, Al-Ain, UAE

Jamil Azzi
Renal Division, Transplantation Research Center, Brigham and Women's Hospital, Harvard Medical School, Boston, MA, USA

Shi-Wei Liu
Department of Endocrinology, Shanxi Bethune Hospital, Shanxi Academy of Medical Sciences, Tongji Shanxi Hospital, Third Hospital of Shanxi Medical University, Taiyuan, China

Fei Sun, Shan-Jie Rong, Ting Wang and Cong-Yi Wang
Department of Respiratory and Critical Care Medicine, The Center for Biomedical Research, National Health Commission (NHC) Key Laboratory of Respiratory Diseases, Tongji Hospital, Tongji Medical College, Huazhong University of Sciences and Technology, Wuhan, China

Jacques C. Mbongue, Jeffrey Rawson, Pablo A. Garcia, Nelson Gonzalez, Kevin Ferreri and Fouad Kandeel
Department of Translational Research and Cellular Therapeutics, Diabetes and Metabolism Research Institute, Beckman Research Institute, City of Hope National Medical Center, Duarte, CA, United States

Ali Alhoshani
Department of Pharmacology and Toxicology, College of Pharmacy, King Saud University, Riyadh, Saudi Arabia

Mohamed I. Husseiny
Department of Translational Research and Cellular Therapeutics, Diabetes and Metabolism Research Institute, Beckman Research Institute, City of Hope National Medical Center, Duarte, CA, United States
Faculty of Pharmacy, Zagazig University, Zagazig, Egypt

Yiman Peng, Xia Li, Yufei Xiang, Xiang Yan, Houde Zhou, Xiaohan Tang, Jin Cheng and Gan Huang
National Clinical Research Center for Metabolic Diseases, Key Laboratory of Diabetes Immunology (Central South University), Ministry of Education, and Department of Metabolism and Endocrinology, The Second Xiangya Hospital of Central South University, Changsha, China

Xiaohong Niu
Department of Endocrinology, Heji Hospital Affiliated to Changzhi Medical College, Changzhi, China

Jing Liu
Department of Endocrinology, Gansu Provincial Hospital, Lanzhou, China

Qiuhe Ji
Department of Endocrinology, Xijing Hospital, Fourth Military Medical University, Xi an, China

Linong Ji
Department of Endocrinology and Metabolism, Peking University People's Hospital, Beijing, China

Tom Eitan Yossipof, Ziva Roy Bazak, Yona Kalechman and Benjamin Sredni
The Mina & Everard Goodman Faculty of Life Sciences, The Safdiè AIDS and Immunology Research Center, C.A.I.R. Institute, Ramat Gan, Israel

Dvora Kenigsbuch-Sredni
Interdisciplinary Department, Bar-Ilan University, Ramat Gan, Israel

Rachel R. Caspi
Laboratory of Immunology, National Eye Institute, National Institutes of Health, Bethesda, MD, United States

Index

www.ingramcontent.com/pod-product-compliance
Lightning Source LLC
LaVergne TN
LVHW082136200926
848484LV00008B/2061